Essentials *of* Pharmacology *for* Health Professions

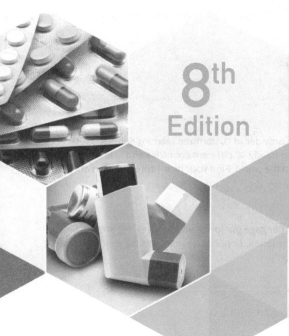

8th Edition

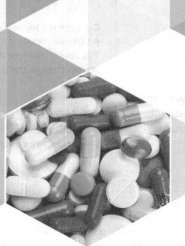

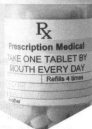

Bruce J. Colbert, MS, RRT

Director of Allied Health Programs
Clinical Associate Professor
University of Pittsburgh at Johnstown
Johnstown, Pennsylvania

Ruth Woodrow, RN, MA

Medical Consultant for Education and Infection Control
Senior Friendship Centers, Inc., Health Services
Sarasota, Florida
Former Director, Staff Development
Plymouth Harbor, Inc.
Sarasota, Florida
Former Instructor, Pharmacology
Coordinator, Continuing Education
Sarasota County Technical Institute
Sarasota, Florida

⁂ Cengage

Australia • Brazil • Canada • Mexico • Singapore • United Kingdom • United States

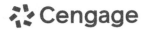

Essentials of Pharmacology for Health Professions, **Eighth Edition**
Bruce J. Colbert, Ruth Woodrow

Senior VP/General Manager, Skills & Global Product Management: Jonathan Lau

Product Director: Matthew Seeley

Senior Product Manager: Laura Stewart

Senior Director, Development: Marah Bellegarde

Senior Product Development Manager: Juliet Steiner

Senior Content Developer: Debra Myette-Flis

Product Assistant: Deborah Handy

Vice President, Marketing Services: Jennifer Ann Baker

Marketing Manager: Jonathan Sheehan

Senior Content Project Manager: Kenneth McGrath

Senior Art Director: Jack Pendleton

Cover Designer: Dave Gink

Interior/Text Designer: Debby Dutton

Cover Image Credits: iStock.com/Merinka; iStock.com/3283197d_273; iStock.com/Nomadsoul1; iStock.com/ziquiu; iStock.com/Jumpeestudio; iStock.com/Sezeryadigar

For product information and technology assistance, contact us at
Cengage Customer & Sales Support, 1-800-354-9706 or support.cengage.com.

For permission to use material from this text or product, submit all requests online at **www.copyright.com.**

Library of Congress Control Number: 2017952877

ISBN: 978-1-337-39589-2

Cengage
200 Pier 4 Boulevard
Boston, MA 02210
USA

Cengage is a leading provider of customized learning solutions with employees residing in nearly 40 different countries and sales in more than 125 countries around the world. Find your local representative at: **www.cengage.com.**

To learn more about Cengage platforms and services, register or access your online learning solution, or purchase materials for your course, visit **www.cengage.com.**

Notice to the Reader

Printed in the United States of America
Print Number: 14   Print Year: 2023

Contents

PART 1 Introduction to Pharmacologic Principles

PART 2   Drug Classifications

CHAPTER 27

Drugs and Older Adults   554

List of Tables

List of Videos on the Online Resources

Dedication

To my loving wife Patty and two fantastic sons, Joshua and Jeremy. Also to Ali, a wonderful daughter-in-law and mother of our latest family addition, baby Lenyx. I'm truly blessed to have such a great family.

Bruce J. Colbert

To my grandchildren, Ashton, Jeff, Samantha, and Eric, may they realize that knowledge is power and seek to grow in knowledge and wisdom all of their lives.

Ruth Woodrow

Preface

This book is designed as:

- A basic text for learners studying nursing, medical assisting, and other health care professions.
- A continuing education update for professionals in health care.
- Part of a refresher program for professionals returning to health care professions.
- A supplemental or reference book for professionals wishing to extend their knowledge beyond basic training in specific health professions.

The purpose of this book is to provide an extensive framework of knowledge that can be acquired within a limited time frame. This book will be especially helpful for learners in one-year training programs with limited time allotted to the study of medications. For those in longer programs, it can be used as the basis for more extensive study. It is appropriate as a required text in training those who will administer medications. This book has been especially designed to meet the needs of learners in nursing and medical assistant programs. However, learners in all health care programs will also find the concise format adaptable to their needs.

This text has been field tested in several classes with learners in various health professions. Learners who have already used this book for updating or supplemental education include registered nurses, licensed practical nurses, medical assistants, surgical technologists, respiratory therapists, and pharmacy technicians.

Those employed in health professions now have increased responsibilities for providing the necessary information to their patients regarding the safe administration of medications, side effects, and interactions. Patient education is presented in every chapter in Part II. Even if you are not involved directly in patient education, it is imperative you understand what information is being conveyed.

ORGANIZATION

The quantity of information could be overwhelming and confusing to the learner unless presented in a reader friendly manner.

The book's comprehensive yet concise format reduces the massive quantity of information and unnecessary detail that may tend to overwhelm or confuse the learner. Outdated or rarely used medications, obsolete information, and complex descriptions are eliminated. The information is both factual and functional.

The textbook is broken down into two specific parts. *Part I* can stand alone as a basic but comprehensive review of pharmacologic principles. *Part I* introduces the learner to the fascinating subject of drugs, their sources, legal concerns, and their medical uses. *Review questions* at the end of each chapter help the learner master the information. Medication preparation, supplies, and specific information on each route of administration are covered. *Administration checklists* allow the learner to put the knowledge into practice. *Illustrations* and *videos* on the *online resources* facilitate the visual learning process.

Part II organizes the drugs according to classifications, arranged in logical order. Each classification is described, along with the characteristics of typical drugs, their purposes, side effects, precautions or contraindications, and interactions. Please note precautions and contraindications are combined as one category since it is clear from the explanation where the drug *is not to be used* in a certain situation (contraindication) and where it *can be used* in a certain situation but should be monitored closely (precautions). A special icon ❗ identifies the most common or most important side effects of drugs. This special icon is meant to serve as a valuable guide for learners. Rather than memorizing every side effect for each drug, the icon emphasizes the side effects with which health care professionals should be most familiar. *Patient education boxes* for each category are highlighted. These special boxes will assist health care professionals to educate patients and answer their questions about the medications they are taking.

Easy-to-use *reference tables* with each classification list the most commonly prescribed drugs according to their generic and trade names, with dosage and available forms.

Reality-based case studies in each chapter in Part II present drug usage scenarios in a variety of settings and stimulate critical thinking by providing practical application of drug information.

Chapter *review quizzes* assist learners to identify areas for further study. *Comprehensive review quizzes* for Part I and Part II encourage learners to practice for the final test.

An extensive *glossary* lists and defines key terms used in the book and defines non-key terms that might not be common knowledge such as unusual side effects. A comprehensive index includes both generic and trade names.

CHANGES TO THE EIGHTH EDITION

Global Textbook Changes

- Each drug classification was updated with the latest and most frequently prescribed drugs available.
- Tables were added and updated to give concise and practical information.

- Patient education boxes were expanded.
- A Clinical Connection feature was added to give a real-life application to the material being discussed to enhance its relevancy.
- Several new illustrations and photos were added to provide learners with a visual connection to the material.
- Additional art was updated to reflect the rapid changes in pharmacology.
- Review questions were updated and new questions were added to cover new material.
- The glossary was expanded to include new terms beyond just the key terms.

The following chapters in the text had significant additions with topics of current interest.

CHAPTER	SPECIFIC CHANGES IN TEXTBOOK
1	Added National Drug Code Directory (NDC) information
	Expansion of discussion on opioid overdose crisis
	Updated Controlled Substances Schedule
	Added medication labels and questions
2	Added discussion of Tall Man Lettering to differentiate look-alike and sound-alike drugs
	Added information of the Over-the Counter (OTC) Drug Advisory Committee
3	Discussed medications that crossed the blood–brain and fetal barriers
	Expanded therapeutic levels, metabolism, and drug interactions
	Added a Clinical Connection on narcotic overdose and treatment
	Expanded images and information on the Epipen and treatment of anaphylaxis
4	Updated IV images and terminology
	Updated needle information
	Expanded the transdermal delivery information
	Discussed implantable medication delivery devices
5	Computerized documentation updates were made, including computerized physician order entry (CPOE) and electronic medication administration records (eMAR)
	Expanded abbreviations for Medication Orders
6	Included a Clinical Connection on the use of reasoning to verify drug dosage calculations
7	Added information on confirming correct dosage forms
	Added a Clinical Connection on confirmation bias
8	Added information on aspiration
	Added eMAR information in relationship to medication administration
	Updated medication administration steps
	Added a Clinical Connection on patient education regarding suppositories
9	Added a new section on IV fluids
	Updated IV administration
	Added a Clinical Connection on proper medication patch disposal
	Provided updated information on insulin pens
	Added a Clinical Connection on site rotation for injections
10	Added a Clinical Connection on contrasting contacting poison control versus emergency services

11	Added a Clinical Connection on Warfarin and Vitamin K
	Added a new section on electrolytes and minerals
	Added a Clinical Connection on Calcium and Vitamin D
12	Updated the photo for oral thrush
	Added a photo for shingles
	Added updated treatment options for shingles
	Added a Clinical Connection on the Shingles vaccine
13	Added information concerning second dose with Epi-Pen
	Added a Clinical Connection on patient compliance with beta blockers
	Added a Clinical Connection on ophthalmic atropine
14	Added an illustration on cancer cell vs normal cell
	Added a photo of Gardasil/Ceravix
	Added extravasation to chemo side effects chart
	Added a Clinical Connection on Methotrexate dosing
	Added a Clinical Connection on Extravasation
15	Added an illustration on urinary tract infections
	Added an illustration on BPH (benign prostatic hyperplasia)
	Updated gout information
	Added a Clinical Connection on urinary tract infections
16	Added an illustration on peptic ulcer
	Added an illustration on *C. diff* and isolation
	Added a Clinical Connection on gastric and duodenal ulcers
	Updated information on diarrhea treatment
	Added a section on mu-opiod receptor antagonists for opioid-induced constipation (OIC)
17	Added the CDC immunization schedule for adults
	Added a Clinical Connection on the duration of antibiotic therapy
	Added information on Z-PAK dosing
	Added a Clinical Connection on Disulfuram-like reactions
18	Added a new section on ear medications
	Added information and an illustration on the anatomy of the ear
	Added a table on otic preparations
	Added a Clinical Connection on eye drops for ear drops
19	Added an illustration of the pain scale
	Added an image on cutting Lidocaine patches
	Added information on PRN dosing for pain versus maintenance dosing
	Added a Clinical Connection on opioid-induced constipation
	Added information on acetaminophen dosing and overdose
	Added information on medical marijuana
20	Added a photo on bipolar disorder
	Added an illustration on alcoholism
	Added information on ADHD treatment
	Added a Clinical Connection on racemic mixtures of drugs
	Added a section on proper disposal and storage of medications

21	Added a photo of Voltaren Gel
	Added an illustration of osteoporosis
	Added a new section on newer drugs for osteoporosis
	Added a new section on muscle relaxants
	Added a Clinical Connection on medication reconciliation
22	Added an illustration on seizures and how to handle them as a bystander
	Added an illustration detailing the symptoms of Parkinson's disease
	Added a Clinical Connection on driving with seizure-related conditions
23	Added illustrations on hypothyroidism and Grave's disease
	Added a corticosteroid equivalency table
	Added a chart on diabetes type I versus type II
	Added information on thyroid replacement dosing and adjustment
	Added a Clinical Connection on narrow therapeutic index drugs
	Added a section on SGLT2 Inhibitor therapy
24	Added an illustration detailing the symptoms of menopause
	Added a photo of oral birth control
	Added a Clinical Connection on deep vein thrombosis prevention
	Updated Plan B availability information
25	Added an illustration on heart failure
	Added a Clinical Connection on patient information interviews
	Added information on INR and warfarin dosing
26	Added a section on cleaning MDI's
	Added a Clinical Connection on rescue inhaler use
	Added information on rinsing the mouth after using inhaled corticosteroids
	Added information on dextromethorphan use in children
	Added information on pseudoephedrine purchasing limits
27	Added photos to illustrate how pill boxes can be used as memory aids for older adults
	Added information on "LOT" benzodiazepines for older adults
	Added a Clinical Connection on the other end of the spectrum
	Added a section on MTM and CMRs to combat polypharmacy
	Added a section on adherence in older adults

STUDENT RESOURCES

Study Guide

The Study Guide offers additional practice with review questions corresponding to each chapter in the text, including multiple choice, fill-in-the-blank, true or false, and matching questions. Case studies encourage students to apply the knowledge learned in Part II about drugs.

Online Resources

Online resources are available to enhance the learning experience. Additional resources include:

- "Treatment of the Opportunistic Infections of AIDS" content
- Medication administration videos that allow learners to "see" concepts in action
- Slide presentations in PowerPoint®

Accessing the online resources:

1. Go to http://www.cengage.com.
2. Register as a new user or log in as an existing user if you already have an account with Cengage Learning or cengage.com.
3. Select **Go to MY Account.**
4. Open the product from the My Account page.

INSTRUCTOR RESOURCES

Learning Lab

The Learning Lab is an **online homework solution** that allows your students to practice the most difficult concepts associated with their Cengage Learning textbooks in a simulated real-world environment.

Developed to help you improve program quality and retention, the Learning Lab prepares your students for their career by *increasing comprehension and critical thinking skills.*

Instructor Companion Site

Powerful resources for instructors are available to assist you with teaching pharmacology, assessing your students' mastery of the material, and elevating students' learning.

- **Cognero online test bank** makes generating tests and quizzes a snap. With over 1,300 questions in a variety of formats to choose from, you can create customized assessments for your students with the click of a button. Adding your own unique questions has never been easier.
  - Also included with the Cognero online test bank are over 500 **NCLEX-style questions.**
- Customizable instructor slide presentations created in **PowerPoint**, including images, focus on the key concepts from each chapter. Medication administration videos that allow learners to "see" concepts in action are available for students on the online resources.

- Electronic Instructor's Manual includes the following tools:
  - Additional review quizzes with answers
  - Comprehensive drug worksheets with answers
  - An alternate Comprehensive Exam for Part II with answers
  - Answers to review quizzes and comprehensive review exams in the text
  - Answers to case studies in Part II in the text
  - Answers to review questions and case studies in the Study Guide

MINDTAP

MindTap is a fully online, interactive learning experience built upon authoritative Cengage Learning content. By combining readings, multimedia, activities, and assessments into a singular learning path, MindTap elevates learning by providing real-world application to better engage students. Instructors customize the learning path by selecting Cengage Learning resources and adding their own content via apps that integrate into the MindTap framework seamlessly with many learning management systems.

The guided learning path demonstrates the relevance of basic pharmacology principles to health care professions through engagement activities, interactive exercises, and procedural videos. The Pronounce activity ensures correct pronunciation of the top 200 drugs, plus additional hospital drugs. Easy-to-use *reference tables* with each classification list the most commonly prescribed drugs according to their generic and trade names, with dosage and available forms, special considerations, and audio to encourage correct pronunciation of the drugs most likely to be encountered in health care. Learners apply an understanding of pharmacology through patient education scenarios. These simulations elevate the study of pharmacology by challenging students to apply concepts to practice.

To learn more, visit www.cengage.com/mindtap.

TO THE LEARNER STUDYING PHARMACOLOGY

Other learners such as you have helped me put this book together. They have learned that the study of medications can be a fascinating one. They have told me that this book has helped them to develop confidence and competence in dispensing medications and sharing information about drugs with their patients. You will find this is only the beginning, a framework upon which you will build a vast store of useful knowledge.

Learners have told me that the objectives, review questions, and case studies were tremendously helpful to them. Organization is the key to acquiring large quantities of information. You will be amazed at all you have learned when you complete this book.

Keep growing and learning and questioning all of your life.

Ruth Woodrow

ACKNOWLEDGMENTS

There are a lot of people to thank in a project of this scope. First and foremost, I would like to thank Ruth Woodrow for her dedication to helping students learn. It is an honor to continue to work on such a quality textbook and with such an inspiring author who maintains her passion for learning, teaching, mentoring, and volunteerism. She truly lives her values and continues to imprint her knowledge and dedication to presenting an engaging, meaningful, and readable pharmacology textbook.

I would also like to thank Adam James who served as the pharmacist consultant on this project to make sure we got it right. I have known Adam for several years and I'm very impressed with his work ethic, knowledge, and professionalism. His updates with the latest and greatest information concerning specific drugs and dosages have been truly appreciated.

Liz Katrancha deserves a big thank you for being the nursing consultant to make sure we keep the project patient centered, clinically applied and up-to-date. I have had the pleasure of working with Liz on several projects and her attention to detail and quality of work are greatly appreciated.

My first editor Matt Seeley deserves a very large thank you for considering me in the first place and believing in me for this project. I also appreciate his forward thinking in adding enhanced digital experiences to an already successful textbook. My current editor Laura Stewart deserves much praise for her dedication in moving this project forward, especially in the digital realms. In addition, she has made the transition a very smooth and pleasant one.

Last but certainly not least, I want to personally thank Debra Myette-Flis, for her tremendous assistance, organizational skills, professional knowledge, and guidance in helping to make this project a joy on which to work. Deb quietly does so much "behind-the-scenes" work that I wanted to especially acknowledge and express my appreciation for keeping me on track and her focus on making this project the best it can be.

Bruce J. Colbert

I would like to acknowledge the support, encouragement, and technical assistance of my husband, Roger.

I am grateful to Bruce Colbert, a dedicated teacher and author, for taking over the edition revisions. Bruce shares my empathy for the student and the ideal of keeping it simple for successful learning. In addition, he continues to share his creative ideas for incorporating technology to enhance the learning experience. A big thanks to Bruce for keeping me involved.

I wish to thank all of those at Cengage Learning who contributed in any way to this text. Appreciation is expressed particularly to Debra Myette-Flis, senior content developer, for all of her guidance and support throughout the editions and especially for her understanding and assistance. She always goes above and beyond expectations.

I also wish to thank Matt Seeley, product team manager, for finding Bruce Colbert, the perfect fit for this book.

Ruth Woodrow

CONSULTANTS/CONTRIBUTING AUTHORS

Adam Joseph James PharmD.
Pharmacy Manager Rite Aid / Duquesne Mylan School of Pharmacy 2014 Graduate
Certified immunizing pharmacist and certified in smoking cessation counselling and medication therapy management

Elizabeth D. Katrancha, DNP, CCNS, RN, CNE
Assistant Professor
Pitt-Johnstown Baccalaureate Nursing Program

REVIEWERS

The authors and Cengage Learning wish to acknowledge and sincerely thank the following reviewers.

Julia Becker, CPhT
Pharmacology Technician Program Director
Western Dakota Tech

Stephen J. Hazelton, RPh
Program Director, Pharmacy Technology
Hennepin Technical College

Tammy McClish, M.Ed., CMA (AAMA)
Medical Assisting Instructor
Wadsworth High School

Diane Rapp
Instructor
Bucks County Community College

Georgette Rosenfeld, PhD., RRT, RN
Professor
IRSC

Lisa Sailor, CMA (AAMA), BS
Program Director and Instructor
Anoka Technical College

Gina Stephens, MSN, RN, CPC-I, CPPM
Assistant Dean
Georgia Northwestern Technical College

PART 1

Introduction to Pharmacologic Principles

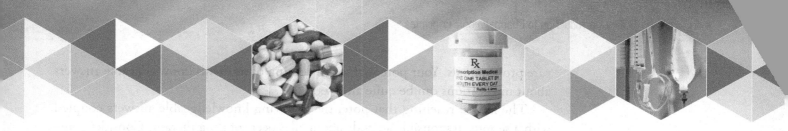

CHAPTER 1

CONSUMER SAFETY AND DRUG REGULATIONS

KEY TERMS AND CONCEPTS

Controlled substances

Drug Enforcement Administration (DEA)

Drug standards

Food and Drug Administration (FDA)

National Drug Code (NDC) Directory

Orphan drugs

Over-the-counter (OTC) medication

OBJECTIVES

Upon completion of this chapter, the learner should be able to

1. Explain what is meant by drug standards

2. Name the first drug law passed in the United States for consumer safety, and give the year it was passed

3. Summarize the provisions of the Federal Food, Drug, and Cosmetic Act of 1938, and identify the government agency that enforces the act

4. Interpret what is meant by USP/NF

5. Summarize the provisions of the Controlled Substances Act of 1970

6. Explain what is meant by a DEA number and the NDC Directory

7. Define schedules of controlled substances, and differentiate between C-I through C-V schedules

8. State several responsibilities you have in administering medications as a direct result of the three major drug laws described in this chapter

9. Define the Key Terms and Concepts

Your decision to pursue a career in the health care field probably took a great deal of thought. No doubt you have questioned whether you will be able to handle the unique situations that arise in a clinic, health care facility, or physician's office. Have you ever stopped to consider the impact *you* will make on the lives of others as a health care professional? Not only can you make a tremendous difference in the facility where you work, but you can also have a positive impact on your friends and family, as well as the patient or client.

It is inevitable that you will receive phone calls and questions about medications, prescriptions, and drug therapy. A great majority of patients are far too inhibited to tell their physicians that there are things they do not understand about their medications. They feel much more at ease discussing their questions with health care professionals. Your potential for informing others with knowledgeable answers about medications can be quite an asset!

The key to reaching that potential is having knowledgeable answers coupled with a serious, responsible attitude about all aspects of drug therapy. Consider yourself a potential prime resource of medication information for your friends, family, and future patients as you begin to examine the foundations of facts about drugs. It may be necessary for you to clarify some of the layperson misunderstandings about the legalities of dispensing medications. Consider the following misconceptions and facts.

Fallacy	Fact
Only nurses can give medications to patients.	Trained and certified health care professionals who may legally give medications include physicians; physician assistants; paramedics; medical office assistants; unlicensed assistive personnel; practical, vocational, and registered nurses; and other allied health specialists such as respiratory therapists and pharmacists.
Only physicians may write prescriptions.	Dentists, physicians, physician assistants, veterinarians, nurse practitioners, and registered pharmacists may write prescriptions for their specific field of work, as governed by state law. For example, veterinarians write prescriptions only for animal use.
Prescriptions are required for narcotics only.	Specific drugs ruled illegal to purchase without the use of a prescription include the following: • Those that need to be controlled *because they are addictive and tend to be abused and dangerous* (e.g., depressants, stimulants, psychedelics, and narcotics). • Those that may cause dangerous health threats from side effects if taken incorrectly (e.g., antibiotics, cardiac drugs, and tranquilizers).
All drugs produced in the United States are made in federally approved laboratories.	Numerous illegal laboratories that produce illicit substances such as methamphetamines exist and operate within the United States today.
All herbal medicines and dietary supplements are safe.	Herbal remedies and other dietary supplements are not approved or manufactured per production standards regulated by the Food and Drug Administration (FDA) and may have serious interactions with prescribed medications. Under the Dietary Supplement Health and Education Act (DSHEA) of 1994, the dietary supplement manufacturer is responsible for ensuring that a dietary supplement is safe before it is marketed. The FDA is responsible for taking action against any unsafe dietary supplement product after it reaches the market and against marketed products that make false or misleading claims. (See Chapter 11.)

DRUG LAWS

Individuals have been using substances and drugs for healing purposes for centuries. Due to scientific advances and changes in our society in the last century, consumer safety has become a critical issue. During the 1900s, laws were passed that specifically addressed the matter of dispensing drugs in the United States.

Drug standards are rules set to assure consumers that they get what they pay for. The law says that all preparations called by the same drug name must be of *uniform strength*, *quality*, and *purity*.

Because of drug standardization, when you take a prescription to be filled, you are assured of getting the same basic drug, in the same amount and quality, regardless of the pharmacy or the part of the country where you take the prescription. According to drug standards, the drug companies must not add other active ingredients or varying amounts of chemicals to a specific drug preparation. They must meet the drug standards (federally approved requirements) for the specified strength, quality, and purity of the drug.

In the market of illegal (illicit) drugs, the lack of enforcement of drug standards poses danger to the consumer. With no controls on the quality of illegal drugs, many deaths have occurred from overdose. Consider the heroin user, accustomed to very poor-quality heroin, who accidentally overdoses when given a much higher quality of heroin from a new source. In general, across the country, opioid and other drug overdoses have become a major problem. This will be highlighted throughout following chapters, but it is important to be aware of the problems that can arise when certain drugs are abused.

The laws that have evolved to provide consumer safety can be summed up by three major acts. They are described in the order they became necessary for consumer safety, beginning with the 1906 Pure Food and Drug Act.

1906 PURE FOOD AND DRUG ACT

First government attempt to establish consumer protection in the manufacture of drugs and foods.

Required all drugs marketed in the United States to meet minimal standards of strength, purity, and quality.

Demanded that drug preparations containing dangerous ingredients have a labeled container indicating the ingredient. Originally there were 11 "dangerous" ingredients, such as morphine.

Established two references of *officially* approved drugs. Before 1906, information about drugs was handed down from generation to generation. No official written resources existed. After the 1906 legislation, two references specified the official U.S. standards for making each drug. These references, listed here, have since been combined into one book, referred to as the *USP/NF.*

- *United States Pharmacopeia (USP)*
- *National Formulary (NF)*

The importance of the timing of the 1938 Federal Food, Drug, and Cosmetic Act should be noted. It came about as the answer to a disastrous occurrence in 1937. A sulfa preparation, not adequately tested for safety, was responsible for 100 deaths that year. Thus, the need was recognized for more proof of the safety of new drugs.

1938 FEDERAL FOOD, DRUG, AND COSMETIC ACT AND AMENDMENTS OF 1951,1962, AND 1972

Established the Food and Drug Administration (FDA) under the Department of Health and Human Services to enforce the provisions of the act.

Established *more specific* regulations to prevent adulteration of (tampering with) drugs, foods, and cosmetics:

- All labels must be accurate and must include a listing of all active and inactive ingredients. Figure 1-1 shows an example of required product information for an over-the-counter (OTC) medication (no prescription [Rx] needed).
- All new products must be approved by the FDA before public release.
- "Warning" labels must be present on certain preparations, for example, "may cause drowsiness," "may cause nervousness," and "may be habit-forming."
- Certain drugs must be labeled with the legend (inscription): "Caution—federal law prohibits dispensing without a

prescription." Thus, the term *legend drug* refers to such preparations. The act also designated which drugs can be sold without a prescription.

- Prescription and nonprescription drugs must be shown to be *effective* as well as *safe*.
- In 1972, the National Drug Code (NDC) Directory was established. This provided the FDA with a list of all drugs manufactured for commercial distribution. Each drug is identified by an NDC number, made up of three parts (see Figure 1-2).
  - The first part is five numbers and identifies the manufacturer.
  - The second part is four numbers and identifies the drug.
  - The third part is two digits and identifies the package size.
    - Example: 00406-0123-01; note it is a common practice to omit a leading zero in the first or second part of the NDC number so this drug could also be written as 0406-123-01.

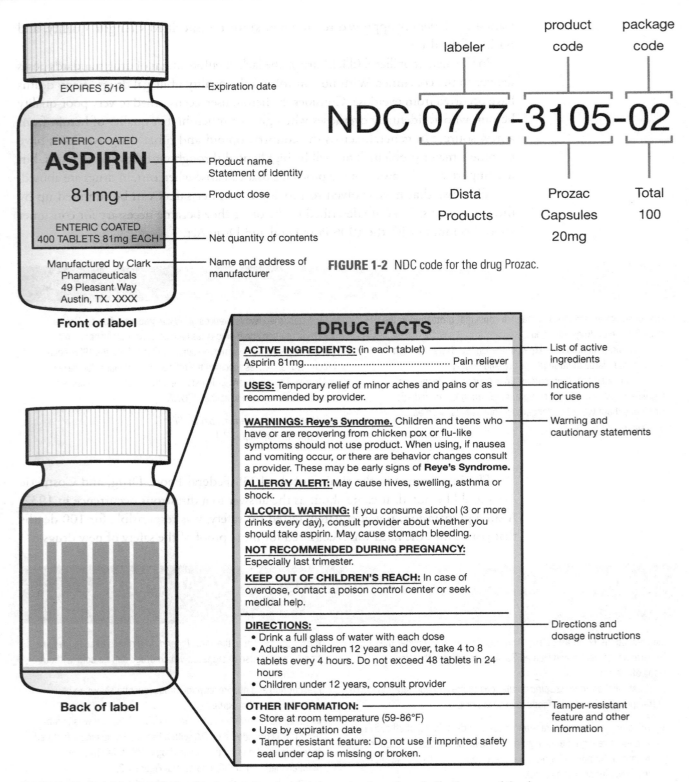

Front of label

EXPIRES 5/16 —— Expiration date

ENTERIC COATED
ASPIRIN —— Product name
Statement of identity

81mg —— Product dose

ENTERIC COATED
400 TABLETS 81mg EACH —— Net quantity of contents

Manufactured by Clark —— Name and address of
Pharmaceuticals   manufacturer
49 Pleasant Way
Austin, TX. XXXX

labeler | product code | package code

NDC 0777-3105-02

Dista
Products

Prozac
Capsules
20mg

Total
100

FIGURE 1-2 NDC code for the drug Prozac.

Back of label

DRUG FACTS

ACTIVE INGREDIENTS: (in each tablet) —— List of active ingredients
Aspirin 81mg................................... Pain reliever

USES: Temporary relief of minor aches and pains or as —— Indications for use
recommended by provider.

WARNINGS: Reye's Syndrome. Children and teens who —— Warning and cautionary statements
have or are recovering from chicken pox or flu-like
symptoms should not use product. When using, if nausea
and vomiting occur, or there are behavior changes consult
a provider. These may be early signs of **Reye's Syndrome.**

ALLERGY ALERT: May cause hives, swelling, asthma or
shock.

ALCOHOL WARNING: If you consume alcohol (3 or more
drinks every day), consult provider about whether you
should take aspirin. May cause stomach bleeding.

NOT RECOMMENDED DURING PREGNANCY:
Especially last trimester.

KEEP OUT OF CHILDREN'S REACH: In case of
overdose, contact a poison control center or seek
medical help.

DIRECTIONS: —— Directions and dosage instructions
• Drink a full glass of water with each dose
• Adults and children 12 years and over, take 4 to 8
  tablets every 4 hours. Do not exceed 48 tablets in 24
  hours
• Children under 12 years, consult provider

OTHER INFORMATION: —— Tamper-resistant feature and other information
• Store at room temperature (59-86°F)
• Use by expiration date
• Tamper resistant feature: Do not use if imprinted safety
  seal under cap is missing or broken.

FIGURE 1-1 Consumer medication labels contain valuable information for safe and effective use of the drug.

The five schedules of controlled substances are arranged with those with the highest potential for abuse at level I and those with the least abuse potential at level V. It should be noted that even those drugs in class level V have more potential for abuse than most drugs. Additionally, the lower the number, the stricter are the restrictions for control by the DEA. Therefore, it makes sense that Schedule I drugs are illegal and are not approved for medicinal purposes in the United States.

Drugs are frequently added, deleted, or moved from one schedule to another. If, for example, the DEA determines that drug A is becoming more of a societal problem, with an increased incidence of overdoses, drug A may be moved from the C-IV schedule to C-III. It is extremely important that the health care professional keep informed of any changes in drug scheduling. For the most part, using the most current drug reference book will keep you up to date.

You will recognize the schedule of a particular controlled substance by noting a *C* with either *I, II, III, IV,* or *V* after it. Some references show the capital C with the Roman numeral inside the curve of the C (Ⓥ). Labels on controlled substances are also designated with a C and a Roman numeral to indicate their level of control. Drug inserts (information leaflets accompanying drugs) are also marked with a C and the appropriate schedule number. (See Table 1-1 and Figure 1-3.)

1970 CONTROLLED SUBSTANCES ACT

Established the Drug Enforcement Administration (DEA) as a bureau of the Department of Justice to enforce the provisions of the act.

Set much tighter controls on a specific group of drugs: *those that were being abused by society;* the name of the act indicates that such *substances needed to be controlled.* These substances include depressants, stimulants, psychedelics, narcotics, and anabolic steroids. The act:

- Isolated the abused and addicting drugs into five levels, or schedules, according to their medical value, harmfulness, and potential for abuse or addiction: C-I, C-II, C-III, C-IV, and C-V.
- Demanded security and accountability of controlled substances; anyone (e.g., pharmacists, hospitals, physicians, and drug companies) who dispenses, receives, sells, or destroys controlled substances must keep on hand special DEA forms, indicating the exact current inventory and a two-year inventory of every controlled substance transaction.
- Set limitations on the use of prescriptions; guidelines were established for each of the five schedules of controlled substances, regulating the number of times a drug may be prescribed in a six-month period as well as for which schedules prescriptions may be phoned in to the pharmacy and so on.
- Demanded that each prescriber of these substances register with the DEA and obtain a DEA registration number, to be present on their prescriptions of controlled substances; drug manufacturers must also be registered and identified with their own DEA numbers, as must pharmacists, physicians, veterinarians, and so on.

MEDIALINK

See It in Action! View a video on *Managing Controlled Substances* on the Online Resources.

Although many other drug laws exist, there are two significant pieces of drug legislation that are important to mention here. The 1983 Orphan Drug Act gives pharmaceutical companies financial incentives to develop medications for diseases that affect only a small number of people. This encourages the companies to develop orphan drugs that would otherwise be of low profitability. The other legislation is the strangely named Omnibus Budget Reconciliation Act (OBRA) of 1990. This act mandates that all OTC drugs a patient is taking must be documented as part of the medical record. OBRA also mandates that pharmacists provide drug use review and patient counseling before dispensing prescriptions to a patient.

TABLE 1-1   **Five Schedules of Controlled Substances**

SCHEDULE NUMBER	ABUSE POTENTIAL AND LEGAL LIMITATIONS	EXAMPLES OF SUBSTANCES
1, ℂ	High abuse potential Not approved for medical use in the United States	Heroin, LSD, mescaline, ecstasy
2, ℂⅠ	High abuse potential May lead to severe dependence Written prescription only (or electronic prescriptions that meet DEA standards) No phoning in of prescription by the office health care professional, in an emergency, physician may phone in, but handwritten prescription must go to the pharmacy within seven days No refills without new written prescription Prescription may be faxed, but original prescription must be handed in to pick up prescription	Morphine, codeine, methadone, Percocet, Dilaudid, Ritalin, Oxycontin, meperidine (Demerol), Hydrocodone with Tylenol
3, ℂⅠ	May lead to moderate dependence Written, faxed, or verbal (phoned in) prescription, by physician only May be refilled up to five times in six months	Codeine and, anabolic (muscle-building) steroids
4, ℂⅤ	Lower abuse potential than the previous schedules Prescription may be written out by the health care professional but must be signed by the physician Prescription may be phoned in by the health care professional or faxed May be refilled up to five times in six months	Valium, Ativan, Xanax, phenobarbital, Librium, Restoril, and Ambien
5, ℂ	Low abuse potential compared to the previous schedules Consists primarily of preparations for cough suppressants containing codeine and preparations for diarrhea (e.g., diphenoxylate) May be refilled up to five times in six months	Promethazine with codeine, Cheratussin AC, Lomotil

Note: Some states may have stricter schedules than the federal regulations. You must be aware of the regulations in your area.

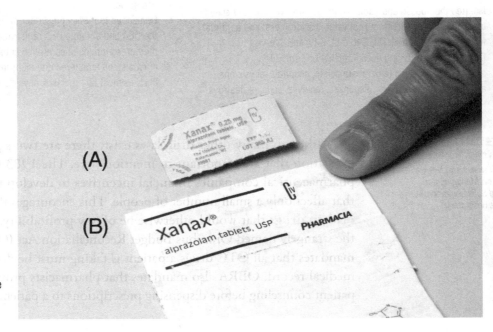

FIGURE 1-3 Controlled substance schedule numbers appear in a variety of drug information resources, including (A) drug packages and (B) drug inserts. Schedule numbers are also found in drug reference sources.

FDA AND DEA

The increase in the number of drugs produced for marketing brought dangers to the public. The federal FDA was established to ensure that some basic standards would be followed. Its responsibilities include:

- Overseeing testing of all proposed new drugs before they are released into the U.S. market
- Inspecting plants where foods, drugs, medical devices, or cosmetics are made
- Reviewing new drug applications and petitions for food additives
- Investigating and removing unsafe drugs from the market
- Ensuring proper labeling of foods, cosmetics, and drugs

When the need for better control of addictive drugs became urgent, the FDA had its hands full just trying to enforce basic drug standards. It became imperative to set up a new department, the DEA, in 1970 to handle all the needs and safety controls for the more dangerous drugs. Thus, the two agencies—FDA and DEA—were established with their own specific areas of drug control.

As a health care professional and an informed citizen, you must be aware of the latest developments concerning these two agencies. Hardly a week goes by without mention of the activities of the FDA or the DEA in the news. You should be able to recognize their separate areas of control.

FDA

Concerned with general safety standards in the production of drugs, foods, and cosmetics.

Responsible for approval and removal of products on the market.

Special note on drug withdrawals: In rare cases, the FDA may need to reassess and change its approval decision on a drug. A conclusion that a drug should no longer be marketed is based on the nature and frequency of the adverse events and how the drug's benefit and risk balance compares with treatment alternatives. When the FDA believes that a drug's benefits no longer outweigh its risks, the agency will ask the manufacturer to withdraw the drug. Interestingly, the FDA does not have the legal authority to withdraw a marketed drug product itself.

DEA

Concerned only with controlled substances.

Enforces laws against drug activities, including illegal drug use, dealing, and manufacturing.

Monitors need for changing the schedules of abused drugs.

HEALTH CARE PROFESSIONALS AND THE LAW AND ETHICS

In some ways, you will be as involved as the physician in observing the restrictions of the drug laws. You will have the responsibility of keeping accurate records of the medications dispensed. You will maintain the supply of drugs at your facility. If you work in a physician's office, a clinic, or an ambulatory care setting, you will also be involved with phoning in prescriptions and securing prescription forms at your facility. You must act ethically to ensure that the ordered medications are given in the appropriate amount to the appropriate patient.

The following guidelines should be followed by the health care professional involved in dispensing medications:

1. Keep a *current* drug reference source available at all times. You should be able to readily identify substances that are controlled by the DEA.

2. Keep controlled substances locked securely. Double-locking is required in most situations. This means:
   a. Placing the drugs in a locked safety box.
   b. Placing the locked box in a cupboard that is also locked.

3. Conceal and secure prescription pads at your office, clinic, or facility. Do not leave pads out in the open, especially in patient examining rooms. The prescription pads, with the physician's DEA registration number, are a possible source of fraud and drug tampering when forged and used illegally. Keep the pads locked up and in a designated location (e.g., a drawer), out of the public areas of the office or nursing station. One of the most common ways prescriptions are forged is through a stolen prescription pad.

4. Keep accurate records of each controlled substance administered, received, or destroyed at your facility. These records, as well as the records from the previous two years, must be available at all times. Properly destroy expired drugs and old records.

5. Be responsible for keeping up to date with current news of the activities of the FDA and the DEA. If working for a physician, monitor the DEA registration renewal date. Keep informed of any changes in the scheduling of controlled substances.

6. Establish a working rapport with a pharmacist. A local pharmacist is an excellent resource for you when you are unsure of your legal responsibilities with drugs or have any uncertainties about drug therapy.

7. If you work in an office, maintain a professional rapport with the pharmaceutical representatives who leave drug samples there. As part of the Affordable Care Act, the Sunshine Act now requires reporting of compensation and gifts paid to physicians by pharmaceutical representatives. It is important that you are aware of the ethical dilemma that may occur when a physician is "rewarded" or compensated for prescribing certain medications.

CHAPTER REVIEW QUIZ

Complete the following statements

1. The first major U.S. drug law was passed in the year _____ and was called the _____.

2. USP stands for _____.

3. NF stands for _____.

4. Which drug law established the USP and NF (which are now one)? _____.

5. The agency that requires you to keep a record of each controlled substance transaction is the _____.

6. Prescriptions for schedule C-_____ drugs may be phoned in by the health care professional.

7. How long must you keep an inventory record of each controlled substance transaction at your office? _____.

8. Three responsibilities of the FDA include:

   _____

   _____

   _____

9. What types of drugs are listed in the C-V schedule? _____.

10. What method is recommended for securing the controlled substances at your office? _____.

11. If a patient calls to request a refill of a Percocet (C-II) prescription, how would you reply? _____.

12. Dawn Vasquez has a rare disease that requires medication for only a small population of patients. Which act has allowed her drug to be produced even though it is not profitable to the pharmaceutical industry?

   _____.

13. A patient calls into the office asking for a new prescription for a narcotic medication that he has been taking for six months. You bring up his chart and notice that he has been requesting new prescriptions every 23 days, whereas the medication should last 30 days. Additionally, the patient also mentions that he feels that he is in need of a higher dose and gets agitated and irritable when you tell him that he will need an appointment. What do you think of this? What should you do?

14. Answer the questions concerning the following three drug labels on the next page.
    a. Which drug(s) requires a prescription?
    b. Which drug(s) can be bought without a prescription?
    c. Which drug(s) requires a DEA number?

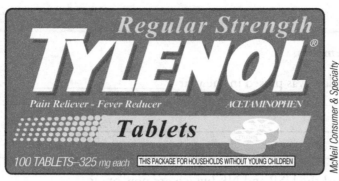

McNeil Consumer & Specialty Pharmaceuticals.

(A)

NDC 46987-410-11

KADIAN®

Morphine Sulfate
Extended-Release Capsules

10 mg KADIAN

10 mg

R only   100 Capsules

ALPHARMA.
Pharmaceuticals

Each capsule contains: 10 mg morphine sulfate as extended-release pellets.
Usual Dosage: See accompanying prescribing information.
The pellets from KADIAN® capsules should NOT be chewed, crushed or dissolved.
Warning: As with all medication, keep out of the reach of children.
Dispense in a sealed, tamper-evident, childproof, light-resistance container. Store at 25°C (77°F); excursions permitted to 15-30°C (59°-86°F). Protect from light and moisture.

Manufactured for:
Alpharma Pharmaceuticals LLC
One New England Avenue
Piscataway, NJ 08854
by: Actavis Elizabeth LLC, 200 Elmora Avenue
Elizabeth, NJ 07207 USA   Rev.04/07

Lot No.:

3 63857-410-11 9

Used with permission from ALPHARMA Pharmaceuticals.

(B)

NDC 0069-2600-66

100 Capsules

Procardia®
(nifedipine)   10

10 mg

Distributed by

Pfizer **Pfizer Labs**
Division of Pfizer Inc, NY, NY 10017

NDC 0069-2600-66

Used with permission from Pfizer, Inc.

(C)

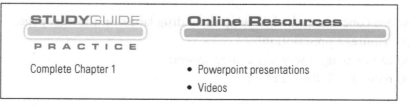

STUDYGUIDE

PRACTICE

Complete Chapter 1

Online Resources

- Powerpoint presentations
- Videos

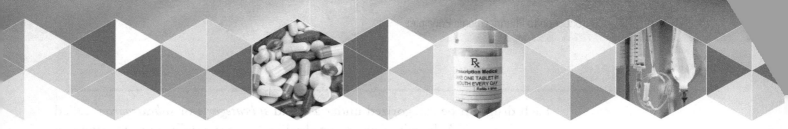

CHAPTER 2
DRUG NAMES AND REFERENCES

KEY TERMS AND CONCEPTS

Actions

Adverse reactions

Cautions

Classifications

Contraindications

Generic names

Indications

Interactions

Legend drug

Official name

Pharmacology

Prototype

Side effects

Tall Man Lettering

Trade names

OBJECTIVES

Upon completion of this chapter, the learner should be able to

1. Describe drug classification systems

2. Differentiate among the following drug names: generic name, official name, trade name, and chemical name

3. Explain what is indicated by a number included in a drug trade name (e.g., Tylenol No. 3)

4. Contrast generic and brand name drugs

5. Define and explain the restrictions of drug sales implied by the following: over-the-counter (OTC) drug, legend drug, and controlled substance

6. Discuss the various terms indicating drug actions contained in reference sources

7. List and describe at least two drug references available today

8. Discuss several characteristics that you consider important in choosing the best drug reference

9. Describe how to evaluate drug information websites

10. Define the Key Terms and Concepts

Pharmacology can be defined as the study of drugs and their origin, nature, properties, and effects on living organisms. We need to know why drugs are given, how they work, and what effects to expect. The thousands of drug products on the market would make this subject difficult to tackle if it were not for:

- Numerous drug references, geared to a variety of levels of readers, from layperson to pharmacist
- Grouping of drugs under broad subcategories
- Continuity in the use of basic identifying terms for the names and actions of drugs

CLASSIFICATIONS

Each drug can be categorized under a broad *subcategory*, or *subcategories*, called classifications. Although drugs can be classified in several different ways, grouping them together according to their therapeutic use is most helpful to the health care professional. Drugs that affect the body in similar ways are listed in the same classification. Drugs that have several types of therapeutic effects fit under several classifications. For example, aspirin has a variety of effects on the body. It may be given to relieve pain (analgesic), to reduce fever (antipyretic), to reduce inflammation of tissues (anti-inflammatory), or as an anti-platelet (anti-thrombotic agent). Therefore, aspirin is categorized under four classifications of drugs (as shown in parentheses).

Another drug, cyclobenzaprine (Flexeril), however, is known to be used for only one therapeutic effect: to relieve muscle spasms. Flexeril, therefore, is listed only under the one classification of muscle relaxant.

Examples of some common drug classifications are listed in Table 2-1. Are you familiar with any of them already?

The second part of this text compares the characteristics of the various major drug classifications. In each chapter, as a classification is explained, you will learn what general information to associate with drugs of that classification, including:

- Therapeutic uses
- Most common side effects
- Precautions to be used
- Contraindications (when *not* to use the drug)
- Interactions that may occur when taken with other drugs or foods
- Some of the most common product names, their usual dosages, and comments on administration

You may also be given a prototype of each drug classification. A prototype is a *model example*, a drug that typifies the characteristics of that classification. For example, propranolol (Inderal) is the prototype of the beta-adrenergic blockers (see Chapter 13).

TABLE 2-1   Top 10 Drug Classifications and Examples

CLASSIFICATION	THERAPEUTIC USE	DRUG EXAMPLE(S)
1) Lipid-lowering agents	Lowers low-density lipoprotein (LDL) cholesterol	simvastatin, atorvastatin, rosuvastatin
2) Antidepressants	Improves symptoms of depression. Also used for anxiety and other neurological disorders	escitalopram, sertraline, paroxetine, venlafaxine
3) Narcotic analgesics	Relieve severe pain	hydrocodone with acetaminophen, oxycodone, oxymorphone, fentanyl
4) Beta blockers	Lowers heart rate and blood pressure	metoprolol, atenolol, propranolol
5) Antihypertensives	Lowers blood pressure	lisinopril, enalapril, valsartan

(continued)

TABLE 2-1   **Top 10 Drug Classifications and Examples (*continued*)**

CLASSIFICATION	THERAPEUTIC USE	DRUG EXAMPLE(S)
6) Diuretics	Increases urinary output	furosemide
7) Antidiabetics	Reduces blood glucose (sugar) levels	insulin, metformin, glipizide, Januvia
8) Antibiotics	Eliminates infection	amoxicillin, cephalexin, doxycycline
9) Proton pump inhibitors	Decreases acidity of stomach	omeprazole, pantoprazole, esomeprazole
10) Anticoagulants	Decreases clotting in blood	warfarin, Xarelto

You can find the classification as well as the various names of a drug by referring to a drug reference source.

IDENTIFYING NAMES

Drug names can seem very complicated because a single drug will have many names attached to it. Four specific names can apply to each approved drug:

1. ***Generic name***.
   a. Common or general name assigned to the drug by the United States Adopted Name (USAN) council
   b. Differentiated from the trade name by initial lowercase letter
   c. Never capitalized
2. ***Trade name*** (also known as proprietary or brand name since owned by company).
   a. The name by which a pharmaceutical company identifies its product
   b. Copyrighted and used exclusively by that company
   c. Distinguished from the generic name by capitalized first letter
   d. Often shown on labels and references with the symbol ® after the name (for "registered" trademark)
3. ***Chemical name***.
   a. The exact molecular formula of the drug
   b. Usually a long, very difficult name to pronounce
   c. Of little concern to the health care professional
4. ***Official name***.
   a. Name of the drug as it appears in the official reference, the *United States Pharmacopeia/National Formulary (USP/NF)*
   b. Generally, the same as the generic name

The use of **generic names** and **trade names** for drugs can be compared to the various names of grocery products. Two examples of generic names are orange juice and detergent. Corresponding trade names for orange juice are Tropicana and Minute Maid, whereas Cheer and Tide are trade names for detergents. Although there is only one generic name, there may be many trade names.

When a company produces a new drug for the market, it assigns a generic name to the product. After testing and approval by the Food and Drug Administration (FDA), the drug company gives the drug a trade name (often something short and easy to remember when advertised). For five years, from the time the company submits a *new drug application (NDA)* to the FDA for approval, the company has the exclusive right to market the drug. Once approved, the drug is listed in the *USP/NF* by an **official name**, which is usually the same as the generic name. After five years have passed and the patent has expired (although patent extensions are requested and frequently granted), other companies may begin to combine the same chemicals to form that specific generic product for marketing. Each company will assign its own specific trade name to the product, or the drug can be offered simply by its generic name and strength, such as acetaminophen 325 mg. See Table 2-2, which compares the names for two drugs.

TABLE 2-2   Comparison of Drug Names

GENERIC NAME	CHEMICAL NAME	TRADE NAMES (DRUG COMPANY)
doxycycline hyclate	2-Naphthacenecarboxamide, 4-(dimethylamino)-1,4,4a,5,5a,6,11,12a-octahydro-3,5,10,12,12a-pentahydroxy-6-methyl-1,11-dioxo-, (4S,4aR,5S,5aR,6R,12aS)-(564-25-0)	Vibramycin (PD-RX Pharmaceuticals) doxycyclinehyclate[a] (West-Ward)
chlordiazepoxide hydrochloride	7-chloro-2 methylamino-5 phenyl-3H-1,4-benzodiazephine 4-oxide hydrochloride	Librium

[a]Some companies simply elect to market the product by the generic name.

Concerning prescription drugs, most states have enacted legislation encouraging physicians to let pharmacists substitute less expensive *generic equivalents* for prescribed brand name drugs. Specific provisions of drug *substitution laws* vary from state to state.

The physician may indicate "no substitutions" on the prescription, usually indicated by a *dispense as written (DAW) order*. Often physicians have preferences for certain products or patients may be difficult to stabilize on a certain class of medications (such as thyroid preparations). Even though the drug contents are the same, the "fillers," or ingredients that are used to hold the preparation together, may be slightly different. This difference in fillers may affect how quickly the drug dissolves or takes effect. Dyes in some products may alter effects in some sensitive patients by leading to an allergic response.

Many products are combinations of several generic components. You will recognize this when you see several generic names (not capitalized) and their corresponding amounts listed under one trade name (capitalized). Examples are given in Table 2-3.

TABLE 2-3   Examples of Combination Drugs

TRADE NAME	GENERIC NAME AND AMOUNT
Dyazide (used to treat high blood pressure)	hydrochlorothiazide 25 mg/triamterene 37.5 mg
Glucovance (used to treat Type 2 diabetes mellitus)	glyburide 1.25 mg/metformin 250 mg
	glyburide 2.5 mg/metformin 500 mg
	glyburide 5 mg/metformin 500 mg
Robitussin DM 5 mL syrup	dextromethorphan10 mg/guaifenesin, 100 mg

PATIENT EDUCATION

Patients may ask you about the difference between generic and trade (brand) name products. The FDA regulates the manufacturing of generic drugs, so patients can be assured that they are safe and cost-effective alternatives. Generally, trade name products are more expensive, although the basic active ingredients (drug contents) are the same as those in the generic. The higher price helps to pay for the costs of drug development and advertisements promoting the trade name. (Can you think of certain trade names that are heavily advertised in television commercials?)

Because generic drug equivalents may exist for both prescription and OTC drug products, it is often economically wise to check for medicines that have the same generic components and strengths. For example, several cough syrups may have exactly the same contents, but the prices may vary widely.

Read and compare all ingredients on the labels.

It should be noted that a number may be part of the trade name. The number often refers to an amount of one of the generic components and helps to differentiate it from an almost identical product. Identify the significance of the numbers in comparing the following trade names:

Trade Name	Generic Name and Amount
Tylenol No. 2	acetaminophen 300 mg codeine 15 mg
Tylenol No. 3	acetaminophen 300 mg codeine 30 mg
Tylenol No. 4	acetaminophen 300 mg codeine 60 mg

Note that each product contains the same amount of acetaminophen, with varying amounts of the controlled substance codeine. *The larger the number in the name, the greater is the amount of controlled substance present.*

Many drug errors have occurred because the trade name was misinterpreted for the number of tablets to be given. So . . .

Be certain you can clearly read and understand the order!

Another type of drug error involves preventable allergic reactions to one of the generic components of a medication. The problem stems from:

- Not consulting the patient's chart for the history of allergies before a new medication is ordered or given
- Not checking a reference to find out if a medication being ordered or given contains any generic components to which the patient has a known allergy

For example, if a patient has an allergy to aspirin, do not administer the first dose of any new medication to the patient without finding out if the product contains aspirin. Although the physician is in error for ordering the medication, you are also in error for administering a medication with which you are unfamiliar. A proficient health care professional should check the history and chart for known allergies and pick up any discrepancies. Alertness is the key to safety in any setting.

According to the Institute for Safe Medication Practices (ISMP) and the FDA, look-alike and sound-alike medications are a leading cause of drug errors. For example, the drug clonidine used for high blood pressure can be confused with the drug clonazepam used for anxiety; Celebrex for arthritis can be confused with Celexa for depression. To help health care professionals differentiate between look-alike and sound-alike drugs, **Tall Man Lettering** is often used to highlight the differences between the two drugs. For example, Celexa would be written CeleXA, whereas Celebrex would be written CeleBREX. This ensures that the health care professional reads and recognizes the correct medication.

These two agencies have created a long-standing relationship with a goal of preventing drug errors. The ISMP has developed tools such as the "List of Confused Drug Names" as a quick drug reference that is available on its website at http://www.ismp.org.

> **Always keep a drug reference handy, and use it when you are unfamiliar with the generic components of a drug ordered for a patient with known drug allergies. With experience, you will learn and remember the names of products most commonly used at your facility.**

LEGAL TERMS REFERRING TO DRUGS

A drug may be referred to by terms other than its classification, generic name, trade name, chemical name, or official name. As mentioned in Chapter 1, the following terms imply the legal accessibility of a drug:

1. ***Over-the-counter (OTC) drug***. No purchasing restrictions by the FDA (with some exceptions, such as pseudoephedrine, which is OTC, but kept behind the pharmacy counter; see Chapter 20)

2. *Legend drug*. Prescription drug; determined unsafe for OTC purchase because of possible harmful side effects if taken indiscriminately; includes birth control pills, antibiotics, cardiac drugs, and hormones

3. ***Controlled substance***. Drug controlled by prescription requirement because of the danger of addiction or abuse; indicated in references by schedule numbers C-I to C-V (see Chapter 1)

In time and with patient research, some prescription drugs can be deemed safe enough to be sold OTC. The OTC Drugs Advisory Committee was formed in 1992 to review prescription or legend drugs and assist the FDA in determining which ones are safe for OTC designation. Some recent examples of previously prescribed medications now available OTC are fexofenadine (Allegra) and triamcinolone (Nasacort) approved for nasal allergies in 2011 and 2014, respectively.

> **The legend drug is so named because it requires a legend or warning statement that says, "Federal law prohibits dispensing without a prescription."**

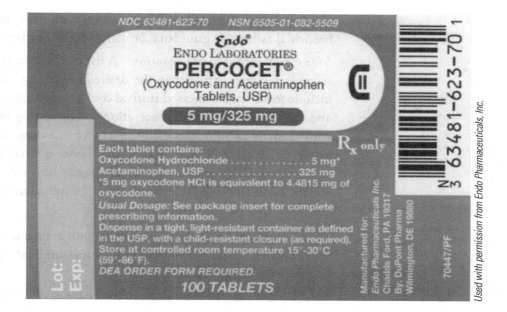

FIGURE 2-1 Information contained on a drug label including the trade name (Percocet) and the generic names of the two drugs (oxycodone and acetaminophen) that it contains.

Figure 2-1 shows the information contained on a drug label including the trade name (Percocet) and the generic names of the two drugs (oxycodone and acetaminophen) that it contains. In addition, can you find the controlled substance marking?

TERMS INDICATING DRUG ACTIONS

Most references follow a similar format in describing drugs. When you research drug information, you will find the following terms as headings under each drug. You will find specific information more quickly if you understand what is listed under each heading.

Indications. A list of medical conditions or diseases for which the drug is meant to be used (e.g., diphenhydramine hydrochloride [Benadryl] is a commonly used drug; indications include allergic rhinitis, mild allergic skin reactions, motion sickness, and mild cases of parkinsonism).

Actions. A description of the cellular changes that occur as a result of the drug. This information tends to be very technical, describing cellular and tissue changes. Although it is helpful to know what body system is affected by the drug, this information is geared more for the pharmacist (e.g., as an antihistamine, Benadryl appears to compete with histamine for cell receptor sites on effector cells).

Contraindications. A list of conditions for which the drug should *not* be given (e.g., two common contraindications for Benadryl are breast-feeding and hypersensitivity).

Cautions. A list of conditions or types of patients that warrant closer observation for specific side effects when given the drug (e.g., due to atropine-like activity, Benadryl must be used cautiously with patients who have a history of bronchial asthma or glaucoma, or with older adults [see Chapter 27]).

Side effects and adverse reactions. A list of possible unpleasant or dangerous secondary effects, other than the desired effect (e.g., side effects of Benadryl include sedation, dizziness, disturbed coordination, epigastric distress, anorexia, and thickening of bronchial secretions). This listing may be quite extensive, with as many as 50 or more side effects for one drug. Because it is difficult to know which are most likely to occur, choose a reference that highlights the most common side effects. Certain drugs may have side effects with which you are not familiar. Note the definitions of the following three side effects associated with specific antibiotics.

- Ototoxicity causes damage to the eighth cranial nerve, resulting in impaired hearing or ringing in the ears (tinnitus). Damage may be reversible or permanent.
- Nephrotoxicity causes damage to the kidneys, resulting in impaired kidney function, decreased urinary output, and renal failure.
- Photosensitivity is an increased reaction to sunlight, with the danger of intense sunburn.

Interactions. A list of other drugs or foods that may alter the effect of the drug and usually should not be given during the same course of therapy (e.g., monoamine oxidase [MAO] inhibitors will intensify the effects of Benadryl; you will find MAO inhibitors listed under interactions for many drugs; the term refers to a group of drugs that have been used for the treatment of depression; it has been found that they can cause serious blood pressure changes, and even death, when taken with many other drugs and some foods).

Other headings often listed under information about a drug include "How Supplied" and "Usual Dosage." "How Supplied" lists the available forms and strengths of the drug. "Usual Dosage" lists the amount of drug considered safe for administration, the route, and the frequency of administration. For example:

How supplied: tablets (tabs): 20 mg and 40 mg; suppository: 20 mg
Usual dosage: 10 mg orally every four hours (q4h)

For a listing of common abbreviations regarding drug administration and medication orders, see Tables 4-1 and 5-1 in the upcoming chapters.

DRUG REFERENCES

Physicians'Desk Reference (PDR) is one of the most widely used references for drugs in current use. It is available online, as a mobile app, and in book form. There are three versions of the *PDR*, one for physicians, one for nurses, and one for consumers. In addition, there are many new choices of references available today. Three are compared here, including the *PDR*. You must find the reference most suitable for you, one that you can interpret quickly and easily. By becoming knowledgeable about the drugs you administer, you may prevent possible drug errors from occurring.

Physician's Desk Reference (PDR)*

PROS	CONS
1. *PDR* for physicians—available for free online, as a mobile app, and for a fee in book form. Benefits include the following: —Product labeling —FDA drug safety communication —Medication guide —Drug alerts, recalls, and approvals —Patient resources —Various tools such as e-Books and mobile *PDR* —Ability to report of adverse reactions —Photographs of many drugs for product identification 2. *PDR* for nurses—available for a fee free mobile apps —Includes 1,500 FDA-regulated drugs —Includes critical black box warnings 3. *PDR* for consumers—written in patient-friendly language —Includes over 300 prescribed drugs —Color images of medications —Comparison tables of OTC drugs —Guide to safe medication use	Contains only those drugs that manufacturers pay to have incorporated Incomplete with regard to OTC drugs, making it necessary to buy *PDR* OTC book

*Published annually by PDR Network, LLC, Montvale, New Jersey.

United States Pharmacopeia and the National Formulary (USP/NF)†

PROS	CONS
Information is available online at http://www.usp.org Provides information on and standards for chemical and biological drug substances, dosage forms, and compounded preparations; medical devices; and dietary supplements	No photographs of drugs Geared for laboratory and manufacturing use No easily identified nursing implications Can be confusing to use

†Published annually by U.S. Pharmacopeial Convention, Inc., Rockville, Maryland.

AHFS Drug Information (American Health-System Formulary Service)‡

PROS	CONS
Distributed to practicing physicians; single paperback volume, includes mobile drug reference and handbook to injectable drugs Good, concise information; easy to read Arranged by classifications, with a general statement about each classification at the beginning of each section Off-label drug indications are listed (not FDA approved) http://www.ashp.org/	Some parts (e.g., "Chemical Information" and "Drug Stability") not necessary for the health care professional No photographs of drugs

‡Published annually by American Society of Health-System Pharmacists, Bethesda, Maryland.

Other references (e.g., *The Pill Book, Handbook of Nonprescription Drugs*) may be found in bookstores, but they may not contain adequate information for the health care professionals. Your school may recommend a specific drug reference other than the three listed in this text. Many new references geared to the nurse or health care professional are currently being published. Electronic drug references such as Lexi-Drugs and/or Epocrates (a free version of this) are also widely used.

THE INTERNET AS REFERENCE

The Internet offers a wealth of information regarding medications and the conditions they treat. However, there can be serious dangers associated with some online sources that may not be reliable, professional, or even legitimate. Therefore, care must be taken to identify and use only websites that are supervised and controlled, such as those under the auspices of government agencies or sponsored by professional pharmacist groups. It is important for the health care professional to obtain accurate information and also be able to direct the patient or client to reliable sources of information regarding medicines. It is the health care professional's responsibility to caution the layperson regarding the controversial and dangerous practices of "online prescribing" without ever evaluating the patient in person, or obtaining medicines without prescriptions through the Internet.

EVALUATING INTERNET DRUG SOURCES

Remember that all websites are not created equal. Pay attention to a few simple rules when seeking the most reputable ones.

1. Check the source. Have scientific studies been done with a large enough sample? Are results reliable and valid? Are there links to a page listing professional credentials or affiliations?

2. Check the date of articles. Medicine is a rapidly evolving field. Information can go out of date quickly.

3. Be wary of information from forums and testimonials. Motivations are unknown. The information is not necessarily valid, and there may be a hidden agenda.

The following websites are reliable professional sources of medical information:

http://www.pharmacist.com	Sponsored by the American Pharmacists Association (APhA), the national professional society of pharmacists.
http://www.fda.gov	U.S. Food and Drug Administration. Includes "Human Drugs" and Center for Drug Evaluation and Research (CDER).
http://www.safemedication.com	Sponsored by the American Society of Health-System Pharmacists. Covers correct dosage, side effects, and optimal use of most prescriptions and OTC drugs. Also offers reports on topics such as antibiotic-resistant bacteria.
http://www.usp.org	U.S. Pharmacopeial Convention (USP/DI). (See United States Pharmacopeia, previous page.)
http://www.cdc.gov/vaccines/	U.S. Centers for Disease Control and Prevention, National Immunization Program. Covers vaccines and immunizations.
http://www.nlm.nih.gov/medlineplus/	A service of the U.S. National Library of Medicine and the National Institutes of Health. A great source for medicine and related health topics.

CHAPTER REVIEW QUIZ

Match the definition with the term.

1. ___ List of conditions for which a drug is meant to be used
2. ___ Subcategories of drugs based on their effects on the body
3. ___ Description of the cellular changes that occur as a result of a drug
4. ___ Conditions for which a drug should not be given

a. Contraindications
b. Precautions
c. Indications
d. Prototype
e. Actions
f. Classifications

Refer to the following drug description to answer questions 5–8.

AZO Standard®
(phenazopyridine HCl tablets, *USP*)
Product of i-Health, a Division of DSM
Description: AZO Standard (phenazopyridine HCl) is a urinary tract analgesic agent, chemically designated 2,6-pyridinediamine, 3-(phenylazo), monohydrochloride.

5. The generic name of the drug is _____.

6. The chemical name of the drug is _____.

7. The trade name of the drug is _____.

8. What is indicated by the ® symbol after the drug name?

_____.

9. Explain when Tall Man Lettering should be used:

_____.

10. Explain the difference between these two medication orders:
    a. Give two Tylenol, PO.
    b. Give one Tylenol No 2 PO.

_____.

_____.

11. An older adult male was found unconscious in his bedroom with several pink and blue pills beside his bed, but no labeled pill bottle can be found. He is rushed to the emergency department for treatment. What drug reference source will be most helpful in this situation?

_____.

STUDYGUIDE
Online Resources

PRACTICE

Complete Chapter 2

• Powerpoint presentations
• Videos

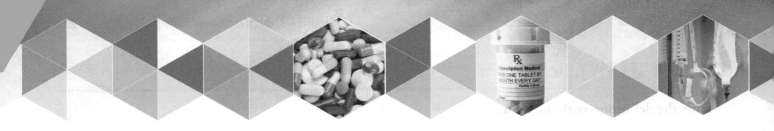

CHAPTER 3
SOURCES AND BODILY EFFECTS OF DRUGS

KEY TERMS AND CONCEPTS

Adverse drug reaction
Anaphylactic reaction
Chemoinformatics
Cumulative effect
Dependence
Dosage
Drug interactions
Drug processes
Hypersensitivity
Idiosyncratic reaction
Keep Vein Open (KVO)
Local effect
Paradoxical reaction
Pharmacogenomics
Placebo effect
Prodrugs
Sources of drugs
Systemic effect
Teratogenic effect
Therapeutic range
Tolerance

OBJECTIVES

Upon completion of this chapter, the learner should be able to

1. Identify the five sources of drugs
2. Differentiate among the following: drug actions and drug effects, systemic effects and local effects, loading dose and maintenance dose, and toxic dose and lethal dose
3. Define the following processes as they relate to the passage of drugs through the body and state conditions that may decrease the effectiveness of each: absorption, distribution, metabolism, and excretion
4. Define the following terms: selective distribution, toxicity, placebo, synergism, potentiation, and antagonism
5. List several variables that may affect the action of drugs
6. Identify and contrast the various routes of drug administration
7. Define adverse drug reactions
8. Define the Key Terms and Concepts

SOURCES OF DRUGS

Any chemical substance ingested or applied on the body for the purpose of affecting body function is referred to as a drug. In earlier times, these substances were found in nature, sometimes accidentally. Plants were the primary **sources of drugs** used on the human body. Berries, bark, leaves, resin from trees, and roots were found to aid the body and are still very important drug sources.

Minerals from the earth also found their way into human use as drugs. Minerals such as iron, sulfur, potassium, silver, and even gold are used to manufacture drugs.

More sophisticated sources of drugs emerged as human beings progressed. Research led to the use of substances from *animals* as effective drugs. Substances lacking in the human body can be replaced with similar substances obtained from the glands, organs, and tissues of animals. Investigation of other animal sources of medicines still remains. For example, an investigational drug to treat Type 2 diabetes by promoting weight loss was recently developed from the saliva of the Gila monster lizard.

Chemists use synthetic sources to make drugs to market for human consumption. The *synthetic* (manufactured) sources evolved with human skills in laboratories and advanced understanding of chemistry. Today, through advances in computers, millions of potential drug candidates can be screened on computers quickly and efficiently using a process called **chemoinformatics**. Chemoinformatics is the application of computer technology, statistics, and mathematics to study information about the structure, properties, and activities of molecules. This method is probably the most actively pursued source of drugs by major companies today. Competitive research is a big industry that involves experimenting with chemicals to discover cures for current medical problems. Numerous antibiotics are synthetic or semisynthetic, the results of researchers meeting the need for better treatment of infections. Someday the cure for cancer or human immunodeficiency virus (HIV) infection may be found from a synthetic source developed in a laboratory.

Genetic engineering of drugs and the recently developed technique of *recombinant DNA technology* has allowed for the production of biologically active substances that are present in the body and that can be used to treat certain diseases. DNA is the genetic material of the cells, and the DNA sequence determines the genetic code. Genetic engineering refers to the alteration of genes in a laboratory setting.

Recombinant DNA techniques involve combining the DNA of two or more different organisms for a desired change or improvement. Some examples of therapeutic agents derived by recombinant DNA technology are hepatitis B vaccine, insulin, and growth hormone. One of the areas of most current interest in recombinant DNA technology is gene therapy. This therapy consists of essentially inserting normal genes into a human chromosome to counteract the effects of an abnormal or a missing gene. This not only has huge implications for preventive medical therapy but also ethical considerations. See Figure 3-1 for examples of sources of drugs.

EFFECTS OF DRUGS

Regardless of the source, the common characteristic of all drugs is the ability to affect body function in some manner. When introduced into the body, all drugs cause cellular changes (drug actions), followed by some *physiological change* (effects of drugs). Generally, drug effects may be categorized as systemic or local:

1. **Systemic effect**. Reaches widespread areas of the body. For example, ibuprofen is often used as an analgesic and anti-inflammatory for pain associated with knee pain due to arthritis. Although you feel the effect in

Sources of Drugs	Example	Trade Name	Classification
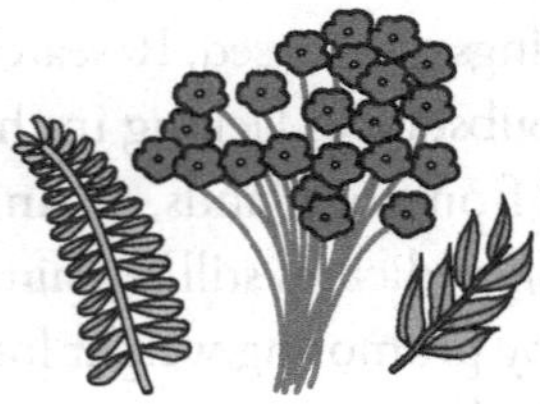 Plants	Cinchona Bark	Quinidine	Antiarrhthymic
	Purple Foxglove Plant	Digitalis	Cardiotonic
	Poppy Plant (Opium)	Morphine, Codeine	Analgesic Analgesic, Antitussive
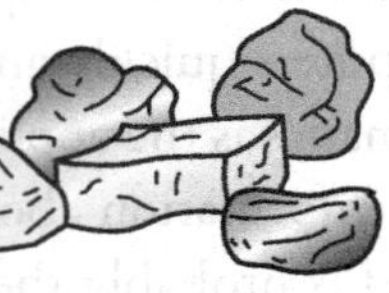 Minerals	Magnesium	Milk of Magnesia	Antacid, Laxative
	Zinc	Zinc Oxide Ointment	Sunscreen, Skin Protectant
	Gold	Auranofin	Anti-inflammatory; Used in the Treatment of Rheumatoid Arthritis
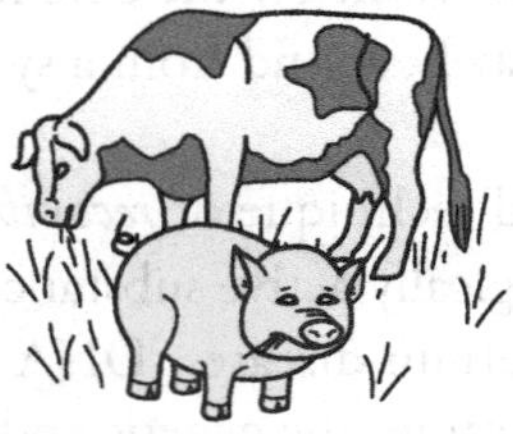 Animals	Thyroid Gland of Animals	Thyroid, USP	Hormone
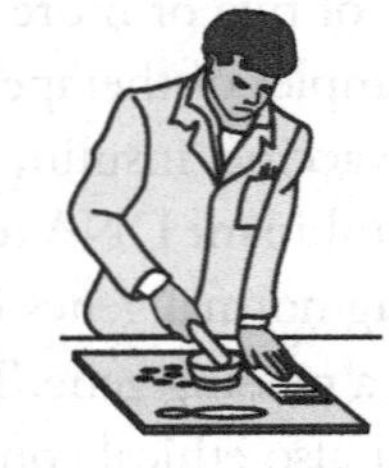 Synthetic	Meperidine	Demerol	Analgesic
	Diphenoxylate	Lomotil	Antidiarrheal
	Co-Trimoxazole	Bactrim, Septra	Anti-infective Sulfonamide; Used in the Treatment of Urinary Tract Infections (UTI) and Some Other Infections
DNA 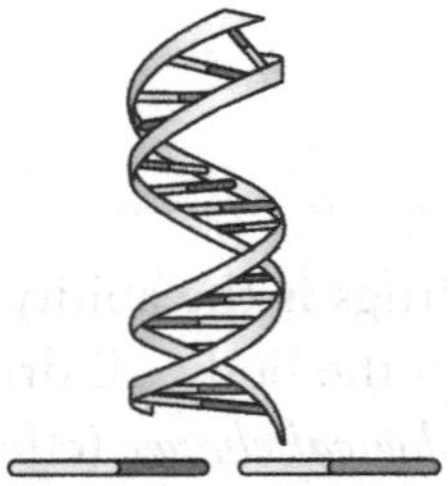 Genetic Engineered	Hepatitis B vaccine	Recombivax HB	Vaccine
	Insulin	Humulin, Novolin	Anti-diabetic
	Growth hormone	Nutropin	Hormone

FIGURE 3-1 Sources of drugs: plants, minerals, animals, synthetic, and genetically engineered.

your knee, the medication is actually providing the same effects all over the body, which is why it can also be used for headaches, cramps, and sunburn just to name a few.

2. **Local effect.** Is limited to the area of the body where it is administered (e.g., dibucaine ointment [Nupercainal], applied rectally, affects only the rectal mucosa to reduce hemorrhoidal pain).

DRUG PROCESSING BY THE BODY (PHARMACOKINETICS)

Kinetics means "movement" and therefore *pharmacokinetics* literally means what happens to the drug as it moves through our body.

Within the body, drugs undergo several changes. From start to finish, the biological changes consist of four **drug processes** (abbreviated as *ADME*):

1. *Absorption.* Passage of a substance through a membrane into the bloodstream
2. *Distribution.* Moving from the bloodstream into the tissues and fluids of the body
3. *Metabolism.* Physical and chemical alterations that the substance undergoes in the body
4. *Excretion.* Eliminating waste products of drug metabolism from the body

Many variables affect how quickly or successfully substances go through the body via these four processes. If any of the four processes are altered, the drug action and effects will be altered, where the medication may have a greater or lesser effect or a longer or shorter duration. Table 3-1 lists conditions that may alter each process.

TABLE 3-1 Processing of Drugs within the Body

PROCESS	PRIMARY SITE OF PROCESS	CONDITIONS THAT MAY ALTER PROCESS
Absorption	Mucosa of the stomach, mouth, small intestine, or rectum; blood vessels in the muscles or subcutaneous tissues; or dermal layers	Incorrect administration may destroy the drug before it reaches the bloodstream or its site of action (e.g., giving certain antibiotics after meals instead of on an empty stomach)
Distribution	Circulatory system, through capillaries and across cell membranes	Poor circulation (impaired flow of blood) may prevent the drug from reaching tissues
Metabolism	Liver, small intestine	Hepatitis, cirrhosis of liver, or a damaged liver may prevent adequate breakdown of the drug, thus causing a build-up of unmetabolized drug
Excretion	Kidneys, sweat glands, lungs, or intestines	Renal damage or kidney failure may prevent passage of drug waste products, thereby causing an accumulation of the drug in the body

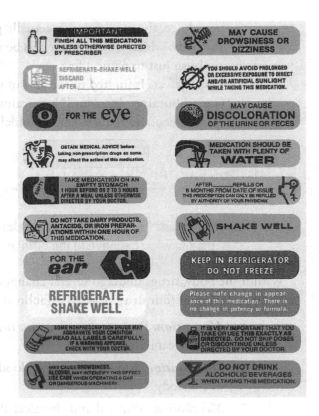

FIGURE 3-2 Warning labels are placed on prescription medication containers. Patients should be advised to read and follow the precautions or instructions.

Directions for the administration of drugs may vary widely because the physical properties of the drugs may vary widely. The specific directions ("Usual Dosage and Administration," "Contraindications," and "Warnings") that accompany each drug are given to enhance the absorption, distribution, metabolism, and excretion of the drug. For example, directions to "Give on an empty stomach" ensure the most effective means of absorption. "Use cautiously in patients with renal dysfunction" implies possible effects on the excretion of a drug. "Decrease dose in patients with hepatic dysfunction" implies possible effects on the metabolism of a drug. *Read all labels carefully, and caution the patient to do so as well* (Figure 3-2).

Absorption

The site of absorption of drugs varies according to the following physical properties of each drug:

1. ***pH.*** Drugs of a slightly acidic nature (e.g., aspirin and tetracycline) are absorbed well within the acidic stomach environment. Drugs of an alkaline pH are not absorbed well through the stomach but are readily absorbed in the alkaline environment of the small intestine. The antibiotic tetracycline is not recommended to be administered with milk, dairy products, or antacids, because it will not be properly absorbed. This is due to *chelation*—the formation of an insoluble complex of tetracycline with calcium in dairy products. pH effect may also play a role. It varies with the specific antacid used. Oral medications for infants (syrups and solutions) may not be absorbed well after infant feedings. The milk or formula neutralizes the acidity of the stomach. Thus,

absorption may be enhanced when the infant is given medications on an empty stomach.

2. *Lipid (fat) solubility.* Substances high in lipid solubility are quickly and easily absorbed through the mucosa of the stomach. Alcohol and substances containing alcohol are soluble in lipids. They are rapidly absorbed through the gastrointestinal (GI) tract. Substances low in lipid solubility are not absorbed well through the stomach or intestinal mucosa and are absorbed best when given by a means other than the GI tract. An exception is the drug neomycin, which is not lipid soluble and yet is given orally. It is indicated for suppression of intestinal bacteria before intestinal or bowel surgery or for the treatment of bacterial diarrhea. By giving neomycin orally, it passes through the GI tract, unable to be absorbed. As a result, it tends to build up and accumulate in the bowel. The trapped antibiotic kills the bacteria in the bowel, for the desired effect.

3. *Presence or absence of food in the stomach.* Food in the stomach tends to slow absorption due to a slower emptying of the stomach. If a fast drug effect is desired, an empty stomach will facilitate quicker absorption. On the other hand, giving some medications on an empty stomach is contraindicated. Medications that are irritating to the stomach can be buffered by the presence of food. Directions may indicate "Give after meals" or "Take with food" to decrease side effects (e.g., nausea and gastric ulcers) on the GI tract.

Distribution

The movement of a drug from the bloodstream into the tissues and fluids of the body is also affected by specific properties of a drug. Reaching sites beyond the major organs may depend on the drug's ability to cross a lipid membrane. Some drugs pass the "blood–brain barrier" to reach the brain or the "placental barrier to reach the developing fetus," whereas others do not. For example, propranolol is the only beta blocker (normally a cardiac medication) that passes the "blood–brain barrier," and this allows it to be used for an adjunct therapy for migraine headaches because it can have an effect in the brain. You may also read about drugs contraindicated for lactating mothers because the drug has the ability to pass through the cell membranes into the milk.

Some drugs have a *selective distribution*. This refers to an affinity, or attraction, of a drug to a specific organ or cell. For example, amphetamines have a selective distribution to cerebrospinal fluid. The human chorionic gonadotropin hormone, which is used as a fertility drug, has a selective distribution to the ovaries.

By virtue of their properties, some drugs are distributed more slowly than others. Thus, although two drugs may be categorized in the same drug classification, one may be known to act on the cells and achieve the effect more quickly than the other.

Metabolism

When transformed in the liver (biotransformation), a drug is broken down and altered to more water-soluble by-products (metabolites). Thus, the drug may be more easily excreted by the kidneys. Some drugs are inactive when administered and only become active when they are metabolized by the liver. This group of drugs is known as **prodrugs** (e.g., clopidogrel [Plavix]).

If hepatic disease is present, a patient may exhibit toxic (poisonous) effects of a drug or the drug may not work as intended. This occurs because the drug is not being broken down properly by the inefficient liver. The drug may accumulate, unchanged by the liver, and may be unable to pass out of the body's excretory system. Metabolism can also be altered by interactions between drugs, between drugs and food, and between drugs and disease states. For example, as mentioned above, clopidogrel is a prodrug, but its metabolism to the active form is inhibited by Nexium (esomeprazole). If these drugs are used together, clopidogrel will not have its intended antiplatelet effect.

It is possible for some drugs to bypass the process of metabolism. They reach the kidneys virtually unchanged and may later be detected in the urine.

Excretion

Although it is possible for some drugs to be eliminated through the lungs (e.g., exhaled gases and anesthetics) or through perspiration, feces, bile, or breast milk, most are excreted by the kidneys via urine.

If a drug is not excreted properly before repeated doses are given, a **cumulative effect** due to a drug build-up may eventually occur. A cumulative effect is an increased effect of a drug demonstrated when repeated doses accumulate in the body. Patients with decreased kidney function may be at risk of drug accumulation. If unnoticed, the cumulative effect may build to a dangerous, or toxic, level. This can be of particular concern with older adults. (See Chapter 27.)

Toxicity refers to a condition that results from exposure to either a poison or a dangerous amount of a drug that is normally safe when given in a smaller amount. In drug therapy, the goal is to give just enough of the drug to cause the desired (therapeutic) effect while keeping the amount below the level at which toxic effects are observed. It should be noted that toxicity can develop even with properly dosed or small amounts of a drug.

Digoxin is a cardiac drug that must be given cautiously because of its potential for causing a cumulative effect. Normally, digoxin slows the heart rate, but if the drug accumulates, the heart rate may slow to a dangerously low level. Circulation and renal function must be adequate, or the digoxin will accumulate, leading to digoxin toxicity.

Keep in mind that the purpose of most medication treatment is to have a desired effect by maintaining a drug level within a **therapeutic range**. The therapeutic range is the range of drug levels in the blood that will give the desired effect without causing serious side effects. The blood can be tested for therapeutic levels and for example the target level for digoxin is 0.8 to 2.0 ng/mL. Lower than this level will not be effective and higher than this range can lead to toxicity.

OTHER VARIABLES AFFECTING DRUG ACTION

Many *variables* affect the speed and efficiency of drugs being processed by the body. The physical properties of the drugs themselves and the condition of the body systems have been discussed. Other variables affecting drug action and effect follow.

Age

Metabolism and excretion are slower in older adults, and therefore attention must be paid to possible cumulative effects. Refer to Chapter 27 for a detailed discussion on how the complex changes of aging affect how drugs are processed in the body. Children have a lower threshold of response and react more rapidly and sometimes in unexpected ways; therefore, frequent assessment is imperative.

Weight

Generally, the bigger the person, the greater the dose should be. However, there is great individual variation in sensitivity to drugs. Many drug dosages are always calculated on the basis of the patient's weight. With certain drugs in patients who are obese, it may be best to calculate their dose based on their ideal body weight rather than their total body weight.

Gender

Women respond differently than men to some drugs. The ratio of fat per body mass differs, and so do hormone levels. If a female is pregnant or nursing, drugs should be selected that are safe to use for both the mother and her child. For example, the common over-the-counter medications ibuprofen and naproxen (Advil and Aleve) should never be used during pregnancy unless under medical supervision.

Psychological State

It has been proven that the more positive the patient feels about the medication being taken, the more positive the physical response. This is referred to as the **placebo effect**.

A *placebo* is an inactive substance that resembles a medication, although no drug is present. For example, a sugar tablet or a saline solution for injection may be used as a placebo in a research study program.

Placebos are most often used in blind study experiments in which groups of people are given either a drug or a placebo. (Needless to say, placebos are not administered if doing so would risk serious or irreversible harm to those taking them.) The individuals, unaware of which they have been given, are studied for the effects. Often, by virtue of strong belief or by the natural fluctuation of a disease (e.g., headaches may get better without treatment), the placebo-administered individuals achieve the desired effect associated with the drug they think they have received.

It is also possible for a drug's effect to decrease when the attitude of a patient toward a medication is negative. Attitudes toward medicines can also be influenced positively or negatively by cultural or religious beliefs. The caregiver needs to understand the importance of these beliefs to the patient.

> The significance of the placebo effect for you, the health care professional, is to recognize that your attitude regarding a medication may be picked up by the patient and indirectly may affect the patient's response to the drug.

Drug Interactions

Often patients are prescribed multiple drugs. Whenever more than one drug is taken, it is possible that the *combination* may alter the normal expected response of each individual drug. One drug may interact with another to increase, decrease, or cancel out the effects of the other.

The following terms are used to describe drug interactions:

Synergism. The action of two drugs working together in which one helps the other simultaneously for an effect that neither could produce alone. Drugs that work together are said to be synergistic.

Potentiation. The action of two drugs in which one prolongs or multiplies the effect of the other. Drug A may be said to potentiate the effect of drug B. This interaction is often used in pain medications.

Antagonism. The opposing action of two drugs in which one decreases or cancels out the effect of the other. Drug A may be referred to as an antagonist of drug B.

It is extremely important for the prescribing physician to know of all medications that a patient is taking to prevent undesirable **drug interactions**. On the other hand, it may be intentionally ordered that two drugs be taken together, because some drug interactions are desirable and beneficial. Compare the following situations, keeping in mind that any of the situations described can be desirable or undesirable based on the drugs and their effects.

Synergism. Simvastatin (Zocor) (lowers high cholesterol) and gemfibrozil (Lopid) (lowers high triglycerides) are very effective in treating patients who have both high cholesterol and triglyceride levels (collectively called high lipids). By giving small amounts of each together, high lipid levels can be treated more effectively. On the other hand, opioid analgesics and benzodiazepines can both cause sedation and drowsiness; when taken together this effect can become severe. To put this in terms of simple numbers, $1 + 1 = 3$, meaning the effect of both drugs together is more than each given separately, where both drugs are contributing to the amount of the effect.

Potentiation. To build up a high level of some forms of penicillin (an antibiotic) in the blood, the drug probenecid (antigout medication) can be given simultaneously. Probenecid potentiates the effect of penicillin by slowing the excretion rate of the antibiotic. To put this in terms of simple numbers, $1 + 0 = 2$, meaning the effect of one drug is increased due to being given with the other, even though the second drug does not contribute to the observed effect.

Antagonism. A narcotic antagonist (e.g., naloxone ([Narcan])) saves lives from drug overdoses by reversing the clinical effect of narcotics. On the other hand, antacids taken at the same time as tetracycline may alter the pH or form chelates, which are insoluble complexes that prevent the absorption of tetracycline. To put this in terms of simple math, $1 + 1 = 0$, meaning that the effect of one drug lowers or eliminates the effects of the other.

CLINICAL CONNECTION

Because of a recent increase in overdoses from both prescription narcotics and illegal opioids such as heroin, naloxone (Narcan) is now being used by prescribers to ensure patients and families are prepared in the case of an overdose. Naloxone works to quickly reverse the effects of opioids by using antagonism at the receptors where the drug is located. It can be administered via injection or nasal inhalation and will revive a person who has stopped breathing due to an overdose. Currently, there is a debate as to whether the use of this drug is ethical in the community and who should have access to the medication.

Dosage

Different dosages of a drug may bring about variations in the speed of drug action or effectiveness. Dosage is defined as the amount of a drug given for a particular therapeutic or desired effect. Terms of various dosage levels are:

1. *Minimum dose.* Smallest amount of a drug that will produce a therapeutic effect.
2. *Maximum dose.* Largest amount of a drug that will produce a desired effect without producing symptoms of toxicity.
3. *Loading dose.* Initial high dose (often maximum dose) used to quickly elevate the level of a drug in the blood (often followed by a series of lower maintenance doses).
4. *Maintenance dose.* Dose required to keep the level of a drug in the blood at a steady state to maintain the desired effect.
5. *Toxic dose.* Amount of a drug that will produce harmful side effects or symptoms of poisoning.
6. *Lethal dose.* Dose that causes death.
7. *Therapeutic dose.* Dose that is customarily given (average adult dose based on body weight of 150 lb); adjusted according to variations from the norm.

You may be familiar with the use of a high loading dose followed by a lesser maintenance dose. If you have taken antibiotics, you may have been instructed to take two tablets or capsules initially and then to take one tablet every 6 hours. It is frequently desirable to give a loading dose of antibiotics to quickly build up a high level of the drug in the blood initially and get the process of killing the bacteria started.

Pharmacogenomics

Did you know that for certain groups of medications the chance of achieving the desired effect is only around 30%–60%? This rather dismal response rate may be due to an individual's genetic background. The term pharmacogenomics is a science that examines how our genes may explain if a drug should work and if it will be toxic to our bodies. For example, the enzymes that metabolize drugs are genetically determined.

Because of this, some of us may metabolize drugs faster or slower than the average person. This may cause the drug to have a greater effect in a slow or poor metabolizer and possibly a poor or no effect in a rapid metabolizer compared to the average person. The hope is that the science of pharmacogenomics will help optimize drug therapy in individual patients by increasing effectiveness, reducing toxicity, and avoiding unnecessary treatment.

Before we dive into a further discussion of pharmacogenomics, we should make sure you understand some basic genetic information. Genes are a piece of DNA (deoxyribonucleic acid) that codes for a single protein; therefore, genes contain instructions for making proteins. Proteins act alone or with other proteins to perform cellular functions. Some genes do not code for proteins but regulate the activity of other genes that do (like a playground cop). These genes reside on chromosomes. Chromosomes are structural units for organizing DNA. Humans normally have 23 pairs of chromosomes (46 chromosomes total) because we inherit one chromosome from each parent.

The basic building blocks of DNA are called nucleotides. There are four nucleotides: adenine (A), guanine (G), thymine (T), and cytosine (C) (http://genomics.energy.gov). Polymorphisms are variations in the DNA sequence that may involve one nucleotide change (single nucleotide polymorphism or SNP, pronounced "snip") or the addition or deletion of an entire gene. These polymorphisms may affect drug pharmacokinetics or pharmacodynamics.

Now we will use a few examples to illustrate how pharmacogenomics may improve patient care. Mercaptopurine is a medication that is used to treat acute lymphoblastic leukemia (a blood cell cancer). It is metabolized by an enzyme abbreviated TMPT. Polymorphisms of this enzyme exist, and some people are poor metabolizers of mercaptopurine. A genetic screening test may be ordered prior to giving a patient this medicine. If the patient is found to be a poor metabolizer, the dose of mercaptopurine will be reduced to avoid increased bone marrow toxic effects (causes red and white blood cells and platelets to be reduced).

CYP2DG is an enzyme found in the liver that is responsible for metabolizing quite a few drugs. Depending on an individuals' genetic makeup, they may have enzyme activity ranging from poor to highly active metabolizers. Recently, the Food and Drug Administration (FDA) issued a warning to health care professionals concerning serious adverse effects including death in children after receiving codeine at a normal dosage after having their tonsils removed. Three children who died had a genetic variation in their CYP2DG enzyme, which caused the codeine to be rapidly metabolized to morphine, possibly leading to an overdose and death. Medications that may be affected by genetic variations in the CYP2DG gene include antidepressants, beta blockers, and tamoxifen, as well as many others.

By now you may be wondering why we do not use pharmacogenomic information more frequently. There are ethical issues to consider such as loss of privacy, genetic profiling, and the potential for discrimination. More research is necessary to prove that pharmacogenomics improves patient outcomes. See Table 3-2 for some examples of pharmacogenomic tests.

TABLE 3-2   **Examples of Pharmacogenomic Laboratory Tests**

DRUG	TEST	SPECIMEN	CLINICAL USE
warfarin	VKORC1, CYP2C9	Blood, buccal swab	Aids in dosing
abacavir	HLA-B 5701	Blood, buccal swab	Detects chance of hypersensitivity
irinotecan	UGT1A1	Blood, buccal swab	Aids in dosing
tamoxifen	CYP2D6	Blood, buccal swab	Determines how fast drug will be metabolized
carbamazepine	HLA-B 1502	Blood, buccal swab	Detects chance of hypersensitivity
azathioprine	TMPT	Blood	Detects chance of toxicity

Routes of Administration

The route of administration is probably the most significant factor in the speed of drug action.

The route of drug administration can be compared to the route of travel. In planning a trip from point A to point B, you may have a map that shows several courses of travel to reach the destination. The course you select is optional, depending on your choice for the quickest, cheapest, safest, or most scenic route.

Options for routes of drug administration are much the same. There are a number of methods by which drugs may be given to reach their destination. Sometimes the route selected is based on the degree of speed, cost, ease, or safety of administration. Sometimes there is no choice of routes because some medications can be given only by one route. Often this is because absorption occurs only by that route, or the substance is dangerous or toxic when given by another route. Insulin, for example, may be given only by injection and more recently via inhalation. Much research has been done to produce an oral form of insulin, but attempts have failed because the drug is destroyed by gastric juices.

The most common routes of administration may be grouped into two main categories as mentioned below:

1. *Enteral or GI tract routes*
   - Oral (PO)
   - Nasogastric tube (NG) and gastric tube
   - Rectal (R) or (PR = per rectum)

2. *Parenteral routes*, which include any route other than the GI tract
   a. Injection routes
   - Intravenous (IV)
   - Intramuscular (IM)
   - Subcutaneous (subcu)
   - Intradermal (ID)
   - Intracardiac, intraosseous, intraspinal, intraventricular, and intracapsular[*]

---

*These five injection routes are less common and are administered by the physician.

b. Non-injectable routes (stand-alone routes)

- Sublingual (SL) (under the tongue) or buccal (cheek: absorbed through mucosa, not swallowed) (*Note*: some classify SL and buccal as oral routes)
  - Transdermal or dermal (D) (skin patches that allow the drug to be slowly absorbed systemically)
  - Topical (T)
  - Ophthalmic (eyes)
  - Otic (ears)
  - Transvaginal
  - Nasal
  - Inhalation

> **The term *enteral* means within or by way of the intestine. The term *parenteral* is derived from the Greek term *para*, "apart from," plus *eneteron*, "the intestine." Therefore, *parenteral* technically means any route other than the gastrointestinal (GI) tract. In medical practice, parenteral is usually used to refer to injectables, whereas the rest of the non injectable routes are referred to as stand- alone routes.**

There are advantages and disadvantages in the use of each route. The physician's choice of a particular route of drug administration may depend on (1) desired effects (e.g., fast or slow, local or systemic); (2) absorption qualities of the drug; and (3) how the drug is supplied. Other general points regarding the effect of the route on the drug absorption are as follows:

1. The oral route is the easiest, but the effects are slower because of the time required for dissolution of the drug product in the alimentary canal before absorption.

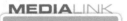

See it in Action! View videos on *Oral Medications and Their Administration* on the Online Resources.

2. The intravenous (IV) route is the fastest: Drugs enter the bloodstream immediately. Doses to be given IV are in small amounts; effects are immediate and can be quite dangerous if given in amounts recommended for other routes. IV drugs can be administered by IV push or bolus (a concentrated drug solution) (see Figure 3-3), or they can be diluted, and solutions are then infused more slowly by IV drip.

   a. IVs are administered by a physician, registered nurse, or paramedic.
   b. IV is the best route for treatment of emergencies because of the speed of action.
   c. IV fluids are used for re-hydration and to replace electrolytes.
   d. **Keep Vein Open** is a slow rate of IV fluid administration used to maintain patency of the IV for quick access for medication delivery

3. Parenteral routes are the choice when:
   a. Patient can take nothing by mouth.
   b. The drug is not suitable for GI absorption.

4. The intramuscular route is fairly rapid because the muscles are highly vascular. If it is desirable to slow the speed of absorption, the drug to be given IM may be added to an oily base.

5. The transdermal route allows for slower consistent drug absorption over time allowing the patient to usually place one patch on in the morning for the entire day.

6. The inhalation route is fast acting due to the large surface area of the lungs and rich blood supply, which allows the drug to enter the bloodstream quickly. This route often requires more involved patient cooperation and therefore education to be effective.

All of these routes will be explained in more detail in upcoming chapters.

MEDIALINK

See it in Action! View a video on *Parenteral Medications and Injections* on the Online Resources.

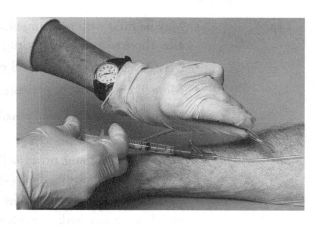

FIGURE 3-3 Intravenous (IV) push or bolus; IV drugs are administered slowly over a specified period of time (usually one to seven minutes).

UNEXPECTED RESPONSES TO DRUGS

Unintended effects from medications are termed side effects and can include a host of reactions such as cough, pain, tremors, headaches, dizziness, change in laboratory values, and photosensitivity. They can also be useful, as when Benadryl causes drowsiness it can be used as a sleep aid in addition to its normal use as an antihistamine. When side effects cause the patient to have a negative reaction, it is termed an **adverse drug reaction**, and many times a change in drug, dose, or frequency is needed to prevent these. Several other terms must be defined to complete your awareness of the bodily effects of drugs. These terms refer to adverse drug effects.

Teratogenic effect. Effect from maternal drug administration that causes physical defects in a fetus. See Table 3-3, which describes the FDA pregnancy categories.

Idiosyncratic reaction. Unique, unusual, and unexpected response to a drug.

Paradoxical reaction. Opposite effect from that expected. For example, a patient may have a paradoxical reaction to a particular tranquilizer if it causes agitation and excitement rather than tranquility.

Tolerance. Decreased response to a drug that develops after repeated doses are given. To achieve the desired effect, the drug dosage must be increased or the drug must be replaced.

Dependence. Acquired need for a drug that may produce psychological or physical symptoms of withdrawal when the drug is discontinued.

- Psychological dependence involves only a psychological craving; no physical symptoms of withdrawal were found other than anxiety.
- Physical dependence exists when cells actually have a need for the drug; symptoms of withdrawal include retching, nausea, pain, tremors, and sweating.

Hypersensitivity. Immune response (allergy) to a drug may be of varying degrees.

- May be mild with no immediate effects; rash or hives may appear after three to four days of drug therapy.
- May develop after uneventful previous uses of a drug.
- More likely to exist in patients with other known allergies.

Anaphylactic reaction. Severe, possibly fatal, allergic (hypersensitivity) response

- Signs include itching, urticaria (hives), hyperemia (reddened, warm skin), vascular collapse, shock, cyanosis, laryngeal edema, and dyspnea.
- Treatment includes cardiopulmonary resuscitation (CPR) if indicated and drugs as required: epinephrine (Adrenalin) and fluids to raise blood pressure; corticosteroid (Solu-Medrol) to reduce inflammation and the body's immunological response; or antihistamine (Benadryl) to suppress histamine, thereby reducing redness, itching, and edema.

Anaphylaxis has been noted often with the following: antibiotics, especially penicillin; X-ray dyes containing iodides (IVP [intravenous pyelogram] dye, angiogram dye, gallbladder dyes, etc.); foods (shellfish, onions, peanuts, etc.); and insect stings (bees and ants).

> **NOTE**
>
> Nausea, vomiting, and diarrhea are not considered signs of allergies.

TABLE 3-3   FDA Drug Pregnancy Categories

CATEGORY	DESCRIPTION
Pregnancy Category A	Drug studies on pregnant women have not demonstrated risk to fetus
Pregnancy Category B	Drug studies not performed on pregnant women; animal studies have not shown fetal risk
Pregnancy Category C	Conclusive drug studies have not yet been performed on pregnant women or animals
Pregnancy Category D	Drug studies have revealed adverse risk to fetus, and the benefit-to-risk ratio must be established before use during pregnancy
Pregnancy Category X	Drug studies have shown teratogenic effects, and the drug is contraindicated during pregnancy

Knowledge of any adverse reactions to drugs should be included in the patient's history. This information can be helpful in preventing repeated episodes. Getting an accurate drug history and clearly listing known allergies is a critical function of the health care professional.

Persons who have had an anaphylactic reaction to a substance should always wear a *Medic-Alert tag* or *bracelet* to identify the substance to which they are extremely allergic. Persons who have had hypersensitivity reactions to a substance are more at risk for reactions to other substances as well. Allergies should be listed on a card and carried in the wallet of the sensitive individual.

Extreme caution should be taken when giving a medication, especially antibiotics, to a patient for the first time, particularly if the patient has a history of other allergies.

CLINICAL CONNECTION

Epi-pens are often provided to patients who have a severe allergy that they may be exposed to unintentionally like a bee sting or peanuts in a baked product. It is important to educate the patient, as well as family and friends, how to properly use the epi-pen in the case of an emergency.

As shown in Figure 3-4, the epi-pen should be injected in a straight downward direction directly into a large muscle. It should be noted that it can be administered through a normal layer of clothing such as a pair of pants or shirt.

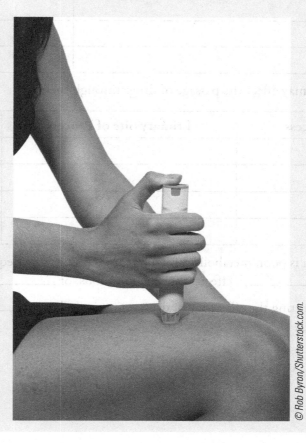

FIGURE 3-4 An epi-pen can be used to treat the severe allergic reaction known as anaphylaxis.

© Rob Byron/Shutterstock.com.

CHAPTER REVIEW QUIZ

Fill in the blanks.

1.

Drug Sources	Example	Trade Name	Classification

2. Drugs that are distributed throughout the body have _____ effects.

3. Drugs whose action is limited to a specific location have _____ effects.

4. As drugs pass through the body, they undergo four processes:

Process	Definition of Process

5. Factors that may affect the passage of drugs through the body:

Process	Primary Site of Process	Conditions Altering Process

6. If circulation is poor, metabolism is faulty, or excretion is inadequate, drugs may build up in the system, leading to _____ effects, causing poisonous, or _____, levels of the drug.

7. Variables affecting the efficiency of drug action include _____, _____, _____, and _____.

Match the term with the definition.

8. Synergism _____

9. Antagonism _____

10. Potentiation _____

11. Lethal dose _____

12. Toxic dose _____

13. Maintenance dose _____

14. Idiosyncrasy _____

15. Tolerance _____

16. Dependence _____

17. Teratogenic _____

a. Amount of drug required to keep drug level steady

b. Amount of drug that can cause death

c. Amount of drug that can cause dangerous side effects

d. One drug making the effect of another drug more powerful

e. Drugs working together for a better effect

f. Drugs working against each other or counteracting each other's effect

g. Acquired need for a drug, with symptoms of withdrawal when discontinued

h. Unusual response to a drug, other than expected effect

i. Effects on a fetus from maternal use of a drug

j. Decreased response after repeated use of a drug, increased dosage required for effect

Fill in the blanks.

18. An allergy or immune response to a drug is called

_____.

19. Allergic reactions to drugs may be *mild*, with symptoms such as

_____.

20. Allergic reactions to drugs are more common in patients with

_____.

21. *Severe* allergic reaction with shock, laryngeal edema, and dyspnea is called

_____.

22. Treatment of severe anaphylactic reactions can include the following: _____, _____, and _____.

STUDYGUIDE	Online Resources
PRACTICE	
Complete Chapter 3.	• Powerpoint presentation
	• Videos

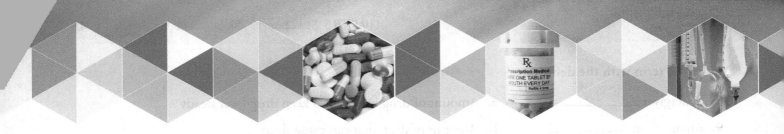

CHAPTER 4
MEDICATION PREPARATIONS AND SUPPLIES

KEY TERMS AND CONCEPTS

Capsule

Drug form

Elixir

Enema

Emulsion

Enteric-coated tablet

Inhalation drug forms

Injectable drug forms

Oral drug forms

Lozenge

Parenteral

Reconstitution

Rectal drug forms

Route of delivery

Solution

Suppository

Suspension

Sustained-release
   capsule or tablet

Syrup

Tablet

Topical drug forms

OBJECTIVES

Upon completion of this chapter, the learner should be able to

1. Differentiate between various oral and rectal drug forms

2. Describe the various injectable drug forms

3. Define the following types of injections and explain how they differ in administration and absorption rate: intravenous (IV), intramuscular (IM), and intradermal (ID)

4. Compare the IV injections referred to as IV push, IV infusion, and IV piggyback

5. Contrast the various topical drug forms

6. Explain the advantages of administering drugs via a transdermal patch

7. Describe inhalable drug forms

8. Identify various supplies used in the preparation of medications

9. Define the Key Terms and Concepts

The forms in which drugs are prepared are as numerous as the routes of administration. **Drug form** refers to the type of preparation in which the drug is supplied. Pharmaceutical companies prepare each drug in the form(s) most suitable for its intended **route of delivery** and means of absorption. *Drug form* and *drug preparation* are synonymous. The *Physicians' Desk Reference* (*PDR*) lists the forms available for each drug under the heading "How Supplied." See Table 4-1 for abbreviations of some of the drug forms and routes of administration.

TABLE 4-1   **Common Abbreviations for Drug Administration**

DRUG FORMS		ROUTES	
cap	capsule	IM	intramuscular
elix	elixir	IV	intravenous
gtt	drop	TOP	topical
supp	suppository	PO, po	oral
susp	suspension	R or PR (per rectum)	rectal
tab	tablet	subcu/sc	subcutaneous

DRUG FORMS AND DEVICES

You probably have received medications in many of the standard forms at some time during your life. Each form is defined and listed in the following sections according to the routes of administration. Figure 4-1 illustrates some examples of oral drug forms. As you read in Chapter 3, drugs may be administered through the gastrointestinal (GI) tract or parenterally. GI routes include oral, nasogastric or gastrostomy tube, and rectal. **Parenteral** refers to any route not involving the GI tract, including injection, topical (skin or mucosal), transdermal and the inhalation route.

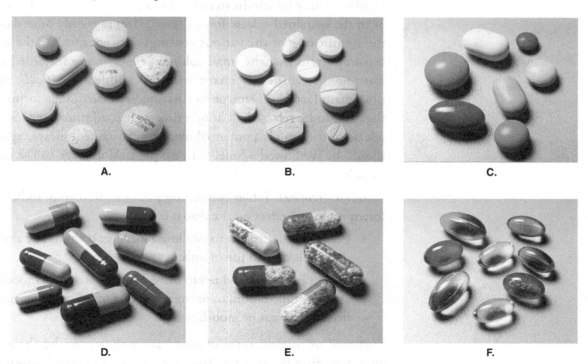

A.   B.   C.

D.   E.   F.

FIGURE 4-1 Oral drug forms. Tablets and capsules vary in size, shape, and color. (A) Tablets, (B) scored tablets, (C) enteric-coated tablets, (D) capsules, (E) sustained-release capsules, and (F) gelatin capsules.

Oral Drug Forms

Oral drug forms include the following:

Tablet. Tablets are disks of compressed drug. They may be of variety of shapes and colors, may be coated to enhance easy swallowing, and may be *scored* (evenly divided in halves or quarters by score lines) to enhance equal distribution of the drug if the tablet has been broken.

Enteric-coated tablet. Tablet with a special coating that resists disintegration by gastric juices. The coating dissolves further down the GI tract in the enteric, or intestinal, region. Some drugs that are irritating to the stomach, such as aspirin, are available in enteric-coated tablets. To be effective, the coating must never be destroyed by chewing or crushing when the tablet is administered. This is why patient education and auxiliary labels are very important to ensure that patients do not crush or split certain medications.

Capsule. Drug contained within a gelatin-type container.

- Easier to swallow than noncoated tablets.
- Double chamber may be pulled apart to add drug powder to soft foods or beverages for patients who have difficulty swallowing (unless specifically contraindicated for absorption).

Sustained-release capsule or tablet. Capsule or tablet containing drug particles that have various coatings (often of different colors) that differ in the amount of time required before the coatings dissolve. This form of drug preparation is designed to deliver a dose of drug over an extended period of time. An advantage of taking a drug in the sustained-release form is the decreased frequency of administration. For example, the antihypertensive Cardizem may be administered in tablet form 60 mg tid (three times daily) or in the sustained-release form (Tiazac, 180 mg) only once daily. Because of the significance of the various coatings that encapsulate the drug particles, it is important that the small colored pellets or any sustained-release dosage form *not* be crushed or mixed with foods unless *specifically allowed* by the drug manufacturer. Damage to sustained-release dosage forms may result in the drug to be released all at one time as it is administered. Such immediate release of the drug is a potential overdose. Sustained-release capsules or tablets should be swallowed whole, with no physical damage to the contents of the capsule.

Lozenge *(troche)*. Tablet containing palatable flavoring, indicated for a local (often soothing) effect on the throat or mouth.

- Patient is advised *not* to swallow a lozenge; it should be allowed to slowly dissolve in the mouth.
- Patient is also advised *not* to drink liquids for approximately 15 minutes after administration, to prevent washing off of the lozenge contents from the throat or mouth.

Suspension. Liquid form of medication that must be shaken well before administration because the drug particles settle at the bottom of the bottle.

The drug is not evenly dissolved in the liquid until properly shaking the mixture.

- A cephalosporin (Cephalexin) suspension is a commonly used antibiotic suspension for children. This form is more easily ingested by children than are capsules of Keflex.
- Flavoring of suspensions is common, as many tend to have a bitter taste, resulting from them being suspended in liquid, rather than dissolved.

Emulsion. Liquid drug preparation that contains oils and fats in water.

Elixir or fluid extract. Liquid drug forms with alcohol base.

- Should be tightly capped to prevent alcohol evaporation.
- Should not be available to alcoholics.
- Caution use in small children.

Syrup. Sweetened, flavored liquid drug form. Cherry syrup drug preparations are common for children.

Solution. Liquid drug form in which the drug is totally and evenly dissolved. Appearance is clear rather than cloudy or settled (as with a suspension).

Many drug forms for the oral route are commonly available over the counter and include thousands of trade name products. The oral route is the easiest and probably the cheapest for administration. It is, however, *not* the route of choice for the treatment of emergencies, acute pain, nothing by mouth (NPO) patients (ordered to have nothing by mouth), or patients who are unable to swallow. Other routes, especially the parenteral routes, produce a more rapid absorption rate and drug effect due to the drug's often direct absorption into the bloodstream.

Rectal Drug Forms

Rectal drug forms include the following:

Suppository. Drug suspended in a substance, such as cocoa butter, that melts at body temperature.

Enema. Drug may be either a suspension (needs to be shaken before administration) or a solution to be administered as an enema.

The rectal route of administration is often the choice if the patient is ordered to have NPO or cannot swallow. The most common classifications of drugs given rectally include laxatives, sedatives, antiemetics (prevent vomiting), and antipyretics (reduce fever). A local analgesic effect may also be achieved by this route.

Injectable Drug Forms

Injectable drug forms include the following:

Liquid. Drug suspended (suspension) or dissolved (solution) in a sterile vehicle.

- Quite often the solutions have a sterile water base and are thus referred to as aqueous (aq) (waterlike) solutions.
- Some solutions have an oil base, which tends to cause a more prolonged absorption time. The oily nature of these solutions makes them thick; thus they are referred to as viscous solutions.

Powder. Dry particles of drugs. The powder itself cannot be injected. It must be mixed with a sterile diluting solution (sterile water or saline solution) to render an injectable solution. This is termed **reconstitution** of a drug. Drugs are supplied undiluted in powder form because of the short period of time they remain stable after dilution.

The various injection routes differ according to the type of tissues into which the drug is deposited and the rate of absorption.

Intravenous. Injected directly into a vein. Immediate absorption and availability to major organs renders this route a dangerous one. IV drugs are usually administered by physicians, paramedics, or registered nurses. Types of IV injections include the following:

- IV push, a small volume of drug (bolus) injected into a peripheral saline lock (PRN adapter), attached to a vein (Figure 4-2A). An IV push medication can also be injected into a port on a primary (continuous) injection line (Figure 4-2B).
- IV infusion or IV drip, a large volume of fluids, often with drugs added, that infuses continually into a vein (Figure 4-2C).
- IV piggyback (IVPB), a drug diluted in moderate volume (50–100 mL) of fluid for intermittent infusion at specified intervals, usually q6–8h; the diluted solution is infused (piggyback) into a port on the main IV tubing or into a rubber adapter on the IV catheter (Figure 4-2D).

Intramuscular. Injected into a muscle by positioning the needle and syringe at a 90-degree angle from the skin (Figure 4-3). Absorption is fairly rapid due to the vascularity (presence of many blood vessels) in muscle. In most cases, a 1-inch needle is used for IM injections, but for a smaller person or a child, a ⅝-inch needle is sometimes more appropriate.

Subcutaneous. Injected into the fatty layer of tissue below the skin by positioning the needle and syringe at a 45-degree angle from the skin (Figure 4-4). Commonly, a ⅝-inch needle is used for subcutaneous injections. This may be the route of choice for drugs that should not be absorbed as rapidly as through the IV or IM routes. Sometimes, especially with self-administration or a shorter needle, a 90-degree angle is used.

Intradermal. Injected just beneath the skin by positioning the needle bevel up and the syringe at a 15-degree angle from the skin (Figure 4-5). This route is used primarily for allergy skin testing. Because of the lack of vascularity in the dermis, absorption is slow. The greatest reaction is in the local tissues rather than systemic. When a small amount (0.1–0.2 mL) of drug is injected intradermally, the amount of redness that develops around the injection site can be

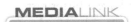

MEDIALINK

See It In Action! View a video on *Powdered Medications* on the Online Resources.

Note

When adding a medication to an IV solution bag through the injection port, take the bag down and invert it a few times to disperse the drug throughout the solution instead of remaining concentrated at the bottom of the bag.

MEDIALINK

See It In Action! View a video on *Preparing an IV Solution* on the Online Resources.

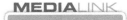

MEDIALINK

See It In Action! View a video on *Parenteral Medications* on the Online Resources.

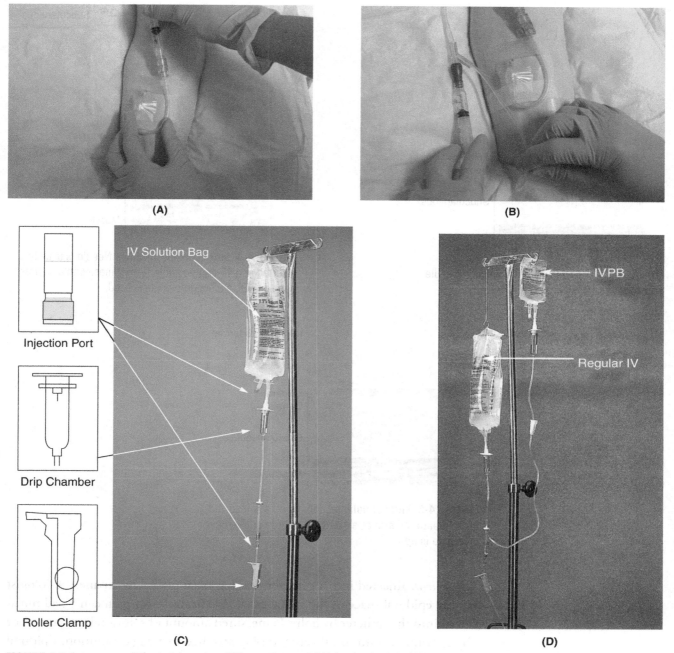

FIGURE 4-2 Intravenous (IV) administration. Different forms of IV injection include (A) IV push, injecting a bolus of medication into a peripheral saline lock; (B) pinch closed the IV tubing of a primary infusion line to administer an IV push medication; (C) IV infusion (continuous); and (D) IV piggyback (IVPB) intermittent.

used to determine whether a person is sensitive to the drug. Tuberculin (TB) skin tests (PPD) are also administered intradermally, and the site is inspected 48–72 h later for hardness (induration) and swelling. Redness (erythema) alone, *without swelling*, does not indicate a positive test result with PPD. The *raised area* (*induration*) is measured with a special ruler and the number of millimeters (mm) is documented. Check with your local Public Health Department regarding appropriate protocol with a positive PPD test result.

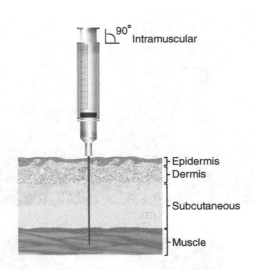

FIGURE 4-3 Intramuscular (IM) injection. Needle is inserted at a 90-degree angle.

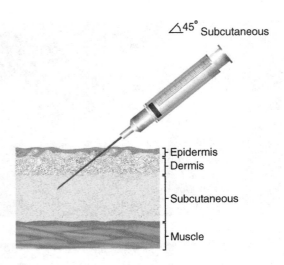

FIGURE 4-4 Subcutaneous injection. Needle is usually inserted at a 45-degree angle. Sometimes, with a shorter needle (3/8), a 90-degree angle is used.

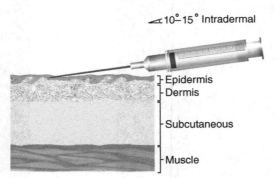

FIGURE 4-5 Intradermal injection. Needle is inserted just beneath the skin at a 10- to 15-degree angle. Bevel of needle is up.

Epidural. Injected into a catheter that has been placed by an anesthesiologist in the epidural space of the spinal canal. Medications for pain can be administered into the catheter by bolus (a measured amount of solution in a syringe) or by continuous infusion through tubing attached to a bag of solution. Epidural catheters have long been used for the administration of opioid analgesics for chronic intractable pain and for chemotherapy. Epidurals have become a popular and widely accepted vehicle for the management of acute postoperative pain.

The less common parenteral routes, which are usually limited to a physician's administration, with some exceptions, are as follows:

Intraosseous. Injected directly into the marrow of long bones. This route may be used to administer medications during a cardiac arrest or other emergency situations when traditional IV access is not available. (The intracardiac route is no longer recommended in Advanced Cardiac Life Support guidelines.)

Intraventricular. Drugs injected directly into the brain via a catheter (called a ventriculostomy) placed in a brain ventricle. In critical care, antibiotics can be given via a ventriculostomy tube.

Intraspinal. Injected into the subarachnoid space, which contains cerebrospinal fluid that surrounds the spinal cord. Drugs injected by this route are frequently anesthetics, which render a lack of sensation to those regions of the body distal to the intraspinal injection.

Intracapsular (intra-articular). Injected into the capsule of a joint, usually to reduce inflammation, as in bursitis. Arthritic or bursitic joints often injected with anti-inflammatory drugs include shoulders, elbows, wrists, ankles, knees, and hips.

Topical Form

Topical drug forms include drugs for dermal application and drugs for mucosal application. Those for *dermal* application include the following:

Cream or ointment. A semisolid preparation containing a drug, for external application. *Note*: Creams and ointments are not the same. The dose used differs for each. Also creams tend to be more aqueous in nature, meaning they are composed of more water-based ingredients than an ointment, which tends to be thicker or more viscous; this affects how they are used with different skin conditions.

Lotion. A liquid preparation applied externally for the treatment of skin disorders. Unlike hand lotions, medicated lotions (e.g., calamine lotion) should be *patted*, not rubbed, on the affected skin.

Liniment. Preparation for external use that is rubbed on the skin as a counterirritant. As such, the liniment creates a different sensation (e.g., tingling or burning) to mask pain in the skin or muscles.

Transdermal patch. Skin patch containing drug molecules that can be absorbed through the skin at varying rates to promote a consistent blood level of the drug between application times (Figure 4-6). Transdermal patches were first taken on the space shuttles during the 1990s for the prevention of nausea. Advantages of this method of administration include:

- Easy application, with minimal discomfort or undesirable taste
- Effectiveness for long periods of time, hours for some drugs, and days for others
- Consistent blood level of drug because the drug is released at varying rates rather than all at one time

Transdermal patches vary in size, shape, and color. They are commonly seen today on patients for the prevention of angina. Current marketing of transdermal patches also includes others for the prevention of motion sickness (may be applied before traveling), management of chronic pain (e.g., Duragesic; see Chapter 19), use as a smoking deterrent (e.g., Nicoderm CQ), and estrogen replacement (e.g., Climara). Research is ongoing for the development of transdermal patches for high blood pressure, ulcers,

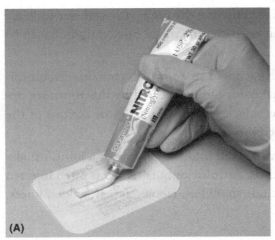
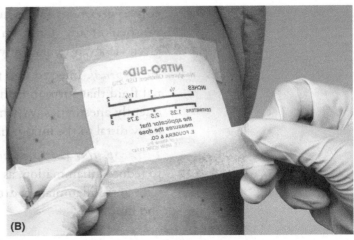

FIGURE 4-6 Topical administration. Dermal application includes creams and liquids placed on the skin. (A) Nitroglycerin ointment is measured on Appli-Ruler paper and (B) paper containing ointment is applied to the skin and taped in place. Mark date and time on tape.

allergies, and heart conditions. Probably not all drug molecules will be adaptable to this drug form, but this form certainly has opened new doors in the area of drug administration.

Both the transdermal patch and ointment are common forms for administration of nitroglycerin. Nitroglycerin is a vasodilator used for the treatment of angina (chest pain related to narrowing of the coronary arteries). The advantage of the external applications of nitroglycerin is their ability to *prevent* angina by the slow, consistent release of the drug over a period of time. Before the external applications became available, nitroglycerin was primarily available in the form of a sublingual tablet to be taken at the time of an angina attack. Now all three forms are used—the tablet, the ointment, and the patch—with the external forms focusing on the prevention of angina. They are applied at regular intervals, as follows:

Ointment. One to two inches measured and applied q8h (every eight hours) on special Appli-Ruler paper (see Figure 4-6).

Transdermal patch. One patch (available in varied doses) usually applied for 12–14 h per day and then removed. Other types of patches are applied every 24–72 h depending on the condition treated (Figure 4-7). (See Chapter 9 for administration instructions.)

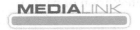

See It In Action! Go to the Online Resources to view a video on *Ointments and their Applications.*

FIGURE 4-7 Nitro-Dur is a transdermal system of delivering medication used for prevention and long-term management of angina pectoris.

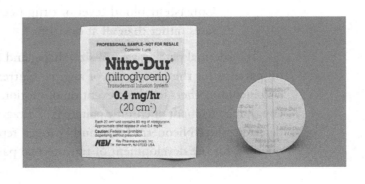

Other drug preparations considered topical are those that are applied to *mucosal membranes*. Some are administered for local effect (at the site of application), and in other cases, a systemic (affecting the whole body) effect is desired. The *mucosal drug forms* include the following:

Eye, ear, and nose drops (gtt). Drugs in sterile liquids to be applied by drops (referred to as instillation of drops).

Eye ointment. Sterile semisolid preparation, often antibiotic in nature, only for ophthalmic use.

Vaginal creams. Medicated creams, often of antibiotic or antifungal nature, that are to be inserted vaginally with the use of a special applicator.

Rectal and vaginal suppositories. Drugs suspended in a substance, such as cocoa butter, that melts at body temperature, for local effect. Some rectal suppositories are also used for systemic effects, for example, Tylenol suppository for fever (Figure 4-8).

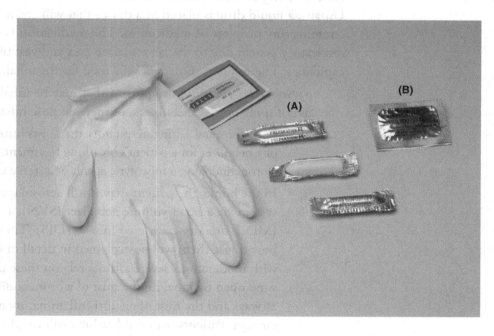

FIGURE 4-8 Topical administration via mucous membranes. Suppositories are available in various shapes and sizes, for example (A) rectal suppositories, wrapped in foil and unwrapped, and (B) vaginal suppository, wrapped in foil. Lubricant and a glove will be needed for administration.

Douche solution. Sterile solution, often an antiseptic such as povidone–iodine solution and sterile water, used to irrigate the vaginal canal.

Buccal tablet. Tablet that is absorbed *via the buccal mucosa* in the mouth.

- Patient should be told *not* to swallow the tablet; it is to be placed between the cheek and gums and allowed to dissolve slowly.
- Not commonly used today. A sublingual tablet is preferable.

Sublingual tablet. Tablet that is absorbed via the mucosa under the tongue.

- Patient should be told *not* to swallow the tablet; it is to be placed under the tongue and allowed to dissolve slowly.
- The most common sublingual tablet is nitroglycerin. Given for the treatment of angina, this drug reaches the bloodstream immediately via the rich vascular supply of sublingual capillaries. Angina may be relieved within one to five minutes after sublingual nitroglycerin is administered.

Implantable Devices

Implantable devices are available in a variety of sizes and are placed just below the skin near blood vessels where the medication can readily be absorbed into the bloodstream. One example is a small infusion pump implanted in a diabetic patient's waist to deliver a continuous supply of insulin. Implantable devices are also used to deliver contraceptives and to administer chemotherapeutic drugs to cancer patients.

Another recent and innovative drug form entails sandwiching the drug between very thin plastic membranes and then placing it under the patient's eyelid. This administration permits a controlled release of medicine over an extended time period. Pilocarpine, which is used to treat glaucoma, has been successfully administered in this manner with little or no discomfort.

Inhalation Drug Forms

The inhalation route is a very fast acting (second to IV route) and effective route for delivering humidification and medication directly into the respiratory system. Usually, a liquid drug is placed in a device that will create a fine mist or aerosol that contains tiny droplets of medication. The medication is rapidly absorbed into the respiratory system due to the large surface area and vast blood supply of pulmonary capillaries. The **inhalation drug forms** used for the inhalation route include:

Spray or mist. Liquid drug forms that may be inhaled as fine droplets via the use of spray bottles, nebulizers, or metered dose inhalers.

- In the hospital setting, respiratory therapists instill a liquid into a chamber of a nebulizer for a patient's breathing treatment. Often the liquid contains a bronchodilator, a mucolytic agent, or a sterile saline solution for moisture.

- In the home, the patient may instill aerosol sprays into the respiratory system via a small-volume nebulizer (SVN), a metered-dose inhaler (MDI), or a dry-powdered inhaler (DPI). These inhaler devices and how to use them will be explained in detail in Chapter 26. Patients with moderate-to-severe asthma rely on these devices to keep their airways open by inhaling the mist of a bronchodilator to open constricted airways and the mist of an anti-inflammatory agent to reduce swollen airways. Patients with mild asthma will use their inhalers when needed (PRN) to treat or prevent mild episodes.

SUPPLIES

Considering the variety of drug forms you may be administering, you must become familiar with various supplies to be used:

Medicine cup. Two types of disposable cups are commonly used. Paper cups are used for dispensing tablets and capsules. Plastic 1-oz medicine cups with measurements (mL, tsp, tbsp, or oz) marked on the side are used for dispensing oral liquid medications. (See Table 5-1 [in Chapter 5] for a list of common abbreviations used in medication orders.)

Individual pill crusher and pill cutter. Used in most institutions (Figure 4-9).

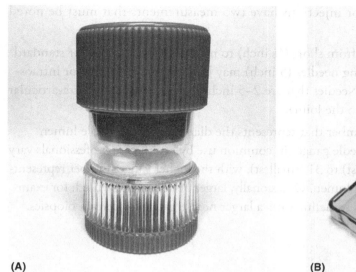

(A)

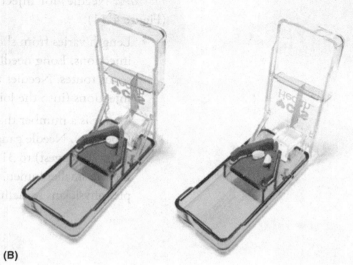

(B)

FIGURE 4-9 (A) A plastic pill crusher. (B) A plastic pill splitter to break scored tablets, if necessary.

Various other pill-crushing devices are available.

Medication for injection is contained in an ampule, a vial, or a prefilled syringe (Figure 4-10):

Ampule. Small glass container that holds a single dose of sterile solution for injection. The ampule must be broken at the neck to obtain the solution.

Vial. Glass container sealed at the top by a rubber stopper to enhance sterility of the contents. Contents may be a solution or a powdered drug that needs to be reconstituted. Vials may be multiple dose or unit dose.

- Multiple-dose vials contain large quantities of solution (up to 50 mL) and may be entered repeatedly through the rubber stopper to remove a portion of the contents. They contain a preservative that prevents microbial growth.

- Unit-dose vials contain small quantities of solution (1–2 mL) that are removed during a single use. Unit-dose vials are widely used today as a means of controlling abuse or removal of excess amounts of solution from a drug vial.

FIGURE 4-10 Medications given parenterally. (A) Ampule, (B) sterile cartridge with premeasured medication, and (C) vial of powder for reconstitution.

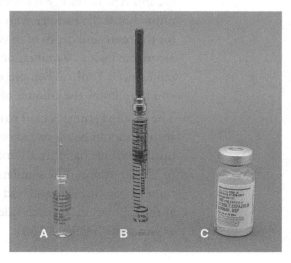

Needles. Needles for injections have two measurements that must be noted (Figure 4-11).

- Length varies from short (⅜ inch) to medium (1–1½ inch) for standard injections. Long needles (5 inch) may be used for intraspinal or intraosseous routes. Needles that are 2–5 inches long are used for intra-articular injections (into the joint).

- Gauge is a number that represents the diameter of the needle lumen (opening). Needle gauges in common use by health care professionals vary from 16 (largest) to 31 (smallest), with the higher gauge number representing the smaller lumen. Occasionally, larger needles may be used; for example, physicians sometimes use a larger needle gauge for certain biopsies.

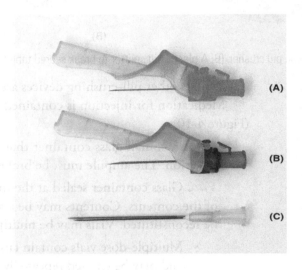

FIGURE 4-11 Examples of some various gauges and lengths of needles. (A) 25-gauge, 1-inch needle with safety cap; (B) 21-gauge, 1-inch needle with safety cap; and (C) 18-gauge, 1½-inch needle.

Syringes. The three most common disposable syringes used for parenteral administration of drugs are the standard hypodermic syringe, the tuberculin (TB) syringe, and the insulin syringe (Figure 4-12).

- The standard hypodermic syringe has a capacity of 2–3 mL. Most companies prepackage this type of syringe with a needle attached. You may use this type of syringe for either subcutaneous or IM injections, so you must choose the package with the needle length and gauge appropriate for the route and depth of injection you will give. All hypodermic syringes are marked with 10 calibrations per milliliter (mL). Thus, each small line represents 0.1 mL. When preparing for an injection with this syringe, you must know the amount of solution needed to the nearest 0.1 mL.

- The insulin syringe is used strictly for administering insulin to diabetics. Insulin should be measured only in an insulin syringe. The standard insulin syringe has only a 1-mL capacity, which is equivalent to 100 units of U-100 insulin. The standard U-100 syringe has a dual scale: even numbers on one side and odd numbers on the other side. Look carefully at the calibrations on each side. Count each calibration (on one side only) as two units (Figure 4-13A).

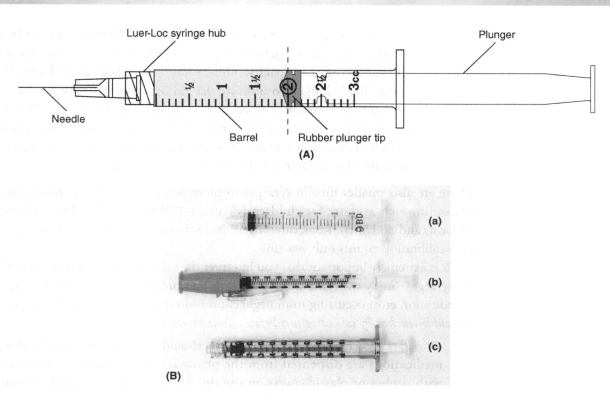

FIGURE 4-12 (A) Parts of a syringe. (B) Types of syringes: (a) 3-mL syringe, (b) standard U-100 insulin, and (c) 1-mL tuberculin with Leur-Lok.

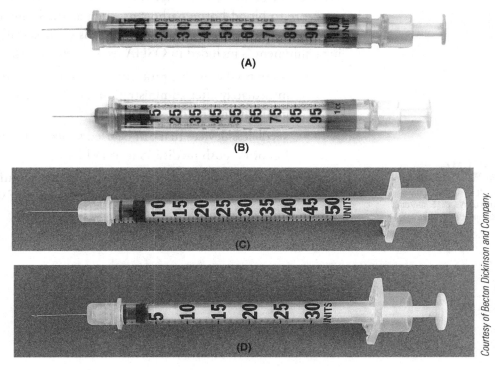

FIGURE 4-13 Insulin syringes. (A) and (B) Opposite sides of the same standard U-100 insulin syringe; note the numbers; (C) Lo-Dose insulin syringes, 50 units; and (D) 30 units.

- The TB syringe is very narrow and is finely calibrated. Like the insulin syringe, the total capacity is only 1 mL. There are 100 fine calibration lines marking the capacity. Thus, each line represents 0.01 mL. Every tenth line is longer, to indicate 0.1 mL increments. Very precise small amounts of solution may be measured with the TB syringe. It is most commonly used for newborn and pediatric dosages and for ID skin tests. When preparing for an injection with this syringe, you must know the amount of solution needed to the nearest 0.01 mL.

There are also smaller insulin syringes to more accurately measure small amounts of insulin, such as those for children (Figure 4-13B for Lo-Dose Insulin Syringes 50 Units and 30 Units). Look carefully at the calibrations. In these Lo-Dose syringes, each calibration counts only *one* unit.

It is extremely important that you interpret the value of the calibrations on each of the syringes. Study the calibrations each time you prepare for an injection to prevent a medication error occurring from negligent misinterpretation. *All insulin dosages must be double-checked by two caregivers before administration.*

Oral syringes. Health care professionals should be aware that some oral liquid medications are dispensed from the pharmacy in disposable plastic syringes with rubber or plastic covers on the tip. These syringes are labeled "Not for injection" or "For oral use only."

Safety Devices

The Occupational Safety and Health Administration (OSHA) has mandated that every effort be made to reduce the risk of needle-stick injuries that could lead to exposure to blood-borne pathogens, such as the human immunodeficiency virus (HIV), hepatitis B virus (HBV), or hepatitis C virus (HCV). Therefore, the following equipment is included in OSHA recommendations:

- Safety needles with a protective sheath that covers the needle automatically immediately after administration, or others that retract into the syringe upon administration.
- Needleless devices that can be used to access IV tubing for the administration of IV push medications or IVPBs.

Safety devices vary depending on the company manufacturing the equipment. Therefore, it is important that you familiarize yourself with the safety equipment used in your facility.

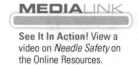

MEDIALINK

See It In Action! View a video on *Needle Safety* on the Online Resources.

CHAPTER REVIEW QUIZ

Fill in the blanks.

1. **a.** Which route of administration is used most often? Why?

   _____.

   b. Which route is fastest? _____.

Complete with the appropriate drug form.

2. A tablet placed under the tongue: _____.

3. A tablet placed in the cheek pouch: _____.

4. A tablet dissolved in the mouth for local action: _____.

5. A coated tablet that dissolves in the intestines instead of in the stomach:

   _____.

6. A tablet or capsule that has delayed action over a longer period of time:

   _____.

7. A liquid drug form with an alcohol base:

   _____.

8. A liquid medication that must be shaken before administration:

   _____.

9. Drugs given by the rectal route include _____.

10. The parenteral route refers to any route other than the GI route. Name four parenteral routes:

    _____

    _____

    _____

    _____.

Fill in the blanks.

11. Topical drug forms include those applied to the _____ and _____.

12. Medicine for injection is contained in two types of glass containers:

    a. With rubber stopper on top: _____.

    b. All glass to be broken at the neck: _____.

13. Needles are selected according to two measurements: _____ and _____.

14. The three most commonly used syringes for injections are _____, _____, and _____.

Labeling.

15. Label the parts of a syringe.

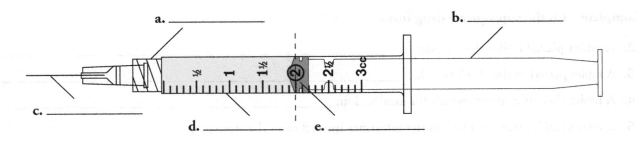

a. _____   b. _____

c. _____

d. _____   e. _____

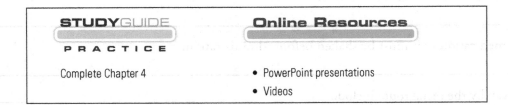

STUDYGUIDE	Online Resources
P R A C T I C E	
Complete Chapter 4	• PowerPoint presentations
	• Videos

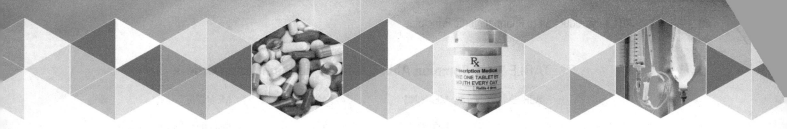

CHAPTER 5

ABBREVIATIONS AND SYSTEMS OF MEASUREMENT

KEY TERMS AND CONCEPTS

Computerized physician order entry (CPOE)

Conversion of units

Electronic medication administration record (eMAR)

e-prescribing (eRx)

Household system

Medical abbreviations

Medication orders

Metric system

Telephone order (TO)

OBJECTIVES

Upon completion of this chapter, the learner should be able to

1. Identify common abbreviations and symbols used for medication orders

2. List the six parts of a medication order and the two additional items required on a prescription blank

3. Describe the responsibilities of a health care professional regarding verbal and telephone orders for medications

4. Interpret medication orders correctly

5. Compare and contrast the three systems of measurement

6. Convert dosages from one system to another by use of the tables for metric and household equivalents

7. Describe appropriate patient education for those who will be measuring and administering their own medications

8. Define the Key Terms and Concepts

ABBREVIATIONS

Interpretation of the medication order is the first responsibility of a health care professional when preparing medication for administration. Knowledge of **medical abbreviations** and symbols is essential for accurate interpretation of the physician's order. The common abbreviations and symbols in Table 5-1 must be memorized. Orders may vary in the use of capital versus lowercase letters. You may occasionally see other abbreviations not included in this list. *When in doubt, always question the meaning. Never guess!*

TABLE 5-1   **Common Abbreviations for Medication Orders**

ABBREVIATION	MEANING	ABBREVIATION	MEANING
a	before	mEq	milliequivalent
ac	before meals	mg	milligram
AD	Right ear	ml, mL	milliliter (equivalent to cc)
AM, am	Morning	mm	millimeter
AS	left ear	NEB	nebulizer
AU	both ears	NG	nasogastric
bid	twice a day	NPO, npo	nothing by mouth
cap	Capsule	NS, N/S, NSS	normal saline (sodium chloride, 0.9%)
cm	centimeter	OD	right eye
c̄	with	ODT	orally disintegrating tablet
D/C, dc	Discontinue	OS	Left eye
D5W	dextrose 5% in water	OU	both eyes
DS	double strength	oz	Ounce
EC	enteric coated	p	After
ER	extended release	pc	after meals
g	Gram	PM, pm	afternoon
gr	grains	po, PO	by mouth, orally
gtt	Drop	PRN, prn	whenever necessary or as needed
h, hr	Hour	q2h	every 2h
Hs	bedtime	qh	every hour
IM	intramuscular	qid	four times a day
IV	intravenous	qs	quantity sufficient
IVPB	intravenous piggyback	R, pr	rectal, per rectum
kg, Kilo	kilogram	RL, R/L	Ringer's lactate
KVO	keep vein open	s̄	without
LA	long acting	sc/subcu[a]	subcutaneous
L	liter	SL	sublingual
LR	Lactated Ringer's	SR	sustained release
mcg	microgram	stat	immediately and once only

ABBREVIATION	MEANING	ABBREVIATION	MEANING
supp	suppository	TO	telephone order
tab	tablet	tsp, t	teaspoon
tbsp, T, tbs	tablespoon	Vag/PV	vaginal
tid	three times daily	VO	verbal order

Note: Abbreviations should be written without periods. Also some abbreviations in this table are on the ISMP's List of Error-Prone Abbreviations, Symbols, and Dose Designations, but it is still important to know them.

ᵃ Although *subcutaneous* can also have the abbreviations of SC, SQ, or subq, these abbreviations are noted on the ISMP's List of Error-Prone Abbreviations, Symbols, and Dose Designations. When handwritten, they can be confused for other terms. Therefore, we will be using "subcu" throughout the chapters. With the expected near-future universal implementation of electronic records and electronic charting, handwritten look-alike errors will hopefully become a thing of the past.

The *Institute for Safe Medication Practices* (*ISMP*) monitors for and categorizes medication errors. Its purpose is to identify practices that have contributed to medication errors. The ISMP has published a list of problematic abbreviations, *ISMP's List of Error-Prone Abbreviations, Symbols, and Dose Designations* (Figure 5-1). In addition, the Joint Commission has approved a minimum list of "dangerous" abbreviations that have been prohibited effective January 1, 2004. Items required to be on an organization's "Do Not Use" list are highlighted with a double asterisk (**) in the ISMP List (Figure 5-1).

Another safety practice requires the avoidance of periods in all medical abbreviations. If poorly written, the period could be mistaken as the number 1, causing an error in dosage. In addition, before giving or taking any medication order, the patient's allergies should be reviewed.

Medication orders contain six parts.

1. Date/time that the order was taken
2. Patient's name
3. Medication name
4. Dosage and/or amount of medication
5. Route or manner of administration (e.g., oral, subcutaneous)
6. Directions for use, including time to be administered and/or frequency

Medication orders must always be written and signed by a physician. In an emergency, the physician may give a verbal order (VO). It is the responsibility of the health care professional to *read back and confirm the order* (i.e., medication and amount) before administration and to write down the medication, amount, and time of administration as soon as they are given. The physician will sign the medication order after the emergency.

Institute for Safe Medication Practices

ISMP's List of *Error-Prone Abbreviations, Symbols,* and *Dose Designations*

The abbreviations, symbols, and dose designations found in this table have been reported to ISMP through the ISMP National Medication Errors Reporting Program (ISMP MERP) as being frequently misinterpreted and involved in harmful medication errors. They should **NEVER** be used when communicating medical information. This includes internal communications, telephone/verbal prescriptions, computer-generated labels, labels for drug storage bins, medication administration records, as well as pharmacy and prescriber computer order entry screens.

Abbreviations	Intended Meaning	Misinterpretation	Correction
µg	Microgram	Mistaken as "mg"	Use "mcg"
AD, AS, AU	Right ear, left ear, each ear	Mistaken as OD, OS, OU (right eye, left eye, each eye)	Use "right ear," "left ear," or "each ear"
OD, OS, OU	Right eye, left eye, each eye	Mistaken as AD, AS, AU (right ear, left ear, each ear)	Use "right eye," "left eye," or "each eye"
BT	Bedtime	Mistaken as "BID" (twice daily)	Use "bedtime"
cc	Cubic centimeters	Mistaken as "u" (units)	Use "mL"
D/C	Discharge or discontinue	Premature discontinuation of medications if D/C (intended to mean "discharge") has been misinterpreted as "discontinued" when followed by a list of discharge medications	Use "discharge" and "discontinue"
IJ	Injection	Mistaken as "IV" or "intrajugular"	Use "injection"
IN	Intranasal	Mistaken as "IM" or "IV"	Use "intranasal" or "NAS"
HS	Half-strength	Mistaken as bedtime	Use "half-strength" or "bedtime"
hs	At bedtime, hours of sleep	Mistaken as half-strength	
IU**	International unit	Mistaken as IV (intravenous) or 10 (ten)	Use "units"
o.d. or OD	Once daily	Mistaken as "right eye" (OD-oculus dexter), leading to oral liquid medications administered in the eye	Use "daily"
OJ	Orange juice	Mistaken as OD or OS (right or left eye); drugs meant to be diluted in orange juice may be given in the eye	Use "orange juice"
Per os	By mouth, orally	The "os" can be mistaken as "left eye" (OS-oculus sinister)	Use "PO," "by mouth," or "orally"
q.d. or QD**	Every day	Mistaken as q.i.d., especially if the period after the "q" or the tail of the "q" is misunderstood as an "i"	Use "daily"
qhs	Nightly at bedtime	Mistaken as "qhr" or every hour	Use "nightly"
qn	Nightly or at bedtime	Mistaken as "qh" (every hour)	Use "nightly" or "at bedtime"
q.o.d. or QOD**	Every other day	Mistaken as "q.d." (daily) or "q.i.d. (four times daily) if the "o" is poorly written	Use "every other day"
q1d	Daily	Mistaken as q.i.d. (four times daily)	Use "daily"
q6PM, etc.	Every evening at 6 PM	Mistaken as every 6 hours	Use "daily at 6 PM" or "6 PM daily"
SC, SQ, sub q	Subcutaneous	SC mistaken as SL (sublingual); SQ mistaken as "5 every;" the "q" in "sub q" has been mistaken as "every" (e.g., a heparin dose ordered "sub q 2 hours before surgery" misunderstood as every 2 hours before surgery)	Use "subcut" or "subcutaneously"
ss	Sliding scale (insulin) or ½ (apothecary)	Mistaken as "55"	Spell out "sliding scale;" use "one-half" or "½"
SSRI	Sliding scale regular insulin	Mistaken as selective-serotonin reuptake inhibitor	Spell out "sliding scale (insulin)"
SSI	Sliding scale insulin	Mistaken as Strong Solution of Iodine (Lugol's)	
i/d	One daily	Mistaken as "tid"	Use "1 daily"
TIW or tiw	3 times a week	Mistaken as "3 times a day" or "twice in a week"	Use "3 times weekly"
U or u**	Unit	Mistaken as the number 0 or 4, causing a 10-fold overdose or greater (e.g., 4U seen as "40" or 4u seen as "44"); mistaken as "cc" so dose given in volume instead of units (e.g., 4u seen as 4cc)	Use "unit"
UD	As directed ("ut dictum")	Mistaken as unit dose (e.g., diltiazem 125 mg IV infusion "UD" misinterpreted as meaning to give the entire infusion as a unit [bolus] dose)	Use "as directed"
Dose Designations and Other Information	**Intended Meaning**	**Misinterpretation**	**Correction**
Trailing zero after decimal point (e.g., 1.0 mg)**	1 mg	Mistaken as 10 mg if the decimal point is not seen	Do not use trailing zeros for doses expressed in whole numbers
"Naked" decimal point (e.g., .5 mg)**	0.5 mg	Mistaken as 5 mg if the decimal point is not seen	Use zero before a decimal point when the dose is less than a whole unit
Abbreviations such as mg. or mL. with a period following the abbreviation	mg mL	The period is unnecessary and could be mistaken as the number 1 if written poorly	Use mg, mL, etc. without a terminal period

FIGURE 5-1 ISMP's List of Error-Prone Abbreviations, Symbols, and Dose Designations. Used with permission from the Institute for Safe Medication Practices, © ISMP 2015. Report actual and potential medication errors to the ISMP National Medication Errors Reporting Program (ISMP MERP) at 1-800-FAIL-SAF(E) or online at, www.ismp.org.

Institute for Safe Medication Practices

ISMP's List of *Error-Prone Abbreviations, Symbols,* and *Dose Designations* (continued)

Dose Designations and Other Information	Intended Meaning	Misinterpretation	Correction
Drug name and dose run together (especially problematic for drug names that end in "l" such as Inderal40 mg; Tegretol300 mg)	Inderal 40 mg Tegretol 300 mg	Mistaken as Inderal 140 mg Mistaken as Tegretol 1300 mg	Place adequate space between the drug name, dose, and unit of measure
Numerical dose and unit of measure run together (e.g., 10mg, 100mL)	10 mg 100 mL	The "m" is sometimes mistaken as a zero or two zeros, risking a 10- to 100-fold overdose	Place adequate space between the dose and unit of measure
Large doses without properly placed commas (e.g., 100000 units; 1000000 units)	100,000 units 1,000,000 units	100000 has been mistaken as 10,000 or 1,000,000; 1000000 has been mistaken as 100,000	Use commas for dosing units at or above 1,000, or use words such as 100 "thousand" or 1 "million" to improve readability

Drug Name Abbreviations	Intended Meaning	Misinterpretation	Correction
To avoid confusion, do not abbreviate drug names when communicating medical information. Examples of drug name abbreviations involved in medication errors include:			
APAP	acetaminophen	Not recognized as acetaminophen	Use complete drug name
ARA A	vidarabine	Mistaken as cytarabine (ARA C)	Use complete drug name
AZT	zidovudine (Retrovir)	Mistaken as azathioprine or aztreonam	Use complete drug name
CPZ	Compazine (prochlorperazine)	Mistaken as chlorpromazine	Use complete drug name
DPT	Demerol-Phenergan-Thorazine	Mistaken as diphtheria-pertussis-tetanus (vaccine)	Use complete drug name
DTO	Diluted tincture of opium, or deodorized tincture of opium (Paregoric)	Mistaken as tincture of opium	Use complete drug name
HCl	hydrochloric acid or hydrochloride	Mistaken as potassium chloride (The "H" is misinterpreted as "K")	Use complete drug name unless expressed as a salt of a drug
HCT	hydrocortisone	Mistaken as hydrochlorothiazide	Use complete drug name
HCTZ	hydrochlorothiazide	Mistaken as hydrocortisone (seen as HCT250 mg)	Use complete drug name
MgSO4**	magnesium sulfate	Mistaken as morphine sulfate	Use complete drug name
MS, MSO4**	morphine sulfate	Mistaken as magnesium sulfate	Use complete drug name
MTX	methotrexate	Mistaken as mitoxantrone	Use complete drug name
NoAC	novel/new oral anticoagulant	No anticoagulant	Use complete drug name
PCA	procainamide	Mistaken as patient controlled analgesia	Use complete drug name
PTU	propylthiouracil	Mistaken as mercaptopurine	Use complete drug name
T3	Tylenol with codeine No. 3	Mistaken as liothyronine	Use complete drug name
TAC	triamcinolone	Mistaken as tetracaine, Adrenalin, cocaine	Use complete drug name
TNK	TNKase	Mistaken as "TPA"	Use complete drug name
TPA or tPA	tissue plasminogen activator, Activase (alteplase)	Mistaken as TNKase (tenecteplase), or less often as another tissue plasminogen activator, Retavase (retaplase)	Use complete drug names
ZnSO4	Zinc sulfate	Mistaken as morphine sulfate	Use complete drug name

Stemmed Drug Names	Intended Meaning	Misinterpretation	Correction
"Nitro" drip	nitroglycerin infusion	Mistaken as sodium nitroprusside infusion	Use complete drug name
"Norflox"	norfloxacin	Mistaken as Norflex	Use complete drug name
"IV Vanc"	intravenous vancomycin	Mistaken as Invanz	Use complete drug name

Symbols	Intended Meaning	Misinterpretation	Correction
ʒ	Dram	Symbol for dram mistaken as "3"	Use the metric system
♏	Minim	Symbol for minim mistaken as "mL"	
x3d	For three days	Mistaken as "3 doses"	Use "for three days"
> and <	More than and less than	Mistaken as opposite of intended; mistakenly use incorrect symbol; "< 10" mistaken as "40"	Use "more than" or "less than"
/ (slash mark)	Separates two doses or indicates "per"	Mistaken as the number 1 (e.g., "25 units/10 units" misread as "25 units and 110" units)	Use "per" rather than a slash mark to separate doses
@	At	Mistaken as "2"	Use "at"
&	And	Mistaken as "2"	Use "and"
+	Plus or and	Mistaken as "4"	Use "and"
°	Hour	Mistaken as a zero (e.g., q2° seen as q 20)	Use "hr," "h," or "hour"
Φ or ⦰	zero, null sign	Mistaken as numerals 4, 6, 8, and 9	Use 0 or zero, or describe intent using whole words

**These abbreviations are included on The Joint Commission's "minimum list" of dangerous abbreviations, acronyms, and symbols that must be included on an organization's "Do Not Use" list, effective January 1, 2004. Visit www.jointcommission.org for more information about this Joint Commission requirement.

© ISMP 2015. Permission is granted to reproduce material with proper attribution for internal use within healthcare organizations. Other reproduction is prohibited without written permission from ISMP. Report actual and potential medication errors to the ISMP National Medication Errors Reporting Program (ISMP MERP) via the Web at www.ismp.org or by calling 1-800-FAIL-SAF(E).

ISMP
INSTITUTE FOR SAFE MEDICATION PRACTICES
www.ismp.org

FIGURE 5-1 Continued

Always determine the policy of the agency before taking a **telephone order (TO)**. Some agencies require a registered nurse to take TOs. In other facilities, licensed practical (vocational) nurses are allowed to take TOs. When taking a TO, always obtain the name of the person calling in the order and write next to the medication ordered the name of that person and the time the call was made, for example, "TO Dr. A. Smith, per Mary Jones, CMA at 1300." Also repeat all of the details regarding the medication, dosage, frequency, and so on as you write down the order. If you are the medical assistant or nurse calling in the prescription to the facility for the physician, be sure to *repeat the name of the drug, dosage, frequency, and route of administration* to the physician as you write it on the patient's office record, adding the time the call was made and the name of the nurse receiving the call in the facility. This documentation is extremely important in preventing medication errors and legal complications. All TOs must be followed by a read-back statement; for example, "TO/RB" means it was a telephone order that was read back for accuracy. The physician must usually sign all VOs and TOs within 24 h.

Medication orders can be written on the patient's record in the physician's office, clinic, or institution or on a prescription blank (Figure 5-2). With the widespread use of the electronic patient records in the physician's office, prescriptions are typed into the system, printed out, and signed or sent directly to the pharmacy. This is referred to as **computerized physician order entry (CPOE)**. In the inpatient setting, **e-prescribing (eRx)** is the way medications are ordered through the electronic health record. The **electronic medication administration record (eMAR)** is how administered medication are electronically recorded in the patient's health record.

It is the responsibility of the health care professional to check the medication order for completeness by noting the six items—date, patient's name, medication name, dosage, route, and frequency (plus additional items if using the prescription blank)—and to question any discrepancy, omission, or unusual order. The prescription blank contains two additional items: the physician's Drug Enforcement Administration registration number if the medication is a controlled substance and the number of times that the prescription can be refilled. If there are to be no refills, write the word "NO," "NONE," or "0" after Refill. Never leave a blank space in that area on the prescription blank.

To reduce the incidence of medication errors due to misinterpretation of the prescription, some states have passed legislation requiring the *name of the medication to be legibly printed or typed*. In addition, these regulations require the *quantity of the drug prescribed to be in both textual and numerical formats*, for example, "ten (10)." *The prescriber must also print his or her name under the signature* (Figure 5-2).

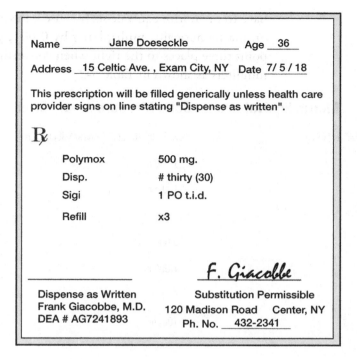

Name _____ Jane Doeseckle _____ Age __36__

Address __15 Celtic Ave. , Exam City, NY__ Date _7/ 5 / 18_

This prescription will be filled generically unless health care provider signs on line stating "Dispense as written".

R̵

Polymox	500 mg.
Disp.	# thirty (30)
Sigi	1 PO t.i.d.
Refill	x3

F. Giacobbe

_____

Dispense as Written
Frank Giacobbe, M.D.
DEA # AG7241893

Substitution Permissible
120 Madison Road   Center, NY
Ph. No. __432-2341__

FIGURE 5-2 Prescription blank. Check for completeness, legibility, and accuracy, including date, patient's name, medication name, dosage, route, frequency or time, number of refills, and the physician's Drug Enforcement Administration (DEA) number for controlled substances. All prescriptions must be printed.

SYSTEMS OF MEASUREMENT

To carry out a medication order accurately, the person administering medications must have an understanding of the different systems of measurement. The original system of weights and measures for writing medication orders was the *apothecary system*. An apothecary is a pharmacist or druggist. The apothecary system has now become obsolete. The **metric system** is the preferred system of measurement and is used at the present time. The third system of measurement is the **household system**, which is the least accurate. However, this system is more familiar to the layperson and is therefore used in prescribing medications for the patient at home. A health care professional must understand systems of measurement for accurate administration of medicines and for patient education as well. Medication orders are concerned with only two types of measurement: (1) measuring fluids, or liquid measure, and (2) measuring solids, or solid weight.

Metric System

Note

The milliliter (mL) is approximately equivalent to the cubic centimeter (cc). Therefore, 1 mL or milliliter is equal to 1 cc or cubic centimeter. However, it is preferred to *not* use the cc designation as it is on the error-prone list.

The metric system was invented by the French in the late eighteenth century and is the international standard for weights and measures. It is based on three basic units of measure: the liter (L) for volume, the meter (m) for length, and the gram (g) for weight. A prefix representing a power of 10 can be placed before each of these basic units to change its value. For example, the prefix *milli* means "one thousandth," and therefore a milligram (mg) would be one thousandth of a gram. Another way of stating this is that 1,000 milligrams equal 1 gram.

Because all prefixes are based on the powers of 10, to convert within the metric system, you simply need to move the decimal point to the correct number of places of the power of 10 that the prefix represents. Notice in Table 5-2, we have placed the most common prefixes you will be working with in the metric system. You do not have to memorize equivalents because knowing that *milli* represents one thousandth or, mathematically, multiplying by 0.001, you simply have to move the decimal point three places to the right when converting grams to milligrams or even liters to milliliters as shown in Table 5-2.

TABLE 5-2   Metric Equivalents for Solid Measurement—Grams to Milligrams

METRIC (GRAMS/LITERS)	METRIC (MILLIGRAMS/MILLILITERS)	METRIC (MICROGRAMS)
1 g	1,000 mg	1,000,000 mcg
0.1 g	100 mg	100,000 mcg
0.001 g	1 mg	1000 mcg
0.000001 g	0.001 mg	1 mcg
1 L	1,000 mL	
0.5 L	500 mL	
0.1 L	100 mL	
0.05 L	50 mL	

Note: Micrograms are used for narrow therapeutic index drugs like levothyroxine and digoxin. These medications have a very high potency and very small range between when they are effective and become toxic and cause side effects, therefore it is important to use micrograms to ensure a proper dose for each patient. Microliters are not commonly used in measurement.

Household System

At times you will find it necessary to convert a dosage from the metric system to the household system, especially in the home care setting. It is important to memorize the few basic equivalents most commonly used. Table 5-3 lists commonly used approximate equivalents for liquid measurement. If it is necessary to convert from one system of measurement to another, always consult a conversion table or a pharmacist to avoid dangerous errors.

TABLE 5-3   Common *Approximate* Equivalents for Liquid Measurement

METRIC	HOUSEHOLD
5 mL	1 tsp
15 mL	1 tbsp
30 mL	1 oz
240 mL	1 measuring cup
473 mL	1 pt
946 mL	1 qt

Equipment most commonly used for measuring medications includes the medicine cup and various syringes calibrated in milliliters.

Common Medical Conversion

Although almost all countries use the metric system as their official measurement system, the United States still uses the English system of measurement, which includes ounces, pounds, feet, miles, and yards. Often a **conversion of units** is needed to properly treat the patient. For example, a patient weighs 150 pounds, but some drugs are ordered on a per-kilogram dose, making it necessary to convert the English unit of pounds to the metric kilogram. Knowing the important conversion factor that 1 kilogram = 2.2 pounds, the conversion becomes an easy process. Any time a weight is given in pounds, simply divide by 2.2 to change it to kilograms. Therefore, a 150 lb individual would weigh 150/2.2 = 68.18 kilograms.

Warning: Be very careful in calculating the weight in kilograms. The slightest error, especially in pediatric doses, could result in serious or fatal consequences.

PATIENT EDUCATION

When explaining dosage preparation, always speak directly to the patient and observe the patient for comprehension. Many older patients have difficulty hearing but are reluctant to admit lack of understanding. Ask them to repeat the directions.

Many older patients also have vision problems. Be sure the directions for dosage preparation are written clearly. If a family member will be assisting in preparation and administration of medications, include that person in the instruction. Be sure that any measuring equipment to be used is clearly marked.

Measuring spoons and clearly marked measuring cups should be used when available for household measurement. Such calibrated utensils are more accurate than tableware (Figure 5-3). Teaspoons, tablespoons, teacups, and drinking glasses vary in size and capacity, and therefore measurements are inaccurate with such utensils.

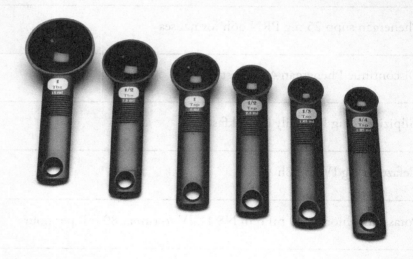

FIGURE 5-3 For accurate household measurement, standard measuring spoons are used versus common utensil spoons.

CHAPTER REVIEW QUIZ

Interpret the following orders

1. Keflex 250-mg cap PO q6h

    _____.

2. Neosporin ophth sol 2 gtt in OU tid

    _____.

3. Feosol 65-mg tab bid pc c̄ orange juice

_____.

4. Diuril 500 mg PO qAM

_____.

5. Dyazide 1 cap bid

_____.

6. Demerol 50 mg IM q4h PRN for pain

_____.

7. Metamucil 1 tsp mixed c̄ 8oz H_2O bid pc

_____.

8. Dulcolax supp R PRN for constipation

_____.

9. Robitussin syr 1 tsp q4h PRN for cough

_____.

10. Nitrostat 1 tab SL PRN for angina attack, may repeat q5min three times

_____.

11. Phenergan supp 25 mg PRN q6h for nausea

_____.

12. Discontinue Phenergan 48 h post-op

_____.

13. Glipizide 5 mg PO daily c̄ breakfast

_____.

14. Cefazolin 1 g IVPB q8h

_____.

15. Potassium chloride 20 mEq in NS 1L IV to run at 80 mL per hour

_____.

16. NPH Insulin 20 units subcu daily ac breakfast

_____.

17. Glyburide 2.5 mg daily c̄ breakfast

_____.

18. Gentamicin ophth sol 1 gtt q3h OD

_____.

19. Cefaclor suspension 20 mg/kg/day in two equal doses q12h

_____.

20. Ambien 5 mg for sleep PRN, may repeat once PRN

_____.

Fill in the blanks

21. Which is the oldest system of measurement for medication?

_____.

22. Which system of drug measurement is used most frequently throughout the world?

_____.

23. Which is the least accurate system for measuring medicine?

_____.

24. Two different types of equipment used to measure drugs are _____ and _____.

Use Tables 5-2 and 5-3 to complete the following conversions and place the correct answer in the blank

25. 1,000 mg = ___ g

26. 75 mg = ___ g

27. 1 kg = ___ lb

28. 150 lb = ___ kg

29. 1 tsp = ___ mL

30. 1 tbsp = ___ mL

31. 100 kg = ___ lb

32. 0.5 g = ___ mg

33. 1 g = ___ mg

34. 100 mcg = ____mg

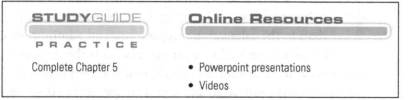

STUDYGUIDE   Online Resources

PRACTICE

Complete Chapter 5   • Powerpoint presentations
                            • Videos

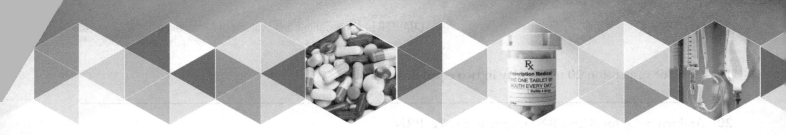

CHAPTER 6
SAFE DOSAGE CALCULATIONS

KEY TERMS AND CONCEPTS

Calculating dosage

Proportion

Ratio

Unit-dose form

Verify your calculations

OBJECTIVES

Upon completion of this chapter, the learner should be able to

1. Identify the three steps for calculation of the dosage ordered when it differs from the dose on hand

2. Write the formula for each of the two methods of dosage calculation presented in this chapter

3. Convert from one system of measurement to another using the ratio and proportion method

4. Solve dosage problems using the basic calculation method

5. Solve dosage problems using the ratio and proportion method

6. List the cautions with the basic calculation method

7. List the cautions with the ratio and proportion method

8. Calculate safe dosages for infants and children

9. List the variables when assessing geriatric patients for safe dosage

10. List five steps to reduce medication errors

11. Define the Key Terms and Concepts

"First, do no harm." Health care professionals are dedicated to the principle of helping others, not harming them. Nowhere is this principle more important than in the calculation, preparation, and administration of safe dosages. One careless mistake can lead to a catastrophe. It is the responsibility of the health care professional to be absolutely certain that the medication administered is exactly as prescribed by the physician *and* is also an *appropriate* dose for that particular patient. Doses for children and older adults can vary significantly from the average dose. Therefore, it may be necessary to calculate a partial dose from the dose on hand for the average patient.

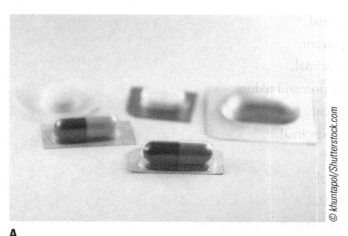

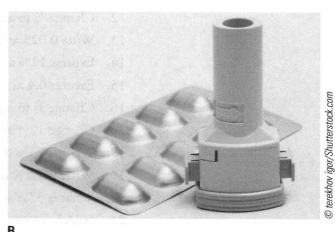

A   **B**

FIGURE 6-1 Examples of unit-dose medications (A) Unit-dose oral medications. (B) Unit-dose capsules for dry powder inhalation device.

Many medications are dispensed by the pharmacist in **unit-dose form,** (Figure 6-1) in which each individual dose of medicine is prepackaged in a separate packet, vial, or prefilled syringe. Although much of the mixing and measuring of medications is now completed by the pharmacist, the person who is administering medications must understand the preparation of dosages to ensure accuracy. On occasion the dosage ordered differs from the dose on hand. Consequently, it may be necessary to calculate the correct dosage. Calculations can be a simple procedure if you follow the necessary steps in sequential order.

A working knowledge of basic arithmetic is required for accurate calculation of drug dosage. To understand the calculation of correct dosage, you must evaluate your basic arithmetic skills by completing the following mathematics pretest.

BASIC ARITHMETIC TEST

1. 6¼ + 3⅔
2. 4⅔ − 2½
3. 2⅔ × 3⅖
4. ⅖ ÷ ¾
5. 2⅔ ÷ 5
6. Write six and a third as a decimal.
7. 6.67 + 0.065 + 0.3
8. 10.4 − 0.037
9. 0.223 × 0.67
10. 46.72 ÷ 6.4
11. Write 8% as a fraction and reduce.

12. Change ⅖ to a decimal.

13. Write 0.023 as a percent.

14. Express 12% as a decimal.

15. Express 0.4 as a fraction and reduce.

16. Change ⅗ to a percent.

17. Change 12½% to a decimal.

18. What is 75% of 160?

19. What is 9.2% of 250?

20. What is 37½% of 192?

21. Which fraction is the largest: ½, ⅖, or ³⁄₁₀?

22. Which is the largest: ⅓, 0.4, or 60%?

23. The label on the bottle reads 0.5 g per tablet. The physician orders 0.25 g. How many tablets should you give?

After completing the quiz, check your answers (see end of chapter for answers). If there is an error, review mathematics for that area until all problems can be solved accurately and easily. A minimum score of 80% is recommended as indicating readiness for dosage calculations. Those not meeting this criterion should seek remedial assistance in review of basics before beginning calculations.

CALCULATION GUIDELINES

Remember, there is no margin of error in administration of medications. It is possible for a small error in arithmetic to seriously harm a patient. A misplaced decimal point could cause a fatality. Safe dosage preparation requires (1) a working knowledge of basic arithmetic and (2) meticulous care with all calculations.

Calculations can be as simple as 1, 2, 3. When the dosage ordered differs from the dose on hand, the problem can be solved simply by completing three basic steps:

1. Check whether all measures are in the same system. Convert if necessary by using known conversion factors or use the ratio and proportion method.

2. Write the problem in equation form *using the appropriate formula and labeling all parts* and complete the necessary calculations.

3. *Check the accuracy* of your answer for reasonableness and have someone else **verify your calculations.**

There are several different methods of **calculating dosage.** Either of the methods presented in this book may be used, or both methods may be used to verify accuracy. The two methods presented here are *basic calculation* and *ratio and proportion*. Basic calculation requires only simple arithmetic; ratio and proportion requires the ability to determine an unknown, *X*.

METHOD 1: BASIC CALCULATION

Use the following formula:

$$\frac{\text{desired dose}}{\text{on-hand dose}} \times \text{quantity of on-hand dose}$$

In short form

$$\frac{D}{OH} \times Q$$

EXAMPLE 1

The physician orders 162 mg of aspirin q4h PRN for fever over 101°. On hand are aspirin 81-mg tablets.

Step 1. Check to see if all measures are in the same system. No conversion is necessary. Both measures are in milligrams.

Step 2. Use the formula $\frac{D}{OH} \times$ Q and label all parts:

$$\frac{162 \text{ mg}}{81 \text{ mg}} \times 1 \text{ tab} = 162 \div 81 = 2 \text{ tabs}$$

Note: The labels of the desired and on-hand doses must be the same. The label of the answer must be the same as the quantity.

Step 3. Check for reasonableness. A drug reference source should be checked to see if this is a reasonable dosage.

If the calculations resulted in an answer such as ¼ tablet or five tablets, the answer may not be reasonable and the calculations should be rechecked. If calculations are correct after recheck, any unusual dosage should be checked with the person in charge: the pharmacist or the physician. *When in doubt, always question.*

EXAMPLE 2

The order reads ampicillin 0.5 g. The unit-dose packet reads 250 mg/cap.

Step 1. Check to see if all measures are in the same system. Convert grams to milligrams:

$$1 \text{ g} = 1,000 \text{ mg}$$
$$0.5 \text{ g} = 0.5 \times 1,000 = 500 \text{ mg}$$

Step 2. Use the formula $\frac{D}{OH} \times$ Q and label all parts:

$$\frac{500 \text{ mg}}{250 \text{ mg}} \times 1 \text{ cap} =$$

Reduce fractions to lowest terms:

$$\frac{500}{250} = 50 \div 25 = 2$$

$$2 \times 1 = 2 \text{ caps}$$

Step 3. Check for reasonableness. A dose of 2 caps or 500 mg is within normal dosage range.

EXAMPLE 3

The narcotics drawer contains vials of meperidine (Demerol) labeled 75 mg in 1 mL. The preoperative order reads Demerol 60 mg IM on call.

Step 1.   Check to see if all measures are in the same system. No conversion is necessary.

Step 2.   Use the formula $\dfrac{D}{OH} \times Q$ and label all parts:

$$\frac{60 \text{ mg}}{75 \text{ mg}} \times 1 \text{ mL} =$$

Reduce fractions to lowest terms:

$$\frac{60}{75} = \frac{12}{15} = \frac{4}{5}$$

Convert fractions to decimals:

$$\frac{4}{5} = 5\overline{)4.0}^{\,0.8}$$

Multiply by quantity.

$$0.8 \times 1 \text{ mL} = 0.8 \text{ mL}$$

Note: Fractions must be converted to decimals and rounded off to one decimal place to coincide with the markings on the syringe.

Step 3.   Check for reasonableness. A dose of 0.8 mL is within normal dosage range.

EXAMPLE 4

The physician orders midazolam (Versed) 3 mg IM preoperatively. On hand are vials labeled 5 mg per mL.

Step 1.   Check to see if all measures are in the same system.

No conversion is necessary.

Step 2.   Use the formula $\dfrac{D}{OH} \times Q$ and label all parts:

$$\frac{3 \text{ mg}}{5 \text{ mg}} \times 1 \text{ mL} = 3 \div 5 = 5\overline{)3.0}^{\,0.6}$$

$$0.6 \times 1 \text{ mL} = 0.6 \text{ mL}$$

Step 3.   Check for reasonableness. A dose of 0.6 mL is within normal dosage range.

EXAMPLE 5

The order reads atropine sulfate 0.6 mg IM on call to surgery. Available ampules are labeled atropine sulfate 0.4 mg/mL.

Step 1.   Check to see if all measures are in the same system.

No conversion is necessary.

Step 2. Use the formula $\frac{D}{OH} \times Q$ and label all parts:

$$\frac{0.6 \text{ mg}}{0.4 \text{ mg}} \times 1 \text{ mL} = 0.6 \div 04 = 0.4\overline{)0.6}^{1.5}$$

$$1.5 \times 1 \text{ mL} = 1.5 \text{ mL}$$

Step 3. Check for reasonableness. A dose of 1.5 mL is within normal dosage range.

Cautions for the basic calculation method

1. *Label* all parts of the formula.
2. Use the *same label* for desired and on-hand doses.
3. Use the *same label* for the quantity and the answer (the amount to be given).
4. *Reduce fractions* to lowest terms before dividing.
5. Multiply by the quantity after dividing.
6. Take extra care with decimals.
7. *Convert* fractions to decimals.
8. *Round off* decimals to one decimal place after computation is complete.
9. *Verify the accuracy* of calculations with an instructor.
10. Question the answer if it is not within normal limits (e.g., less than ½ tab, more than 2 tabs, or more than 2 mL for injection).

METHOD 2: RATIO AND PROPORTION

A **ratio** describes a relationship between two numbers. Example:

$$1 \text{ g} : 15 \text{ gr}$$

A **proportion** consists of two ratios that are equal. Example:

$$1 \text{ g} : 15 \text{ gr} = 2 \text{ g} : 30 \text{ gr}$$

Always label each term in the equation. The terms of each ratio must be in the same sequence. In the previous examples, the first term of each ratio is labeled g and the second term of each ratio is labeled gr.

To solve a problem with the ratio and proportion method, set up the formula with the known terms on the left and the desired and unknown terms on the right. Use X to represent the unknown. Label all terms.

For example, we know that 1,000 mg is equal to 1 g (known). We need to administer 500 mg (desired) and do not know how many grams are equivalent (unknown X). To convert a dosage from one system to another when a table of metric and apothecary equivalents (such as Table 5-4) is unavailable, set up the problem as a proportion

$$\underset{\text{of measure}}{\textit{known unit}} : \underset{\text{equivalent}}{\textit{known}} = \underset{\text{of measure}}{\textit{desired} \text{ unit}} : \underset{\text{equivalent}}{\textit{unknown}}$$

$$1{,}000 \text{ mg} : 1 \text{ g} = 500 \text{ mg} : X\text{g}$$

means

extremes

To solve the problem, multiply the two outer terms, or extremes, and then multiply the two inner terms, or means. Using our example

$$1{,}000X = 500 = 1{,}000\overline{)500.0}^{\,0.5}$$

$$X = 0.5 \text{ g}$$

We now know that our desired dose, 500 mg, is equal to 0.5 g.

When the dose ordered differs from the dose on hand, the problem can be solved simply by completing three basic steps:

1. Verify that all measures are in the same system. Convert if necessary by using a table of metric equivalents if available or by using the ratio and proportion method if the equivalent is unknown.

2. Set up the problem as a proportion, *label all terms*, and complete the calculations. Use the following formula:

$$\underset{\text{on hand}}{\text{dose}} : \underset{\text{quantity}}{\text{known}} = \underset{\text{desired}}{\text{dose}} : \underset{\text{quantity}}{\text{unknown}}$$

Note: The answer should be stated as a whole number or a decimal. Convert fractions to decimals and round them off to one decimal place.

3. Check the accuracy of your answer for reasonableness and also have someone else verify your calculations.

EXAMPLE 1

The preoperative order reads Demerol 60 mg IM on call. The narcotics drawer contains vials labeled meperidine (Demerol) 100 mg/2 mL.

Step 1.   Verify that all measures are in the same system.

No conversion is necessary.

Step 2.   Set up the problem as a proportion and label all terms:

$$\underset{\text{on hand}}{\text{dose}} : \underset{\text{quantity}}{\text{known}} = \underset{\text{desired}}{\text{dose}} : \underset{\text{quantity}}{\text{unknown}}$$

$$100 \text{ mg} : 2 \text{ mL} = 60 \text{ mg} : X \text{ mL}$$

$$100X = 120 = 100\overline{)120.0}^{\,1.2}$$

$$X = 1.2 \text{ mL}$$

Step 3.   Check for reasonableness. A dose of 1.2 mL is within the normal dosage range.

EXAMPLE 2

The physician is treating a child weighing 44 pounds for epilepsy. The order reads phenobarbital elixir 3 mg/kg at bedtime. Phenobarbital elixir is labeled 15 mg/5 mL. How many milliliters will the child receive?

Step 1.   Verify that all measures are in the same system. Pounds must be converted to kilograms (kg). To convert lb to kg, divide the number of pounds by 2.2.

The child weighs 20 kg.

The order reads 3 mg/kg. Therefore, 3 mg/kg × 20 kg = 60-mg dose.

Step 2.   Set up the problem as a proportion. Label all terms.

$$\begin{array}{ccccc} \text{dose} & : & \text{known} & = & \text{dose} & : & \text{unknown} \\ \text{on hand} & & \text{quantity} & & \text{desired} & & \text{quantity} \end{array}$$

$$15 \text{ mg} : 5 \text{ mL} = 60 \text{ mg} : X \text{ mL}$$

$$15X = 300 = 15\overline{)300}^{\,20}$$

$$X = 20 \text{ mL}$$

Step 3.   Check for reasonableness. An oral dose of 20 mL is a large amount for a young child to take at one time. The physician might want to divide the daily dose. If so, the order would be written: phenobarbital 30 mg BID.

EXAMPLE 3

Meperidine oral solution is available as Demerol solution 50 mg/5 mL. The order reads Demerol liquid 150 mg PO q6h PRN.

Step 1.   Verify that all measures are in the same system.

No conversion is necessary.

Step 2.   Set up the problem as a proportion. Label all terms.

$$\begin{array}{ccccc} \text{dose} & : & \text{known} & = & \text{dose} & : & \text{unknown} \\ \text{on hand} & & \text{quantity} & & \text{desired} & & \text{quantity} \end{array}$$

$$50 \text{ mg} : 5 \text{ mL} = 150 \text{ mg} : X \text{ mL}$$

$$50X = 750 = 50\overline{)750}^{\,15}$$

$$X = 15 \text{ mL}$$

Step 3.   Check for reasonableness. An oral dose of 15 mL is appropriate for an adult.

EXAMPLE 4

An 88-lb child with cancer has an order for pain medication that reads morphine liquid PO 0.2 mg/kg q4h PRN. Available morphine solution is labeled 20 mg/5 mL.

Step 1. Verify that all measures are in the same system. Pounds must be converted to kilograms (kg). To convert lb to kg, divide the number of pounds by 2.2. The child weighs 40 kg.

Σ The order reads 0.2 mg/kg. Therefore, 0.2 mg/kg × 40 kg = 8-mg dose.

Step 2. Set up the problem as a proportion. Label all terms.

$$\underset{\text{on hand}}{\text{dose}} : \underset{\text{quantity}}{\text{known}} = \underset{\text{desired}}{\text{dose}} : \underset{\text{quantity}}{\text{unknown}}$$

$$20 \text{ mg} : 5 \text{ mL} = 8 \text{ mg} : X \text{ mL}$$

$$20X = 40 = 20\overline{)40}^{\,2}$$

$$X = 2 \text{ mL}$$

Step 3. Check for reasonableness. An oral dose of 2 mL is appropriate for a terminally ill child when consulting a drug reference source.

EXAMPLE 5

The physician orders Benadryl elixir 25 mg q12h. The bottle in the medicine cupboard is labeled 12.5 mg/5 mL.

Step 1. Verify that all measures are in the same system. No conversion is necessary.

Step 2. Write the problem as a proportion and label each term

$$12.5 \text{ mg} : 5 \text{ mL} = 25 \text{ mg} : X \text{ mL}$$

$$12.5X = 125 = 12.5\overline{)125.00} = 12.5\overline{)125.00}^{\,10}$$

$$X = 10 \text{ mL}$$

Step 3. Check for reasonableness. The dose 10 mL is within normal limits for oral solution.

Cautions for the Ratio and Proportion Method

1. *Label* all parts of the equation.
2. The ratio on the *left* contains the *known* quantity, and the ratio on the *right* contains the *desired* and *unknown* quantities.
3. Terms of the second ratio must be in the same sequence as those in the first ratio.
4. *Multiply* the *extremes first* and then the means.
5. Take extra care with decimals.

6. *Convert* fractions to decimals. *Round off* decimals to one decimal place.

7. *Label* the answer.

8. *Verify the accuracy* of calculations with an instructor.

9. *Question* any unusual dosage that is not within normal limits (e.g., less than ½ tab, more than 2 tabs, or more than 2 mL for injection).

PEDIATRIC DOSAGE

Children are not miniature adults. You cannot merely take a portion of an adult dose and give it to a child. There are many other variables to consider. There are numerous formulas available for computing an *approximate* child's dose based on body surface area, weight, or age. However, other factors must be taken into consideration as well. In neonates, renal function and some enzyme systems needed for drug absorption and metabolism are not fully developed. The neonate's blood–brain barrier is more permeable, and his or her total body water contributes to a greater percentage of body weight, also affecting drug absorption.

Appropriate dosage for children, as well as adults, must take into consideration variables such as age, weight, sex, and metabolic, pathological, or psychological conditions. Recommended pediatric drug dosages are derived from data obtained in clinical trials utilizing sick children. When preparing drug dosages for children, it is important to always refer to recommended dosages as listed in drug inserts, *Physicians' Desk Reference (PDR)* or *AHFS Drug Information (AHFS DI)*.

Recommended dosages of drugs are often expressed in the references as a number of milligrams per unit of body weight, per unit of time. For example, the recommended dose for a drug might be 6 mg/kg/24 h. This information can then be used to

1. Calculate the dose for the individual patient

2. Check on the appropriateness of the prescribed dose, watching particularly for possible overdoses

EXAMPLE 1

The recommended dose of meperidine (Demerol) is 6 mg/kg/24 h for pain, in divided doses every 4–6 h, as necessary. Demerol is available in ampules or cartridges labeled 50 mg/mL. How much Demerol would be appropriate for a 33-lb child as a single dose every 6 h?

Step 1.   Convert pounds to kilograms (divide the number of pounds by 2.2).

$$33 \text{ pounds} = 15 \text{ kg}$$

6 mg/kg in 24 h is recommended.

$$6 \text{ mg} \times 15 \text{ kg} = 90 \text{ mg in 24 h}$$

(*continued*)

Step 2.   Calculate the number of *milliliters needed in 24 h.* Write the problem as a proportion and label each term.

$$\begin{array}{c} \text{dose} \\ \text{on hand} \end{array} : \begin{array}{c} \text{known} \\ \text{quantity} \end{array} = \begin{array}{c} \text{dose} \\ \text{desired} \end{array} : \begin{array}{c} \text{unknown} \\ \text{quantity} \end{array}$$

$$50 \text{ mg} : 1 \text{ mL} = 90 \text{ mg} : X \text{ mL}$$

$$50X = 90 = 50\overline{)90.0}^{\;1.8}$$

$$X = 1.8 \text{ mL in 24 Hours}$$

Then, calculate the number of *milliliters* needed in 6 h. Remember, the unknown quantity is always the last term in the equation.

$$24 \text{ h} : 1.8 \text{ mL} = 6 \text{ h} : X \text{ mL}$$

$$24X = 10.8 = 24\overline{)10.80}^{\;0.45}$$

$$X = 0.45 \text{ mL dose every 6 h}$$

Step 3.   The appropriateness of this dose can be checked by applying *Clark's rule:*

$$\frac{\text{child's wt in lb}}{\text{average adult wt}} \times \text{adult dose} = \text{child's } \textit{approximate} \text{ dose}$$

$$\frac{33}{150} \times 100 \text{ mg} = 22 \text{ mg approximate child's dose}$$

Note: The average adult weight is 150 pounds.

Demerol is available in ampules labeled 100 mg/2 mL.

$$100 \text{ mg} : 2 \text{ mL} = 22 \text{ mg} : X \text{ mL}$$

$$100X = 44 = 100\overline{)44.00}^{\;0.44}$$

$$X = 0.44 \text{ mL dose to be administered}$$

Remember, this is a *general* rule and other variables must be considered when assessing for appropriateness of dosage.

GERIATRIC DOSAGE

Special consideration must be given to preparation and administration of safe dosage to older adults. As with children, the dose frequently needs to be reduced. Factors leading to possible dangerous cumulative effects can include slower metabolism; poor circulation; or impairment of liver, kidneys, lungs, or central nervous system. Any chronic disease, debility, dehydration, or electrolyte imbalance can affect assimilation of drugs and interfere with therapeutic effect. Many drugs can impair the mental status of older adults, leading to confusion. Any older adult taking many drugs is also at risk for potentially lethal interactions. There is no formula to guide you in safe geriatric dosage. Start low and go slow is a good general approach to follow. Careful assessment on an *individual* basis, constant monitoring, and reduction of dosage whenever possible are the rules to follow. Each individual reacts differently to drugs, and changes occur over time. You have the responsibility to question the appropriateness of any drug, and especially as the patient's condition changes. See also Chapter 27, "Drugs and Older Adults."

PREVENTION OF MEDICATION ERRORS

Medication errors can occur for a number of reasons: administering the wrong drug, in the wrong amount, at the wrong time, by the wrong route, or to the wrong patient or improperly documenting drug information. The Rights of Medication Administration will be discussed in the next chapter. However, we will consider here errors that can occur when the drug order is misinterpreted.

- Never leave the decimal point naked. Writing .2 instead of 0.2 could cause the decimal point to be missed and could result in an overdose. Always place a zero *before* a decimal point, for example, 0.2, 0.5.

- Never place a decimal point and zero after a whole number. The decimal point could be missed, and the zero could be misinterpreted; for example, 5.0 mg could be read as 50 mg. The correct way is to write 5 mg.

- Avoid using decimals whenever whole numbers can be used as alternatives; for example, 0.5 g can be expressed as 500 mg.

- Have a second qualified person double-check any calculations for accuracy.

- If you have difficulty interpreting the spelling of a drug name or the number used for the dosage, or the dosage seems inappropriate, *always question* the order. Not only is this your duty, but you also have an ethical and a legal responsibility to be sure that the drugs you administer are safe. If a medication error results in legal action, you could be held accountable, even though the order was written incorrectly. You are expected to recognize inappropriate dosage, to check reference books for unfamiliar drugs, and to ask the physician or pharmacist about any questionable dosage.

CLINICAL CONNECTION

Use reasoning to verify and check your calculations: When doing a calculation, it is easy to make a simple math error or to use an incorrect method, often times this will result in not only a wrong answer, but also an unreasonable one. This is why it is important to always check your answer to see if it is reasonable compared to the common dose and to the dosage available. For instance, if you calculate a dose that requires you to use many units of an available dose (like 10 capsules for one dose) or a small fraction of an available dose (like 0.01 vials) this is indicative of an incorrect calculation.

Note: when necessary use references to obtain normal dosing ranges.

CHAPTER REVIEW QUIZ

Section A

The available dosages are listed with each drug. Choose the most appropriate available form to deliver the dosage ordered. Use only *one* form of each drug. Indicate the *amount* and *which drug form* you should give for the following orders. *Use the smallest number of tablets possible.*

Drug and Dose Ordered	Amount to Administer
1. atenolol (Tenormin) 75·mg	_____ of _____ mg tab
Available 50-mg and 100-mg tablets of Tenormin	
2. buspirone (Buspar) 25 mg	_____ of _____ mg tab
Available 5-mg and 10-mg tablets of Buspar	
3. alprazolam (Xanax) 0.75 mg	_____ of _____ mg tab
Available 0.25-mg, 0.5-mg, and 1-mg tablets of Xanax	
4. bumetanide (Bumex) 2 mg	_____ of _____ mg tab
Available 0.5-mg and 1-mg tablets of Bumex	
5. cimetidine (Tagamet) 200 mg	_____ of _____ mg tab
Available 300-mg and 400-mg tablets of Tagamet	
6. furosemide (Lasix) 60 mg	_____ of _____ mg tab
Available 20-mg, 40-mg, and 80-mg tablets of Lasix	
7. levothyroxine (Synthroid) 0.3 mg	_____ of _____ mg tab
Available 0.05-mg, 0.1-mg, and 0.15-mg tablets of Synthroid	
8. propranolol (Inderal) 15 mg	_____ of _____ mg tab
Available 10-mg, 20-mg, and 40-mg tablets of Inderal	
9. prednisone 15 mg	_____ of _____ mg tab
Available 5-mg, 10-mg, and 20-mg tablets of prednisone	
10. sertraline (Zoloft) 75 mg	_____ of _____ mg tab
Available 50-mg and 100-mg tablets of Zoloft	

Section B

Show your work. Label and circle your answers.

1. The physician orders Lovenox 1 mg/kg subcu q12h. The patient weighs 176 lb. Lovenox is available as 100 mg in 1 mL.

  a. What is the patient's weight in kilograms? _____.

  b. What is the dose of Lovenox to be administered? _____ mg in _____ mL.

2. The medication order reads Demerol 60 mg IM. The narcotic drawer contains syringes labeled meperidine (Demerol) 75 mg/mL.

   a. How many milliliters would you administer? _____.

   b. How many milliliters would you discard and mark as "wasted" on the narcotic record? _____

   _____.

3. Lasix is available in 40-mg tablets. The order reads Lasix 60 mg PO qAM. How many tablets should you give?

4. Phenergan 12.5 mg IV is ordered. Available vials of phenergan are labeled 25 mg/mL. How many milliliters would you administer?

5. Acetaminophen elixir 650 mg PO is ordered. The container is labeled 325 mg/5 mL.

   a. How many milliliters would you administer? _____.

   b. How many teaspoons per dose? _____.

6. Morphine sulfate PO 30-mg liquid is ordered. Morphine oral solution is labeled 20 mg/mL. How many milliliters would you administer?

7. The medication order reads heparin 5,000 units. Vials available in the medication cupboard are labeled heparin 10,000 units/mL. How many milliliters should you draw into the syringe?

8. Digoxin elixir is available in 50 mcg/mL. The physician orders 125 mcg PO daily. How many milliliters should you give?

9. The physician orders prednisone PO 7.5 mg daily. Prednisone is available in 5-mg and 10-mg scored tablets, which can be broken in half. Which strength tablet and how many tablets should you give?

10. Amoxicillin suspension 750 mg PO q8h is ordered. Liquid medication available is labeled 250 mg/5 mL. How many milliliters should you give?

11. Calcium carbonate 1,000 mg PO daily is prescribed, to be given in divided doses bid. Available tablets contain calcium 250 mg/tab. How many tablets should be taken each time?

12. Cheratussin AC contains 10 mg of codeine in each teaspoon (5 mL). If 2 tsp Cheratussin AC PO is prescribed q4h, how much codeine would be contained in each dose?

13. The physician orders ivermectin tablets for a 200-lb adult with scabies. The recommended dose is 0.2 mg/kg. Ivermectin tablets are labeled 3 mg. How many tablets should be given for the dose?

14. The physician orders cefaclor (Ceclor) suspension 200 mg PO q8h for a 44-lb child. Ceclor suspension is available in 250 mg/5 mL.

   a. How many milliliters should be administered each time? _____.

   b. Recommended dosage of Ceclor is 30 mg/kg/daily. How many milligrams would be appropriate for this child daily? _____.

15. List five variables to consider in determining a child's dose:

   _____, _____, _____, _____,

   and _____.

16. List five factors that could lead to serious cumulative effects with medicines in the older adults:

_____, _____, _____, _____,

and _____.

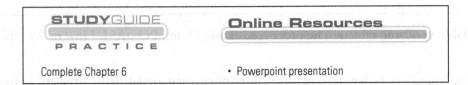

STUDYGUIDE

P R A C T I C E

Complete Chapter 6

Online Resources

• Powerpoint presentation

Answers to Basic Arithmetic Test

1. $9^{11}/_{12}$
2. $2^{1}/_{6}$
3. $9^{1}/_{15}$
4. $^{8}/_{15}$
5. $^{8}/_{15}$
6. 6.333
7. 7.035
8. 10.363

9. 0.14941
10. 7.3
11. $^{2}/_{25}$
12. 0.4
13. 2.3%
14. 0.12
15. $^{2}/_{5}$
16. 60%

17. 0.125
18. 120
19. 23
20. 72
21. ½
22. 60%
23. ½

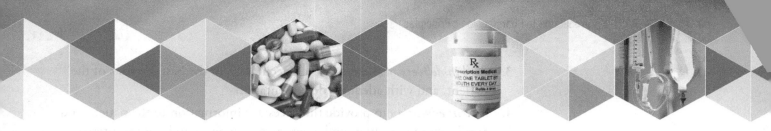

CHAPTER 7

RESPONSIBILITIES AND PRINCIPLES OF DRUG ADMINISTRATION

KEY TERMS AND CONCEPTS

Documentation of drug administration

Medication Errors Reporting (MER) program

Medication reconciliation

Reporting of medication errors

Responsibilities

Responsibilities of drug administration

Six Rights of Medication Administration

MedWatch

OBJECTIVES

Upon completion of this chapter, the learner should be able to

1. Describe four responsibilities of the health care provider in safe administration of medications

2. List the Six Rights of Medication Administration

3. Explain moral, ethical, and legal responsibilities regarding medication errors

4. Cite three instances of medication administration that require documentation

5. Explain the rights of the health care professional to question or refuse to administer medications

6. Define the Key Terms and Concepts

RESPONSIBLE DRUG ADMINISTRATION

The safe and accurate administration of medications requires knowledge, judgment, and skill. The **responsibilities of drug administration** of the health care professional in this vital area are as follows:

1. Adequate, up-to-date *information* about all medications to be administered, including their purpose, potential side effects, cautions and contraindications, and possible interactions.

2. *Wisdom* and judgment to accurately *assess* the patient's needs for medications, to *evaluate* the response to medications, and to *plan* appropriate interventions as indicated.

3. *Skill in delivery* of the medication accurately, in the best interests of the patient, and with adequate documentation.

4. *Patient education* to provide the necessary information to the patient and family about why, how, and when medications are to be administered and their potential side effects and precautions with administration by the layperson.

Responsibility for safe administration of medications requires that the health care professional be familiar with every medication before administration. Knowledge of the typical and most frequently used drugs of the systems (as described in Part II of this text) is imperative. However, this is only a framework upon which to build and add other knowledge of new drugs or new effects as changes in medicine become known. Unfamiliar drugs should never be administered. Resources such as the *PDR,* the *AHFS Drug Information,* the *USP/DI,* package inserts, and pharmacists must be consulted *before* administration of a drug to become familiar with its desired effect, potential side effects, precautions and contraindications, and possible interactions with other drugs or with foods.

Responsibility for safe administration of medications requires *complete planning* for patient care, including prior *assessment, interventions,* and *evaluations* of the results of drug therapy. Assessment involves taking a complete history, including all medical conditions (e.g., pregnancy or illness), allergies, and all other medications in use, including over-the-counter drugs, vitamins, and herbal remedies. Assessment also involves careful observation of the patient's vital signs, posture, skin temperature and color, and facial expression before and after drug administration. Appropriate interventions require judgment in timing, discontinuing medicine if required, and taking steps to counteract adverse reactions, as well as knowing what and when to report to the physician. Evaluation and documentation of results also play a vital role for all health care providers, including the physician, in planning effective drug therapy.

The safe administration of medications necessitates training to develop skills in the delivery of medications. The goal is to maximize the effectiveness of the drug with the least discomfort to the patient. Sensitivity to the unique needs of each patient is encouraged (e.g., awareness of difficulty swallowing or impaired movement that could affect administration of medications).

Patient education is an essential part of the safe administration of medicines. If patients are to benefit from drug therapy, they must understand the importance of taking the medicine in the proper dosage, on time, and in the proper way. Information for patients should be in the language they understand, with both verbal and written instructions as well as demonstrations of techniques when indicated. If the medication administration requires extra equipment or has multiple steps, a return demonstration should be required.

Administration of medication carries moral, ethical, and legal responsibilities. Some rules and regulations vary with the institution, agency, or office. When in doubt, consult those in authority—supervisors or administrators—and/or policy and procedure books. However, documentation on the patient's record is always required for all medicines given as well as for patient education. In addition, controlled substances given must also be recorded in a narcotics record as explained in Chapter 1.

MEDICATION ERRORS

Medication errors can and do occur in all health care settings. More errors are reported from acute care settings, where the risk is greatest. However, outpatient facilities, ambulatory care sites, home health care, and long-term care facility professionals have challenges unique to their practice as well. Patients in these settings often are older adults and likely to have several chronic conditions requiring multiple medications (see Chapter 27, "Drugs and Older Adults"). Increasing the number of medications an individual receives not only increases the risk of interactions and adverse side effects but also increases the risk of error.

Medication errors can occur in the following situations:

1. Administering a drug to the *wrong* patient
2. Administering the *wrong* drug or drug form
3. Administering a drug via the *wrong* route
4. Administering a drug at the *wrong* time
5. Administering the *wrong* dosage
6. *Wrong* documentation: improperly documenting drug administration information on a patient's medical record

Meticulous care in preparation and administration of medications reduces the chances of error. However, if a mistake is made, it is of the utmost importance to *report it* immediately to the one in charge so that corrective action can be taken for the patient's welfare. The patient's record should reflect the corrective action taken for justification in case of legal proceedings. An incident report must also be completed as a legal requirement. Failure to report errors appropriately can jeopardize the patient's welfare, as well as increase the possibility of civil suits against the health care provider and/or the risk of loss of professional license or certificate. Honesty is not only the best policy, but it is also the *only* policy for moral, ethical, and legal reasons.

Health care professionals have a responsibility to provide quality care and provide for patient safety at all times. Remember, "*First, do no harm.*" This challenge includes prevention of medication errors and also reporting of medication errors so that corrective steps can be taken. As part of this goal, the *U.S. Pharmacopeia (USP)* has established a Medication Errors Reporting (MER) program.

In addition, the Agency for Healthcare Research and Quality has federally certified the Institute for Safe Medication Practices (ISMP) as a Patient Safety Organization (PSO) to operate a national error-reporting program for both vaccine and medication errors. Health care professionals and the public should be encouraged to report errors to ISMP because a PSO confers both privilege and confidentiality to the information reported. Error reporting by health care professionals and hospitals is necessary to develop safety alerts and quality improvement programs.

Medication reconciliation is a method used to compare the medications a patient is taking to the medications ordered by the patient's physician. This comparison is done every time there is a change in the patient's care. For example, medication reconciliation is done whenever a patient is admitted, transferred, or discharged. Medication reconciliation is done to prevent medication errors caused by omissions, duplications, errors in doses, or medication interactions (The Joint Commission, October 2012).

According to the Joint Commission, medication reconciliation consists of five steps:

1. Develop a list of current medications
2. Develop a list of medications to be prescribed
3. Compare the medications on the two lists
4. Make clinical decisions based on the comparison
5. Communicate the new list to appropriate caregivers and to the patient

PRINCIPLES OF ADMINISTRATION

When preparing to administer medications, several basic principles should always be kept in mind:

1. *Cleanliness:* Always wash hands before handling medicines, and be sure preparation area is clean and neat.
2. *Organization:* Always be sure medications and supplies are in the appropriate area and in adequate supply. When stock drugs are used, they should be reordered immediately.
3. *Preparation area:* Should be well lighted and away from distracting influences.

Guidelines to review before administering medicines are called the **Six Rights of Medication Administration** (Figure 7-1):

1. Right medication
2. Right amount
3. Right time
4. Right route
5. Right patient
6. Right documentation

Right Medication and Dosage Form

You can confirm that you have the right medication by carefully comparing the name of the drug prescribed (on the physician's order sheet, prescription blank, medication record, or medicine card) with the label on the package, bottle, or unit-dose packet (medications with each dose separately sealed in an individual paper, foil, plastic, or glass container). *Never* give medication when the name of the medication is obscured in any way. Some drugs have names that sound or look similar (e.g., Novolin 70/30 and Novolog Mix 70/30), and therefore it is essential to scrutinize every letter in the name when comparing the medicine ordered with the medicine on hand. Accuracy can be facilitated by placing the unit-dose packet next to the name of the drug ordered on the patient's record, while comparing the drug ordered with the drug on hand. (See Figure 8-2 in Chapter 8.)

Always confirm that you have the correct dosage form. The most common mistake made regarding dosage forms is substituting a capsule for a tablet or vice versa, but you should always double check the dosage form for all medications. Choosing the incorrect dosage form may not seem like a major issue, but it can cause vastly different pharmacological effects for the patient. Tablets are often intended to dissolve in the acidic stomach, whereas some capsules are specifically designed to not dissolve until they reach the more basic small intestine. Selecting the wrong dosage form could lead to a decreased efficacy of the drug. Some medications that have both a capsule and tablet form are actually used completely different in practice. For example, hydroxyzine in tablet form is generic for the brand name Atarax, but in capsule form is generic for the brand name Vistaril. Atarax is primarily used for acute puritis (itching), whereas Vistaril is often used as an adjunct therapy for depression and anxiety. Additionally, medications that come in both a capsule and in a tablet are much different in cost, meaning selecting the correct dosage form is important to the financial costs to the patient.

If there is any question about the drug order because of handwriting, misspelling, inappropriateness, allergies, or interactions, you have the *right* and *responsibility to question* the physician and/or the pharmacist.

Never give medications that someone else has prepared. *Never* leave medications at the bedside unless specifically ordered by the physician (e.g., nitroglycerin tablets and contraceptives are frequently ordered to be left with the patient for self-administration). If the patient is unable to take a medication when you present it, the medication must be returned (in an unopened packet) to the patient's drawer in the medicine cart or medicine room. Never open the unit-dose packet until the patient is prepared to take the medicine.

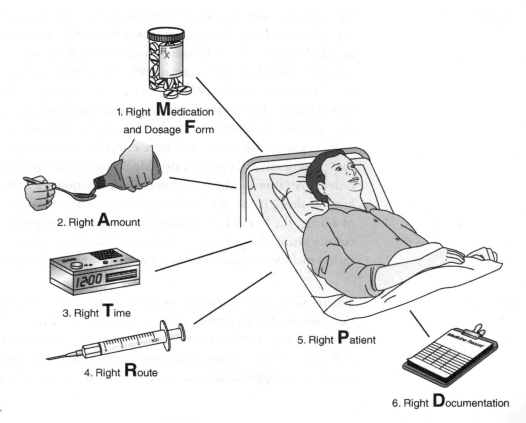

1. Right **M**edication and Dosage **F**orm

2. Right **A**mount

3. Right **T**ime

4. Right **R**oute

5. Right **P**atient

6. Right **D**ocumentation

FIGURE 7-1 The Six Rights of Medication Administration.

Right Amount

Administering the right amount of drug is extremely important. The drug dosage ordered must be compared *very carefully* with the dose listed on the label of the package, bottle, or unit-dose packet. Here again, accuracy can be facilitated by placing the unit-dose packet next to the written order on the patient's record while comparing the dose ordered with the dose on hand.

The three different systems of measurement (household, apothecary, and metric) were discussed in Chapter 5. It is important to consult a table of equivalents if necessary to convert from one system to another. Directions for calculation of different drug doses were presented in Chapter 6. Drug calculations are infrequent with unit-dose packaging. However, if it is necessary to compute calculations, such calculations must be checked by another trained health care professional, pharmacist, or physician to verify accuracy. Be especially careful when the dose is expressed in decimals or fractions. Always recheck the dose if less than ½ tablet or more than two tablets or more than 2 mL for injection is required. An unusual dosage should alert you to the possibility of error. Those who administer medications have the right, as well as the responsibility, to question any dosage that is unusual or seems inappropriate for the individual patient. Remember that drug action is influenced by the condition of the patient, metabolism, age, weight, sex, and psychological state (see Chapter 3). The health care professional has the responsibility of reporting the results of careful assessment and observations to assist the physician in prescribing the right dosage for each patient.

Directions for measurement and preparation of the right dose are described in Chapters 8 and 9. An important part of the patient education includes complete instructions about the importance of preparing and taking the right amount of medicine prescribed by the physician.

Right Time

The time for administration of medications is an important part of the drug *dosage,* which includes the amount, frequency, and number of doses of medication to be administered. For maximum effectiveness, drugs must be given on a prescribed schedule. The physician's order specifies the number of times per day the medicine is to be administered (e.g., BID, or twice a day). Some medications need to be maintained at a specific level in the blood (*therapeutic level*) and are therefore prescribed at regular intervals around the clock (e.g., q4h or every four hours). Some medications, such as some antibiotics, are more effective on an empty stomach and are therefore prescribed *ac* (before meals). Medications that are irritating to the stomach are ordered *pc* (after meals). Drugs that cause sedation are more frequently prescribed at hour of sleep. If the physician does not prescribe a specific time for administration of a drug, the health care professional arranges an appropriate schedule, taking into consideration the purpose, action, and side effects of the medication. Patient education includes instruction about the right time to take specific medicines and why.

Right Route

The route of administration is important because of its effect on degree of absorption, speed of drug action, and side effects. Many drugs can be administered in a variety of ways (see Chapter 4). The physician's order specifies the route of administration. Those administering medications have the right and responsibility to question the appropriateness of a route based on assessment and observation of the patient. Change of route may be indicated because of the patient's condition (e.g., nausea, vomiting, or difficulty swallowing). However, the route of administration may not be changed without the physician's order.

Right Patient

The patient who is to receive the medication must be identified by use of certain techniques to reduce the chance of error. In health care facilities, the patient's wrist identification band should be checked *first*, and then the patient should be called by name or asked to state her name, *before* administering the medication. In the ambulatory care setting, the patient can be asked to give name and date of birth; this can be verified with the chart before administering medications. If the patient questions the medication or the dosage, recheck the order and the medicine before giving it.

Right Documentation

Another essential duty is **documentation of drug administration**. Every medication given must be recorded on the patient's record, along with *dose, time, route,* and *location* of injections. In addition, any unusual or adverse patient reactions must be noted. If the medication is given on a PRN (as necessary) basis (e.g., for pain), notation should also be made on the patient's record regarding the effectiveness of the medication. The person administering the medication must also sign or initial the record after administration (the policy of each facility determines the exact procedure to be followed). The accuracy of medication documentation is a very important legal responsibility. At times, patients' records are examined in court, and the accuracy of medication documentation can be a critical factor in some legal judgments.

Documentation also includes the recording of narcotics administered on the special controlled substances record kept with the narcotics. If narcotics are destroyed because of partial dosage, cancellation, or error, two health care professionals must sign as witnesses of the disposal of the drug (the policy about documentation of narcotics may vary with the agency).

CLINICAL CONNECTION: CONFIRMATION BIAS

As a health care professional each day you might be responsible for reviewing many medication orders for correctness before administering them to a patient. Often times when a person is in a routine, they will read a medication order and see what they expect to see. For example, an order reads: metformin 1000 mg TID. Metformin is almost always given twice daily, so it would be easy for a person to expect to see "BID" and read it as such. This type of mistake most often results from seeing the same thing multiple times and is more common when a person is hurried or stressed. This phenomenon is known as *confirmation bias*. Confirmation bias accounts for many medication-related errors, but it can be easily avoided if you are diligent in checking the six rights.

In summary, safe and effective administration of medications involves current drug information; technical and evaluation skills; and moral, ethical, and legal responsibilities. Guidelines include the Six Rights of Medication Administration. In addition, the health care professional has the right and responsibility to question any medication order that is confusing or illegible or that seems inappropriate and the right to refuse to administer any medication that is not in the best interests of the patient. The welfare of the patient is the primary concern in the administration of medications.

MedWatch

The Food and Drug Administration (FDA) issued a form in 1993 to assist health care professionals in reporting serious, adverse events or product quality problems associated with medications, medical devices, or nutritional products regulated by the FDA, for example, dietary supplements or infant formulas. Even the large, well-designed clinical trials that precede FDA approval cannot uncover every problem that can come to light once a product is widely used. For example, a drug could interact with other drugs in ways that were not revealed during clinical trials. Reports by health care professionals can help ensure the safety of drugs and other products regulated by the FDA.

In response to these voluntary reports from the health care community, the FDA has issued warnings, made labeling changes, required manufacturers to do postmarketing studies, and ordered the withdrawal of certain products from the market. Such actions can prevent injuries, suffering, disabilities, congenital deformities, and even deaths.

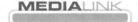

MEDIALINK

See it in Action! View a video on *Medication Errors, Documentation, and Administration* on the Online Resources.

You are not expected to establish a connection or even wait until the evidence seems overwhelming. The agency's regulations will protect your identity and the identities of your patient and your facility. With your cooperation, MedWatch can help the FDA to monitor product safety and, when necessary, take swift action to protect you and your patients. MedWatch encourages you to regard voluntary reporting as part of your professional responsibility. See Figure 7-2 for a partial MEDWATCH form and for instructions for completing and submitting this form to the FDA. In addition, you can complete a MEDWATCH online voluntary reporting form (3500) by visiting www.fda.gov/medwatch/.

U.S. Department of Health and Human Services

MEDWATCH

The FDA Safety Information and Adverse Event Reporting Program

For VOLUNTARY reporting of adverse events, product problems and product use errors

Page 1 of 2

Form Approved: OMB No. 0910-0291, Expires: 6/30/2015
See PRA statement on reverse.

FDA USE ONLY
Triage unit sequence #

PLEASE TYPE OR USE BLACK INK

A. PATIENT INFORMATION

1. Patient Identifier	2. Age at Time of Event or Date of Birth:	3. Sex	4. Weight
In confidence		☐ Female ☐ Male	_____ lb or _____ kg

B. ADVERSE EVENT, PRODUCT PROBLEM OR ERROR

Check all that apply:

1. ☐ Adverse Event   ☐ Product Problem (e.g., defects/malfunctions)
   ☐ Product Use Error   ☐ Problem with Different Manufacturer of Same Medicine

2. Outcomes Attributed to Adverse Event (Check all that apply)
   ☐ Death: _____ (mm/dd/yyyy)
   ☐ Life-threatening
   ☐ Hospitalization - initial or prolonged
   ☐ Required Intervention to Prevent Permanent Impairment/Damage (Devices)
   ☐ Disability or Permanent Damage
   ☐ Congenital Anomaly/Birth Defect
   ☐ Other Serious (Important Medical Events)

3. Date of Event (mm/dd/yyyy)	4. Date of this Report (mm/dd/yyyy)

5. Describe Event, Problem or Product Use Error

6. Relevant Tests/Laboratory Data, Including Dates

7. Other Relevant History, Including Preexisting Medical Conditions (e.g., allergies, race, pregnancy, smoking and alcohol use, liver/kidney problems, etc.)

C. PRODUCT AVAILABILITY

Product Available for Evaluation? (Do not send product to FDA)

☐ Yes   ☐ No   ☐ Returned to Manufacturer on: _____ (mm/dd/yyyy)

D. SUSPECT PRODUCT(S)

1. Name, Strength, Manufacturer (from product label)
#1 Name:
   Strength:
   Manufacturer:
#2 Name:
   Strength:
   Manufacturer:

2.	Dose or Amount	Frequency	Route
#1			
#2			

3. Dates of Use (If unknown, give duration) from/to (or best estimate)	5. Event Abated After Use Stopped or Dose Reduced?
#1	#1 ☐ Yes ☐ No ☐ Doesn't Apply
#2	#2 ☐ Yes ☐ No ☐ Doesn't Apply

4. Diagnosis or Reason for Use (Indication)	8. Event Reappeared After Reintroduction?
#1	#1 ☐ Yes ☐ No ☐ Doesn't Apply
#2	#2 ☐ Yes ☐ No ☐ Doesn't Apply

6. Lot #	7. Expiration Date	9. NDC # or Unique ID
#1	#1	
#2	#2	

E. SUSPECT MEDICAL DEVICE

1. Brand Name

2. Common Device Name	2b. Procode

3. Manufacturer Name, City and State

4. Model #	Lot #	5. Operator of Device
		☐ Health Professional
Catalog #	Expiration Date (mm/dd/yyyy)	☐ Lay User/Patient
Serial #	Unique Identifier (UDI) #	☐ Other:

6. If Implanted, Give Date (mm/dd/yyyy)	7. If Explanted, Give Date (mm/dd/yyyy)

8. Is this a Single-use Device that was Reprocessed and Reused on a Patient?
☐ Yes ☐ No

9. If Yes to Item No. 8, Enter Name and Address of Reprocessor

F. OTHER (CONCOMITANT) MEDICAL PRODUCTS

Product names and therapy dates (exclude treatment of event)

G. REPORTER (See confidentiality section on back)

1. Name and Address
Name:
Address:

City:	State:	ZIP:

Phone #	E-mail

2. Health Professional?	3. Occupation	4. Also Reported to:
☐ Yes ☐ No	▼	☐ Manufacturer ☐ User Facility ☐ Distributor/Importer
5. If you do NOT want your identity disclosed to the manufacturer, place an "X" in this box: ☐		

FORM FDA 3500 (2/13)   Submission of a report does not constitute an admission that medical personnel or the product caused or contributed to the event.

FIGURE 7-2 MedWatch form. (A) The FDA Medical Products Reporting Program for voluntary reporting by health care professionals of adverse events and product problems. (B) MedWatch form. The FDA Medical Products Reporting Program for voluntary reporting by health professionals of adverse events and product problems. Partial MED WATCH form. The FDA Medical Products Reporting Program for voluntary reporting by health professionals of adverse events and product problems. Visit www.fda.gov for the complete, interactive MED WATCH form and instructions for completing.

ADVICE ABOUT VOLUNTARY REPORTING

Detailed instructions available at: http://www.fda.gov/medwatch/report/consumer/instruct.htm

Report adverse events, product problems or product use errors with:

- Medications *(drugs or biologics)*
- Medical devices *(including in-vitro diagnostics)*
- Combination products *(medication & medical devices)*
- Human cells, tissues, and cellular and tissue-based products
- Special nutritional products *(dietary supplements, medical foods, infant formulas)*
- Cosmetics
- Food *(including beverages and ingredients added to foods)*

Report product problems - quality, performance or safety concerns such as:

- Suspected counterfeit product
- Suspected contamination
- Questionable stability
- Defective components
- Poor packaging or labeling
- Therapeutic failures (product didn't work)

Report SERIOUS adverse events. An event is serious when the patient outcome is:

- Death
- Life-threatening
- Hospitalization - initial or prolonged
- Disability or permanent damage
- Congenital anomaly/birth defect
- Required intervention to prevent permanent impairment or damage (devices)
- Other serious (important medical events)

Report even if:

- You're not certain the product caused the event
- You don't have all the details

How to report:

- Just fill in the sections that apply to your report
- Use section D for all products except medical devices
- Attach additional pages if needed
- Use a separate form for each patient
- Report either to FDA or the manufacturer *(or both)*

Other methods of reporting:

- 1-800-FDA-0178 - To FAX report
- 1-800-FDA-1088 - To report by phone
- www.fda.gov/medwatch/report.htm - To report online

If your report involves a serious adverse event with a device and it occurred in a facility outside a doctor's office, that facility may be legally required to report to FDA and/or the manufacturer. Please notify the person in that facility who would handle such reporting.

If your report involves a serious adverse event with a vaccine, call 1-800-822-7967 to report.

Confidentiality: The patient's identity is held in strict confidence by FDA and protected to the fullest extent of the law. FDA will not disclose the reporter's identity in response to a request from the public, pursuant to the Freedom of Information Act. The reporter's identity, including the identity of a self-reporter, may be shared with the manufacturer unless requested otherwise.

-Fold Here-

The information in this box applies only to requirements of the Paperwork Reduction Act of 1995

The burden time for this collection of information has been estimated to average 36 minutes per response, including the time to review instructions, search existing data sources, gather and maintain the data needed, and complete and review the collection of information. Send comments regarding this burden estimate or any other aspect of this collection of information, including suggestions for reducing this burden to:

Department of Health and Human Services *Food and Drug Administration* *Office of Chief Information Officer* *Paperwork Reduction Act (PRA) Staff* *PRAStaff@fda.hhs.gov*	*Please DO NOT* *RETURN this form* *to the PRA Staff e-mail* *to the left.*	*OMB statement:* *"An agency may not conduct or sponsor, and a person is not required to respond to, a collection of information unless it displays a currently valid OMB control number."*

U.S. DEPARTMENT OF HEALTH AND HUMAN SERVICES
Food and Drug Administration

FORM FDA 3500 (2/13) (Back)   **Please Use Address Provided Below -- Fold in Thirds, Tape and Mail**

**DEPARTMENT OF
HEALTH & HUMAN SERVICES**

Public Health Service
Food and Drug Administration
Rockville, MD 20857

Official Business
Penalty for Private Use $300

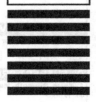

NO POSTAGE
NECESSARY
IF MAILED
IN THE
UNITED STATES
OR APO/FPO

BUSINESS REPLY MAIL

FIRST CLASS MAIL PERMIT NO. 946 ROCKVILLE MD

POSTAGE WILL BE PAID BY FOOD AND DRUG ADMINISTRATION

MedWatch
The FDA Safety Information and Adverse Event Reporting Program
Food and Drug Administration
5600 Fishers Lane
Rockville, MD 20852-9787

FIGURE 7-2 continued

CHAPTER REVIEW QUIZ

Complete the statements by filling in the blanks.

1. According to the Joint Commission, medication reconciliation consists of what five steps?

   _____

   _____

   _____

   _____

   _____

2. Before administering any medication, you should have the following three pieces of information about the patient:

   _____

   _____

   _____

3. When preparing to administer medications, what three principles should be kept in mind?

   _____

   _____

   _____

4. Patient education about medication should include the following four pieces of information:

   _____

   _____

   _____

   _____

5. When administering a controlled substance, documentation is necessary in what two places?

   _____

   _____

6. Documentation of an injection given for pain should include the following five pieces of information:

   _____

   _____

   _____

   _____

   _____

7. Name the Six Rights of Medication Administration:

_____

_____

_____

_____

_____

_____

8. Medication errors must be reported immediately, and documentation includes recording the information in the following two areas:

_____

_____

STUDYGUIDE	**Online Resources**
P R A C T I C E	
Complete Chapter 7	• Powerpoint presentations
	• Videos

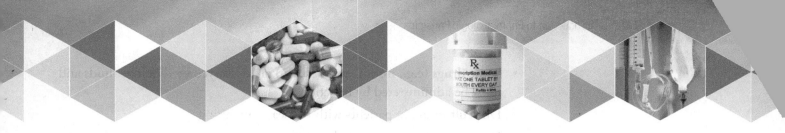

CHAPTER 8

ADMINISTRATION BY THE GASTROINTESTINAL ROUTE

KEY TERMS AND CONCEPTS

Aspiration

Dysphagia

Gastric tube administration

G-tube or PEG tube

Nasogastric tube administration

Oral medication administration

Rectal medication

Retention enema

OBJECTIVES

Upon completion of this chapter, the learner should be able to

1. Describe the advantages and disadvantages of administering medications orally, by nasogastric or gastrostomy tube, and rectally

2. Explain the appropriate action to be taken when patient is NPO (ordered to have nothing by mouth), has dysphagia, refuses medication, vomits medication, or has allergies

3. List the special precautions to be followed in the preparation of sustained-release capsules, enteric-coated tablets, and oral suspensions

4. Demonstrate the measurement of liquid medications using medicine cup and syringe

5. Demonstrate the proficiency in administering medications orally, by nasogastric or gastric tube, and rectally

6. Satisfactorily complete all of the activities listed on the checklists

7. Define the Key Terms and Concepts

Medications are administered by the gastrointestinal route more often than any other way. Gastrointestinal administration includes four categories: oral, nasogastric tube, gastric tube, and rectal.

Advantages of the **oral medication administration** include the following:

- Convenience and patient comfort
- Safety, because some medication can be retrieved in case of error or intentional overdose
- Economy, because there are few equipment costs and most medications are formulated for this route.

Disadvantages of the oral route include:

- Slower onset of absorption and action
- Rate and degree of absorption vary with gastrointestinal contents and motility

- Some drugs (e.g., insulin and heparin) are destroyed by digestive fluids and must be administered by injection
- Difficult to use in patients with nausea or vomiting
- Dangerous to use if patient has difficulty swallowing (**dysphagia**), because of possible **aspiration**; aspiration is the inhalation of a foreign substance or regurgitated gastric contents, which can cause severe lung damage.
- Cannot be used for unconscious patients
- Cannot be used if patient is NPO (e.g., before surgery or because of an acute medical condition). May not be able to be used if a patient is fasting for a test such as a lipid panel or scan, although often maintenance medications can still be taken with clear liquids.
- Administration of medications by nasogastric tube, small-bore silicone gastric tube, or percutaneous endoscopic gastrostomy (PEG) tube is sometimes ordered when the patient is unable to swallow for periods of time because of illness, trauma, surgery, or unconsciousness. Medications are usually administered intravenously when these conditions exist for short periods of time.

*Advantages of the **nasogastric tube** include:*

- Ability to bypass the mouth and pharynx when necessary
- Elimination of numerous injections

The *disadvantage of the nasogastric tube* with a conscious patient is the discomfort of the tube in the nose and throat for prolonged periods of time.

When a patient is unable to take nourishment by mouth for a long period of time, the surgeon will sometimes insert a *gastric tube* through the skin of the abdomen, directly into the stomach. This **G-tube, or PEG tube**, as it is sometimes called, is secured in place and can remain there for feeding purposes indefinitely. Medication can be administered via the PEG tube directly into the stomach.

Medications are sometimes administered by the rectal route when nausea or vomiting is present, or the patient is unconscious or unable to swallow. *Advantages of the **rectal route** include:*

- Bypassing the action of digestive enzymes
- Avoidance of irritation to the upper GI tract
- Usefulness with dysphagia

Disadvantages of the rectal route include:

- Many medications are unavailable in suppository form
- Some patients have difficulty retaining suppositories (e.g., older adults and children)
- Prolonged use of some rectal suppositories can cause rectal irritation (e.g., bisacodyl)
- Absorption may be irregular or incomplete if feces are present

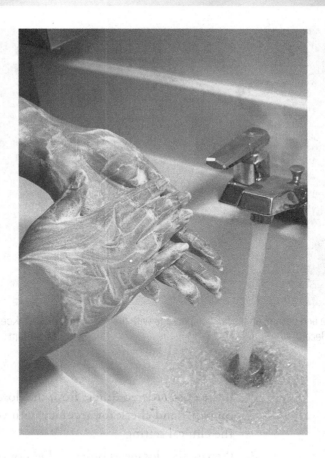

FIGURE 8-1 Medical asepsis handwash.

ADMINISTRATION OF MEDICATIONS ORALLY

Guidelines for Oral Medications Administration

1. Wash your hands (Figure 8-1).

2. Locate the appropriate medication order, medication sheet or, if using an eMAR, scan the patient's wristband and check for completeness of the order (i.e., date, patient's name, medication name, dosage, route, and time).

3. Check for special circumstances (e.g., allergies or NPO).

4. Be sure that you know the purpose of the drug, possible side effects, contraindications, cautions, interactions, and normal dosage range. If unfamiliar with the drug, consult a reference source for this information.

5. Select the appropriate receptacle in which to place the medication (i.e., paper medicine cup for tablets or capsules and plastic medicine cup for liquids).

6. Locate medication in the medication cupboard or medication cart drawer. If using an eMAR, scan it and compare the label screen, if using a paper record compare the medication to the chart, for the Six Rights of Medication Administration: right medicine, right amount, right time, right route, right patient, and right documentation (Figure 8-2). Also be sure to check the drug's expiration date.

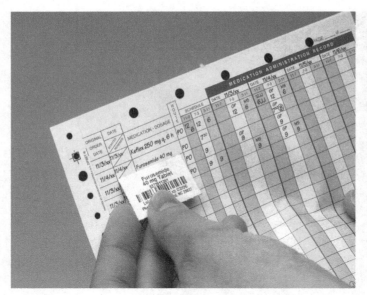

FIGURE 8-2 Compare name and dosage on medication package with the Medication Administration Record.

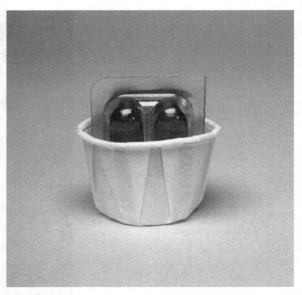

FIGURE 8-3 Keep the unit-dose packet intact until you are with the patient.

7. If the dose ordered differs from the dose on hand, complete calculations on paper and check for accuracy with your instructor or a co-worker in the clinical setting.

8. Prepare the dosage as ordered. Do not open unit-dose packages until you are with the patient (Figure 8-3). If medication is liquid, see "Preparation of Liquid Medications" later in this section.

9. Take medication in a cup to the patient and place it on a table nearby.

10. Check the patient's identification bracelet (Figure 8-4). Ask the patient to *tell you* his or her name and date of birth (DOB). Compare this information with the medication administration record to verify that you have the right patient. If the patient is unable to provide his or her

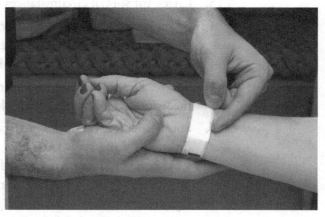

FIGURE 8-4 Check identification to be sure it is the right patient. Also ask the patient for name and date of birth and verify with the Medication Record. Always check for allergies.

name and/or DOB, use an alternate method to identify the patient such as a photograph or identity confirmation by a family member, friend, or coworker.

11. Call the patient by name and explain what you are doing. Answer any questions. Recheck the medication order if the patient expresses any doubts. Use this opportunity for patient education about the medication.

12. Monitor the patient's vital signs if required for specific medication (e.g., blood pressure, apical pulse, or respiration). Blood pressure should always be taken and recorded *before* administering antihypertensives.

13. Open the unit-dose package and place the container in the patient's hand. Avoid touching the medication (Figure 8-5).

14. Provide a full glass of water and assist the patient as necessary (e.g., raise the head of the bed and provide drinking straw if required).

15. Stay with the patient until the medication has been swallowed. Make the patient comfortable before you leave the room.

16. Discard the used medicine cup and wrappers in a wastebasket.

17. Record the medication, dosage, time, route, and your signature or initials in the correct place on the patient's record according to the rules of the facility.

18. Document on the patient's record and report if a medication is withheld or refused and the reason. Record and *report* any unusual circumstances associated with administration or any adverse side effects.

Special Considerations for Oral Administration

1. If patient is NPO, check with the person in charge regarding the appropriate procedure, based on the reason for NPO. If patient is fasting for tests, medication can usually be given at a later time with possible modification of time schedule or with clear liquids if the physician approves. If patient is NPO for surgery, nausea, or dysphagia, it may be necessary to consult the doctor regarding a change of route. Do not omit the medications completely without specific instructions to that effect. Abrupt withdrawal of

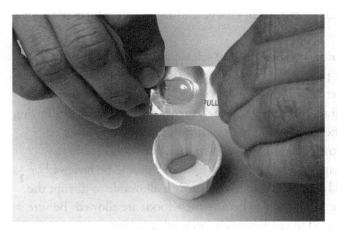
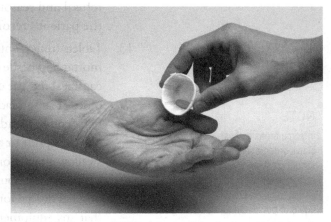

FIGURE 8-5 Do not touch medicine. (A) Open the unit-dose packet and drop the tablet in a cup. (B) Place the medicine in the patient's hand.

some medications, for example, phenytoin (Dilantin) or diazepam (Valium), may lead to dangerous conditions, such as seizures.

2. *Always check the patient's record carefully for allergies* and be aware of the components of combination products. Patients with a history of allergy should be watched carefully for possible drug reactions when any new medication is administered.

3. Give the most important medicine first; for example, cardiac medicine before a vitamin.

4. Elevate the patient's head, if not contraindicated by the patient's condition, to aid in swallowing.

5. Stay with the patient until the medication is swallowed. *Do not* leave the medication at the bedside or in the patient's possession unless ordered by the physician.

6. Administer oral medications with water unless ordered otherwise. *Do not* give medicine with fruit juice, milk, or any other liquid unless indicated by specific directions. The absorption of many medicines (e.g., antibiotics) is inhibited by interaction with acid or alkaline products.

7. Medications whose action depends on contact with the mucous membranes of the mouth or throat (e.g., topical anesthetics or fungicides) *should not* be administered with any fluid or food.

8. If tablets must be divided, *do not* break by hand. If available, a pill-cutter may be used. In home care setting, cut with a knife on score marks only.

9. When removing tablets or capsules from a stock bottle, pour into the lid and from there into the medicine cup. *Do not* touch tablets or capsules.

10. *Do not* administer any medication that is discolored, has precipitated, is contaminated, or is outdated.

11. If a patient is NPO, refuses the medication, or vomits within 20–30 min of taking the medication, always report this to the person in charge. An order from the physician is required to change either the medication or the route of administration. Document on the patient's record the time of emesis and appearance of the emesis to check whether the medication remained intact.

12. If the patient refuses a medication, determine the reason. Report the refusal and reason to the person in charge and record all information on the patient's record.

13. Tablets (unless enteric coated or sustained-release) may be crushed with mortar and pestle or pillcrusher. Some capsules (even sustained-release capsules) may be opened and the contents mixed with applesauce, pudding, or ice cream to facilitate administration for patients with difficulty swallowing (e.g., children and the elderly). Do not crush the contents of a sustained-release capsule or allow patients to chew them. If a patient is unable to swallow a tablet or capsule whole, the package insert should be reviewed or a pharmacist should be consulted to make sure it is allowable to disrupt the original dosage form. Check diet to be sure these foods are allowed. Be sure that any equipment used to crush medication is wiped clean.

NOTE

In some areas a physician's order is required for pill crushing. If available, ask for the medication to be ordered in liquid or powdered form.

Preparation of Liquid Medications

Follow the "Guidelines for Administration of Oral Medications" at the beginning of this section. Preparation of *liquid medications* requires these additional steps:

1. Shake bottle if indicated. Remove cap and place cap upside down on table.

2. Hold the medicine bottle with the label side upward to prevent smearing of label while pouring (Figure 8-6).

3. Place medicine cup at eye level. You may place your thumbnail on level to which medication will be poured (Figure 8-6).

4. While holding the medicine cup straight at eye level, pour the prescribed amount of medication.

5. Replace the cap on the bottle.

6. Compare the information on the medication sheet against the label on the stock bottle and the quantity of drug in the cup.

7. Replace the medication bottle in the cupboard or the medicine cart.

8. Recheck the Six Rights of Medication Administration.

9. Proceed with the "Guidelines for Administration of Oral Medications."

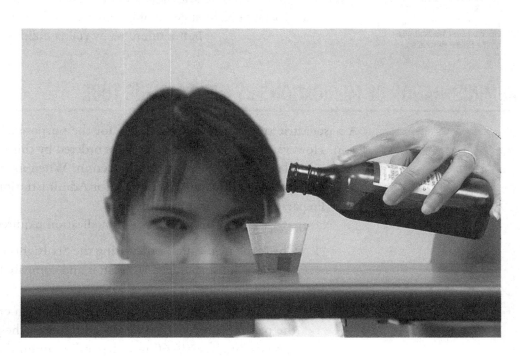

FIGURE 8-6 Hold the medicine bottle with label side up and medicine cup at eye level.

When administering liquid medication to someone who is unable to drink from a cup (e.g., infants and persons with wired jaws), a syringe may be used. Follow the "Guidelines for Administration of Oral Medications." Administration of *liquid medications orally via syringe* requires these additional steps:

1. Pour the prescribed medication into the medicine cup. If automated, scan it and compare the label against the medication sheet or automated screen for the Six Rights of Medication Administration: right medicine, right amount, right time, right route, right patient, and right documentation.

2. Withdraw the prescribed amount with a syringe.

3. Check the medication and order using the Six Rights of Medication Administration.

4. Identify the patient and scan wristband if using an eMAR, verify name and date of birth (DOB), and elevate the patient's head.

5. Be sure the patient is alert and able to swallow.

6. Place the syringe tip in the pocket between the cheek and the gums. (When administering large amounts of liquid via a syringe, it helps to fit a 2-inch length of latex tubing on the syringe tip to facilitate instillation of the medication into the cheek pocket.)

7. Instill the medication slowly to lessen chances of aspiration.

8. Be sure the patient swallows all the medication completely.

9. Proceed with "Guidelines for the Administration of Oral Medications."

10. Remember the "sixth right" and document appropriately.

NOTE

Never mix two liquids together in the same medicine cup. When pouring medication, never touch the medicine cup with the medication bottle. If too much medication is poured into the medicine cup, discard the extra medication. Do not pour the extra medication back into the bottle.

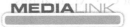

See it in Action! View a video on *Oral Medications* on the Online Resources.

Administration of liquid oral medications is the preferred form for children less than 5 years old. In addition, flavored medications are often preferred and better tolerated by young children.

ADMINISTRATION OF MEDICATIONS BY NASOGASTRIC TUBE

A nasogastric tube is not inserted solely for the purpose of administering medication. However, medications are sometimes ordered by this route when a nasogastric tube is in place for tube feeding or for suction. When medications are ordered by nasogastric tube, follow the "Guidelines for Administration of Oral Medications" and "Preparation of Liquid Medications."

Nasogastric tube administration of medication requires these additional steps:

1. Check the medication order using the Six Rights of Medication Administration. If using an eMAR, scan it and compare the label against the medication sheet or automated screen.

2. If the medication must be administered on an empty stomach and the patient is receiving a tube feeding, hold the medication, stop the tube feeding for 30–60 min depending upon the medication being administered, and return at the appropriate time to administer the medication.

3. If the patient is not receiving a tube feeding or the medication can be administered with the tube feeding, continue with medication administration.

4. Wash hands. Wear gloves when handling tubes.

5. Prepare the medication as ordered and take it to the patient's room. Be sure the medication is at room temperature.

6. Check the identification bracelet and, if automated, scan the patient's wristband, ask the patient his or her name and verify it, and explain the procedure. Elevate the head of the bed, if not contraindicated.

7. Hold the end of the tube up and remove the clamp, plug, or adapter.

8. Verify that the tube is properly placed in the stomach and verify that the tube is taped at the appropriate centimeter marking. Aspirate with bulb or piston syringe for stomach contents and check the pH of the aspirated fluids. Gastric juice is acidic (pH of 0.9–1.5). If the aspirate does not meet these parameters or if there is any question, do *not* instill any liquids. Instead, report to the person in charge. If the criteria are met, flush the tube with normal saline solution or with water (see Figure 8-7).

9. Clamp the tube with your fingers by bending it over upon itself or by pinching it. After the tube is closed, remove the plunger or the bulb from the syringe, leaving the syringe attached firmly to the tubing. Flush the tube with water (Figure 8-8).

10. Pour the medication into the syringe. Release or unclamp the tubing and let the medication flow through by gravity. Never force fluids down a nasogastric tube (Figure 8-8). Watch the patient during the procedure and stop immediately at any sign of discomfort, coughing, or shortness of breath by pinching the tube. Holding the syringe too high causes fluid to run in too quickly, possibly causing nausea and vomiting. The syringe should be at the level of the patient's shoulder.

11. Before the syringe empties completely, flush the tube by adding 60–100 mL of water to the syringe or the amount ordered. If the

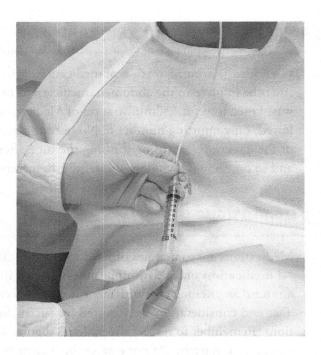

FIGURE 8-7 Test for correct placement of small-bore silicone gastric tube. Aspirate with syringe and check the pH.

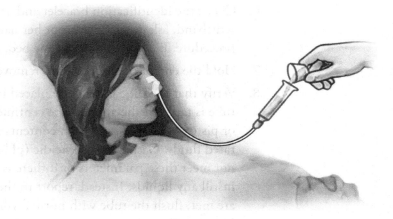

FIGURE 8-8 Pinch tube shut before filling syringe. Let fluid flow in by gravity. Hold syringe at level of patient's shoulder. Flush tube with water.

patient's input and output are being monitored, be sure to add this amount to the patient's record.

12. After the water has run in, pinch the tube, remove the syringe, and clamp or plug the tube. If the patient is ordered suction, be sure to leave the suction turned *off* for at least 30 min until medication is absorbed, then restart suction as ordered. If the patient is receiving a tube feeding, be sure to leave the tube feeding turned *off* for 30–60 min, depending upon the medication, until the medication is absorbed; then restart the tube feeding.

13. Position the patient on the right side and/or elevate the head of the bed to encourage the stomach to remain empty. Make the patient comfortable.

14. Proceed with "Guidelines for the Administration of Oral Medications" for documentation.

ADMINISTRATION OF MEDICATIONS BY GASTRIC TUBE

Gastric tube administration of medications is a simple matter. If a patient has a gastric tube in place in the abdomen, medications can be administered per order in this way. Directions for "Administration of Medications by Nasogastric Tube" can be followed, only omitting number 8. No test for placement of tube is necessary. The rest of the directions regarding flushing the tube afterward and positioning the patient, and so on, should be followed carefully. Remember to document appropriately.

ADMINISTRATION OF MEDICATIONS RECTALLY

Medications are sometimes ordered to be administered by the rectal route. The **rectal medication** may be in suppository form or in liquid form to be administered as a **retention enema**. This treatment is more effective with the patient's cooperation. Tact and consideration are required for successful administration of rectal medications. Remember to respect the patient's dignity and privacy by closing the door and curtains completely. Do not expose the patient unnecessarily.

The retention enema is administered in the same way as a cleansing enema. However, the retention enema must be retained approximately 30 min or more for absorption of the medication. Therefore, the patient is instructed to lie quietly on either side to aid in retention. If the patient is uncooperative, unconscious, or has poor sphincter control, the buttocks can be taped together with 2-inch paper adhesive for 30 min. Do not use this method unless absolutely necessary. Remember to treat the patient with dignity. Always explain everything you are doing and why. Even if patients are unconscious or unable to speak, they may be able to hear and cooperate in some way if they understand.

CLINICAL CONNECTION: PATIENT EDUCATION OF SUPPOSITORIES

When a patient receives a medication for self-administration it is very important to ensure that you educate them on the route of administration. Although to a health care professional this may seem arbitrary, many times patients assume all medications are to be taken orally. This would of course be a problem if the prescribed medication is a suppository meant to be administered per rectal. Common suppositories that are prescribed for self-administration are hydrocortisone suppositories used for hemorrhoids and acetaminophen suppositories used for pain and fever. Ensure that the patient understands that the suppository needs to be unwrapped prior to administration. Although this may seem like common sense, to an uneducated patient it may not be. To be safe, always assume that the patient needs as much information as you can provide.

ADMINISTRATION OF RECTAL SUPPOSITORY

1. Wash hands.
2. If using an eMAR, scan and compare the label against the medication sheet or screen. Check the medication order using the Six Rights of Medication Administration.
3. Identify the medication (purpose, side effects, contraindications, cautions, and normal dose range). Research information, if necessary.
4. Assemble supplies: disposable glove and water-soluble lubricant.
5. Select the medication as ordered, checking medication name and dosage again. Some suppositories are stored in a refrigerator, and some may be stored at room temperature, according to the manufacturer's instructions.
6. Check the patient's identification bracelet and, if automated, scan the patient's wristband, ask patient for name and DOB, and explain the procedure. Answer any questions.
7. Close the door and curtain completely.
8. Lower the head of the bed if necessary and position the patient on the left side with the upper knee bent. Keep the patient covered, exposing only the rectal area (Figure 8-9).
9. Put on disposable gloves.
10. Remove the suppository from the wrapper and lubricate the tapered end with a water-soluble lubricant.
11. With the nondominant hand, separate the patient's buttocks gently so you can see the anus.

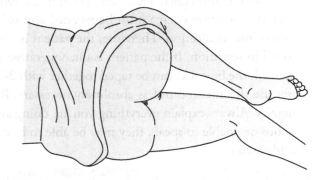

FIGURE 8-9 Drape and position patient on side with upper knee bent.

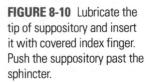

FIGURE 8-10 Lubricate the tip of suppository and insert it with covered index finger. Push the suppository past the sphincter.

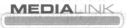

See It In Action! View a video on *Administering Rectal Medications* on the Online Resources.

NOTE

Although this video emphasizes the five rights of medication administration, keep in mind the recently added sixth right of "proper documentation."

12. Ask the patient to take a deep breath. Insert the lubricated suppository gently into the rectum and push gently with gloved index finger until the suppository has passed the internal sphincter (Figure 8-10). With infants, use the gloved *little* finger.

13. Urge the patient to retain the suppository for at least 20 min. If the patient is unable to cooperate, hold the buttocks together as required.

14. Remove and dispose of gloves, turning them inside out as you remove them.

15. Be sure the patient is comfortable, with covers and bed adjusted appropriately.

16. Wash hands.

17. Record the medication in the appropriate place.

CHAPTER REVIEW QUIZ

1. Name six disadvantages of oral administration compared with administration by injection.

_____

_____

_____

_____

_____

_____

Match the column on the left with the appropriate action on the right. Actions may be used more than once.

2. ____ To facilitate swallowing

3. ____ If NPO for laboratory tests

4. ____ Patient vomits 15 min after

5. ____ Most medications

6. ____ Patient is allergic to penicillin

7. ____ Most important medicine

8. ____ Tablet cannot be swallowed

9. ____ Sustained-release capsules

10. ____ Dilantin ordered PO, patient NPO for surgery

a. Watch closely for drug reactions

b. Crush tablet, mix with applesauce

c. Administer first

d. Usually cannot be opened

e. Elevate patient's head

f. Notify person in charge

g. Modify schedule, give medicine later

h. Administer with water

i. Leave medication at bedside

Complete the following statements by filling in the blanks.

When pouring liquid medicine:

11. The bottle should be held ____.

12. The medicine cup should be held ____.

13. The bottle cap should be placed ____.

14. If medication is in suspension, the bottle should first be _____.

When administering medication by nasogastric tube:

15. Check tube placement first with which two tests:

_____

_____

Check the appropriate answer.

When administering medication by nasogastric tube:

16. _____   **a.** Medication should be pushed through the nasogastric tube by pressure on the barrel of a syringe.

     _____   **b.** Medication should flow through the nasogastric tube by gravity.

17. _____   **a.** Medication should be cold.

     _____   **b.** Medication should be at room temperature.

18. _____   **a.** Patient's head should be elevated.

     _____   **b.** Patient should be placed in the Trendelenburg position.

19. Name four steps in administration of a rectal suppository that are different from PO administration.

_____

_____

_____

_____

20. Medication documentation should include:

_____

_____

_____

_____

CHECKLIST FOR ADMINISTRATION OF ORAL MEDICATIONS

Activity	Rating	
	S	U
1. Washed hands	_____	_____
2. Checked medication sheet/automated screen for date, dosage, time, route, and allergies	_____	_____
3. Identified medication: purpose, side effects, contraindications, cautions, interaction, and normal dosage range	_____	_____
4. Selected appropriate medicine cup	_____	_____
5. Selected correct medication/scan barcode and checked label against medication sheet for Six Rights of Medication Administration	_____	_____
6. Calculated correct dosage on paper if necessary and verified calculations with instructor	_____	_____
7. Placed medication as ordered in cup without opening packet or touching medication; prepared liquid medication by shaking if necessary, pouring away from label and measuring at eye level	_____	_____
8. Identified patient by checking/scanning bracelet and asking patient for name and DOB. Use alternate method for verifying identity if necessary. To prevent aspiration, make sure head of bed is elevated unless otherwise ordered	_____	_____
9. Explained procedure to patient and answered any questions about medication	_____	_____
10. Checked patient's vital signs if necessary for specific medicine	_____	_____
11. Opened unit-dose packages and offered medication in container to patient	_____	_____
12. Provided drinking water and assisted patient as necessary	_____	_____
13. Made patient comfortable and left unit in order	_____	_____
14. Recorded medication, dosage, time, and signature or initials on patient's record (the sixth right)	_____	_____

Note: S, satisfactory; U, unsatisfactory.

CHECKLIST FOR ADMINISTRATION OF RECTAL SUPPOSITORY

Activity	Rating	
	S	U
1. Washed hands		
2. Checked the medication order for date, dosage, time, route, and allergies		
3. Identified medication: purpose, side effects, contraindications, cautions, and normal dosage range		
4. Assembled supplies: gloves and lubricant		
5. Selected/scanned correct medication and checked label with medication order for Six Rights of Medication Administration		
6. Identified patient by checking bracelet or scanning and asking patient for name and DOB. Used alternate method for verifying identity if necessary		
7. Explained procedure to patient and answered any questions about medication		
8. Closed door and curtain		
9. Positioned patient on left side with upper knee bent and only rectal area exposed		
10. Put on disposable gloves		
11. Removed wrapping from suppository and lubricated tapered end		
12. With nondominant hand, separated buttocks gently		
13. Instructed patient to take a deep breath and inserted suppository gently, pushing it past the sphincter		
14. Instructed patient about retaining the suppository		
15. Removed gloves correctly and disposed of them appropriately		
16. Made patient comfortable and left unit in order		
17. Washed hands		
18. Recorded medication, dosage, time, and signature or initials on patient's record		

Note: S, satisfactory; U, unsatisfactory.

STUDYGUIDE

PRACTICE

Complete Chapter 8

Online Resources

- Powerpoint presentations
- Videos

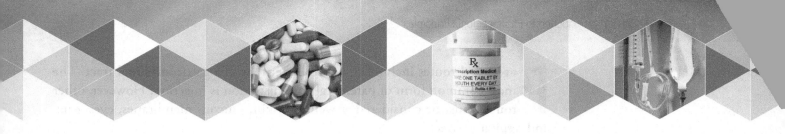

CHAPTER 9

ADMINISTRATION BY THE PARENTERAL ROUTE

KEY TERMS AND CONCEPTS

Bolus

Buccal administration

Continuous IV infusion

Dry-powder inhalers (DPIs)

Inhalation route

Injections

Intermittent IV infusion

Intradermal

Intramuscular

Local effects

Metered-dose inhalers (MDIs)

Parenteral

Piggyback

Small-volume nebulizer (SVN)

Subcutaneous

Sublingual administration

Systemic effects

Topical

Transdermal

Transcutaneous

Z-track method

OBJECTIVES

Upon completion of this chapter, the learner should be able to

1. Name four parenteral routes with systemic effects

2. Explain administration via the sublingual and buccal routes, including instructions to the patient

3. Demonstrate application of nitroglycerin ointment and the transdermal patch

4. Identify three conditions treated with transcutaneous delivery systems

5. Compare and contrast the advantages and disadvantages of the inhalation route

6. Describe patient education for those receiving inhalation therapy with hand-held nebulizers

7. Contrast small-volume nebulizers (SVNs), metered-dose inhalers (MDIs), and dry-powder inhalers (DPIs)

8. Identify the three parts of the syringe and the three parts of the needle

9. Select appropriate-length and correct-gauge needles for various types of injections

10. List the three types of syringes and a purpose for each

11. Demonstrate drawing up medications from a vial and an ampule

12. Describe and demonstrate an intradermal injection

13. Describe and demonstrate a subcutaneous injection

14. Describe three sites for intramuscular (IM) injection and demonstrate IM injection

15. Give the purpose and a demonstration of Z-track injection

16. List the two types of IV administration and various types of IV fluids that can be prescribed

17. List four types of administration for local effects

18. Define the Key Terms and Concepts

Parenteral routes include any route other than the gastrointestinal tract. The most common form of parenteral administration is injection. However, other routes must be considered as well: the skin, mucous membranes, eyes, ears, and respiratory tract.

Parenteral administration can be understood more easily if the *purpose* of administration or the effects desired are considered in two categories: systemic and local. **Systemic effects** are those affecting the body as a whole, the entire system. The goal of administering drugs for systemic effects is to distribute the medication through the circulatory system to the area requiring treatment. Parenteral routes with systemic effects include (1) sublingual or buccal, (2) transcutaneous (transdermal), (3) inhalations, and (4) injections.

Local effects are those limited to one particular part (location) of the body with very little, if any, effect on the rest of the body. Medications in this category include:

1. Medications applied to the skin for skin conditions, sometimes called **topical** medications
2. Drugs applied to the mucous membranes to treat that specific tissue
3. Medications instilled in the eyes for eye conditions
4. Medications instilled in the ears for ear conditions

SUBLINGUAL AND BUCCAL ADMINISTRATION

With **sublingual administration**, the medication is placed under the tongue. The drug is absorbed directly into the circulation through the numerous blood vessels located in the mucosa of this area. With **buccal administration**, the medication is placed in the pouch between the cheek and the gum at the back of the mouth. The sublingual route is used more commonly than the buccal. Medications absorbed in this way are unaffected by the stomach, intestines, or liver. Absorption via this route is quite rapid, and therefore, this method is used frequently when a quick response is required (e.g., with nitroglycerin to treat acute angina pectoris). The constricted coronary blood vessels are usually dilated within a few minutes, bringing quick relief from pain.

PATIENT EDUCATION

For the sublingual or buccal route, include the following instructions:

1. Hold the tablet in place with mouth closed until medication is absorbed.

2. Do not swallow the medication.

3. Do not drink or take food until the medication is completely absorbed (~15 min.).

TRANSCUTANEOUS DRUG DELIVERY SYSTEM

Note

To reduce the occurrence of headaches sometimes the physician will order the nitroglycerin ointment or patch to be applied at bedtime and removed the next day at noon.

Transcutaneous, or **transdermal** systems deliver the medication to the body by absorption through the skin. Nitroglycerin ointment, for example, is applied to the skin in prescribed amounts every few hours for prevention of angina pectoris. The absorption is slower, and therefore this method is not effective in the treatment of acute angina attacks. Other transcutaneous delivery systems utilize a patch impregnated with a particular medication, applied to the skin, and left in place for continuous absorption. Examples of transcutaneous drug delivery systems include nitroglycerin (Nitro-Dur), in which the patch is sometimes left in place for 12h daily (e.g., on in the morning and removed at night to reduce development of nitrate tolerance) for treatment of chronic angina; scopolamine (Transderm-Scop), in which the patch is placed behind the ear and left in place up to 72h, as necessary, to prevent motion sickness; and fentanyl (Duragesic), applied on the skin and changed every 72h in the management of chronic pain in patients requiring opiate analgesia. (See Analgesics, Chapter 19.) Other medications delivered transdermally include estrogen (Climara) and nicotine replacement for smoking cessation therapy. Absorption by this method is slower, but the action is more prolonged than with other methods of administration, and most important the drug is released at a constant rate so that the concentration of the drug is kept at a certain level in the body.

CLINICAL CONNECTION

Medication patches such as fentanyl (Duragesic) must be disposed of properly because they still contain medication when removed. In the acute care setting, the health care professional must verify the patch is in place once per shift and when removing the patch to place a new one, must have a witness to the disposal. They should be disposed of in a designated area such as a "sharps" container that cannot be re-accessed. When educating a patient about disposal at home, warn patients that the discarded patch can be dangerous to children and animals if it is handled or chewed.

PATIENT EDUCATION

For those applying transcutaneous systems of administration, include the following instructions. With nitroglycerin ointment (Figure 9-1):

1. Squeeze the prescribed amount of ointment onto dose-measuring application paper (Appli-Ruler). When the ointment reaches the correct marking, give the tube a slight twist to cut off the ointment and recap the tube.

2. *Do not* touch the ointment! Absorption of ointment through the skin of the fingers can cause a severe headache. Wearing gloves eliminates this risk.

3. Carefully fold the Appli-Ruler paper lengthwise with the ointment inside.

4. Flatten the folded paper carefully to spread the ointment inside. *Do not* allow the ointment to reach the edges of the paper. Keep the paper folded.

5. Rotate the sites for application. Appropriate areas include chest, back, upper arms, and upper legs. *Do not* shave the area. Be sure the area is clean, dry, and free of irritation, rash, and abrasion.

6. After the area for application is exposed, open the paper carefully and apply paper to the skin, ointment side down. *Do not* touch the ointment. Fasten paper in place with paper tape. Write the date, time, and your initials on the tape.

7. Remove the previous paper carefully, without touching the inside, and discard it in the trash container. Cleanse area and inspect skin for any sign of irritation. Report and record any skin changes.

8. Wash hands immediately.

9. Report and record any skin changes or complaints of headache.

(*continued*)

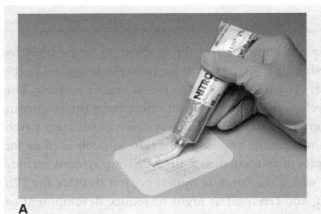
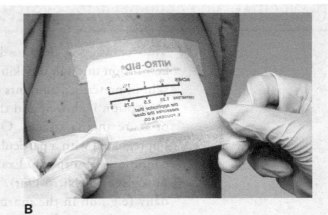

A   **B**

FIGURE 9-1 Transdermal administration of nitroglycerin ointment. (A) Ointment is measured on Appli-Ruler paper. (B) Paper containing ointment is applied to the skin and fastened with paper tape. Write date and time on tape.

With transdermal sealed drug delivery systems (Figure 9-2):

1. Remove the previous patch carefully, without touching the inside, and discard it in the designated container. Cleanse area and inspect skin for irritation.

2. Select site for new administration, rotating areas. Be sure the skin is clean, dry, and free of irritation.

3. Open the packet carefully, pulling the two sides apart *without touching the inside.*

4. Apply the side containing the medication to the skin. Press the adhesive edges down firmly all around. If for any reason

the adhesive edges do not stick, fasten in place with paper tape. This is usually unnecessary. Write date, time, and initials on patch.

5. Wash hands immediately.

6. Certain patches must be removed prior to cardioversion or defibrillation to prevent burns to the patient. Also, removal of certain patches (i.e., Catapres-TTS) before undergoing magnetic resonance imaging (MRI) is recommended because the patch contains aluminum.

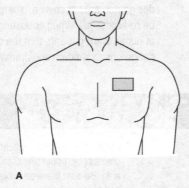
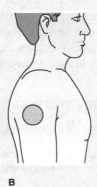

A   **B**

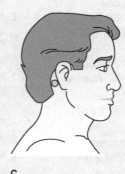

FIGURE 9-2 Transdermal drug delivery. Dermal patches vary in size and shape. (A, B) For prevention of angina pectoris. (C) For prevention of motion sickness. Other patches are also available for analgesia, estrogen replacement, and smoking cessation.

C

INHALATION ROUTE

Medications are frequently administered by the inhalation route, especially to those with chronic pulmonary conditions, such as asthma. Patients may self-administer the medication with a metered-dose inhaler (MDI), dry-powder inhaler (DPI), or small-volume nebulizer (SVN) (Figure 9-3), or the physician may prescribe inhaled medications to be administered by trained personnel such as respiratory therapists.

Advantages of the **inhalation route** include:

1. Rapid action of the drug, with local effects within the respiratory tract.

2. Potent drugs may be given in small amounts, minimizing the side effects.

3. Convenience and comfort of the patient.

Disadvantages of inhalation therapy include:

1. Requires cooperation of the patient in proper breathing techniques for effectiveness.

2. Adverse systemic side effects may result rapidly because of extensive absorption capacity of the lungs.

3. Improperly administered, or too frequently administered, inhalations can lead to irritation of the trachea or bronchi, or bronchospasm.

4. Asthmatic and chronic obstructive pulmonary disease (COPD) patients sometimes become dependent on an SVN, DPI, or MDI.

5. If not cleaned properly, the SVN can be a source of infection.

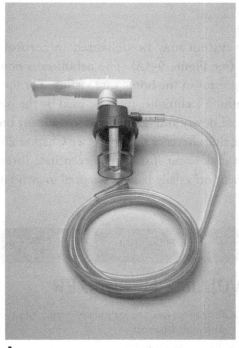

A

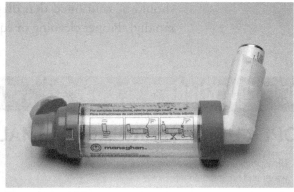

B

FIGURE 9-3 (A) Small-volume aerosol nebulizer (SVN). (B) Metered-dose inhaler (MDI) with spacer.

Metered-Dose Inhaler (MDI)

Metered-dose inhalers (see Figure 9-3B) deliver a measured (metered) dose via a propellant within a canister. MDIs are portable and easy to use, however, proper administration by the patient is essential for drug effectiveness. Older adult patients may have difficulty coordinating the depression of the canister and inhaling at the same time. A *spacer* may be added to act as a reservoir for the aerosol, allowing the patient to first depress the canister and then inhale. Many spacers have an audible horn or whistle to signal the patient if inspiration is too rapid. MDIs may be used in pediatric patients with a mouthpiece or a mask. A full MDI canister provides approximately 200 puffs of medication. See Chapter 26 for more information on respiratory medications and for variations of the MDI.

PATIENT EDUCATION

HOW TO USE A METERED-DOSE INHALER (MDI)

1. Sit upright or stand.
2. Assemble the inhaler and shake for 10 sec. (For consistent dosing, it is recommended to discharge a waste dose if it has been 24h since you last used your inhaler.)
3. Remove the upper dentures if dentures are loose.
4. Exhale slowly and completely.
5. Place the mouthpiece between the lips, forming a seal, or preferably use a spacer prescribed by your physician.
6. Push down on the inhaler while breathing in slowly and deeply to full capacity.

7. Hold your breath for at least 5–10 sec.
8. Exhale slowly through pursed lips.

If your prescription is for more than 1 puff, rest for 1 or 2 min before the second dose.

Note: If a bronchodilator and an inhaled steroid medication are to be given at the same time, administer the bronchodilator first and then the steroid.

Important: If using an inhaled steroid (such as Asmanex, Flovent, Pulmicort, or QVAR), rinse your mouth out with a mouth wash or water after using the inhaler to reduce risk of developing an oral fungal infection such as thrush.

Small-Volume Nebulizers (SVNs, MINI-NEBs, MED-NEBs)

Many drugs for the respiratory system may be delivered in aerosol form via a small-volume nebulizer (SVN) (see Figure 9-3A). The nebulizer is powered by a gas source, usually a small air compressor in the home care setting. For optimal drug deposition in the lung, proper breathing techniques must be used by the patient. The patient should be instructed to inhale slowly and deeply, perform a short breath hold, and exhale slowly. In addition to the side effects of the drugs (see Chapter 26), patients should be cautioned that dizziness may occur if they hyperventilate (breathing too rapidly). Proper cleaning of equipment on a daily basis is essential to avoid infection.

PATIENT EDUCATION

PROPER HOME CLEANING OF SMALL-VOLUME NEBULIZER

1. Disassemble the pieces of the nebulizer. Wash in mild soapy water and rinse thoroughly.
2. Place in a solution of one-part vinegar to two parts water. Soak for 20–30 min.
3. Wash your hands with soap and water.

4. Remove the nebulizer parts from vinegar solution and rinse with warm tap water.
5. Allow to dry completely.
6. Reassemble pieces for next use.

PATIENT EDUCATION

With use of an inhaler or nebulizer, include the following instructions:

1. Name of the medication, dosage, and how often it is to be administered.

2. Desired effects and possible adverse side effects (e.g., palpitations, tremor, nervousness, dizziness, headache, nausea, dry mouth, irritated throat, hoarseness, or coughing).

3. Notify the physician if any adverse side effects occur or if the medication seems ineffective. The doctor may want to change the dosage or the medication.

4. Caution *not* to take any other medication, including over-the-counter drugs, without the physician's permission. Many drugs and alcohol can interact with these drugs, causing serious side effects.

5. Rising slowly from a reclining position will help prevent dizziness.

6. Rinsing the mouth before inhalation to moisten the mouth.

7. Rinsing the mouth after inhalation to counteract dry mouth or unpleasant taste.

8. Step-by-step demonstration with the patient, answering all questions.

9. Rinsing equipment after use and storage of medication as indicated on the package.

10. Importance of not smoking.

11. Importance of handwashing before treatments.

Dry-Powder Inhalers (DPIs)

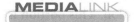

See it in Action! Go to the Online Resources to view videos on showing a patient how to use an inhaler and administering nebulized medications.

In recent years, **dry-powder inhalers (DPIs)** have become popular to use, especially with children. DPIs are devices that deliver a drug in powder form into the lung with no propellant or external power source. The patient must generate a sufficient inspiratory flow rate for the powder to aerosolize properly, and therefore DPIs are used for prophylactic treatment and not for acute breathing problems. The advantages of a DPI are that it is small and relatively easy to use and eliminates timing of inspiration technique problems encountered with an MDI. It also can be used in very cold environments such as ski slopes where propellants may not work as effectively. The disadvantages are fewer drugs are available in powder form, and the patient must be able to generate a significant inspiratory effort for proper drug delivery.

PATIENT EDUCATION

HOW TO USE A DRY-POWDER INHALER (DPI)

1. Sit upright or stand.

2. Break the dry powder capsule (if applicable) according to the device being used.

3. Remove the upper dentures if dentures are loose.

4. Exhale slowly and completely.

5. Place the mouthpiece between the lips, forming a seal.

6. Breathe In FAST and DEEP.

7. Hold your breath for at least 5–10 sec.

8. Exhale slowly through pursed lips.

Note: DPIs are NOT to be used in respiratory distress or emergency situations. The patient must be able to generate adequate inspiratory flow rates, and this device is used for maintenance or prophylactic treatment only.

Intermittent Positive Pressure Breathing (IPPB)

Intermittent positive pressure breathing treatments, although not commonly used, may be ordered by the physician. IPPB combines administration of an aerosol with a mechanical breather to assist patients who are unable to take a deep breath on their own. Health care personnel, such as respiratory therapists or nurses, are specifically trained in the use of this equipment.

Cautions with IPPB therapy include:

1. Monitor vital signs closely, watching for a sudden drop in blood pressure, tachycardia, and decreased or shallow respirations.

2. Observe for nausea or distended abdomen.

3. Watch for tremors or dizziness.

4. Assure the patient that coughing after the treatment is to be expected. The goal of the treatment is to aid in coughing up the loosened secretions.

5. Record effectiveness of therapy and any side effects observed or reported by the patient.

INJECTIONS

To administer **injections**, you must be familiar with the equipment.

Syringes

The syringe has three parts (Figure 9-4):

1. ***Barrel.*** The outer, hollow cylinder that holds the medication. It contains the calibrations for measuring the quantity of medication. This portion is not sterile.

2. ***Plunger.*** The inner, solid rod that fits snugly into the cylinder. Pulling back on the plunger allows solution to be drawn into the syringe. Pushing forward on the plunger ejects solution or air from the syringe. The inner portion of the plunger is sterile.

3. ***Tip.*** The portion that holds the needle. Most tips have a system called a Luer-Lok, which locks the needle in place. The tip is sterile.

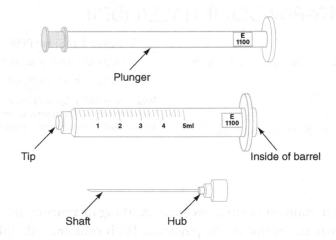

FIGURE 9-4 Parts of a syringe and needle that must remain sterile during preparation and administration of medication.

Most syringes are plastic and disposable after one use. Some syringes for special procedures are glass and must be resterilized after use.

Needles

The needle has three parts:

1. *Hub.* The flared end that fits on the tip of the syringe. This is sterile.
2. *Shaft.* The long, hollow tube embedded in the hub. Needles have shafts with different lengths. Shorter needles (1/2, 3/8, and 5/8 inches) are used for intradermal (into the skin) or subcutaneous (into the tissue just below the skin) injections. Longer needles (1½ and 2 inches) are used for intramuscular (into the muscle) injections. The length of the needle depends on the type of injection and the size of the patient (i.e., shorter needles for children and thin adults and longer needles for larger adults). The gauge is the size of the lumen, or hole, through the needle, or the diameter of the shaft. The gauge is numbered in reverse order (i.e., the thinner needle with the smaller diameter has the larger number, for example, 25 gauge for subcutaneous injections, and 19–21 gauge, a thicker needle with a larger opening, for IM or IV injections. The size of the gauge is determined by the site of the injection and the viscosity of the solution (e.g., blood and oil require a thicker-gauge needle, e.g., 15–18). The shaft of the needle is sterile.
3. *Tip.* The pointed end with a beveled edge. The tip is sterile.

Three main types of syringes are used for injections. The type used is determined by the medication and the dosage. The three types are:

1. *Standard syringe.* Used most frequently for subcutaneous or IM injections, calibrated or marked in cubic centimeters (cc) or milliliters (mL) (Figure 9-5). The most commonly used size is 3 mL or 2½ mL. Larger sizes of 5–60 mL are available for other purposes (e.g., irrigations, withdrawing fluids from the body, and intravenous [IV] injections).

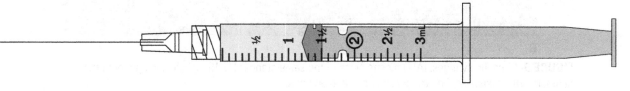

FIGURE 9-5 3-mL syringe.

2. *Tuberculin (TB) syringe.* Used for intradermal injections of very small amounts of a substance (e.g., testing for tuberculosis or for allergies). The TB syringe is also used for subcutaneous injections when a small amount of medication, up to 1 mL, is ordered (e.g., in pediatrics). The TB syringe is calibrated in tenths of a milliliter and holds only a total of 1 cc, or 1 mL (Figure 9-6).

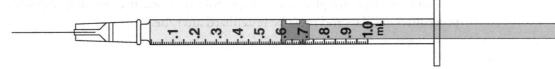

FIGURE 9-6 Tuberculin syringe with 1-mL capacity.

3. ***Insulin syringe.*** Used only for injection of insulin and calibrated in units. The size in common use today is U-100, in which 100 units of insulin is equal to 1 mL. The standard U-100 syringe has a dual scale: even numbers on one side and odd numbers on the other side. Look carefully at the calibrations on each side. Count each calibration (on one side only) as two units (Figure 9-7A). The insulin pen is another popular option for diabetics. There is a dial at the end in which you "dial in" the desired amount of insulin that eliminates the need to withdraw insulin from a vial, thus limiting errors (Figure 9-8).

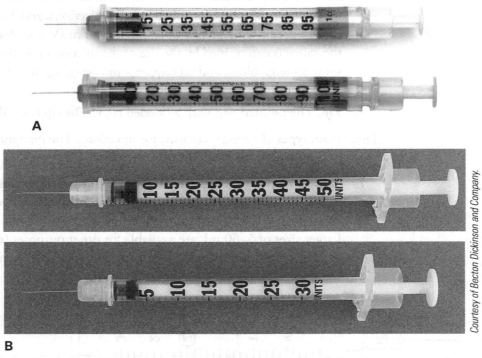

FIGURE 9-7 Insulin syringes. (A) Opposite sides of the same standard U-100 insulin syringe; note the numbers. (B) Lo-dose insulin syringes, 50 units and 30 units.

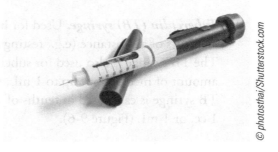

FIGURE 9-8 Insulin pen.

Courtesy of Becton Dickinson and Company.

© photosthai/Shutterstock.com

There are also smaller insulin syringes to more accurately measure small amounts of insulin, such as for children (Figure 9-7B for Lo-Dose Insulin Syringes 50 Units and 30 Units). Look carefully at the calibrations. In these Lo-Dose syringes, each calibration counts *only one* unit. It is extremely important that you study the calibrations carefully each time you prepare for an insulin injection, to prevent a medication error from misinterpretation. **All insulin dosages should be double-checked by two caregivers before administration.**

When instructing new diabetics in self-administration or administration by a family member, be sure that they can see and understand the calibrations and what they represent.

Prefilled syringes are available for certain medications (Figure 9-9). A premeasured amount of the drug is contained in the syringe. Check the dose ordered, compare with the dose in the syringe, and adjust if necessary. After injection, discard the syringe with needle attached and uncapped in the disposal bin.

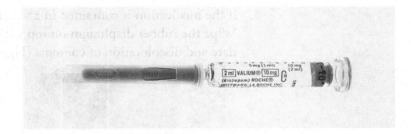

FIGURE 9-9 Prefilled, single-dose syringe. Courtesy of Roche Laboratories, Inc.

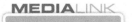

See it in Action! Go to the Online Resources to view a video on the *Cartridge Injection System.* Although this video emphasizes the five Rights of Medication Administration, keep in mind the recently added sixth right of "proper documentation."

Prefilled cartridges are also available, in which a premeasured amount of a medication is contained in a disposable cartridge. These prefilled units are made ready for injection by placing the cartridge in a holder. This unit can then be used to access a needleless IV system, or a needle can be attached to administer IM or subcutaneous injections. After administration, the used cartridge is released from the holder and dropped into the disposal bin. If a needle is attached, it is released *uncapped* along with the cartridge into the bin. An example of such a unit is the *Carpuject*, produced by Hospira (Figure 9-10). Other units are also available. Follow the manufacturer's direction regarding assembly of the cartridge unit.

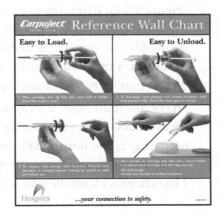

FIGURE 9-10 Carpuject prefilled cartridge. Carpuject Syringe System reprinted with permission from Hospira, Inc., Lake Forest, IL.

CLINICAL CONNECTION SITE ROTATION

When administering a medication through the skin on a consistent basis it is important to rotate administration sites. This is particularly important with insulin injections, transdermal patches, and topical creams and ointments. In all three cases, not rotating sites can lead to irritation and redness at the administration site. Insulin, if injected in the same spot repeatedly can cause growths (fatty deposits) to form. These growths are both undesirable for the patient and can affect the way insulin is absorbed. In the case of patches and topical preparations, not rotating sites can also lead to saturation of the skin by the medication, which changes its permeability resulting in decreased absorption of the drug.

Drawing Up Medications

1. Wash hands.

2. Assemble equipment (i.e., syringe, needle, packaged alcohol wipes, and medication ampule or vial).

3. Check the order using the Six Rights of Medication Administration. If there is an eMAR system in place, scan the patient and medication.

4. If the medication is contained in a vial, first remove the protective cap. Wipe the rubber diaphragm on top with an alcohol wipe. Check vial for date and discoloration of contents (Figure 9-11).

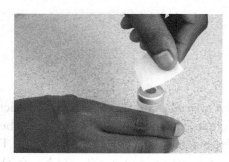

FIGURE 9-11 Preparing to withdraw medication from a vial. Cleanse the top with alcohol wipe.

5. Seat the needle securely on the syringe by pressing firmly downward on the top of the needle cover. Pull the needle cover straight off. *Note:* Luer-Loks require a half-turn to lock the needle in place.

6. Draw air into the syringe equal to the amount of solution you will be withdrawing from the vial. Insert the needle into the center of the rubber diaphragm and inject air into the vial above the medication (Figure 9-12). Invert the vial and withdraw the prescribed dosage (Figure 9-13). Be sure the syringe is filled to the proper level with solution and no bubbles are present. Withdraw the needle from the vial. For IM injections, a small bubble (0.2 mL) of air may now be added to the correct dose of medicine already in the syringe.

7. The needle must now be recapped *carefully* to maintain sterility and prevent needle sticks. After withdrawing the solution from an ampule or vial, the needle cap is laid horizontally on a flat surface. The syringe is held in the dominant hand, and the sterile needle is inserted carefully into the cap. The syringe with needle attached is then used to scoop up the cap without

Note

If two drugs are to be combined in a syringe, you must first check for compatibility of the drugs.

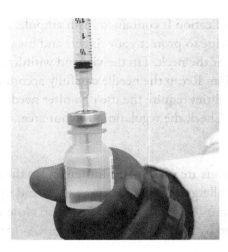

FIGURE 9-12 Injection of air into vial. Vial is upright so air is not injected into fluid.

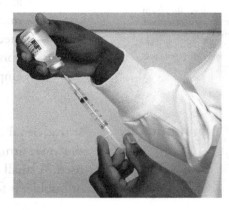

FIGURE 9-13 Withdrawal of prescribed amount of medication. Invert the vial. Be sure needle point is in fluid, not in the air.

touching it. *Do not contaminate the needle* by touching it to the outside of the cap. Remember, *only sterile needles are to be recapped* (Figure 9-14). An alternative method would be to remove the needle from the syringe carefully and discard the needle in the sharps container, replacing it with a sterile, capped needle.

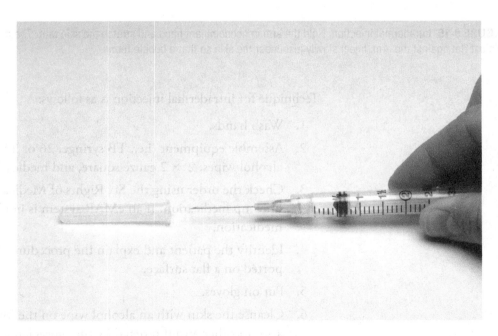

FIGURE 9-14 Recapping sterile needle. After withdrawing solution from an ampule or a vial, the needle cap is laid horizontally on a flat surface. The syringe is held in the dominant hand, and the sterile needle is inserted carefully into the cap. The syringe with needle attached is then used to scoop up the cap without touching it. Contaminated needles are never recapped but are discarded uncapped in sharps container.

MEDIALINK

See it in Action! Go to the Online Resources to view videos on *filling a syringe from a vial and drawing meds from two vials.*

8. If the medication is contained in an ampule, hold the tip with an alcohol wipe to protect your fingers and break open along the scored marking at the neck. Tip the vial and withdraw the prescribed amount of medication. Recap the needle carefully according to previous directions. Some facilities require the use of a filter needle to withdraw fluid from an ampule. Check the regulations in your area.

Administration by Injection

Intradermal injections are usually administered into the skin on the inner surface of the lower arm. For allergy testing, the upper chest and upper back areas may also be used. A small amount (0.1–0.2 mL) is injected so close to the surface that a wheal, or bubble, is formed by the skin expanding (Figure 9-15).

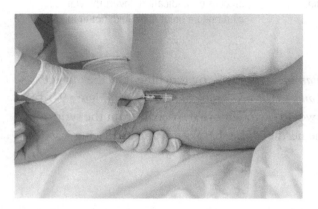
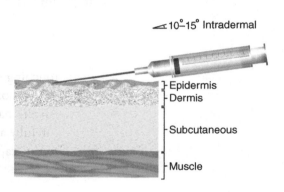

FIGURE 9-15 Intradermal injection. Hold the arm in nondominant hand and stretch the skin taut. *The needle bevel is up.* The needle is almost flat against the arm. Inject slowly just under the skin so that a bubble forms.

Technique for intradermal injection is as follows:

1. Wash hands.
2. Assemble equipment (i.e., TB syringe, 26 or 27 gauge, 3/8-inch needle, alcohol wipes, 2 × 2 gauze square, and medication).
3. Check the order using the Six Rights of Medication Administration and draw up medication. If an eMAR system is in place, scan the patient and medication.
4. Identify the patient and explain the procedure. The arm should be supported on a flat surface.
5. Put on gloves.
6. Cleanse the skin with an alcohol wipe on the inner surface of the forearm (or other area if ordered by the physician). Allow the skin to dry thoroughly. Do *not* blow or fan the skin to assist drying because this can foster infection. (If you inject before the skin is dry, you might introduce alcohol into the skin and interfere with test results.) Avoid areas with hair or blemishes.

7. Hold the patient's arm in your nondominant hand and *stretch the skin taut.*

8. Hold the syringe so that *the bevel* is *up* and the needle is almost flat against the patient's arm. Slowly insert the needle only far enough to cover the lumen or opening in the needle. The point of the needle should be visible through the skin.

9. Inject the medication *very slowly.* You should see a small, white bubble in the skin forming immediately. If no bubble forms, withdraw the needle slightly; it may be too deep. If the solution leaks out as you inject, the needle is not deep enough.

10. After the correct amount of medication is injected, withdraw the needle and apply gentle pressure with a 2 × 2 gauze. *Do not* massage the area or you may interfere with test results.

11. Discard the syringe with needle *uncapped* into the sharps container immediately without touching the needle. Remove gloves. Wash hands.

12. Note drug name, dosage, time, date, and site of injection on the patient's record.

13. Instruct the patient not to scrub, scratch, or rub the area. Provide written instructions regarding the time to return for reading. Tell the patient to contact the physician immediately or report to an emergency facility if breathing difficulty, hives, or a rash appears.

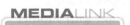

See it in Action! Go to the Online Resources to view a video on *Intradermal Injection.* *NOTE:* Although this video emphasizes the five Rights of Medication Administration, keep in mind the recently added sixth right of "proper documentation."

> **Caution**
>
> Do not start allergy testing unless emergency equipment is available nearby and personnel are trained in emergency care in case of anaphylactic response. Patients receiving allergy testing should remain in office or clinical facility for 30 min after injection to be observed for possible anaphylactic reaction.

Subcutaneous injections are administered into the fatty tissues on the upper outer arm, front of the thigh, abdomen, or upper back (Figure 9-16). A 2½–3-mL syringe is usually used with a 24–26-gauge, ⅜–⅝-inch needle. No more than 2 mL of medication may be administered subcutaneously.

Technique for subcutaneous injection is as follows:

1. Wash hands.

2. Assemble the equipment (correct-size syringe and needle, alcohol wipes, 2 × 2 gauze square, and medication).

3. Check the order with the Six Rights of Medication Administration and draw up medication. If an eMAR system is in place, scan the patient and medication.

4. Identify the patient, ask the patient's name, check the armband, and explain the procedure.
Use an alternate method to identify the patient if necessary.

5. If the patient is receiving frequent injections, be sure to rotate the injection sites.

6. Put on gloves.

7. Cleanse the skin with an alcohol wipe.

8. Pinch the skin into a fat fold of at least 1 inch (Figure 9-16).

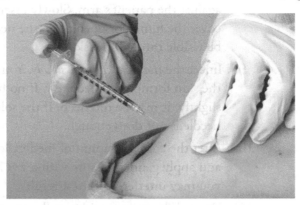

FIGURE 9-16 Subcutaneous injection. The tissue is pinched, and the needle is held at a 45-degree angle.

9. Insert the needle at a 45-degree angle. A 90-degree angle may be used with a ⅜ needle, if there is sufficient subcutaneous tissue, and also for insulin and heparin injections.

10. Discard the syringe with needle *uncapped* into the sharps container immediately. You will then have to draw up fresh solution with another sterile syringe and needle.

11. Inject the medication *slowly*, pushing the plunger all the way. Too rapid injection may cause pain.

12. Place a dry 2 × 2 gauze over the entry site, applying pressure with it, as you withdraw the needle rapidly. Do not push down on the needle while withdrawing it.

13. Massage the site gently with the dry 2 × 2 gauze to speed absorption. (*Do not* massage with heparin or insulin injection.) Be sure that there is no bleeding.

14. Discard the syringe with needle *uncapped* into the sharps container immediately.

15. Remove gloves and discard.

16. Wash hands.

17. Note the medication, dosage, time, date, site of injection, and your signature on the patient's record.

18. Observe the patient for effects and record observations.

Subcutaneous injection of heparin includes these steps:

1. Administer the heparin subcutaneously in the fat pad of the abdomen, at least 2 inches (approximately three fingers) away from the umbilicus. Use a ⅝- or ⅞-inch needle. Grasp the skin to form a fat pad, but do not pinch the tissues. Insert the needle with a dart-like motion at a 90-degree angle in the average size adult, in very thin patients a 45-degree angle may be used.. Release fingers holding the fat pad and inject *slowly*.

MEDIALINK

See it in Action! Go to the Online Resources to view a video on *Subcutaneous Injections.*

2. Rotate the injection sites and document the site of injection.

3. Do not rub the site with an alcohol sponge. Merely hold the sponge on the site gently for approximately 10 sec.

4. Be sure that there is no bleeding from the site.

IM injections are administered deep into large muscles (Figure 9-17). There are three recommended sites. Previously, there were two additional sites (dorsogluteal and rectus femoris) that are no longer recommended according to the new CDC guidelines owing to close proximity of nerves and resultant nerve damage.

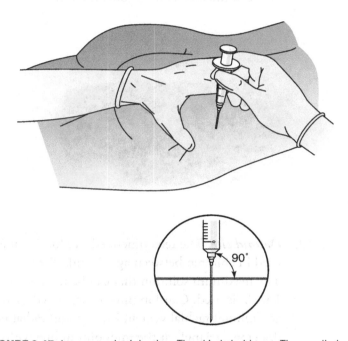

FIGURE 9-17 Intramuscular injection. The skin is held taut. The needle is at a 90-degree angle.

1. *Ventrogluteal.* Above and to the outside of the buttock area, on the hip

2. *Deltoid.* Upper outer arm above the axilla

3. *Vastus lateralis.* Front of the thigh toward the outside of the leg

The IM route has two advantages over the subcutaneous route:

1. A larger amount of solution can be administered (up to 3 mL, or a maximum of 1 mL in children).

2. Absorption is more rapid because the muscle tissue is more vascular (i.e., contains many blood vessels).

The needle must be long enough to go through the subcutaneous tissue into the muscle. The length of the needle varies with the size of the patient. With a child or very thin, emaciated adult, a 1-inch needle is usually adequate. For most adults, a 1½-inch needle is appropriate. However, for an obese person, a 2-inch needle might be required. The needle is inserted at a 90-degree angle with the skin spread taut (Figure 9-17).

Because there are more large blood vessels and nerves in this deeper tissue, the site for injection must be chosen more precisely. Using the illustrations as a guide, follow these steps in selecting the site:

1. ***Ventrogluteal site.*** Can be used for all patients. Position the patient on the back or side (Figure 9-18). Identify the site by placing the palm of your hand on the patient's greater trochanter (use your left hand for the patient's right hip or your right hand for the patient's left hip). Place the index finger on the anterior superior iliac spine and the middle finger on the iliac crest. The injection is made into the center of the V formed between the index and middle fingers.

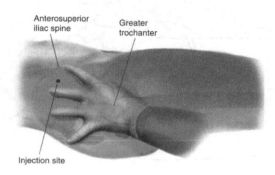

Anterosuperior iliac spine

Greater trochanter

Injection site

FIGURE 9-18 Ventrogluteal site for IM injection. Can be administered with patient on back or side.

2. ***Deltoid site.*** The recommended site for vaccines for adults and may be used in children between ages 1 and 18 years for vaccines (Figure 9-19). The maximum solution that can be used is 1 mL; and a shorter needle, 1 inch, is used. Caution must be exercised to avoid the clavicle, humerus, acromion, brachial vein and artery, and radial nerve. Identify the site by drawing a triangle at the midpoint in line with the axilla on the lateral aspect of the upper arm, with the base of the triangle at the acromion process. The injection is made in the center of the triangle

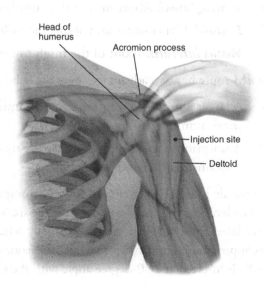

Head of humerus

Acromion process

Injection site

Deltoid

FIGURE 9-19 Deltoid site for IM injection. Maximum of 1-mL of medication and 1-inch needle is used. Injected above the level of the armpit.

3. ***Vastus lateralis.*** Located on the anterior lateral thigh, the preferred site for infants, since these muscles are the most developed for children under the age of three years (Figure 9-20). In the older, nonambulatory, and emaciated adult, this muscle may be wasted and insufficient for injection. Identify site by dividing the thigh into thirds horizontally and vertically and administer the injection in the middle outer third.

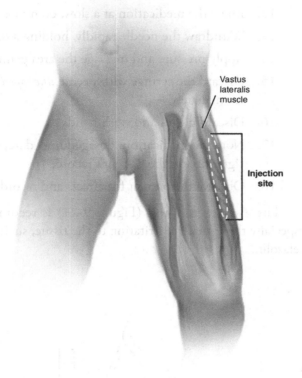

Vastus
lateralis
muscle

Injection
site

FIGURE 9-20 Vastus lateralis site for IM injection, preferred for infants. Injected on the anterior lateral thigh.

Technique for IM injection is as follows:

1. Wash hands.

2. Assemble the equipment (i.e., correct-size syringe, needle, alcohol wipes, 2 × 2 gauze square, and medication). If an eMAR system is in place, scan the patient and medication.

3. Check the order with the Six Rights of Medication Administration and draw up the medication, or insert the appropriate prefilled cartridge into the Carpuject holder.

4. After measuring the correct amount of medication in the syringe, draw 0.2 mL of air into the syringe to clear the needle. Recap carefully using the method illustrated in Figure 9-14.

5. Identify the patient, ask the patient's name and check the armband, and explain the procedure. Use an alternate method to identify the patient if necessary.

6. If the patient is receiving frequent injections, be sure to rotate sites.

7. Put on gloves.

8. Position the patient and expose the area to be used for injection.

9. Cleanse the skin with an alcohol wipe.

10. With your nondominant hand, stretch the skin taut at the injection site.

11. Insert the needle at a 90-degree angle with a quick, dart-like motion of your dominant hand.

12. Inject the medication at a slow, even rate.

13. Withdraw the needle rapidly, holding a dry 2 × 2 gauze over the site.

14. Apply pressure and massage the area gently with an alcohol wipe.

15. Discard the syringe with needle *uncapped* into the sharps container immediately.

16. Discard gloves and wash hands.

17. Note the medication, dosage, time, date, site of injection, and your signature on the patient's record.

18. Observe the patient for effects and record observations.

The **Z-track method** (Figure 9-21) is recommended for all IM injections especially those that are irritating to the tissue, such as iron dextran, hydroxyzine, or cefazolin.

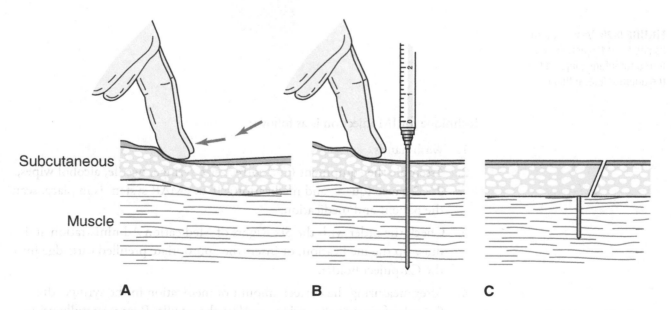

Subcutaneous

Muscle

A   B   C

FIGURE 9-21 Z-track method of IM injection of iron preparations. (A) Skin and subcutaneous tissue pulled to one side and held there. (B) Needle is placed in muscle. (C) Z-track sealed when tissue released.

Technique for the Z-track method is as follows:

1. Draw up the medication and then add 0.3–0.5 mL of air to the syringe. Then replace the needle with a sterile one, 2 to 3 inches long.

2. Stretch the skin as far as you can to the outer side and hold it there.

3. After cleansing the site, insert the needle with a dart-like motion, and then inject the medication *slowly*. Wait 10 sec before withdrawing the needle.

4. Withdraw the needle and allow the skin to return to the normal position. This seals off the needle track.

5. Press firmly on injection site with a 2 × 2 gauze square. Do not massage the site because this could spread the medication to the subcutaneous tissue, causing irritation.

6. Advise the patient that walking will aid absorption and to avoid tight fitting garments that cause pressure on the site.

MEDIALINK

See it in Action! Go to the Online Resources to view videos on *Administering an IM Injection and the Z-track Method*

IV MEDICATIONS

The IV route involves injecting liquids (medications or fluids) into a vein. The therapeutic effect of this route is immediate. The IV route is used for the following:

- To administer medications,
- Correct body fluid imbalances (i.e., dehydration from vomiting),
- Correct electrolyte imbalances (i.e., low potassium),
- Provide some nutritional support to patients who are NPO for a short time
- To administer blood and blood products.

There are two types of IV administration: **continuous IV infusion or intermittent IV infusion (piggyback or bolus/push).** Both types require similar equipment; an IV catheter inserted in the vein and either a bag of IV fluid, a small bag of medication (piggyback) or medication in a syringe. See Chapter 4, Figure 4-3 that illustrates IV administration.

A physician, registered nurse, or licensed practical nurse are typically responsible for administering IV medications of any type. However, it is important for others on the health care team to have an understanding of IV therapy.

Continuous IV infusion

Continuous infusion is administered slowly over long periods of time. The IV solution may or may not contain added medications prescribed by the physician. The bag is hung from an IV pole and typically infused via an infusion pump at a prescribed rate. There are three types of IV solutions classified based on the effect they have on the cell. They are isotonic (cells remain the same), hypotonic (cells swell) and hypertonic (cells shrink). Table 9-1 lists examples of common IV solutions.

TABLE 9-1   **Types of IV Fluids**

TYPE	EXAMPLES AND INDICATIONS
Isotonic	Normal Saline (NSS or 0.9% NSS) Lactated Ringers (LR) Whole Blood Indicated for fluid replacement
Hypotonic	½ Normal Saline (½ NS) Dextrose 5% in Water (D5W) Indicated to raise total fluid volume, helpful in rehydrating
Hypertonic	Dextrose 5% in 0.9% saline (D5NS) Dextrose 5% in 0.45% saline (D5½NS) Dextrose in 5% Lactated Ringer's (D5LR) Indicated for daily maintenance of body fluids, minimal nutrition support and rehydration, hypertonic fluids are most commonly used postoperatively.

Intermittent IV infusion

Piggyback is the term used for medication mixed in an additional bag that contains a small amount (50–100 mL) of IV fluid that is administered over a short period of time at a prescribed interval (e.g., every 4 h). These are most often antibiotics. Again an infusion pump is used and set at the prescribed rate. The piggyback is often attached to the main continuous IV infusion.

IV bolus/push is when a medication is not diluted in IV fluid but is injected directly into the IV catheter. It is important that the health care professional administering a bolus or push know the correct rate of administration because giving a medication too fast could cause serious adverse effects.

SKIN MEDICATIONS

Topical medications for the skin are prescribed for a great variety of conditions and are available in a variety of forms: ointments, lotions, creams, solutions, soaks, and baths. Administration of topical medications requires knowledge of the condition being treated and the purpose of the treatment, and strict adherence to directions as prescribed by the physician or provided by the pharmacist, or to instructions on the medication container or in a package insert. *When in doubt regarding administration techniques, always ask a qualified person for advice.* Some specific principles for skin medications are outlined in Chapter 12. In addition, good judgment is also required.

Several suggestions for applying topical medications include:

1. For burns, use sterile gloves to apply, and cover with sterile dressings because of the danger of infection. Use a gentle, light touch because of pain.

2. For skin conditions in which there is irritation or itching, use a cottonball or snug-fitting gloves to apply. *Never* use gauze, which can cause additional irritation and discomfort.

3. Follow the physician's order regarding covering or leaving open to the air.

4. Wash old medication off before applying new, unless specifically directed to do otherwise.

APPLICATION TO THE MUCOUS MEMBRANES

Medications applied to the mucous membranes also come in a variety of forms: suppositories, ointments, solutions, sprays, gargles, and so on. Always follow the specific directions that accompany the individual medication, unless directed to do otherwise by the physician. When in doubt, always ask questions.

EYE MEDICATIONS

Technique for instillation of eye medications is as follows:

1. Wash hands.

2. Assemble eye medication (ophthalmic solution or ointment).

3. Check the order with the Six Rights of Medication Administration. If an eMAR system is in place, scan the patient and medication. Pay particular attention to *percentage* on the medication label and to *which eye* is to be treated (right eye, left eye, or both eyes).

4. Identify the patient, ask the patient's name, and explain the procedure. Use an alternate method to identify the patient if necessary.

5. Put on gloves.

6. Position the patient flat on the back or upright with the head back. Ask the patient to look up.

7. Carefully instill the ophthalmic solution, correct number of drops, or ointment into the lower conjunctival sac, using caution to avoid contamination of the tip of the dropper or ointment tube (Figure 9-22). Do not let the solution run from one eye to the other.

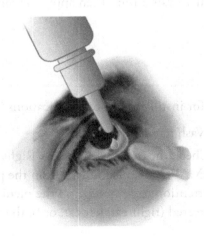

FIGURE 9-22 Instilling eye medication. Gently press the lower lid down and have the patient look upward. Ophthalmic solution is dropped inside lower eyelid.

8. Tell the patient to close the eye gently so as not to squeeze out the solution.

9. Press gently on the inner canthus following administration of eye drops (Figure 9-23). Systemic absorption is thus minimized with medications such as corticosteroids, miotics, and mydriatics.

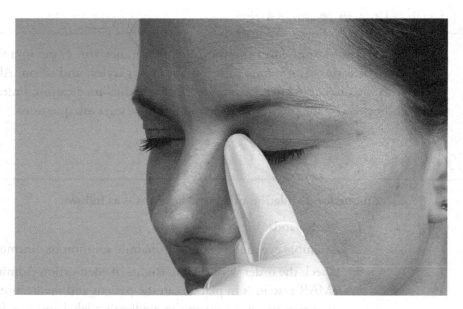

FIGURE 9-23 Gentle pressure on the inner canthus following administration of ophthalmic medications. Systemic absorption is thus minimized with medications such as corticosteroids, miotics, and mydriatics.

10. Remove gloves.

11. Wash hands. Replace the medication in an appropriate place.

12. Record the medication, dosage, time, date, and which eye was treated on the patient's record.

13. When more than one eye medication is ordered, wait at least 5 min before instilling the second medication.

14. If eye drops and ointment are ordered for the same time, instill eye drops first, wait 5 min, then apply the ointment.

MEDIALINK

See it in Action! Go to the Online Resources to view a video on Administering Eye Medications.

EAR MEDICATIONS

Technique for instillation of ear medications is as follows:

1. Wash hands.

2. Check the order with the Six Rights of Medication Administration. If an eMAR system is in place, scan the patient and medication. Pay particular attention to *percentage* on the medication label and to *which ear* is to be treated (right ear, left ear, or both ears).

3. Identify the patient, ask the patient's name, and explain the procedure. Use an alternate method to identify the patient if necessary.

4. Put on gloves.

5. Position the patient lying on their side or so that their head is tilted to one side with the desired ear upward, Figure 9-24.

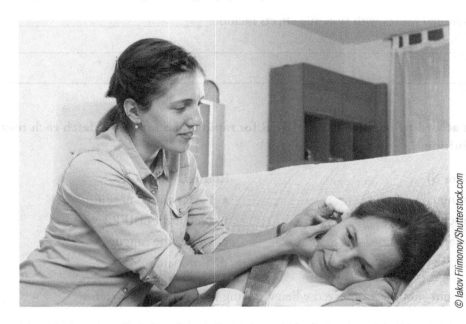

FIGURE 9-24 Instilling ear drop medication.

6. Gently shake the bottle; most ear drops are suspensions that need to be shaken. Allow drops to warm in your hands to prevent dizziness and nausea.

7. Grasp just above the earlobe (pinna) and gently pull the ear up and back. For children younger than 3, pull gently down and back.

8. Place the dropper over the ear canal; **DO NOT** touch the dropper to the ear.

9. Carefully instill the correct number of drops to the ear canal.

10. Press gently on the ear flap and instruct the patient to stay in the sideways position for 1–2 min.

11. Remove gloves.

12. Wash hands. Replace the medication in an appropriate place.

13. Record the medication, dosage, time, date, and which ear was treated on the patient's record.

When in doubt about administration of any medication, always ask a qualified person for advice. Never guess! Remember that the patient who is receiving the medication could be you or your loved one. By thinking of yourself in the patient's place you will have the proper attitude to administer medications with competence, good judgment, and compassion.

MEDIALINK

See it in Action! Go to the Online Resources to view a video on Administering Ear Drops

CHAPTER REVIEW QUIZ

Fill in the blanks.

1. Parenteral includes any routes other than the _____.

2. Systemic effects are those affecting _____.

3. The four parenteral routes with systemic effects include:_____

   _____

   _____.

Label the routes according to their action. Use R for rapid and S for slow. Match each route with the appropriate definition.

Action (R or S)		Route Definition
4. _____ Sublingual	_____	**a.** Given with a needle
5. _____ Transcutaneous	_____	**b.** Nebulizer or IPPB
6. _____ Inhalation	_____	**c.** Under the tongue
7. _____ Injection	_____	**d.** Skin patch

8. What precautions should be observed when applying transcutaneous systems?

   _____.

9. DPI refers to _____.

Select the correct needle for the purpose. Needle size may be used for more than one purpose.

Purpose	Needle
10. _____ Subcutaneous injection	**a.** 21 gauge, 1½ inch
11. _____ Intravenous injection	**b.** 25 gauge, 5/8 inch
12. _____ Allergy testing	**c.** 18 gauge
13. _____ IM injection	**d.** 27 gauge, 3/8 inch

14. What are the two purposes of the tuberculin syringe?

    _____

    _____.

15. The insulin syringe is calibrated in _____, and 1 mL is equal to _____ in an insulin syringe.

16. On a standard insulin syringe, each calibration represents _____ unit/s.
    On a Lo-Dose insulin syringe, each calibration represents _____ unit/s.

Match the injection with the proper technique.

	Injection		Technique
17.	_____ Intramuscular	**a.**	Needle 45-degree angle, skin pinched up
18.	_____ Subcutaneous	**b.**	Needle flat, bevel up, skin taut
19.	_____ Intradermal	**c.**	Needle 90-degree angle, skin taut

20. List the three sites for IM injections and when each is used.

_____

_____

_____

21. Why is the Z-track method used? _____

Describe Z-track administration. _____

_____

_____

22. Define local effects. _____

_____

List four areas to administer medication for local effects.

_____

_____

23. What are the two types of IV administration?

_____   _____

24. List two examples of IV solutions in each of the categories:
Isotonic solution types

_____   _____

Hypotonic solution types

_____   _____

Hypertonic solution types

_____   _____

STUDYGUIDE

P R A C T I C E

Complete Chapter 9

Online Resources

- Powerpoint presentations
- Videos

CHECKLIST FOR INTRADERMAL INJECTION

Activity	Rating	
	S	**U**
1. Washed hands	_____	_____
2. Checked medication order for date, dosage, time, route, and allergies	_____	_____
3. Identified medication: purpose, side effects, cautions, and normal dosage range	_____	_____
4. Assembled supplies: TB syringe, 27-gauge, 3/8-inch needle, alcohol wipes, and medication	_____	_____
5. Checked medication vial against medication sheet using the Six Rights of Medication Administration. If eMAR system is in place, scanned patient and medication	_____	_____
6. Withdrew correct dose from vial after cleansing top with alcohol and injecting equivalent amount of air into vial	_____	_____
7. Recapped needle using sterile technique (see Figure 9-14 for technique)	_____	_____
8. Identified patient by checking bracelet and asking the patient's name and DOB. Used an alternate method to identify patient if necessary	_____	_____
9. Explained procedure to patient and answered any questions regarding procedure	_____	_____
10. Positioned patient with inner forearm exposed and supported on a flat surface	_____	_____
11. Put on gloves	_____	_____
12. Selected area without hair or blemish, cleansed skin with alcohol wipe, and allowed skin to dry	_____	_____
13. Held patient's arm with nondominant hand, stretching the skin taut	_____	_____
14. Expelled any air bubbles from syringe	_____	_____
15. Inserted needle point slowly, bevel side up, only enough to cover needle opening; point of needle visible through skin	_____	_____
16. Injected medication very slowly, with immediate formation of small bubble	_____	_____
17. Withdrew needle and applied gentle pressure to injection site with dry gauze (no massage)	_____	_____
18. Discarded syringe with needle *uncapped* into sharps container	_____	_____
19. Removed gloves	_____	_____
20. Washed hands	_____	_____
21. Recorded drug name, dosage, time, date, and site of injection on patient's record and signed or initialed entry	_____	_____
22. Observed patient for 30 min for possible anaphylactic reaction; identify location of emergency equipment and medication if required	_____	_____
23. Provided written instructions regarding time to return for reading; instructed patient to avoid scrubbing, scratching, or rubbing the area and to report to emergency facility with dyspnea, hives, or rash	_____	_____

Note: S, satisfactory; U, unsatisfactory.

CHECKLIST FOR SUBCUTANEOUS INJECTION

Activity	Rating S	U
1. Washed hands		
2. Checked medication order for date, dosage, time, route, and allergies		
3. Identified medication: purpose, side effects, contraindications, interactions, and normal dosage range		
4. Assembled supplies: 2½–3-mL, TB, or insulin syringe; 24–26-gauge, 3/8–5/8-inch needle; alcohol wipes; and medication vial or ampule		
5. Checked medication against medication sheet using the Six Rights of Medication Administration; also checked drug for date and discoloration. If eMAR system is in place, scanned patient and medication		
6. Calculated correct dosage on paper if necessary and checked calculations with instructor		
7. If drug is contained in vial, withdrew correct amount after cleansing top with alcohol wipe and injecting equivalent amount of air into vial. If drug is contained in ampule, held tip with alcohol wipe while breaking it at neck. Withdrew correct amount of drug without bubbles in syringe. Used a filtered needle to administer dose drawn from ampule		
8. Recapped needle using proper sterile technique (see Figure 9-14 for technique)		
9. Identified patient by checking identification bracelet and asking the patients' name and DOB. Used an alternate method to identify patient if necessary		
10. Explained procedure to patient and answered any questions		
11. Selected appropriate site, using rotation for frequent injections		
12. Put on gloves		
13. Cleansed skin with alcohol wipe		
14. Pinched skin into fold with nondominant hand		
15. Expelled any air bubbles from syringe		
16. Inserted needle at 45-degree angle and released skin fold		
17. Injected medication slowly		
18. Placed alcohol wipe over entry site and applied pressure as needle was withdrawn; massaged site gently (with heparin, pressure only, no massage)		
19. Disposed of syringe and needle uncapped in sharps container		
20. Removed and discarded gloves		
21. Washed hands		
22. Recorded drug name, dosage, time, date, site of injection, and signature on patient's record; also recorded effects after appropriate time		

Note: S, satisfactory; U, unsatisfactory.

CHECKLIST FOR IM INJECTION

Activity	Rating S	U
1. Washed hands		
2. Checked medication order for date, dosage, time, route, and allergies		
3. Identified medication: purpose, side effects, cautions, and normal dosage range		
4. Assembled supplies: 2½, 3-mL syringe; 1½–2 inch-needle, usually 21-gauge; alcohol wipes; and medication		
5. Checked medication against medication sheet using the Six Rights of Medication Administration; if PRN medication, checked time of last dose. If eMAR system in place, scanned patient and medication		
6. If narcotic, signed and checked time of last dose on controlled substance sheet; calculated correct dosage on paper if necessary and double checked calculations with instructor		
7. If drug is contained in *vial*, withdrew correct amount after cleansing top with alcohol wipe and injecting equivalent amount of air into vial. If drug is contained in *ampule*, held tip with alcohol wipe while breaking it at neck. Withdrew correct amount of drug without bubbles in syringe. Used filtered needle to administer dose drawn from ampule		
8. *After* measuring the drug accurately in syringe, drew 0.2 mL air into syringe		
9. Recapped needle using sterile technique (see Figure 9-14 for techniques)		
10. Identified patient by checking bracelet and asking name and DOB. Used an alternate method to identify patient if necessary		
11. Explained procedure to patient and answered any questions		
12. Closed door to room and/or curtain around bed		
13. Selected appropriate site, using rotation for frequent injections		
14. Put on gloves		
15. Positioned patient appropriately, exposing only the area for injection		
16. Cleansed skin with alcohol wipe		
17. With forefinger and thumb of nondominant hand, spread the skin *taut* at injection site		
18. Inserted needle at a 90-degree angle with a quick, dart-like motion of dominant hand		
19. Injected medication at a slow, even rate		
20. Applied pressure with alcohol wipe over entry site as needle was withdrawn rapidly; massaged site gently with alcohol wipe unless medication irritating (with cefazolin, hydroxyzine, or iron dextran, pressure only, no massage)		
21. Made sure there was no bleeding before covering patient and making patient comfortable		
22. Disposed of syringe and needle *uncapped* in sharps container		
23. Discarded gloves appropriately; washed hands		
24. Recorded drug, name, dosage, time, date, site of injection, and signature on patient's record		

Note: S, satisfactory; U, unsatisfactory.

CHECKLIST FOR INSTILLATION OF EYE MEDICATION

	Rating	
Activity	S	U
1. Washed hands	_____	_____
2. Checked the order with the Six Rights of Medication Administration; noted percent of strength of drug, which eye, and allergies. If eMAR system is in place, scanned patient and medication	_____	_____
3. Identified medication: purpose, side effects, and cautions	_____	_____
4. Identified patient by checking bracelet and asking the patient's name and DOB. Use an alternate method to identify patient if necessary	_____	_____
5. Explained procedure to patient and answered any questions regarding procedure	_____	_____
6. Positioned patient on back or upright with head back	_____	_____
7. Asked the patient to look up	_____	_____
8. Used aseptic technique to instill correct number of drops or ointment dosage into lower conjunctival sac	_____	_____
9. Gently closed the eyelid and applied pressure to the inner canthus (eye drops only)	_____	_____
10. Washed hands and replaced medication in appropriate place	_____	_____
11. Recorded medication, dosage, time, date, and which eye was treated, on patient's record	_____	_____

Note: S, satisfactory; U, unsatisfactory.

Procedural Note: If more than one eye medication is ordered, wait at least 5 min before instilling the second medication. If eye drops and ointment are ordered for the same time, instill eye drops first, wait 5 min, and then apply the ointment.

CHECKLIST FOR INSTILLATION OF EAR MEDICATION

	Rating	
Activity	**S**	**U**
1. Washed hands	____	____
2. Checked the order with the Six Rights of Medication Administration; noted percent of strength of drug, which ear, and allergies. If eMAR system is in place, scanned patient and medication	____	____
3. Identified medication: purpose, side effects, and cautions	____	____
4. Identified patient by checking bracelet and asking the patient's name and DOB. Use an alternate method to identify patient if necessary	____	____
5. Explained procedure to patient and answered any questions regarding procedure	____	____
6. Positioned patient on side or with head tilted sideways	____	____
7. Pulled the pinna in the correct direction based on patient age	____	____
8. Used aseptic technique to instill correct number of drops	____	____
9. Gently pressed on the ear flap and ensured the patient remained sideways for 1–2 min.	____	____
10. Washed hands and replaced medication in appropriate place	____	____
11. Recorded medication, dosage, time, date, and which ear was treated, on patient's record	____	____

Note: S, satisfactory; U, unsatisfactory.

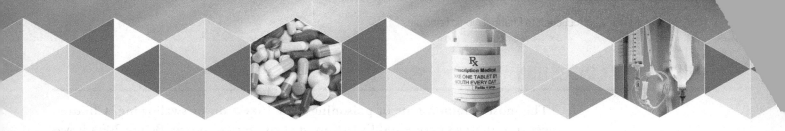

CHAPTER 10
POISON CONTROL

KEY TERMS AND CONCEPTS

Antidotes

Antivenom injections

Emetic

Ingestion

Poison

OBJECTIVES

Upon completion of this chapter, the learner should be able to

1. Identify four routes by which poisons may be taken into the body

2. List five conditions in which vomiting, after the ingestion of poisons, could be injurious to the patient

3. Describe the first step to take in the event of any poisoning and the procedure to follow

4. Explain the purpose of activated charcoal and when it is given

5. Name three clinical procedures required when caring for patients who have been poisoned

6. Describe appropriate therapy for poisoning by inhalation, external poison, and insect sting

7. Identify two groups of people at risk for poisoning

8. List 10 recommendations for patient education to help prevent poisoning

9. Define the Key Terms and Concepts

A **poison** is a substance taken into the body by ingestion, inhalation, injection, or absorption that interferes with normal physiological functions. In some cases, only a small amount of a substance can cause severe tissue damage directly (e.g., corrosives). In other cases, the substance can be beneficial in small amounts but lethal in excessive amounts (e.g., overdose of medication).

In a case of suspected poisoning, the best policy is to contact a Poison Control Center directly or through an emergency care facility. Instructions can then be given by phone for appropriate emergency treatment based on the type of poison and the patient's condition, age, and size.

POISONING BY INGESTION

The most common type of poisoning is by ingestion or swallowing. Children between the ages of one and five are most at risk for poisoning. Before 2004 it was recommended that children who had ingested poisons be given the emetic ipecac syrup to induce vomiting. However, extensive research conducted through the American Association of Poison Control Centers, Toxic Exposure Surveillance System, identified several concerns regarding ipecac, which are as follows:

1. Outcomes failed to justify its effectiveness.
2. Adverse effects, such as persistent vomiting could interfere with other treatment.
3. There has been evidence of widespread abuse of ipecac by people with anorexia and bulimia.

Therefore, in early 2004, the American Academy of Pediatrics (AAP) issued a policy statement on poison treatment in the home. The AAP recommended against keeping ipecac in the home and further recommended that ipecac presently in the home be disposed of safely.

The first step to take in any poisoning is to contact your local Poison Control Center. This number can be obtained by calling the national toll-free Poison Control number: **1-800-222-1222**. This number should be programmed into your phone for quick access in time of /emergency. Callers should be prepared to give details regarding the poison and the age, weight, and health status of the individual who took the poison. Mention allergies and asthma if present.

CLINICAL CONNECTION: POISON CONTROL CENTER VERSUS 911 EMERGENCY SERVICES

Poison Control Centers are absolutely the best resource for finding out information about the exposure to poisons and other harmful substances and what to do in these situations. That being said, patients should be properly educated that this should not be the first phone call in a medical emergency. If a person is unconscious, has severe changes in vital signs, cognition, or behavior after ingesting a substance, the quickest way to get them help is to call 911. Additionally, this is especially important if you are not absolutely certain what substance was ingested, which is often the case when a person is found unconscious. In a medical emergency, after calling 911 it is then okay to call a Poison Control Center to get more information. Educating patients to make this distinction could be the difference between saving a life and permanent damage or death.

Under the following conditions, vomiting could be injurious to the patient and should be avoided if possible:

1. Ingestion of corrosive substances such as mineral acids or caustic alkalis (e.g., carbolic acid, ammonia, drain cleaners, oven cleaners, dishwasher detergent, and lye). Check also for burns around or in the mouth. If the ingested substance burned tissue on the "way down," it is likely it will also burn and damage tissue on the "way back up" and therefore vomiting can cause additional tissue damage.

2. Ingestion of volatile petroleum products (e.g., gasoline, kerosene, lighter fluid, and benzene). Vomiting can cause aspiration and/or asphyxiation (suffocation).

3. Ingestion of convulsants (e.g., strychnine or iodine). Vomiting can precipitate seizures.

4. If patient is semiconscious, severely inebriated, in shock, convulsing, or has no gag reflex, vomiting could cause choking, aspiration, and/or asphyxiation.

5. If patient is less than one-year old.

6. In patients with cardiac or vascular disease, vomiting can increase blood pressure and precipitate a stroke, cardiac arrhythmias, or an atrioventricular block.

If any of these conditions exist, the patient should be transported *immediately* to an emergency care facility. Trained personnel can remove the stomach contents by gastric lavage, if appropriate, and administer appropriate antidotes as indicated.

Antidotes, such as flumazenil or naloxone and/or CPR (cardiopulmonary resuscitation), may be required in poisoning with central nervous system depressants. The routine use of gastric lavage is no longer recommended by the American Academy of Clinical Toxicology and is *not* used in patients who have ingested corrosives because of the danger of perforating the damaged tissue of the esophagus. If perforation exists, surgery is required. Observation is required in an acute care facility.

Sometimes a substance such as activated charcoal is administered by mouth to minimize systemic absorption of the ingested poison. If indicated, gastric lavage followed by or preceded and followed by activated charcoal may be more effective than activated charcoal alone. However, if activated charcoal is given, it may interfere with antidotes given via the gastric route as well (e.g., *n*-acetylcysteine for Tylenol poisoning), but the clinical significance of this is unknown.

Personnel caring for poisoning victims should observe the following cautions:

- *Be sure to save emesis.* It may be necessary to send it to a laboratory to determine the type of poison. In addition, save any evidence of what may have caused the poisoning such as plant parts, mushrooms, pills, and so on. If there is doubt about the poison, the physician may also order urine and blood tests for toxicology.

- Closely monitor the vital signs of patients who have taken poison of any kind.

- Observe closely for possible confusion, tremors, convulsions, visual disturbances, loss of consciousness, respiratory distress, or cardiac arrhythmias.

POISONING BY INHALATION

Poisoning by inhalation requires symptomatic treatment: fresh air, oxygen, and CPR if indicated. Incomplete combustion and fires can produce carbon monoxide. Carbon monoxide poisoning can quickly rob the tissues of vital oxygen, and high-percentage oxygen therapy or even oxygen under pressure (hyperbaric oxygen) in severe cases may be needed. Inhaling insect spray may require administration of an antidote such as atropine.

EXTERNAL POISONING OF SKIN OR EYES

External poisons should be flushed from the skin for 20 min or eyes for 30 min with a continuous stream of water. The patient should then be transported to an emergency care facility for further treatment as required. Systemic absorption of poisons through the skin may require administration of an antidote.

POISONING BY STING AND SNAKEBITE

Poisoning by insect sting (e.g., bee, wasp, scorpion, or fire ant) should be treated by cleansing the area, immediately removing the stinger, and applying an icepack to the site of the sting. If the patient is allergic, watch closely for possible anaphylactic reaction. CPR and administration of epinephrine and corticosteroids may be required. Transport the patient to an emergency care facility immediately if indicated. Some allergic persons carry a kit with medication prescribed by their physician (e.g., an epinephrine auto-injector for self-injection or injection by someone else).

After emergency care is completed, aftercare to lessen the pain, discomfort, and redness associated with stings can include application of topical corticosteroid ointment. (See Topical Corticosteroids in Table 12-1.)

Do not apply ice or apply a tourniquet to a snakebite. Venom is very irritating and may cause sloughing of the tissues. Keep the patient quiet to slow circulation, and transport the patient, lying down, to an emergency care facility for **antivenom injections**. If possible, take the snake along, in a closed container, for identification purposes. It may be nonpoisonous.

MEDIALINK

See it in Action! Go to the Online Resources to view a video on How to Manage an Obstructed Airway.

PATIENT EDUCATION

Patients with known allergies should be instructed on the following:

1. Be particularly careful when working outdoors and do not approach any insect nests or hives. Have lawn areas and shrubbery periodically inspected for insect nests and colonies.
2. Always wear shoes and light-colored clothing when outside. If possible wear long sleeves and pant legs.
3. Remove stinger by scraping it off with the edge of something rigid such as a credit card. Pulling a stinger out with tweezers may actually cause more poison to be injected into the body as you squeeze the stinger.
4. If epinephrine or a self-injected device is prescribed, the patient should be instructed on its use.

PEOPLE AT RISK

Poisonings are the leading cause of health emergencies for children in the nation and a major cause of death among young children because of their natural curiosity and active lifestyle. The danger is particularly great with flavored medications, such as aspirin or iron tablets. Great care must be taken to prevent poisoning of young children. The child between the ages of one and five years old is most at risk.

Keep all chemicals in a locked cupboard. Keep infrequently used drugs, for example, pain medications, in a lockable box such as a tackle box or file box. Be sure that medications taken daily by adults are always in childproof containers. Be particularly vigilant when visiting with older adult friends or relatives who may not have childproof containers for their pills. Be aware that the most common sources for poisoning in children under six are cosmetics and personal care products. In 2011, these accounted for 2,706 reported cases in the United States.

The health care professional can play a major role in reducing the number of accidental poisonings in children by stressing preventive measures to parents. One educational program teaches the child to stay away from dangerous products by labeling them with a "Mr. Yuk" sticker. Figure 10-1 is a warning label for children who cannot read. These stickers are available from many poison information centers throughout the United States.

Another group at risk for poisoning is older adults. Overdoses of medication can result in toxicity, with symptoms of confusion, dizziness, weakness, lethargy, ataxia, tremors, or cardiac irregularities. Toxic reactions from medications taken by older adults can possibly result from the following:

1. Slower metabolism, impaired circulation, and decreased excretion causing medication to remain in the body longer and build up to dangerous levels

2. Wrong dosage caused by impaired vision or poor memory (patients may forget that they have taken medicine and take a double dose)

3. Interactions when many different medications are taken and over-the-counter medications or herbal remedies are self-administered with inadequate medical supervision

4. Medical conditions affecting absorption

(See Chapter 27: Drugs and Older Adults.)

FIGURE 10-1 Mr. Yuk and similar stickers may be obtained from many Poison Control Centers throughout the United States. The telephone number of the nearest Poison Control Center is frequently printed on these stickers. Permission to reproduce Mr. Yuk has been granted by Children's Hospital of Pittsburgh.

Many medicines and common household products resemble candy or food. Children may be attracted to the unique shapes and bright colors used in packaging. Impaired vision may contribute to mistakes by adults, especially older adults. It is important to keep medicines and dangerous chemicals in an area separate from food and medicines. Don't be fooled by look-alikes (Figure 10-2).

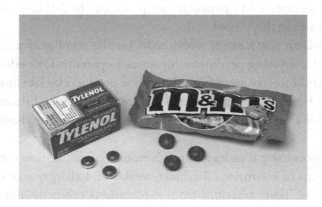
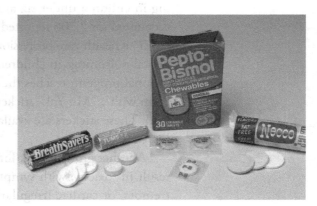
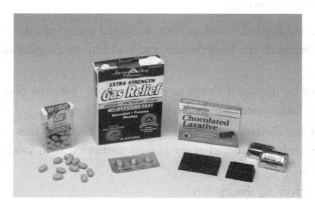
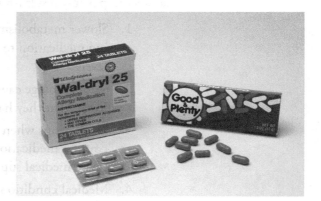

FIGURE 10-2 Look-alikes: Don't be fooled! Many common household products and medicines resemble candy or food. Keep these products in separate areas. The compared products are chosen for illustration purposes only. The manufacturers do not intend any misuse of their products.

PATIENT EDUCATION

POISONS

Public education is of paramount importance in preventing poisoning. The general public must be instructed in precautions with medications, and it is especially important to inform the parents and caretakers of young children and older adults. It is the responsibility of all health care professionals to provide the necessary information to help prevent poisoning.

To prevent poisoning, the American Medical Association recommends the following precautions:

1. Keep all medicines, household chemicals, personal care products, cleaning supplies, and pesticides in a locked cupboard. There is no place that is "out of reach of children."

2. Never transfer poisonous substances to unlabeled containers or to food containers such as milk or soda bottles or cereal boxes. Keep in original labeled container.

3. Never store poisonous substances in the same area with food. Confusion could be fatal.

4. Never reuse containers of chemical products.

5. Do not give or take medications in the dark.

6. Never leave medications on a bedside stand. Confusion while a person is sleepy could result in a fatal overdose.

7. Always read the label before taking any medication or pouring any solution for ingestion.

(continued)

8. Never tell children the medicine you are giving them is candy. Explain to children that medication is taken for your well-being and that all medication is to be taken only as directed by a physician.

9. When preparing a baby's formula, taste the ingredients. Never store boric acid, salt, or talcum near the formula ingredients.

10. Never give or take any medication that is discolored, has a strange odor, or is outdated.

11. Do not take medicine in front of children.

12. Keep pocketbooks, purses, and pillboxes out of reach of children. Do not allow children access to cosmetic products.

13. Rinse out containers thoroughly before disposing of them.

Note: In the past, most people flushed old medicines down the toilet to prevent accidental poisonings of children and animals who may find medicines in the trash. Drugs such as powerful narcotic pain relievers and other controlled substances carry instructions for flushing to reduce the danger of unintentional use or overdose and illegal abuse.

Despite the safety reasons for flushing drugs, some people are questioning the practice because of concerns about trace levels of drug residues found in surface water, such as rivers and lakes, and in some community drinking water supplies. However, the main way drug residues enter water systems is by people taking medications and then naturally passing them through their bodies.

To address this concern, the Food and Drug Administration (FDA) recommends mixing most other medicines with kitty litter or used coffee grounds, placing the mixture in a sealed container or plastic bag, and disposing of it in your household trash. In addition, many cities and towns have medicine take-back programs or household hazardous waste facilities where you can bring your old medicines. When in doubt, ask your pharmacist about proper disposal in your area. FDA's recommendations regarding disposal of unused medicines can be found at their website.

Obtain the number of your nearest Poison Control Center and place it on or near your telephone along with programming into your cell phone. There are more than 72 Poison Control Centers throughout the United States and Canada with computerized data to give you the latest information about poisons. Remember, *the wrong treatment is often more dangerous than none.* You can obtain the number of the Poison Control Center in your area of the United States by calling 1-800-222-1222 or the nearest emergency care facility, by logging on to the website (http://www.aapcc.org) of the American Association of Poison Control Centers, or by checking the emergency numbers in your phone book or online. Canada does *not* have a national poison control center number. Obtain the number of your nearest Poison Control Center in Canada by logging on to the website (http://www.capcc.ca) of the Canadian Association of Poison Control Centers. The Poison Control Center is also a good source of information regarding poisonous plants, insects, snakes, reptiles, and poisonous marine organisms such as stingray and jellyfish.

CHAPTER REVIEW QUIZ

Complete the statements by filling in the blanks:

1. Poisons can be taken into the body in four different ways:

   _____

   _____

   _____

   _____

2. In cases of poison ingestion, vomiting is to be avoided under the following five conditions:

   _____

   _____

   _____

   _____

   _____

3. Gastric lavage is contraindicated when a patient has ingested what type of substance?

   _____

4. When is activated charcoal administered?

   _____

5. Why are gastric contents saved after emesis or gastric lavage?

   _____

6. What is the treatment for poisons that contact skin or eyes?

   _____

7. What two groups of people are most at risk for poisoning?

   _____

   _____

8. Name four conditions that may lead to toxic medication reactions in older adults.

   _____

   _____

   _____

   _____

9. What is the leading cause of poisoning deaths in children under six years of age?

_____

10. What is the number of the National Poison Control Center?

_____

11. In what scenarios is it appropriate to call 911 before poison control?

_____

Note

A Comprehensive Review Exam for Part I can be found at the end of the text following the Summary.
Answers to this comprehensive exam are available from your instructor.

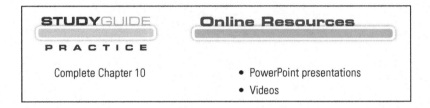

STUDYGUIDE

P R A C T I C E

Complete Chapter 10

Online Resources

- PowerPoint presentations
- Videos

PART 2
Drug Classifications

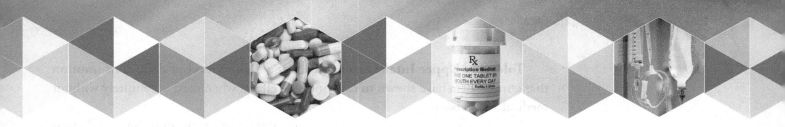

CHAPTER 11
VITAMINS, MINERALS, AND HERBS

KEY TERMS AND CONCEPTS

Antioxidants

Dietary Reference
Intakes (DRIs)

Deficiency

Electrolytes

Fat-soluble vitamins

Herbal

Hyperkalemia

Minerals

Overdoses

Supplements

Symptoms of overdose

Toxicity

U.S. Recommended
Dietary Allowances
(U.S. RDAs)

Water-soluble vitamins

OBJECTIVES

Upon completion of this chapter, the learner should be able to

1. Categorize vitamins as water soluble or fat soluble

2. List vitamins and their sources, functions, signs of deficiency, and symptoms of overdose if known

3. Describe common electrolytes in the body and list their normal blood chemistry values

4. Identify vitamins by name and letter

5. List minerals and their sources, functions, and signs of deficiency

6. Identify the chemical symbol for each mineral

7. Describe conditions that may require vitamin or mineral supplements

8. Explain the role of antioxidants in nutrition therapy

9. Describe why and how consumers should be more vigilant in the use of herbal products

10. Define the Key Terms and Concepts

ietary requirements for vitamins and other nutrients may be listed in several ways:

U.S. Recommended Dietary Allowances (U.S. RDAs) of vitamins and minerals necessary for the maintenance of good nutrition in the average healthy adult under normal living conditions in the United States. The Food and Drug Administration (FDA) uses RDAs to develop daily values (seen on most product labels) to help consumers compare the nutrient content of products.

Adequate intake (AI) is based on observed or experimentally determined estimates of nutrient intake by healthy people and used when data to calculate an RDA are insufficient.

Tolerable Upper Intake level (UL) is the highest level of daily consumption that current data have shown to cause no side effects when used indefinitely without medical supervision.

Dietary Reference Intakes (DRIs) are a system of nutrition recommendations from the Institutes of Medicine of the U.S. National Academy of Sciences composed of RDAs, AIs, and ULs listed here. The National Academies issue periodic reports, such as those released in April 2000, urging caution with megadoses of antioxidant supplements that can cause adverse side effects.

Under special circumstances, vitamin and mineral supplements are required for a person's optimal function and health. *Indications for vitamin and mineral supplements include the following:*

Inadequate diet. Because of anorexia, weight reduction, or other special diets, illness, alcoholism, or poor eating habits

Malabsorption syndromes. Chronic gastrointestinal (GI) disorders or surgery that results in chronic diarrhea

Increased need for certain nutrients. As in pregnancy and lactation (especially iron, folic acid, and calcium), infants under one year of age, adolescence, older adults, debilitation, illness, unusual physical activity, and postmenopausal women (calcium)

Deficiency due to medication interactions. For example, potassium deficiency with the use of diuretics

Nutrients function in groups or teams. Therefore, if diet supplementation is warranted, it is likely that both vitamins and some additional minerals are needed. An example of this teamwork is bone growth, development, and strength, which depend on calcium, magnesium, vitamin A, vitamin D, and several other nutrients (fluoride, etc.). However, patients should be advised to avoid self-medication with large doses of vitamins or minerals, which may not be indicated if the diet is well balanced and the individual is in good health. Overdoses of some vitamins, especially A and D, and some minerals, for example iron, can be injurious to health. A need or deficiency should be established by a physician's diagnosis or blood test before exceeding the RDA. Supplementary (prophylactic) multivitamin preparations may reasonably contain 50%–150% of the RDA of vitamins (except that the amount of vitamins A and D and folic acid should not exceed the RDA). Combination vitamin preparations containing iron should not be used unless a deficiency has been established with a blood test or physician's diagnosis.

It is important to differentiate between water-soluble and fat-soluble vitamins to avoid their build-up in the body with possible symptoms of overdose. Megadoses of vitamins (more than the RDA) should be taken only if prescribed by a physician and/or approved by the FDA. *Remember, the RDA includes the amount of vitamins from foods you eat as well as supplements.* Research reports have indicated a possibility of damage to tissues with large quantities of vitamins (above the RDA), especially those stored in the fat cells of the body.

The RDAs and DRIs listed on the following pages are established for average, normal, healthy adults. Larger amounts are required with certain conditions (e.g., pregnancy, lactation, and some illnesses). Larger amounts are required for males than females. Smaller amounts are required for children (consult references). However, megadoses should *never* be taken except under the direct supervision of a physician.

The RDA and DRI are presented here only for reference. You are not expected to remember these figures. However, before taking any supplements or educating patients on supplements, it is wise to consult references for appropriate doses and to avoid overdosage. Overdosage can sometimes cause severe adverse effects and even acute toxicity, especially with the fat-soluble vitamins.

FAT-SOLUBLE VITAMINS

The **fat-soluble vitamins** are vitamins A, D, E, and K.

Vitamin A (Retinol, Retinal, Beta Carotene)

Vitamin A is processed in the body from the carotene of plants, especially yellow-orange and dark-green leafy vegetables, fruits, oily saltwater fish, dairy products, and eggs (RDA 800–1,000 units per day, DRI 700–3,000 mcg per day). Beta carotene is an antioxidant. (See "Antioxidants" later in this chapter.)

Necessary for:

Resistance to infection

Proper visual function at night

Normal growth and development of bones and soft tissues, and maintenance of healthy epithelial tissues (skin and mucous membranes)

Healing of wounds (sometimes prescribed for acne)

Reproduction

Deficiencies may result from:

Malabsorption of fats

Diarrhea

Obstruction of bile

Presence of mineral oil in the intestines

Overcooking of vegetables in an open container (heat and air cause oxidation)

Prolonged infection or fever

Signs of deficiency include:

Night blindness

Slow growth, anorexia, weight loss, bone and teeth deformities

Dry eyes and skin, pruritus (itching)

Supplements of vitamin A (e.g., Aquasol A) may be necessary for:

Infants fed unfortified skim milk or milk-substitute formulas

Those with prolonged infection or fever

Those with diabetes or hypothyroidism

Those with liver disease

Vitamin A has been used as a screening test for fat absorption.

Some dermatological disorders are treated with retinoids (synthetic vitamin A products). One retinoid product, isotretinoin, is prescribed for severe acne; another is acitretan, used for severe psoriasis. Retinoids can cause fetal abnormalities and are therefore contraindicated in pregnancy. They have also caused increased intracranial pressure, possible liver injury, and other adverse side effects associated with hypervitaminosis A. (See Chapter 12, "Skin Medications.") It is sad to note that vitamin A deficiency is the leading cause of blindness in children worldwide.

Symptoms of overdose (hypervitaminosis A) from greater than 50,000 units (15,000 mcg of retinol) in adults and 2,000 units (6,000 mcg of retinol in infants and children) include:

> ❗ Irritability, psychiatric symptoms
>
> Fatigue, lethargy
>
> Headache, insomnia
>
> ❗ Brittle nails, dry skin, and hair
>
> ❗ Anorexia, nausea, diarrhea, jaundice
>
> Acute toxicity with increased intracranial pressure, vertigo, coma
>
> ❗ Joint pain, myalgia
>
> Stunted growth, fetal malformations

Caution should be used with kidney or liver problems or diabetes.

> ❗ Long-term use of large doses of vitamin A is *contraindicated* for women who are, or may become, pregnant. *Fetal malformations* have been reported following maternal ingestion of large doses of vitamin A, either before or during pregnancy. Many medications that are vitamin A derivatives, such as tretinoin cream, are also contraindicated during pregnancy.

Vitamin D (D₂-Calciferol, D₃-Cholecalciferol, D₂-Ergocalciferol)

Vitamin D is synthesized in the body through the action of sunlight on the skin. Other sources include fish oils (especially salmon, tuna, and mackerel) and food products fortified with vitamin D, such as milk and cereals (RDA 400 units per day, DRI 5–15 mcg per day). Vitamin D_3 is the form seen in products containing 10,000 units or less of vitamin D; D_2 is the form seen in products containing 50,000 units of vitamin D. Cholecalciferol or D_3 is more proficient in raising vitamin D serum concentrations.

Earlier research studies have shown that people with low vitamin D levels are twice as likely to develop coronary artery disease, heart failure, stroke, high blood pressure, and diabetes as those with normal levels. Vitamin D deficiency is common in the northern latitudes where people do not get much sunlight and spend much of their time indoors.

The National Institute of Health (NIH) compiled a list of individuals who need increased vitamin D, and they include:

- Breast-fed infants
- People who are 50 years or older

- Those with limited sun exposure
- Dark-skinned people
- People with obesity (BMI greater than 30)

Consequently, several researchers suggested that the use of vitamin D supplements be increased; however, the risk of overdose and toxicity must be considered. Vitamin D is fat soluble and stays in the system longer and can accumulate to toxic levels. Those taking large doses must be assessed carefully for symptoms of toxicity, which are listed shortly.

Necessary for:

Maintenance of normal nerves and muscles

Regulating the absorption and metabolism of calcium and phosphorus for healthy bones and teeth

Pregnancy and lactation, when it is especially important

Signs of deficiency include:

Poor tooth and bone structure (rickets)

Skeletal deformities

Osteoporosis, osteomalacia

Tetany (muscle spasms)

Vitamin D supplements are prescribed as calcitriol (Rocaltrol) or ergocalciferol (Drisdol) to prevent or treat rickets or osteomalacia and to manage hypocalcemia in cases of renal disease or parathyroid malfunction. The difference between the therapeutic dosage and that causing hypercalcemia is very small; therefore, dosage must be carefully regulated and monitored.

Symptoms of vitamin D overdose and toxicity include:

⚠ Nausea, anorexia, weight loss

⚠ Muscle and/or bone pain

⚠ Kidney damage and kidney stone formation

⚠ Heart rhythm abnormalities

⚠ Hypercalcemia with convulsions or confusion

⚠ Fetal disorders

Caution not to exceed the RDA of vitamin D especially with:

Cardiovascular disorders

Kidney diseases

Pregnancy (possible fetal malformations or mental retardation)

Lactation

Interactions may occur (overdose may antagonize) with:

Digoxin

Mineral oil may interfere with intestinal absorption of vitamin D.

Vitamin E (Tocopherol)

Vitamin E is abundant in nature, found especially in cereals, wheat germ, seeds, nuts, vegetable oils, eggs, meat, and poultry (RDA 30 units per day, DRI 15–1,000 mg per day). Vitamin E has antioxidant properties (see "Antioxidants" later in this chapter).

Necessary for:

Normal metabolism

Protection of tissues of the eyes, skin, liver, breasts, muscles, and lungs

Protecting red blood cells (RBCs) from damage

Decreasing platelet clumping

Off-label uses included vitamin E supplements as one of the treatment protocols for management of early Alzheimer's disease and for possibly slowing the progress of such symptoms as memory loss. However, such supplements will neither cure nor prevent the disease.

Deficiencies are found in those with:

Alcohol abuse

Malabsorption syndromes, for example, celiac disease, sprue, cystic fibrosis

Pathological conditions of liver and pancreas

Sickle-cell anemia

Also found in premature infants or low-birth-weight neonates

Signs of deficiency are not firmly established. Premature infants may show irritability, edema, or hemolytic anemia. Adults who are vitamin E deficient may show muscle weakness and some abnormal laboratory values, such as low RBC count.

⚠ **Vitamin E overdose** (1,200 units) can result in bleeding in patients who are vitamin K deficient or on oral anticoagulants.

Interactions: Excessive use of mineral oil may decrease the absorption of vitamin E.

> **Note**
>
> In general, vitamin E supplements should be taken at the lowest dosage necessary and especially while on anticoagulant therapy because of increased risk of bleeding (including cerebral hemorrhage).

Vitamin K (Phytonadione)

Vitamin K is found in green or leafy vegetables, cabbage, vegetable oils, cheese, eggs, and liver and is absorbed in the small intestine in the presence of bile salts (RDA 60–80 mg per day, DRI 90–120 mcg per day).

Necessary for blood clotting. Unlike other fat-soluble vitamins, the body does not store vitamin K, but recycles it in less significant amounts.

Deficiencies may result in low blood clotting factor levels caused by:

Insufficient vitamin K stores in the newborn

Inadequate dietary intake

Malabsorption syndromes, ulcerative colitis, prolonged diarrhea

warfarin overdose

Prolonged use of salicylates, quinine, long-term parenteral nutrition, and broad-spectrum antibiotics

Signs of deficiency include:

Increased clotting time

Petechiae and bruising

Blood in the urine (hematuria)

Blood in the stool (melena or hematochezia)

Note

Patients receiving anticoagulant therapy should be consistent in the amount of vitamin K–rich foods they eat daily to keep the levels of prothrombin and other vitamin K–dependent clotting factors stable. Large amounts of vitamin K–rich foods can counteract anticoagulant therapy. See Chapter 25, "Cardiovascular Drugs," for more information regarding anticoagulant therapy.

Vitamin K is usually administered orally or intravenously. Injectable vitamin K package inserts warn against intravenous (IV) administration due to the possibility of severe allergic reactions. However, IV administration is recommended as the route of choice by the American College of Chest Physicians for serious bleeding related to vitamin K deficiency or as an antidote for bleeding complications during warfarin therapy. Vitamin K is effective only for bleeding disorders caused by low concentrations of vitamin K–dependent blood clotting factors. It is not effective for bleeding from other causes such as heparin overdose or the newer oral anticoagulants.

The American Academy of Pediatrics recommends that vitamin K (phytonadione) be routinely administered to infants at birth to prevent hemorrhagic disease of the newborn. Some state regulations currently require this prophylaxis.

Adverse effects are rare, but hypersensitivity reactions have occurred with IV injections. **Toxicity** in infants can cause jaundice or hemolytic anemia.

CLINICAL CONNECTION

Warfarin and Vitamin K

Currently, warfarin is one of the oldest anticoagulants used. It was assumed that as newer medications (Pradaxa and Xarelto) came on to the market, warfarin would be used less and become obsolete due to its interactions with food and variable effectiveness. It turns out that this is not the case, and warfarin is still used as a primary anticoagulation treatment. This is because it is much cheaper than newer options and has a readily available antidote (vitamin K), which is a major advantage over other anticoagulants when serious bleeding occurs.

WATER-SOLUBLE VITAMINS

The **water-soluble vitamins** include the B-complex vitamins and vitamin C.

Vitamin B$_1$ (Thiamine)

Vitamin B$_1$ is a coenzyme utilized in carbohydrate metabolism. It is found in whole grains; wheat germ; peas; beans; nuts; yeast; meat, especially pork and organ meats; oysters; collard greens; oranges; and enriched cereals (DRI 1.1–1.4 mg per day).

Necessary for normal function of the nervous and cardiovascular systems.

Deficiencies in the United States may be due to:

Chronic alcoholism and substance abuse

Malabsorption and liver disease

Signs of deficiency (beriberi; symptoms are sometimes vague) include:

Anorexia and constipation, GI upset, nausea

Neuritis, pain, tingling in extremities, loss of reflexes

Muscle weakness, fatigue, ataxia

Mental depression, memory loss, confusion

Cardiovascular problems

Hypersensitivity reactions have occurred mainly following repeated IV administration of the drug.

Vitamin B$_2$ (Riboflavin)

Vitamin B$_2$ is a coenzyme utilized in the metabolism of glucose, fats, and amino acids. It is found in milk; eggs; nuts; meats, especially liver; yeast; enriched bread; and green leafy vegetables (DRI 1.3–1.6 mg per day).

Necessary for:

Cell growth and metabolism, with the release of energy from carbohydrates, proteins, and fats in food

Regulation of certain hormones and formation of RBCs.

Deficiencies of vitamin B$_2$ in the United States may be due to:

Chronic alcoholism

Poor diet

Signs of deficiency include:

Glossitis (inflammation of the tongue)

Cheilosis (cracking at corners of the mouth)

Dermatitis, photophobia, vision loss, burning or itching eyes

Vitamin B$_6$ (Pyridoxine)

Vitamin B$_6$ is a coenzyme utilized in the metabolism of carbohydrates, fats, proteins, and amino acids. It is found in meats, fish, poultry, legumes, peanuts, soybeans, wheat germ, whole-grain cereals, and bananas (DRI 1.3–1.9 mg per day). There is significant loss of vitamin B$_6$ when foods are frozen.

Deficiencies may be due to:

Chronic alcoholism

Cirrhosis

Malabsorption syndromes

Signs of deficiency include:

Seizure activity in infants

Neuritis, dermatitis, nausea, vomiting, and depression in adults

Peripheral neuropathy

Caution

Overdose in pregnant women may result in newborns with seizures who have developed a need for greater than normal amounts of pyridoxine.

Vitamin B_{12} (Cobalamin, Cyanocobalamin)

Vitamin B_{12} is found in meats (especially organ meats), poultry, fish and shellfish, milk, cheese, and eggs (DRI 2.4 mcg per day). Absorption of vitamin B_{12} depends on intrinsic factor, which is normally present in the gastric juice of humans. Absence of this factor leads to vitamin B_{12} deficiency and pernicious anemia.

The National Academy of Sciences now suggests that all Americans over the age of 50 begin taking a low-dose vitamin B_{12} supplement or regularly eat breakfast cereals that are fortified with the vitamin. The problem in older adults results from a reduced ability to absorb vitamin B_{12}. This is especially true for those taking medications that reduce gastric acid, for example, cimetidine (Tagamet) or omeprazole (Prilosec).

Necessary for maturation of RBCs and maintenance of the nervous system.

Deficiencies can be associated with:

> Vegetarian diets without meat, eggs, or milk products
>
> Gastrectomy or intestinal resections
>
> Malabsorption syndromes
>
> Pernicious anemia

Signs of deficiency include:

> Anemia and weakness first symptoms of clinical deficiency
>
> Poor muscle coordination
>
> Numbness of hands and feet (paresthesia)
>
> Mental confusion, disorientation, memory loss, and irritability

Treatment for pernicious anemia consists of vitamin B_{12}, cyanocobalamin, 100–1,000 mcg intramuscularly (IM) monthly for life to prevent neurological damage.

Side effects include:

> Transient diarrhea
>
> Itching and urticaria
>
> Anaphylaxis (rare)

Interactions may occur (decreased absorption of B_{12}) with:

> Neomycin

Folic Acid (Folate, Vitamin B₉)

Folic acid is a vitamin included in the B-complex group and is found in leafy and green vegetables (broccoli), avocado, beets, orange juice, kidney beans, and organ meats (DRI 400 mcg per day). Folic acid is lost with overcooking and reheating.

Necessary for protein synthesis, production of RBCs, cell division, and normal growth and maintenance of all cells. Deficiency during pregnancy can result in neural tube defects, such as spina bifida, in the newborn.

Deficiencies can be associated with:

Improper diet

Chronic alcoholism

Liver pathology

Intestinal obstruction

Malabsorption syndromes, malnutrition

Renal dialysis or prolonged use of some medicines (see listed interactions)

Signs of deficiency include:

Anorexia, weight loss, weakness, and fatigue

Irritability and behavior disorders

Anemia

Interactions of folic acid, over the DRI, could interfere with the action of the following drugs:

Phenytoin (Dilantin)

Methotrexate

Trimethoprim

Triamterene

> **Caution**
>
> Folic acid *should not be given to anyone with undiagnosed anemia,* because it may mask the diagnosis of pernicious anemia. Over-the-counter (OTC) vitamin supplements should contain no more than 0.4 mg; however, 1-mg doses are available by prescription.

PATIENT EDUCATION

Patients should avoid taking folic acid supplements without consulting a physician first.

Niacin (Nicotinic Acid, Niacinamide, Vitamin B₃)

Niacin is a vitamin included in the B-complex group and is found in meat, chicken, milk, eggs, fish, green vegetables, cooked dried beans and peas, soybeans, nuts, peanut butter, and enriched cereal products (DRI 14–18 mg per day).

Necessary for lipid metabolism and nerve functioning, especially in the circulation and maintenance of all cells.

Deficiency results in pellagra, a severe skin and mucous membrane disorder that progresses to systemic and central nervous system disorders.

Signs of niacin deficiency include:

Peripheral vascular insufficiency

Dermatitis and varicose ulcers

Diarrhea

Dementia, hallucinations, depression

Mouth sores

Lethargy, weakness, anorexia, indigestion

Niacin is used primarily to prevent and treat pellagra. Other treatment conditions (usually as an adjunct with other medications) include:

Many vascular disorders (e.g., vascular spasm, arteriosclerosis, Raynaud's disease, angina, varicose veins, pressure ulcers)

Circulatory disturbances of the inner ear, Ménière's syndrome

Lower blood lipid levels (see Chapter 25)

Daily doses of up to 1,000 mg appear to be safe.

Side effects of niacin, especially over 1,000 mg daily, can include:

❗ Headache, flushing, and burning sensations of face, neck, and chest

❗ Postural hypotension

❗ Jaundice

❗ Nausea, diarrhea, vomiting

❗ Increased blood glucose and uric acid

Caution for patients with liver disease, gallbladder disease, gout, or diabetes

PATIENT EDUCATION

Patients should be instructed regarding possible side effects, especially flushing and a burning sensation, and should be cautioned to rise slowly from a reclining position. They should be told that the flushing usually resolves within two weeks. Taking niacin in divided doses or extended-release products can sometimes lessen this effect. Sometimes aspirin is prescribed to counteract flushing.

Vitamin C (Ascorbic Acid)

Vitamin C is a water-soluble vitamin found in fresh fruits and vegetables, especially citrus fruits, cantaloupe, tomatoes, cabbage, green peppers, and broccoli (DRI 75–90 mg per day). It is unstable when exposed to heat or air or combined with alkaline compounds (e.g., antacids). Adding baking soda to vegetables for color retention destroys vitamin C. Vitamin C is considered an antioxidant. (See "Antioxidants" later in this chapter.)

Necessary for:

Formation of intracellular substances (collagen)

Normal development of teeth, gums, and bones

Absorption of iron

Healing of wounds and bone fractures

Deficiencies are associated with:

Diet lacking fresh fruit and vegetables

Alcoholism

Infections and hemodialysis

Smoking

Signs of the vitamin C deficiency (scurvy) include:

Muscle weakness and cramping

Sore and bleeding mouth and gums, loose teeth

Capillary fragility (bruising); dry, scaly skin

Poor healing

Supplements of ascorbic acid are available in capsules, tablets (extended-release), solution, chewables, or injection form. They are indicated for:

Treatment of scurvy (adults 100–250 mg bid, children 100–300 mg per day divided doses)

Hemodialysis patients (100–200 mg daily)

Infants beginning at two to four weeks of age (20–50 mg per day)

Dosages larger than those recommended are to be avoided because of the potential for side effects. In addition, because ascorbic acid is water soluble, more than 50% of the dose is excreted in the urine of normal subjects. Excretion of less than 20% of the dose over 24h suggests vitamin C deficiency.

Side effects of large doses of vitamin C, more than the RDA, can include:

⊘ Heartburn, abdominal cramps, nausea, vomiting, diarrhea

⊘ Increased uric acid levels; may precipitate gouty arthritis

⊘ Increased urinary calcium; may precipitate kidney stone formation

⊘ Scurvy in neonates following large amounts taken during pregnancy

Interactions may occur with:

Aspirin, causing elevated blood levels of aspirin

Iron (excess iron absorption with excess supplementation)

PATIENT EDUCATION

Patients should be given the following information concerning vitamin C:

- Vitamin C is destroyed by heat and air; therefore, raw fresh fruits and vegetables are the best sources of vitamin C.
- Large quantities of supplemental vitamin C are to be avoided, unless prescribed by a physician, because of potential side effects, such as gastric irritation, increased uric acid, and kidney stone formation.

- Antacids should not be taken at the same time as vitamin C supplements because the alkaline compound neutralizes the ascorbic acid.
- Megadoses of vitamin C taken during pregnancy may cause the newborn to require larger-than-average amounts of ascorbic acid.

See Table 11-1 for a summary of water- and fat-soluble vitamins.

TABLE 11-1 Summary of Fat-Soluble and Water-Soluble Vitamins

NAME	FOOD SOURCES	FUNCTIONS	DEFICIENCY/TOXICITY

Vitamin A (Retinol, beta carotene)	Animal
	    Oily saltwater fish
	    Dairy products
	    Eggs
	Plants
	    Dark-green leafy vegetables
	    Deep-yellow or orange fruit and vegetables
		Dim light vision
		Maintenance of mucous membranes
		Growth and development of bones
		Healing of wounds
		Resistance to infection
		Antioxidant (beta carotene)
			Deficiency
			Retarded growth
			Faulty bone and tooth development
			Night blindness
			Dry skin
			Xerophthalmia (dry eyes)
			Xerosis (dry mouth)
			
			Toxicity
			(hypervitaminosis A)
			Irritability, lethargy, headache
			Joint pain, myalgia
			Stunted growth, fetal malformations
			Jaundice, nausea, diarrhea
			Dry skin and hair

Vitamin D (cholecalciferol)	Animal
	    Fish oils
	    Fortified milk
	Plants
	    Fortified cereals
	    Sunlight
		Development of healthy bones and teeth
		Muscle function
		Absorption of calcium
			Deficiency
			Softening bones:
			    Rickets (in children)
			    Osteomalacia (in adults)
			Poorly developed teeth
			Muscle spasms
			Toxicity (Hypercalcemia)
			Convulsions
			Kidney stone formation, kidney damage
			Muscle/bone pain
			Nausea, anorexia
			Fetal disorders

Vitamin E (tocopherol)	Plants
	    Vegetable oils
	    Seeds, nuts
	    Wheat germ, cereals
		Antioxidant
		Decreases platelet clumping
		Normal metabolism and tissue protection
			Deficiency
			Destruction of RBCs, muscle weakness
			Toxicity
			Prolonged bleeding time
			Cerebral hemorrhage
			Increased risk of prostate cancer

(*continued*)

TABLE 11-1 **Summary of Fat-Soluble and Water-Soluble Vitamins (*continued*)**

NAME	FOOD SOURCES	FUNCTIONS	DEFICIENCY/TOXICITY
Vitamin K (phytonadione)	Animal 　Egg yolk, cheese 　Liver Plants 　Vegetable oil 　Green leafy vegetables 　Cabbage, broccoli	Blood clotting Bone maintenance	**Deficiency** Prolonged blood clotting time Blood in urine and stool **Toxicity** Jaundice in infants
Vitamin B$_1$ (thiamine)	Animal 　Pork, beef, liver 　Oysters Plants 　Yeast 　Whole and enriched grains, wheat germ 　Beans, peas, collard greens, nuts, asparagus 　Oranges	Normal function of nervous and cardiovascular systems	**Deficiency** GI upset, constipation Neuritis, mental disturbance Cardiovascular problems Muscle weakness, fatigue **Toxicity** None known
Vitamin B$_2$ (riboflavin)	Animal 　Milk 　Meat, liver Plants 　Green vegetables 　Cereals 　Enriched bread 　Yeast	Aids in energy metabolism of glucose, fats, and amino acids	**Deficiency** Cheilosis Glossitis Photophobia, vision problems, itching eyes Dermatitis, rough skin **Toxicity** None
Vitamin B$_6$ (pyridoxine)	Animal 　Pork, beef, chicken, tuna, salmon Plants 　Whole-grain cereals, wheat germ 　Legumes, peanuts, soybeans 　Bananas	Synthesis of amino acids Antibody production Maintenance of blood glucose level	**Deficiency** Anorexia, nausea, vomiting Dermatitis Neuritis, depression **Toxicity** Seizures in newborns
Vitamin B$_{12}$ (cyanocobalamin)	Animal 　Seafood/shellfish 　Meat, poultry, liver 　Eggs 　Milk, cheese Plants 　None	Synthesis of RBCs Maintenance of nervous system	**Deficiency** Nerve, muscle, mental problems Pernicious anemia **Toxicity** None

(continued)

TABLE 11-1   **Summary of Fat-Soluble and Water-Soluble Vitamins (*continued*)**

NAME	FOOD SOURCES	FUNCTIONS	DEFICIENCY/TOXICITY

Niacin (nicotinic acid, vitamin B$_3$)	Animal
	    Milk
	    Eggs
	    Fish
	    Poultry
	Plants
	    Legumes, nuts
	    Green vegetables
		Lipid metabolism
		Nerve functioning
			Deficiency
			Pellagra
			Toxicity
			Headache, flushing
			Increased blood glucose and uric acid

Folate (folic acid, vitamin B$_9$)	Animal
	    Organ meats
	Plants
	    Green leafy vegetables
	    Avocado, beets
	    Broccoli, kidney beans
	    Orange juice
		Synthesis of RBCs, leukocytes, DNA, and RNA
		Needed for normal growth and reproduction
			Deficiency
			Increased risk of neural tube defects
			Macrocytic and megaloblastic anemias
			Irritability, behavior disorders
			Toxicity
			None

Vitamin C (ascorbic acid)	Fruits
	    All citrus, cantaloupe
	Plants
	    Broccoli
	    Tomatoes
	    Brussels sprouts
	    Cabbage
	    Green peppers
		Development of normal teeth, gums, and bone
		Prevention of scurvy
		Formation of collagen
		Healing of wounds
		Absorption of iron
		Antioxidant
			Deficiency
			Scurvy
			Poor healing
			Muscle cramps/weakness
			Ulcerated gums/mouth, loose teeth
			Capillary fragility (bruising)
			Toxicity
			Raise uric acid level, gout
			GI distress
			Kidney stone formation
			Rebound scurvy in neonates

MINERALS

Minerals are chemical elements occurring in nature and in body fluids. The correct balance of each is required for the maintenance of health. Minerals dissolved in the body fluids are called **electrolytes** because they carry positive or negative electrical charges required for body activities, such as conduction of nerve impulses, beating of the heart, skeletal muscle contraction, absorption of nutrients from the GI tract, protein synthesis, energy production, blood formation, and many other body processes. The most common electrolytes are sodium (Na), potassium (K), and chloride (Cl). These electrolytes can be measured via a blood sample. The normal ranges for these electrolytes can be found in Table 11-2. When the electrolytes become imbalanced in the body due to dietary issues or disease processes, the patient develops symptoms that are directly related to the function of the electrolyte in the body. Table 11-2 lists common symptoms related to electrolyte imbalances.

TABLE 11-2 Ranges for Select Electrolytes in the Body

NORMAL RANGE	ELECTROLYTE ABNORMALITIES
Sodium (Na) 135-145 mEq/L	Hyponatremia (Na <135 mEq/L) • Nausea/vomiting • Headache • Confusion • Seizures Hypernatremia (Na >145 mEq/L) • Anorexia • Lethargy • Irritability • Coma
Potassium (K) 3.5-5.5 mmol/L	Hypokalemia (K <3.5 mmol/L) • Weakness, cramping • Tingling/numbness • Constipation • Palpitations Hyperkalemia (K > 5.5 mmol/L) • Abnormal heart rhythms • Muscle fatigue • Paralysis • Nausea
Chloride (Cl) 96-106 mEq/L	Hypochloremia (Cl <96 mEq/L) • Often none until very low • Headache • Nausea Hyperchloremia (Cl > 196 mEq/L) • Often no symptoms • Anorexia • Irritability • Coma

Necessary for:

Numerous body functions and maintaining homeostasis (body balance).

The correct ratio of fluids to electrolytes must be maintained for normal functioning of the body. Fluids and minerals are excreted every day and must be replaced with fluid and food intake.

The principal minerals in the body and their chemical symbols are sodium (Na), chloride (Cl), potassium (K), calcium (Ca), and iron (Fe).

Sodium and Chloride (NaCl)

Sodium and chloride are the principal minerals in the extracellular body fluids. The best source of sodium and chloride is table salt (NaCl).

Deficiencies of sodium and chloride are associated with:

Excessive fluid loss: bleeding, diarrhea, vomiting, or excessive perspiration

Insufficient oral intake (starvation or extended fasting)

Alkalosis (chloride deficiency)

Treatment consists of oral or IV therapy with sodium chloride (NaCl) according to needs:

Normal saline solution (0.9% sodium chloride)

Potassium (K)

Potassium (DRI 4.7 g per day) is another of the principal minerals within cells. Natural sources of potassium include citrus fruits, bananas, tomatoes, potato skin, cantaloupe, avocadoes, dried fruits, cooked dried beans, and peas.

Necessary for:

Acid–base and fluid balance

Normal muscular irritability (heartbeat regulation)

Deficiencies are associated with:

Insufficient oral intake due to surgery, anorexia, or weight-reduction diets

Diarrhea or vomiting

Diabetic ketoacidosis

Diaphoresis (excessive perspiration)

Use of diuretics, especially thiazides and loop diuretics

Digoxin toxicity

Long-term use of corticosteroids or long-term use of laxatives

Kidney disease

Signs of deficiency include:

Muscular weakness, paralysis

Cardiac arrhythmias

Lethargy and fatigue, mental apathy, and confusion

Treatment consists of:

KCl given IV postoperatively or for severe dehydration (diluted according to directions)

One of the numerous oral products available, usually in effervescent tablet or powder form, to be dissolved in water or juice and taken after meals, or capsules to be swallowed (e.g., Micro-K), extended-release tablets (e.g., Klor-Con), or oral liquid preparations.

Side effects of potassium overdose can include:

Nausea, vomiting, or diarrhea

GI bleeding, or abdominal pain

Cardiac arrest

Pain at the injection site or phlebitis may occur during the IV administration of solutions containing 30 mEq or more potassium per liter when infused via a peripheral vein. IV solutions containing potassium should always be run at a slow rate (max of 10 mEq/h) to prevent pain or hyperkalemia.

Hyperkalemia (excessive potassium in the blood) is not likely to result from oral administration, except in the case of severe renal impairment. Care must be taken when adding potassium to IV solutions that the dilute solution is thoroughly mixed, inverted, and agitated, before the solution is hung for administration. Never add potassium to hanging IV solution. Some medications can have an effect on potassium levels. Angiotensin-converting enzyme inhibitors and angiotensin receptor blockers can increase the amount of potassium in the body and cause possible hyperkalemia.

Symptoms of potassium overdosage can include:

> ❗ Fall in the blood pressure and/or *cardiac arrhythmias* from hyperkalemia
> Confusion

Caution with the use of potassium in the following conditions:

Cardiac disease

Renal impairment

Gastric or intestinal ulcers (extended-release products contraindicated)

Mental confusion (unable to follow directions properly)

PATIENT EDUCATION

Patients taking potassium supplements should be instructed regarding:

Natural sources of potassium-rich foods

Conditions requiring potassium supplements

Directions for taking potassium supplements with or after meals to avoid GI distress and the importance of following directions on package carefully

The importance of following specific directions carefully with certain formulations that need to be dissolved in water

Notifying a physician immediately of any side effects

Calcium (Ca)

Calcium is a mineral component of bones and teeth. It is absorbed in the small intestine with the help of vitamin D. Natural sources include milk and dairy products (RDA 1,000–1,200 mg per day). In postmenopausal women not receiving estrogen therapy, the RDA is about 1,500 mg per day. Those who are lactose intolerant (unable to take milk) should include in their diet dark-green leafy vegetables (except spinach), broccoli, and canned fish with the bones. (DRI 1,000–1,300 mg per day, with the higher figure recommended for adolescents of both sexes and postmenopausal women.) The normal blood calcium level is 8.8–10.4 mg/dL.

Necessary for:

Strong bones and teeth

Contraction of cardiac, smooth, and skeletal muscles

Nerve conduction

Blood coagulation, capillary permeability, and normal blood pressure

The balance between *dietary* calcium and magnesium is important in the prevention of heart disease.

Deficiencies (supplements required) are associated with:

Pregnancy and lactation

Postmenopausal women (or those with estrogen deficiency)

Hypoparathyroidism

Long-term use of corticosteroids, some diuretics, or anticonvulsants

Chronic diarrhea, pancreatitis, renal failure

Lack of weight-bearing exercise

Signs of deficiency may include:

Osteoporosis, or osteomalacia (softening of bones), including frequent fractures, especially in older adults

Rickets in children (softening of bones)

Muscle pathology, including cardiac myopathy or tetany (muscle spasm) and leg cramps

Increased clotting time

Treatment consists of taking calcium supplements 400–600 mg daily PO. A higher-dosage supplement is required for those not including calcium-rich foods in the diet (e.g., without dairy products). The RDAs, *including foods,* are 1,200 mg per day for adults and 1,500 mg per day for postmenopausal women not taking estrogen. Many products and combinations are available including calcium gluconate, calcium carbonate, or calcium lactate. Of these three, calcium carbonate delivers the highest amount of elemental calcium per tablet.

Adding vitamin D for calcium metabolism may be necessary for people without exposure to sunlight (see "Vitamin D").

Side effects of calcium salts can include:

❗ Constipation from oral products

Tissue irritation from IV products

When injected IV, calcium salts should be administered *very slowly* to prevent tissue necrosis or *cardiac arrhythmias.*

Emerging evidence has raised concerns (and confusion) about potential adverse effects of high calcium intake on cardiovascular health. Several recent large studies have shown that women who use *calcium supplements* had a statistically significant increase in MIs; men experienced a significantly elevated risk of heart disease mortality. These risks have not been reported with dietary calcium, suggesting that the rapid rise in calcium concentrations with supplements may be a factor.

Caution: Calcium should be used cautiously, if at all, with:

Cardiac disease

Renal disease

Respiratory conditions (e.g., sarcoidosis)

Administration: The most common oral calcium supplement, calcium carbonate, is best taken with meals, whereas other calcium supplements should be administered 1–1.5 h after meals. Remember to always check the label.

Interactions may occur with:

Digoxin, resulting in potentiation (may cause arrhythmias)

CLINICAL CONNECTION

Patient Counseling

Vitamin D and calcium carbonate are regularly used to treat or prevent osteoporosis. Patients usually take two to three doses per day. It is important to counsel patients that the bones absorb calcium best when they are resting. This means that the most important dose is at bedtime, when the patient will be lying down (sleeping) for the next 6–8 h. This is important because patients often forget doses, but reminding them that the nighttime dose is the most important can be helpful.

PATIENT EDUCATION

Patients taking calcium should be instructed regarding:

Calcium-rich diet, especially dairy products and vitamin D milk, which can be low fat

Necessity for calcium supplements (including discussion of risk versus benefits), usually recommended for women beginning at age 35, and especially for postmenopausal women not on estrogen therapy

Importance of upright exercise, for example walking at least three to four times per week to preserve bone mass

Importance of outdoor activity because sunlight helps create vitamin D necessary for calcium metabolism

Taking calcium supplements as specified on the label

Not taking calcium at the same time as other medicines

Iron (Fe)

Iron is vital for the oxygen carrying and the delivery component of blood. Iron is a mineral found in meat (especially liver), egg yolk, beans, spinach, enriched cereals, dried fruits, prune juice, and poultry. The DRI for iron is 8–18 mg per day.

Necessary for hemoglobin formation and 70% of the body's iron is bound to hemoglobin.

Deficiencies (supplements recommended) are associated with:

Hemorrhage and excessive menstrual flow

Internal bleeding, ulcers, and GI tumors

Pregnancy

Infancy

Puberty at the time of growth spurt

Patients undergoing hemodialysis

Signs of deficiency may include:

Paleness of the skin and/or mucous membranes

Lethargy and weakness

Vertigo (dizziness, lightheadedness)

Air hunger

Decline in mental skills

Irregular heartbeat and function

Cravings for nonfood items, for example ice, clay, or starch (called pica)

Treatment of anemia due to iron deficiency consists of administration of iron preparations

Side effects of taking iron preparations can include:

- ❗ Black stools
- ❗ Nausea and vomiting (GI effects can be minimized by taking iron after or with meals, *but not with coffee, tea, or milk*)
- ❗ Constipation or diarrhea

Anaphylactic reactions or phlebitis with IV administration of iron dextran

Contraindicated in patients with peptic ulcer, regional enteritis, or ulcerative colitis

Parenteral iron should *not* be administered concomitantly with oral iron therapy.

Iron should *not* be administered without confirming a diagnosis of deficiency with a blood test and determining the cause of deficiency.

Interactions may occur with:

Vitamin C or orange juice, taken at the same time, which *enhances* iron absorption

Symptoms of acute overdose of iron may occur within minutes or days and include:

Lethargy

- ❗ Shock

PATIENT EDUCATION

Patients taking iron supplements should be instructed regarding:

Avoidance of self-medication without established need (blood test) and without medical supervision to determine why hemoglobin level is low. Taking iron when not prescribed could mask the symptoms of internal bleeding or GI malignancy.

Black stools to be expected

Taking iron at meals to minimize GI distress and with orange juice for better absorption

Interactions (i.e., avoidance of coffee, tea, milk, or antacids at the same time)

Caution with flavored children's tablets (overdosage can be dangerous, even fatal)

Taking liquid iron preparations with drinking straw to avoid temporary stain of dental enamel

The iron in meats is called heme iron and is better absorbed than nonheme iron in vegetables and fruits

Nonheme iron is absorbed better if consumed with meat proteins or a rich source of vitamin C (e.g., orange juice)

Zinc (Zn)

Zinc is a component of numerous enzymes and is an essential element in metabolism. It is usually found in adequate amounts in a well-balanced diet. Rich sources include lean meat, organ meats, oysters, poultry, fish, and whole-grain breads and cereals (DRI 8–11 mg per day). Zinc is an antioxidant.

Necessary for:

Wound healing

Mineralization of bone

Insulin production and glucose regulation

Normal taste

Deficiencies (supplements recommended) are associated with:

Inadequate or vegetarian diet

Chronic, nonhealing wounds

Major surgery or trauma

Deficiency symptoms can include:

Poor wound healing

Reduced taste perception

Poor alcohol tolerance, glucose intolerance

Anemia, slowed growth, sterility

Dermatitis and hair loss

Toxicity (more than 2 g per day) may cause:

Nausea, GI distress, vomiting

Treatment consists of tablets or capsules administered with meals TID to minimize gastric distress. Standard supplement of zinc is no more than 11 mg/24 h. If a zinc supplement is required for more than 90 days, blood levels should be monitored. Chronic consumption of high levels of zinc may cause copper deficiency.

Many combinations of various vitamins and minerals are available in OTC products with various strengths and forms.

PATIENT EDUCATION

Vitamins and Minerals

Patients should be instructed regarding:

Well-balanced diets and natural sources of vitamins and minerals

Food preparation to avoid loss of vitamins

Information regarding signs of deficiency and overdose/toxicity

Caution taking supplements without established need or without medical supervision, especially megadoses, fat-soluble vitamins, and iron

Proper administration to minimize side effects

See Table 11-3 for a summary of major minerals.

TABLE 11-3   **Summary of Major Minerals**

NAME	FOOD SOURCES	FUNCTIONS	DEFICIENCY/TOXICITY
Calcium (Ca) (DRI 1,000–1,300 mg per day)	Milk, cheese, yogurt Sardines Salmon Green vegetables except spinach	Development of bones and teeth Contraction of cardiac, smooth, and skeletal muscles Nerve conduction Blood clotting	**Deficiency** Osteoporosis, osteomalacia Rickets (in children) Muscle pathology Heart disease Increased clotting time **Toxicity** Kidney stones
Potassium (K) (DRI 4.7 g per day)	Oranges, bananas Dried fruits Tomatoes	Contraction of muscles Heartbeat regulation Transmission of nerve impulses Maintaining fluid balance	**Deficiency** (*Hypokalemia*) Muscle weakness Cardiac arrhythmias Lethargy, mental confusion **Toxicity** (hyperkalemia) Weakness Cardiac arrhythmias

Sodium (Na) (DRI 1,300–1,500 mg per day)	Table salt
	    Beef, eggs
	    Milk, cheese
		Maintaining fluid balance in blood
		Transmission of nerve impulses
			Deficiency
			Low blood pressure
			Toxicity
			High blood pressure

Chloride (Cl) (DRI 1.8–2.3 g per day)	Table salt	Gastric acidity Regulation of osmotic pressure Activation of salivary amylase	**Deficiency** Imbalance in gastric acidity Imbalance in blood pH **Toxicity** Diarrhea
Magnesium (Mg) (DRI 320–420 mg)	Green vegetables Whole grains	Synthesis of ATP (adenosine triphosphate) Transmission of nerve impulses Relaxation of skeletal muscles	**Deficiency** (seldom) Imbalance Weakness **Toxicity** Diarrhea
Iron (Fe) (DRI 8–18 mg per day)	Meat Liver Eggs Poultry Spinach Dried fruits Dried beans Prune juice	Hemoglobin formation	**Deficiency** (anemia) Paleness Lethargy Air hunger Irregular heartbeat **Toxicity** Lethargy, shock Vomiting, diarrhea Erosion of GI tract Liver or kidney damage

(*continued*)

TABLE 11-3 **Summary of Major Minerals (*continued*)**

NAME	FOOD SOURCES	FUNCTIONS	DEFICIENCY/TOXICITY
Iodine (I) (DRI 150 mcg per day)	Freshwater shellfish and seafood Iodized salt	Major component of thyroid hormones Regulating rate of metabolism Growth, reproduction Nerve and muscle function Skin and hair growth	Deficiency Goiter Hypothyroidism *Toxicity* "Iodine goiter" Hyperactive, enlarged goiter
Zinc (Zn) (DRI 8–11 mg per day)	Meat Liver Oysters Poultry Fish Whole-grain bread and cereal	Wound healing Mineralization of bone Insulin and glucose regulation Normal taste Antioxidant	*Deficiency* Poor wound healing Reduced taste perception Alcohol/glucose intolerance *Toxicity* GI distress Copper deficiency with extended use of high levels of zinc

PATIENT EDUCATION

Food labels provide a nutritional analysis of the food product. The Percentage (%) Daily Value is the amount of the nutrient obtained by eating the equivalent of one serving of the product. The amount is given in a percentage based upon a 2,000-calorie daily diet. See Figure 11-1.

Nutrition Facts

Serving Size 5 oz. (144g)
Servings Per Container 4

Amount Per Serving

Calories 310   **Calories** from Fat 100

	% Daily Value*
Total Fat 15g	**21%**
Saturated Fat 2.6g	**17%**
Trans Fat 1g	
Cholesterol 118mg	**39%**
Sodium 560mg	**28%**
Total Carbohydrate 12g	**4%**
Dietary Fiber 1g	**4%**
Sugars 1g	
Protein 24g	

Vitamin A 1% • **Vitamin C** 2%
Calcium 2% • **Iron** 5%

*Percent Daily Values are based on a 2,000 calorie diet. Your daily values may be higher or lower depending on your calorie needs:

	Calories	2,000	2,500
Total Fat	Less Than	65g	80g
Saturated Fat	Less Than	20g	25g
Cholesterol	Less Than	300mg	300mg
Sodium	Less Than	2,400mg	2,400mg
Total Carbohydrate		300g	375g
Dietary Fiber		25g	30g

Calories per gram:
    Fat 9 • Carbohydrate 4 • Protein 4

FIGURE 11-1 Nutrition facts.

ANTIOXIDANTS

No discussion of nutrition would be complete without an explanation of the antioxidants, as we know them. **Antioxidants**, sometimes referred to as "anticancer foods" or "natural drugs," inhibit cell destruction in damaged or aging tissues caused by unstable molecules known as free radicals. Although free radical damage may lead to cancer and laboratory evidence suggests that antioxidants may slow or possibly prevent cancer, several large-scale clinical trials have not shown a decrease in the risk of cancer (or heart disease and other risks).

Free radicals attack the cells, causing damage, which prevents the transport of nutrients, oxygen, and water into the cell and the removal of waste products. This damage affects the nucleic acids in their function of growth and repair of tissues. Free radical damage is associated with several age-related diseases. For example, damage to the nucleic acids might initiate the growth of abnormal cells, the first step in cancer development. Also, free radical attack to the cell membranes of the tissues lining the blood vessels can lead to cholesterol accumulation in the damaged arteries, the initial state of atherosclerosis and heart disease. In addition, free radicals are associated with inflammation, drug-induced organ damage, immunosuppression, and possibly other disorders as well.

The body has developed an antioxidant system response to defend itself from free radicals. An antioxidant is defined as any compound that fights against the destructive effects of free radical oxidants. This system is comprised of enzymes, vitamins, and minerals. Antioxidants function in the prevention of free radical formation by binding to, and neutralizing, destructive substances before they damage cells and tissues.

The antioxidant vitamins—*vitamin C, vitamin E,* and *beta carotene*—can function independently of enzymes. Antioxidant minerals include copper, manganese, selenium, and zinc. These minerals work with antioxidant enzymes and are essential for proper enzyme function. If the diet is inadequate in these minerals, the enzymes are not produced or are ineffective.

Caution

Taking antioxidants while undergoing chemotherapy or radiation treatments could be contraindicated. Chemotherapy and radiation generate free radicals, and they need an oxidative process to actually kill tumor cells. By giving antioxidants concurrently with chemotherapy or radiation, you actually can increase the tumor cell's life. It is recommended that patients stop taking antioxidants two days before chemotherapy or radiation and avoid them during the treatment and for two days after completion of the treatment.

PATIENT EDUCATION

Patients asking about antioxidants should be instructed regarding:
- Foods that provide antioxidant action
- Natural antioxidants in certain foods, which are more effective than synthetic products

When antioxidants are contraindicated and the health problems with megadosing.

ALTERNATIVE MEDICINES

Herbs and Other Dietary Supplements

As a health care professional, you may be asked about dietary supplements and, in particular, about herbal remedies. It is important for you to be able to answer these questions effectively and refer your patients to reliable sources of information. There are many books on the market and articles on the Internet describing the use of herbal remedies. In assessing the value of these resources, question the source, the credentials of the author, the research involved in collecting the data, and the reliability and validity of the statistics. Be sure that the information is based on fact, not opinion. You have a responsibility to caution your patients regarding the dangers of taking remedies not approved by the FDA and especially the risk of possible interactions between "natural products" and prescription drugs.

In April 2005 (updated April 7, 2012) the FDA published a report entitled *Guidance for Industry: A Dietary Supplement Labeling Guide,* which answers many questions on the labeling of dietary supplements. In February 2009 (updated March 2013), the National Center of Complementary and Alternative Medicine at the National Institutes of Health published a fact sheet entitled *Get the Facts: Using Dietary Supplements Wisely.* The following information is taken from these materials.

Congress passed the Dietary Supplement Health and Education Act (DSHEA) of 1994, which amended the Food, Drug, and Cosmetic Act to recognize dietary supplements as distinct from food additives and drugs, which are monitored and regulated by the FDA. *Food supplements are not subject to the same scrutiny and restrictions,* so consumers and manufacturers have the responsibility for checking the safety of dietary supplements and determining the truthfulness of label claims.

Dietary Supplements

Dietary supplements have traditionally referred to products made of one or more of the essential nutrients, such as vitamins, minerals, and proteins. DSHEA broadens the definition to include, with some exceptions, any product intended for ingestion as a supplement to the diet. This includes vitamins; minerals; herbs; botanicals; other plant-derived substances; amino acids (the individual building blocks of protein); and concentrates, metabolites, constituents, and extracts of these substances.

It is easy to spot a supplement because DSHEA requires manufacturers to include the words *dietary supplement* on product labels. Also, since March 1999, a "Supplement Facts" panel is required on the labels of most dietary supplements. The supplement manufacturers are required to document substantiation of their claims. They must also include a disclaimer on their labels that the dietary supplements *are not drugs and receive no FDA premarket approval.* The rule, published in the January 6, 2000, *Federal Register,* also prohibits "structure/function" claims (claims that the products affect the structure or function of the body) without prior FDA review. Supplement labels also *may not, without prior FDA review, bear a claim that they can prevent, treat, cure, mitigate, or diagnose a disease.*

Drugs used as traditional medicines are sometimes derived from plants. However, before marketing, they must undergo extensive clinical studies to determine their effectiveness, safety, possible interactions, and appropriate dosages before FDA approval. *The FDA does not authorize or test dietary supplements.*

Dietary supplements are available in many forms, including tablets, capsules, powders, softgels, gelcaps, and liquids. Though commonly associated with health food stores, dietary supplements also are sold in grocery, drug, and national discount chain stores, as well as through mail-order catalogs, TV programs, the Internet, and direct sales.

Under DSHEA, once a dietary supplement is marketed, the FDA has the responsibility for showing that a dietary supplement is *unsafe* before it can take action to restrict the product's use. This was the case when, in June 1997, the FDA proposed, among other things, to limit the amount of ephedrine alkaloids in dietary supplements (marketed as, e.g., ephedra, ma huang, and epitonin) and provide warnings to consumers about the hazards associated with the use of dietary supplements containing these ingredients. The hazards ranged from nervousness, dizziness, and changes in blood pressure and heart rate to chest pain, heart attack, hepatitis, stroke, seizures, psychosis, and death. The proposal stemmed from the FDA's review of adverse event reports it had received, scientific literature, and public comments. Finally, in 2004, the FDA announced a ban on the weight-loss aid ephedra. However, there are numerous other dangerous supplements still on the market.

In September 2010, *Consumer Reports* identified a dozen supplements that according to government warnings and adverse-event reports were too dangerous to be on the market. However, the following unsafe supplements were still available at that time in retail stores or by shopping online: *germanium* (linked to kidney failure and death); *yohimbe* (linked to heart and blood pressure problems); *bitter orange* (linked to arrhythmias, heart attacks, and stroke); and *chapparal, comfrey,* and *kava* (linked to liver failure). These products and others listed in *Consumer Reports'* "dirty dozen" (*Dangerous Supplements*) can have many other trade names. For details, consult *Natural Medicines Comprehensive Database.*

Fraudulent Products

Consumers need to be on the lookout for fraudulent products. These are products that don't do what they say they can or don't contain what they say they contain. At the very least, they waste consumers' money, and they may cause physical harm. Fraudulent products often can be identified by the types of claims made in their labeling, advertising, and promotional literature. Some possible indicators of fraud, says Stephen Barrett, M.D., a board member of the National Council Against Health Fraud, are as follows:

- Claims that the product is a secret cure and use of such terms as *breakthrough, magical, miracle cure,* and *new discovery.* "If the product were a cure for a serious disease, it would be widely reported in the media and used by health care professionals," he says.

- Claims that a product is backed by scientific studies, but with no list of references or references that are inadequate. For instance, if a list of references is provided, the citations cannot be traced, or if the references are traceable, the studies are out of date, irrelevant, or poorly designed.

Quality Products

The growing market for supplements, with fewer regulations, creates the potential for quality-control problems. For example, the FDA has identified several manufacturers that were buying herbs, plants, and other ingredients without first adequately testing them to determine whether the product they ordered was actually what they received or whether the ingredients were free from contaminants and were of the strength stated.

To help protect themselves, consumers should:

- Look for ingredients in products with the U. S. Pharmacopeia (USP) notation, which indicates that the manufacturer followed the standards established by the USP.
- Realize that the label term *natural* doesn't guarantee that a product is safe. "Think of poisonous mushrooms," says Elizabeth Yetley, Ph.D., Director of FDA's Office of Special Nutritionals. "They're natural."
- Consider the name of the manufacturer or distributor. Supplements made by a nationally known food and drug manufacturer, for example, have been made under tight controls because these companies already have in place manufacturing standards for their other products.
- Write to the supplement manufacturer for more information. Ask the company about the conditions under which its products were made.
- Avoid products sold for considerably less money than competing brands.

Reading and Reporting

Consumers who use dietary supplements should always read product labels, follow directions, and heed all warnings.

Supplement users who suffer from a serious harmful effect or illness that they think is related to the use of supplements should call a physician or other health care professional. He or she, in turn, can report it to the FDA MedWatch by calling 1-800-FDA-1088 or on the MedWatch website at https://www.accessdata.fda.gov /scripts /medwatch/medwatch-online.htm. Patients' names are kept confidential.

Much regarding the health benefits and potential risks about many dietary supplements remains unknown. Therefore, consumers who decide to take advantage of the expanding market should do so with care, making sure to have the necessary information and consulting with their physicians regarding any health conditions that could be compromised or any medications they are taking that may interact adversely with the herbs. "The majority of supplement manufacturers are responsible and careful," FDA's Yetley says. "But, as with all products on the market, consumers need to be discriminating. FDA and industry have important roles to play, but consumers must take responsibility, too."

Your responsibility as a health care professional includes warning your patients, and others who may seek your advice, regarding the dangers of taking products not approved by the FDA and not adequately tested. You must also caution them about the possibility of fraudulent products and lack of quality control. Most important, you must warn them about possible interactions with the medicines they are taking and the potential for serious adverse reactions. All of the herbal remedies on the market are too numerous to mention in this book. However, you will find some of the more popular ones, along with cautions or interactions known at this time, listed in Table 11-4. See Table 11-4 for a list of some herbs, possible uses, cautions, and interactions.

TABLE 11-4 **Herbs**

HERBS	POSSIBLE USES	POSSIBLE SIDE EFFECTS, CAUTIONS, AND INTERACTIONS
Ashwagandha	Used to improve thinking ability, decrease pain and swelling (inflammation), and prevent the effects of aging. Also used for fertility problems in men and women and to increase sexual desire	Short-term use only. Large doses may cause stomach upset, vomiting, and diarrhea. Interacts with thyroid medication. May increase the symptoms of autoimmune diseases. Do not use during pregnancy or lactation. Stop taking at least two weeks before surgery
Astragalus	Used alone or with other herbs to support or enhance the immune system	May interact with medications that suppress the immune system; may affect blood sugar levels and blood pressure. Some *Astragalus* species, normally not used in dietary supplements, may be toxic
Cascara sagrada	Relieves occasional constipation	Do not use if appendicitis, rectal bleeding, diarrhea, or a history of stomach or intestinal problems (e.g., blockage, inflammation, ulcers, Crohn's disease, bleeding, severe constipation) are present; if recent abdominal surgery has been performed; if pregnant or breast feeding; or if heart problems are present. Interacts with digoxin
Cat's claw	Anti-inflammatory used for osteoarthritis and rheumatoid arthritis; antiviral used for treatment of viral infections such as shingles and cold sores	Affect medications changed by the liver, medications that suppress the immune system, and antihypertensive medications. Take with caution; may cause hypotensive episodes. May worsen leukemia. May increase the symptoms of autoimmune diseases. Do not use if pregnant or breast-feeding. Stop taking two weeks before surgery
Cinnamon	Lowers blood sugar; alleviates gas and muscle and stomach spasms; prevents nausea, vomiting, diarrhea; used to treat infections, such as the common cold	Short-term use only. Unsafe when taken in large amounts or long term. May cause skin irritation or allergic reaction when applied to skin. Do not use if pregnant or breast-feeding. May affect blood sugar levels. Observe for hypoglycemia. Monitor blood sugar. May damage the liver. Do not use with liver disease. Interacts with antidiabetic medications. Stop taking two weeks before surgery
Cranberry	Antibacterial, prevents urinary tract infections (UTIs)	Do not use with active UTI
Chamomile	Sedative tea, prevents insomnia nausea	Those allergic to pollens, for example, ragweed, may be allergic to it

(continued)

TABLE 11-4 Herbs (*continued*)

HERBS	POSSIBLE USES	POSSIBLE SIDE EFFECTS, CAUTIONS, AND INTERACTIONS
Echinacea	Proven ineffective in 2005 studies for prevention and treatment of colds	Can cause allergies and rashes Contraindicated in those with autoimmune diseases, for example, human immunodeficiency virus, MS , or lupus, and chronic use, longer than eight weeks
Elderberry	Treatment of the flu; may reduce inflammation	Possibly safe when used for up to five days. Not for long-term use. Raw and unripe fruit may cause nausea, vomiting, and severe diarrhea. Do not use if pregnant or breast-feeding. May increase the symptoms of autoimmune diseases. May interact with medications that suppress the immune system
Fenugreek	May lower blood sugar, cholesterol, and triglycerides. May reduce symptoms of heart burn	Interacts with antidiabetic medications, warfarin, anticoagulants, and antiplatelets. Likely safe for people when taken by mouth in amounts normally found in foods. Side effects include diarrhea, stomach upset, bloating, gas, a "maple syrup" odor in urine. Likely unsafe for children or women who are pregnant or breast-feeding. Might cause early labor. May affect blood sugar levels in people with diabetes. Observe for signs of hypoglycemia. Monitor blood sugar carefully
Garlic	Taken to lower blood pressure and cholesterol Anti-infective, immune enhancing	Risk of bleeding with anticoagulants Nausea, vomiting, diarrhea, heartburn, and flatulence
Ginger	Prevents nausea, motion sickness	Doses higher than 6 g can cause gastric irritation
Ginkgo (GBE)	Used as antidepressant, anxiolytic, and antioxidant Proven ineffective in a 2008 study for prevention or slowing of dementia or Alzheimer's disease	May interact with anticoagulants to cause bleeding and strokes Rare GI upset, headache
Ginseng	Antistress, antifatigue agent	Not for long-term use May cause hypertension, nausea, vomiting, diarrhea, nervousness, mental changes Contraindicated in pregnancy
Glucosamine	Anti-inflammatory for arthritis	Elevated cholesterol Insulin resistance, higher blood glucose
Goldenseal	Antibacterial, antiparasitic agent	Short-term use only May cause nausea and vomiting May alter the way body processes medications Use with caution
Kava	FDA warning March 2002 Banned in Canada, Germany, South Africa, and Switzerland	Possible liver damage, often irreversible; deaths reported

(*continued*)

TABLE 11-4 **Herbs (*continued*)**

HERBS	POSSIBLE USES	POSSIBLE SIDE EFFECTS, CAUTIONS, AND INTERACTIONS
Milk thistle	Anti-inflammatory, liver protectant, aids in regeneration of liver cells	No harmful effects if taken at normal recommended doses
Peppermint	Treats indigestion and stomach upset, treats colds and congestion, and relieves pain when applied topically	Do not use in babies for it may cause choking Do not inhale for prolonged periods of time
Saw palmetto	Taken for benign prostatic hyperplasia (BPH) Antiandrogen	Rare GI upset See a physician for diagnosis and treatment
Turmeric	Taken for stomach upset, osteoarthritis	Usually does not cause significant side effects. May make gallbladder problems worse. May interact with anticoagulant/antiplatelet drugs. Do not take if pregnant or breast-feeding. Stop taking two weeks before surgery
Valerian	Taken for anxiety, insomnia	Morning-after drowsiness Avoid during pregnancy Short-term use only

PATIENT EDUCATION

Dietary Supplements

Patients should be instructed regarding the following:

- Consulting a physician or pharmacist before taking any "herbal remedies." Some herbs may be contraindicated with certain diagnoses.
- Taking a list of all products you are using, including herbal remedies, herbal teas, vitamins and minerals, OTC (nonprescription) medicines, and prescription drugs, to a physician or pharmacist. Many of these products can interact, with dangerous, even life-threatening, results. Consulting a physician is important before starting any "alternative medicines." Do not mix prescription drugs and herbal remedies for the same condition.
- The fact that "natural" does not mean "safe."
- Not taking more than the recommended amount listed on the label. Even vitamins and minerals in excess of the RDA or DRI can cause serious problems. Herbs that may be safe in small

doses could be harmful at larger doses or over a prolonged period of time. Products without dosage recommendations should be avoided.
- All products should carry a lot number, expiration date, and manufacturer's name, address, and phone number. Products should be *avoided* that lack this information or that claim an effect on the body's structure or function, or claim to be able to cure a disease or condition.
- Storing herbal products away from young children and pets.
- Not using herbal products for children without the approval of a pediatrician.
- Not using herbal remedies if you are pregnant, trying to become pregnant, or nursing.
- Not taking these products with alcohol without first determining the safety of such a combination.
- Not using these products as a substitute for proper rest and nutrition. A balanced diet is necessary for good health.

SUGGESTED READINGS

Medical Corps Pharmacy. *Common herbal medications: Cranberry*. Retrieved November 5, 2012, from http://www.medicalcorps.org/pharmacy/Herbals.htm

Medical Corps Pharmacy. *Common herbal medications: Peppermint*. Retrieved November 5, 2012, from http://www.medicalcorps.org/pharmacy/Herbals.htm

National Center for Complementary and Integrative Health. *Complimentary, alternative or integrative health: What's in a name?* Retrieved August 1, 2016 from https://nccih.nih.gov/health/integrative-health

National Center for Complementary and Alternative Medicine. *Get the facts: Using dietary supplements wisely*. Retrieved November 5, 2012, from http://nccam.nih.gov /health/supplements/wiseuse.htm

U.S. Food and Drug Administration (April 2005). *Dietary supplements*. Retrieved August 1, 2016, from http://www.fda.gov/Food/DietarySupplements/default .htm / WebMD. *Find a vitamin or supplement: Ashwagandha*. Retrieved November 12, 2012, from http://www.webmd.com/vitamins-supplements /ingredientmono-953-ASHWAGANDHA.aspx?activeIngredientId=953&active IngredientName=ASHWAGANDHA&source=3

WebMD. *Find a vitamin or supplement: Cassis cinnamon*. Retrieved November 9, 2012, from http://www.webmd.com/vitamins-supplements/ingredientmono-1002-CASSIA+CINNAMON.aspx?activeIngredientId=1002&activeIngredient Name= CASSIA+CINNAMON&source=3

WebMD. *Find a vitamin or supplement: Cat's claw*. Retrieved November 9, 2012, from http://www.webmd.com/vitamins-supplements/ingredientmono-395-CAT'S+CLAW.aspx?activeIngredientId=395&activeIngredientName=CAT'S+ CLAW&source=3

WebMD. *Find a vitamin or supplement: Elderberry*. Retrieved November 12, 2012, from http://www.webmd.com/vitamins-supplements/ingredientmono-434-ELDERBERRY.aspx?activeIngredientId=434&activeIngredientName=ELDER-BERRY&source=3

WebMD. *Find a vitamin or supplement: Fenugreek*. Retrieved November 12, 2012, from http://www.webmd.com/vitamins-supplements/ingredientmono-733-FENUGREEK.aspx?activeIngredientId=733&activeIngredientName=FENU-GREEK&source=3

WebMD. *Find a vitamin or supplement: Turmeric*. Retrieved November 12, 2012, from http://www.webmd.com/vitamins-supplements/ingredientmono-662-TURMERIC.aspx?activeIngredientId=662&activeIngredientName= TURMERIC&source=3

CASE STUDY A

Water-Soluble Vitamins

Jeanne Kim is a 37-year-old pregnant female. She is at her OB-GYN physician's office for a 16-week checkup.

1. The physician is reviewing Jeanne's diet and inquires about her intake of folic acid. She explains that a deficiency in folic acid during pregnancy can result in which condition in newborns?
   a. Cerebral palsy
   b. Cardiac malformations
   c. Spina bifida
   d. Seizures

2. Which of the following foods is richest in folic acid?
   a. Radishes
   b. Black beans
   c. Broccoli
   d. Alfalfa sprouts

3. Why is folic acid a necessary supplement for Jeanne?
   a. For the production of RBCs
   b. For fat metabolism
   c. For cell mitosis
   d. For the destruction of white blood cells (WBCs)

4. Which of the following is a sign that Jeanne might have a folic acid deficiency?
   a. Weight gain
   b. Muscle cramps
   c. Pale sclera
   d. Weight loss

5. The physician cautions Jeanne about the amount of daily folic acid supplementation. What should she recommend as the maximum amount of folic acid intake per day?
   a. 0.4 mg
   b. 0.8 mg
   c. 1.2 mg
   d. 5 mg

CASE STUDY B

Minerals

Seventy-three-year old Jose Velasquez has started taking a loop diuretic to reduce his elevated blood pressure.

1. While taking this specific high blood pressure medication, Jose is at risk for developing a deficiency in which mineral?
   a. Potassium (K)
   b. Chloride (Cl)
   c. Calcium (Ca)
   d. Iron (Fe)

2. Which of the following may result from a deficiency of K?
   a. Anorexia
   b. Muscular weakness
   c. Hypothermia
   d. Constipation

3. The physician determines that Jose needs a potassium supplement but emphasizes that Jose should take the correct dose of K to avoid a potassium overdose. What is one symptom of K overdose?
   a. Hypokalemia
   b. Shortness of breath
   c. Urinary retention
   d. Cardiac arrest

4. While taking a potassium supplement, Jose experiences some GI distress. When should he take the K+ to minimize these GI side effects?
   a. With or after meals
   b. Just before bed
   c. Upon rising in the morning
   d. Two hours prior to a meal

5. Which of the following will provide Jose with the best source of K?
   a. Carrot salad
   b. Broccoli rabe saute
   c. Fruit salad
   d. Green beans

CHAPTER REVIEW QUIZ

Multiple Choice

1. Antioxidants
   a. Are safe to take in megadoses
   b. Consist of proteins, carbohydrates, and fats
   c. Are found only in synthetic products
   d. Fight against the destructive effects of free radicals

2. Free radical damage can be associated with
   a. Stunted growth
   b. Glaucoma
   c. Heart disease
   d. Grand mal seizure

3. Which of the following is an antioxidant vitamin?
   a. Calcium
   b. Beta carotene
   c. Folate
   d. Niacin

4. Which of the following is an antioxidant mineral?
   a. Potassium
   b. Sodium
   c. Zinc
   d. Iron

5. Signs of a vitamin A deficiency may include which of the following?
   a. Watery eyes
   b. Night blindness
   c. Weight gain
   d. Accelerated growth

6. When buying dietary supplements, you should look for which term on the label?
   a. Natural
   b. FDA
   c. USP
   d. New discovery

7. Which of the following herbs can interact with anticoagulants to cause bleeding?
   a. Cranberry and milk thistle
   b. Garlic and ginkgo
   c. Saw palmetto and glucosamine
   d. Ginseng and echinacea

8. Glucosamine
   a. Is always combined with chondroitin
   b. Has no known side effects
   c. Can elevate cholesterol level
   d. Counteracts thyroid medicine

9. Garlic
   a. Lowers blood pressure and cholesterol level
   b. Helps to control menopause symptoms
   c. Alleviates symptoms of depression
   d. Was banned by the FDA due to the danger of heart problems and stroke

10. Ginseng
    a. Interacts with oral contraceptives
    b. Has no known side effects
    c. Causes liver damage
    d. May cause hypertension, mental changes, and nervousness

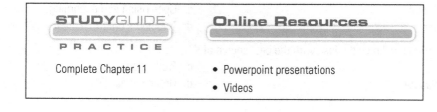

STUDYGUIDE	Online Resources
PRACTICE	
Complete Chapter 11	• Powerpoint presentations
	• Videos

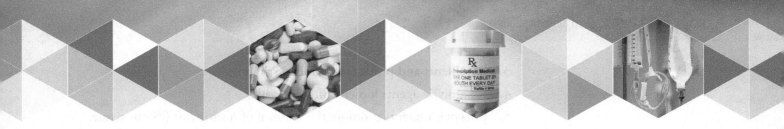

CHAPTER 12
SKIN MEDICATIONS

KEY TERMS AND CONCEPTS

Antifungals

Antipruritics

Antiseptics

Antiviral

Bactericidal

Emollients

Keratolytics

Protectants

OBJECTIVES

Upon completion of this chapter, the learner should be able to

1. Describe application procedures for various skin medications
2. Identify indication, side effects, and precautions or contraindications of the nine major categories of skin medications
3. Compare and contrast scabicides and pediculicides
4. Explain the factors that influence the absorption of skin medications
5. Classify drugs according to their action: antipruritic, emollient, keratolytic, enzymatic, antifungal, anti-infective, or agents to treat burns and acne
6. List five possible side effects of long-term topical corticosteroid therapy
7. List five precautions or contraindications for topical corticosteroid therapy
8. Describe proper selection and application of sunscreen products
9. Describe important patient education for all skin medications described in this chapter
10. Define the Key Terms and Concepts

The skin is the largest organ of the body. Because such a great area is involved, many conditions can affect the skin, causing annoyance and discomfort. Skin ailments can range from minor ones, such as pruritus (itching), to major ones, such as severe burns. Treatment is usually topical or local (applied to the affected area), but skin conditions are sometimes treated internally with oral medications or injections for their systemic effects.

This chapter primarily explains topical medications. Medications given parenterally or orally to relieve inflammation or itching, such as corticosteroids and antihistamines, are discussed more extensively in other chapters.

Topical skin preparations can be classified into nine principal categories according to their action:

1. Antipruritics relieve itching.
2. Corticosteroids treat dermatological disorders associated with allergic reactions.

3. Emollients and protectants soothe irritation.

4. Keratolytic agents loosen epithelial scales.

5. Enzymatic agents promote the removal of necrotic or fibrous tissue.

6. Scabicides and pediculicides treat scabies or lice.

7. Local anti-infectives prevent and treat fungal, bacterial, and viral infections.

8. Burn medications to prevent or treat infections.

9. Agents that treat acne.

Factors that influence the rate of absorption of topical medication include condition and location of the skin, heat, and moisture. If the skin is thick and callused, absorption will be slower. If the skin is moist, macerated (raw), or warm, absorption will be more rapid. Sometimes, the physician will order that the skin be premoistened or a plastic wrap be applied over the ointment to aid absorption; in other cases, the skin must be left exposed to the air to slow absorption and reduce systemic effects. At times, the length of time for the medication to remain on the skin is very important. Complete understanding of appropriate directions for each topical medication is vital before administration.

ANTIPRURITICS

Antipruritics are used short term to relieve discomfort from dermatitis (rashes) associated with allergic reactions, poison ivy, hives, and insect bites. They relieve itching by the use of products, singly or in combination, containing:

- Local anesthetics (e.g., the "-caines," such as benzocaine, dibucaine).
- Drying agents (e.g., calamine).
- Anti-inflammatory agents (e.g., corticosteroids) applied locally or given PO for systemic effect. Use should be avoided in patients with pruritus without inflammation. Topical agents are preferred because of fewer adverse effects.
- Antihistamines administered PO for systemic effect (antihistamines applied topically can cause hypersensitivity reactions—use only a few days).

See Chapter 26 for further information on antihistamines.

Side effects of antipruritics can include:

⊘ Skin irritation, rash

    Stinging and a burning sensation

⊘ Allergic reactions (especially with the "-caines")

    Seizures and heart rhythm problems with topical anesthetics when used on broken skin or in large amounts.

⊘ Sedation from antihistamines PO or paradoxical agitation in children.

    Nonsedating antihistamines may be as effective as sedating antihistamines in the treatment of pruritus.

Precautions or contraindications for antipruritics include:

>   Delayed healing—on open wounds for corticosteroids

>   Prolonged use (especially corticosteroids)

>   Hypersensitivity (severe allergic) reaction to the active drug or any component of the formulation

Figure 12-1 shows contact dermatitis conditions where antipruritics would be indicated.

FIGURE 12-1 (A) Allergic contact dermatitis and (B) poison ivy with fluid-filled vesicles. Courtesy of the Centers for Disease Control and Prevention/Richard S. Hibbits.

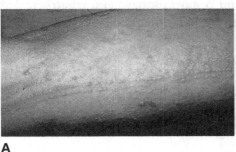
A

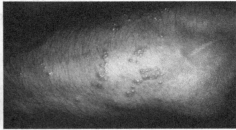
B

PATIENT EDUCATION

Patients being treated with antipruritics should be instructed to:

  Clean area thoroughly before application

  Rub in gently until the medication vanishes

  Use caution if they have allergies

  Avoid contact of the medication with eyes or mucous membranes

  Avoid covering the area with dressings unless directed by the physician

  Avoid prolonged use (not longer than one week)

  Discontinue if condition worsens or irritation develops

  Trim children's fingernails to reduce the possibility of infection from scratching

CORTICOSTEROIDS

The corticosteroids are used *both topically and systemically* to treat dermatological disorders associated with allergic reactions. Most topical steroids are available in a variety of dosage forms and potencies (low, medium, high, and very high); the choice depends upon the area affected and the condition being treated. Topical corticosteroids are also used to treat psoriasis and seborrheic dermatitis.

See Chapter 23, "Endocrine System Drugs," for more in-depth information regarding corticosteroids.

Side effects of corticosteroid ointments and creams, especially used long term (e.g., psoriasis), can include:

>   ❗ Epidermal thinning, with frequent skin tears, increased risk of infection, and frequent bruising

>   ❗ Increased fragility of cutaneous blood vessels

>   Irritation, burning, or stinging

>   Ulceration, especially with occlusive dressings

>   ❗ Activation of latent infections and slow healing

>   Hyperglycemia, glycosuria, and Cushing's syndrome, with *prolonged use* of *very high-potency* products

Precautions or contraindications for corticosteroids include:

Skin infections, bacterial or fungal, and cutaneous (skin) or systemic viral infections

Open wounds

Abrupt discontinuation of very high-potency products used for a long period of time

Hypersensitivity (severe allergic) reaction to the active drug or any component of the formulation

Figures 12-2A and B show psoriasis and seborrheic dermatitis conditions where topical corticosteriods would be indicated.

FIGURE 12-2 (A) Psoriasis, a chronic skin disorder with red papules and covered with silvery scales. (B) Seborrheic dermatitis of the face showing crusting over of a red scaly, itchy rash (seborrhea) of the face. Christine Langer-Pueschel/www.Shutterstock.com. Dr. P. Marazzi/Science Source.

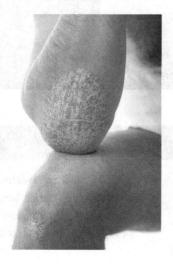

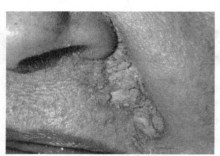

A   **B**

EMOLLIENTS AND PROTECTANTS

Emollients and **protectants** are used topically to soothe, soften, protect, and seal out wetness in minor dermatological conditions, such as diaper rash, irritation, abrasions, and minor burns. Their purpose is to moisten the skin; this is achieved by utilizing a lipid barrier that does not let moisture out of the skin. In many cases, emollients are used as first-line therapy in eczema and other conditions, which helps to avoid the need for corticosteroid or other medication use.

KERATOLYTICS

Keratolytic agents, for example salicylic acid, are used to control conditions of abnormal scaling of the skin, such as dandruff, seborrhea, and psoriasis, or to promote peeling of the skin in conditions such as acne, hard corns, calluses, and warts.

Antifungals are also used at times for seborrheic dermatitis and dandruff.

Side effects can include:

❗ Severe skin irritation, pruritus, or stinging

❗ Irritation to eyes or mucous membranes

! Photosensitivity

! Systemic effects in allergic individuals or with multiple applications and prolonged use (e.g., headache and gastrointestinal [GI] symptoms)

Precautions or contraindications for keratolytics include:

Open areas of the skin

Hypersensitivity (severe allergic) reaction to the active drug or any component of the formulation

Figures 12-3A and B show common and plantar warts, conditions where keratolytic agents would be indicated.

FIGURE 12-3 (A) Common wart. (B) Plantar wart. Courtesy of Robert A. Silverman, M.D., Clinical Associate Professor, Department of Pediatrics, Georgetown University.

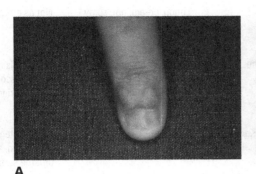

A

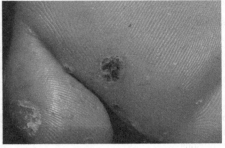

B

PATIENT EDUCATION

Patients being treated with keratolytics should be instructed to:

Use only as directed, and for the entire treatment period, even if the condition improves

Avoid contact with eyes and mucous membranes

Avoid prolonged use

Discontinue and seek medical aid if irritation occurs

Avoid contact with surrounding tissues when applied as a caustic agent to warts, corns, or calluses

ENZYME PREPARATIONS

Bedridden patients are prone to decubitus ulcers (pressure sores), and diabetic patients are prone to develop foot ulcers. These ulcerations produce necrotic (dead) skin that must be removed to promote proper healing. Collagenase (Santyl) is a topical enzyme ointment used for the chemical debridement (removal of dead or damaged tissue) of dermal ulcers and burns. Collagenase should be used only on wounds associated with necrotic material. If a topical antibiotic is to be applied to an infected site, the antibiotic is applied before collagenase. Avoid using detergents, povidone–iodine, and heavy metal (e.g., mercury, silver)–containing agents, which will inhibit the enzymatic activity of collagenase.

See Table 12-1 for antipruritics, emollients and protectants, keratolytics, and enzyme preparations.

TABLE 12-1 Topical Medications for the Skin: Antipruritics, Emollients and Protectants, Keratolytics, and Enzymatics

GENERIC NAME	TRADE NAME	AVAILABLE AS	COMMENTS
Antipruritics			
Local anesthetics			
benzocaine	Lanacane, Americaine, Orajel	Ointment, spray, gel, lotion, cream, liquid, lozenge	Can cause hypersensitivity reaction
dibucaine	Nupercainal	Ointment	Potential for hypersensitivity
Antihistamine			
diphenhydramine	Benadryl	Lotion, cream, gel, spray	Not as effective as oral
Corticosteroids			
Very high potency betamethasone	Diprolene, Temovate, others	Ointment, cream, lotion, solution, gel, foam, shampoo (formulations available in all potencies)	Duration is maximum two to four weeks—do not discontinue abruptly if used for a long period of time; avoid occlusive dressings
Various other potencies (high, medium, low) hydrocortisone	Cortaid, Topicort, Lidex, Kenalog, Synalar, others	Ointment, cream	Lower potency agents preferred for the face, groin, armpits, skin folds, or treatment of large surface area
Emollients and protectants			
ammonium lactate	AmLactin, Lac-Hydrin	Cream, lotion	Moistening, rehydrating agent; also used in sunscreen products
vitamins A and D	A & D Ointment	Ointment	
	Desitin (with zinc oxide)	Ointment	
zinc oxide	Balmex	Cream, ointment	
Keratolytics			
coal tar	Balnetar, Polytar, Neutrogena T/Gel	Shampoo, oil, cream, lotion, ointment, soap, solution	For dandruff, seborrheic dermatitis, or psoriasis (stains clothing)
salicylic acid	Clearasil, Fostex, Compound W	Cream, liquid, gel, patches	For dandruff, psoriasis, acne, warts, corns, calluses
sulfur	Many combinations with other keratolytics	Cream, lotion, soap, gel, solution, pads	For acne, scabies, seborrheic dermatitis
Enzyme preparations			
collagenase	Santyl	Ointment	For use only on necrotic skin tissue

Note: This table lists only typical medications and does not include all of those on the market.

SCABICIDES AND PEDICULICIDES

MEDIALINK

See it in Action! View
the **Ointments** video on
the Online Resources.

Scabies is caused by an itch mite that burrows under the skin. Pediculosis is caused by infestation of lice on the hairs of the scalp, pubic area, and trunk. Both are easily transmitted from one person to another by direct contact or through contact with contaminated clothing or bed linens. Effective treatment includes laundering in hot water or dry cleaning all clothing and bedding. Sometimes concurrent treatment of close contacts is recommended.

Scabicides (permethrin 5% or lindane lotion) must be applied *according to directions* on the package insert, left in place the required period of time (usually 8–14 h), and then rinsed thoroughly. One application is generally curative although some experts recommend two applications separated from the first by one or two weeks. This second application serves to eliminate any remaining scabies, or any that were retransmitted from linens that were missed or not thoroughly washed.

Pediculicides, for example, permethrin 1% and lindane shampoo, are used in the topical treatment of lice infestations. Pyrethrins (e.g., RID shampoo) are considered safer for pediculosis, although a repeat treatment after 7–10 days is needed.

Side effects, rare when applied topically according to directions, may include:

Slight local irritation, rash, or conjunctivitis

Dermatitis with frequent application

However, with excessive or prolonged use, or with oral ingestion or inhalation of vapors, central nervous system (CNS) symptoms and hepatic or renal toxicity may occur. Anemia and seizures have been reported, especially with the use of lindane. Therefore, lindane should be used only in patients who cannot tolerate or have failed first-line treatment for lice with safer medications.

Precautions or contraindications include:

Acutely inflamed, raw, or weeping surfaces

Because lindane can be absorbed systemically following topical application, it should be avoided during pregnancy and lactation or with infants, children, older adults, those who weigh less than 110 pounds; or those with known uncontrolled seizure disorders.

However, permethrin is a safer alternative under these conditions for scabies. Pyrethrins (e.g., RID) are a safer alternative than lindane for pediculosis.

Because of the toxicity of lindane, the oral antiparasitic agent ivermectin (Stromectol) has been used successfully as an alternative (off-label) to treat mass scabies outbreaks in an institutional setting and to treat head lice resistant to standard therapies. It is given orally as a single dose (weight-based), with a repeat dose 10–14 days later. Recently, the Food and Drug Administration (FDA) approved a topical ivermectin lotion (Sklice) for the treatment of head lice in patients age six months or older. The lotion treats lice in most patients with a single 10-min application to dry hair without nit combing.

Figure 12-4A shows scabies, a condition where scabicides would be indicated, and Figure 12-4B shows the scabies mite. Figure 12-4C shows lice infestation, a condition where pediculicides would be indicated.

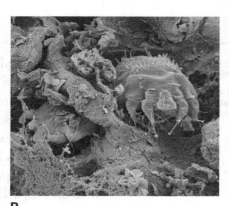

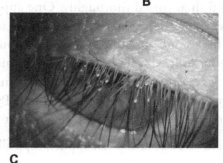

FIGURE 12-4 (A) Scabies skin infection (B) and the scabies mite. (C) Lice infestation of the eyelash hairs. Courtesy of the Centers for Disease and Prevention/Joe Miller; Eye of Science/Science Source; and Paul Parker/Science Source.

PATIENT EDUCATION

Patients being treated with scabicides or pediculicides should be instructed to:

Follow directions carefully (read and understand the medication guide dispensed with the lindane prescription); itching may still occur after the successful killing of lice and is not necessarily an indication for retreatment with lindane shampoo

Thoroughly launder (130°F) clothing and bedding and dry using the hot cycle of a dryer for at least 20 min

Large items (e.g., pillows, comforters) may be bagged in plastic for two weeks

Use caution to prevent accidental oral ingestion

Use caution with infants who might suck their thumbs

Inform sexual partner if the condition is present in the pubic area

Alert the school if head lice infestation occurs

LOCAL ANTI-INFECTIVES

Local anti-infectives are used to treat diseases caused by microorganisms. These diseases include fungal, viral, and bacterial diseases of the skin.

Antifungals

Antifungals, for example, nystatin, are useful in the treatment of fungal infections (candidiasis), such as thrush, diaper rash, and vaginitis. Other antifungals such as clotrimazole (Lotrimin) are used to treat fungal infections such as athlete's foot, body ringworm, and jock itch. Antifungals are also combined with corticosteroids, for example, Lotrisone (betamethasone/clotrimazole) and Mycolog II (nystatin/triamcinolone), but these products are not recommended by dermatologists.

Effective treatment includes topical administration according to directions on the package insert and good hygiene practices, including washing, drying, and exposing to air when possible.

For the treatment of candidiasis of the oral cavity, a nystatin oral suspension administered four times daily or clotrimazole oral lozenges administered five times daily for 14 days are equally effective. Additionally, fluconazole oral tablets can be used, which would be dosed at 200 mg on the first day then 100 mg daily for two weeks. For infants, administer after the feeding, which is followed by water to rinse the mouth *before therapy*. Place one-half dose in each side of the mouth. For adults, apply *after meals* and *after rinsing* of the mouth. Then, the entire dose should be used to thoroughly coat inside the mouth, holding it for as long as possible (e.g., several minutes) before swallowing. In both cases, the patient should be NPO (nothing by mouth) for at least 1h after treatment.

With inadequate response to treatment, cultures should be obtained to confirm the diagnosis and assist in selecting the most appropriate medication.

Side effects, although rare, may include:

Contact dermatitis

Itching, burning, and irritation

Contraindication or caution applies to the use of vaginal preparations during pregnancy. Use these preparations only under medical supervision. Some products can cause fetal abnormalities.

PATIENT EDUCATION

Patients being treated with antifungals should be instructed to:

Carefully wash and *dry* affected areas.

Expose the affected areas to air whenever possible.

With genital fungus, avoid tight undergarments, pantyhose, and wet bathing suits.

With athlete's foot, use open sandals instead of sneakers.

Follow application instructions carefully. Use for the entire time, even if asymptomatic.

Remove any stains with soap and warm water.

Continue prescribed vaginal treatment even during menstruation, or if symptomatic relief occurs, until the entire regimen is completed.

Consult a physician before vaginal preparations are used during pregnancy.

For oral suspensions or lozenges, apply after meals and after thorough rinsing of mouth. No food or liquids should be taken for at least 1h after treatment.

For vaginal infections, refrain from intercourse until treatment is complete.

Consider treating partner if reinfection occurs.

Figure 12-5 shows various fungal infections where antifungals would be indicated.

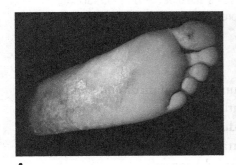
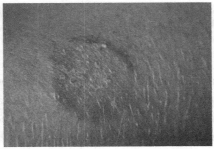
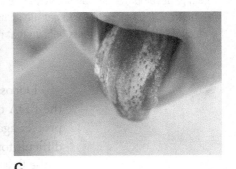

A   **B**   **C**

FIGURE 12-5 (A) Athlete's foot; medically known as tinea pedis. (B) Body ringworm; medically known as tinea corporis. (C) Thrush (yeast infection) of the tongue; medically known as candidiasis. Courtesy of the Centers for Disease Control and Prevention/Dr. Lucille K. Georg; Victoria 1/www.Shutterstock.com.

Antivirals

Acyclovir has an **antiviral** effect on herpes simplex (cold sores or genital herpes), herpes zoster (shingles), and varicella zoster (chickenpox) viruses. Acyclovir (Zovirax) is available in oral and parenteral preparations (see Chapter 17) or applied topically. Zovirax *cream* is indicated *only* for the treatment of cold sores. Topical therapy is substantially less effective than systemic therapy (parenteral or oral). Topical acyclovir therapy is *not a cure* and does not reduce the frequency or delay the appearance of new lesions. However, topical therapy generally decreases the duration of viral shedding, the duration of pain and itching, and the time required for crusting and healing of lesions. It is effective in first-episode genital herpes infection, but recurrent infections have shown little, if any, therapeutic benefit from topical therapy. The ointment should be applied as soon as possible following the onset of signs and symptoms of infections. Take care not to get the ointment in the eyes. It is *not effective in preventing infections.*

For more effective treatment of herpes zoster (shingles), acyclovir (Zovirax) is available orally. Valacyclovir (Valtrex) and famciclovir (Famvir) are derivatives of acyclovir and can be dosed less frequently, improving patient compliance. *All oral antivirals need to be started within 72h of rash onset and are most effective if started within the first 48h of onset.* (See Chapter 17 for a discussion regarding oral antivirals and a vaccine to prevent shingles.) If antivirals are not effective, or if the time frame for their effective use has passed, other oral medications can be used to treat the pain associated with the shingles rash. These range from anti-inflammatories like ibuprofen to opioids like Percocet or tramadol, and even medications that treat nerve pain such as Lyrica and gabapentin.

CLINICAL CONNECTION

Patient Education for Shingles

Shingles is a disease that is frequently misunderstood by patients. It is often believed that shingles rash can only occur once in a person's lifetime. This is not true. Therefore, it is important to educate patients who have had shingles that they are still at risk (and possibly greater risk) to develop the rash again. With this information, patients will be more likely to get the shingles (Zostavax) vaccine. Also, many patients believe that if they did not have (or do not remember having) the chicken pox, that they are not at risk to develop the shingles rash. Again, this is not true. Even in the unlikely case that they have not been exposed, receiving the Zostavax vaccine is still recommended and safe. Currently, the recommendation is that all patients 60 years and older receive the vaccine, but the FDA has approved it for use in all those 50 years and older.

Docosanol (Abreva) is the only over-the-counter (OTC) medication approved by the FDA to shorten the healing time and duration of cold sore symptoms. It helps protect against the herpes simplex virus by modifying the cell membrane, making it difficult for the virus to combine with and penetrate the cell. Apply docosanol as soon as the first symptoms (tingling, redness, bump, or itch) appear.

Figure 12-6 shows various viral skin infections where antivirals would be indicated.

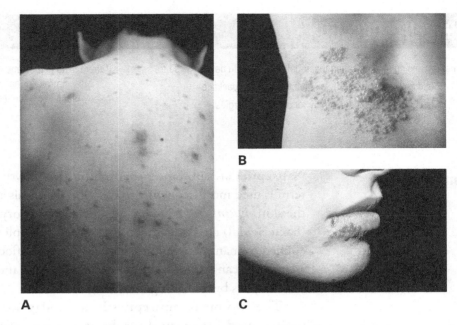

FIGURE 12-6 (A) Chickenpox caused by varicella zoster. (B) Shingles, a later eruption of the chickenpox virus as the herpes zoster virus. Note the characteristic "band" shape of the rash around the rib and trunk area. (C) Cold sores of the mouth caused by herpes simplex virus. Courtesy of the Centers for Disease Control and Prevention. adtapon duangnim/www.Shutterstock.com. Courtesy of the Centers for Disease Control and Prevention/Joe Miller.

Antibacterial Agents

Mupirocin (Bactroban) is an antibiotic that is structurally unrelated to any other topical or systemic antibiotics. Mupirocin ointment is used topically to treat impetigo caused by *Staphylococcus aureus* and certain species of *Streptococci*. The ointment is used to treat secondarily infected traumatic skin lesions. Mupirocin nasal ointment is applied intranasally to reduce the risk of infection in patients with high risk during institutional outbreaks of MRSA (methicillin-resistant strains of *S. aureus*).

There are many other prescription and OTC topical antibacterial agents on the market, including ointments, creams, and solutions too numerous to mention here. These products have the potential for adverse side effects, including local, hypersensitivity, and systemic reactions. Overuse or extended use of antibacterial agents can also lead to *resistance*. For further information regarding antibacterial agents, see Chapter 17, "Anti-Infective Drugs."

Figure 12-7 shows an impetigo infection, a condition where an antibacterial agent would be indicated.

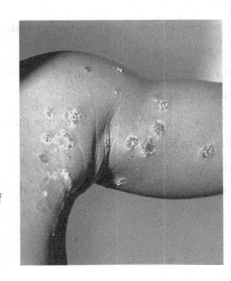

FIGURE 12-7 Impetigo is a highly contagious bacterial skin infection commonly found in children. Courtesy of Robert A. Silverman, M.D., Clinical Associate Professor, Department of Pediatrics, Georgetown University.

Antiseptics

Antiseptics are substances that inhibit the growth of bacteria (bacteriostatic). The term is used most frequently to describe chemicals applied to body tissues, especially the skin. *Disinfectants* are included in this category, but chemicals that kill bacteria (**bactericidal**) are frequently too strong to be applied to body tissues and are *usually* applied to inanimate objects, such as furniture, floors, and instruments. Sometimes a chemical can be used as an antiseptic on skin and also as a disinfectant on inanimate objects by increasing the strength.

The two major antiseptics in use today are chlorhexidine and povidone–iodine, used for surgical scrubs and as bacteriostatic skin cleansers. Prior to surgery, skin cleansing with chlorhexidine is preferred because of lower rates of surgical site infections compared to povidone–iodine. Some iodine preparations are also bactericidal and are used to treat superficial skin wounds and to disinfect the skin preoperatively. Chlorhexidine (Hibiclens) should not be used on wounds involving more than the superficial layers of the skin. It is important to rinse thoroughly after use.

Side effects of chlorhexidine can include:

- Dermatitis and irritation
- Photosensitivity (increased reaction such as burn from brief sun exposure)
- Allergic reactions, especially in the genital area

Side effects of povidone–iodine (Betadine) can include:

- Skin irritation or burns
- Allergic reactions

Precautions or contraindications for chlorhexidine include:

Pregnancy category B
Not for frequent use for total body bathing
Not for use in eyes and ears

Precautions or contraindications for povidone–iodine include:

Not for those allergic to iodine
Not for use on open wounds
Not for use in newborns (risk of iodine absorption)

PATIENT EDUCATION

Patients being treated with local anti-infectives should be instructed to:

Rinse chlorhexidine *thoroughly*

Avoid chlorhexidine for total body bathing or frequent use

Avoid use of chlorhexidine on open skin lesions, mucous membranes, and genital areas

Take care to avoid chlorhexidine or povidone–iodine in the eyes or ears; flush thoroughly

Use caution with povidone–iodine in anyone with allergies

See Table 12-2 for a summary of scabicides, pediculicides, antifungals, antivirals, antibacterials, and antiseptics.

TABLE 12-2 Medications for the Skin: Scabicides, Pediculicides, Antifungals, Antivirals, Antibacterials, and Antiseptics

GENERIC NAME	TRADE NAME	AVAILABLE	COMMENTS
Scabicides and Pediculicides			
permethrin	Acticin, Elimite	5% Cream (Rx)	Apply from head to feet, wash off after 8–14 h
		1% Lotion (OTC)	Apply to damp hair, to remain on for 10 min
lindane	Argocide	Lotion, shampoo	Second-line therapy due to toxic potential
pyrethrins	RID	Shampoo	For head lice only
ivermectin	Stomectol	3-mg tabs	For scabies/head lice
	Sklice	0.5% lotion	10-min application to dry hair
ANTI-INFECTIVES			
Antifungals[a]			
clotrimazole	(Mycelex)[b] Lotrimin Gyne-Lotrimin	Troches, cream, lotion, sol, vaginal cream	For oral, topical, or vaginal application
ketoconazole	Nizoral	Cream, 2% shampoo (Rx)	Topical antifungal, shampoo for dandruff
	Nizoral A-D	1% shampoo (OTC)	
miconazole	Monistat Lotrimin AF	Cream, gel, ointment Powder, spray	Also vaginal cream and suppositories
nystatin	(Mycostatin)[b]	Oral suspension, tabs, cream, ointment, vaginal tab, powder	Apply oral suspension or lozenges PC, then NPO 1 h
terbinafine	Lamisil AT Lamisil (Rx)	Cream, gel, spray tabs, granules	Oral form very effective for nail infections (onychomycosis)
tolnaftate	Tinactin	Aerosol spray, cream, powder, solution	Avoid inhaling spray or powder contact with eyes

(continued)

TABLE 12-2 **Medications for the Skin: Scabicides, Pediculicides, Antifungals, Antivirals, Antibacterials, and Antiseptics (*continued*)**

GENERIC NAME	TRADE NAME	AVAILABLE	COMMENTS
Antivirals			
acyclovir	Zovirax	Cream	For cold sores only: five times per day for four days
		Ointment, orally[a]	six times per day (q3h) for seven days
docosanol	Abreva	Cream	five times per day for 10 days max; wash hands before/after
Antibacterials			
mupirocin	Bactroban	2% cream, ointment	Avoid contact with eyes
Antiseptics			
chlorhexidine	Hibiclens	Solution, liquid, foam	Antimicrobial skin cleanser, surgical scrub; rinse thoroughly
	Peridex	Oral rinse for Tx of gingivitis	
povidone-iodine	Betadine	Aqueous solution, ointment, liquid scrub, spray	Bactericidal, antiseptic, surgical scrub; watch for allergies

[a]Oral preparations and dosing are discussed in Chapter 17.
[b]Brand name is no longer marketed, but the name is still commonly used.
Note: Other preparations are available. This is a representative list.

BURN MEDICATIONS

Burns are injuries to the skin and tissues below the skin that are caused by heat from flames, hot liquids, steam, heated objects, chemicals, friction, electricity, radiation, or the sun. They are usually classified as first-, second-, or third-degree burns, depending upon their severity and the depth to which tissues have been damaged (Figure 12-8). In addition, another classification method describes their depth of penetration of the skin layers.

Burn treatments include topical application of medications to prevent or treat infections associated with the damaged skin. The two most commonly used agents for this purpose in second- and third-degree burns are silver sulfadiazine (Silvadene) and mafenide (Sulfamylon). These agents should be applied with a sterile-gloved hand.

Side effects of burn medications can include:

- ❗ Pain, burning, and itching
- ❗ Allergic reactions
- Staining of the skin temporarily

Precautions or contraindications apply to newborns or to patients with:

Impaired kidney or liver function (cumulative effects)

History of allergy, especially to sulfa drugs

Do not use silver sulfadiazine with collagenase or trypsin-containing enzymatic debriding agents—silver will inactivate these enzymes

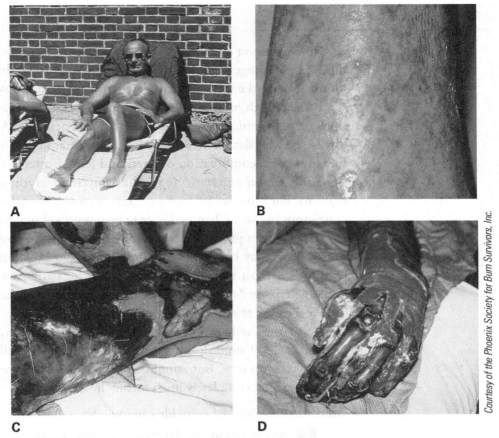

Courtesy of the Phoenix Society for Burn Survivors, Inc.

FIGURE 12-8 Examples of varying degrees of burns. (A) first degree, superficial; (B) second degree, partial thickness; (C) third degree, full thickness; and (D) third degree, full thickness.

PATIENT EDUCATION

Patients using burn medications should be instructed to:

Use aseptic technique to prevent infection

Watch for allergic reactions

Keep careful intake and output record

Keep the affected area covered at all times with cream and sterile dressing

Sunscreens

Nearly every person has experienced the pain of sunburn at some point. Overexposure to the sun is considered to be the primary cause of skin cancer, which is the most common form of all cancers in the United States, with more than one million new cases diagnosed each year. Ultraviolet (UV) radiation is a type of invisible light emitted by the sun and can be divided into two types: UVA and UVB.

Sun protection factor (SPF) is a measure of the protection a sunscreen offers. Only broad-spectrum sunscreens (both UVA and UVB) with an SPF value ≥30 can claim to reduce the risk of skin cancer and early skin aging if used as directed with other skin protection measures. Those measures include applying sunscreen to dry skin at least 15 to 30 min prior to sun exposure, limiting sun exposure (especially between 10 A.M. and 4 P.M.), wearing sun-protective clothing, use of water-resistant sunscreens when swimming or sweating, and reapplying at least every 2h (even on cloudy days).

AGENTS USED TO TREAT ACNE

Acne is a common condition of the skin that affects almost everyone to some degree during the teenage years and even some people into adulthood. Acne is most commonly seen on the face, scalp, neck, chest, back, and shoulders.

Patients with mild acne may choose from several *nonprescription topical* medications such as sulfur, salicylic acid, and benzoyl peroxide. A patient with more severe disease or who desires treatment from a dermatologist may be prescribed topical therapy with a combination of a retinoid (e.g., isotretinoin—decreases oil production) and *topical antibiotics* (e.g., clindamycin or erythromycin—decrease inflammation). For more severe forms of acne, a course of *oral antibiotics* (tetracyclines or erythromycin—see Chapter 17) may be prescribed in addition to topical products. For patients who produce too much male hormones, *systemic female hormones* (*birth control pills*) may be of benefit. Retinoids taken by mouth (e.g., isotretinoin) are used for the most severe forms of acne and for patients who fail other treatments. (The *Isotretinoin Medication Guide* describes treatment with cautions regarding possible severe side effects.)

Accutane, a retinoid prescribed to treat type 4 acne, was taken off the market in November 2009 amid signs the drug may be linked to inflammatory bowel disease. Generic versions (e.g., isotretinoin) are still available; however, they may be removed from the market completely upon further investigation.

Side effects of benzoyl peroxide can include:

⚠ Skin irritation, mild stinging, redness, dry skin

Precautions for benzoyl peroxide include:

Pregnancy, breast-feeding

Use in patients with skin diseases (dermatitis, eczema, sunburn, etc.) may increase the risk of skin irritation

Benzoic acid or paraben hypersensitivity

Avoid exposure to the eyes or mucous membranes; can cause severe irritation

See Table 12-3 for burn medications and acne medications.
Figure 12-9 shows the skin condition of acne.

PATIENT EDUCATION

Patients being treated with acne agents should be instructed to:

Use preparations every day as directed; often these agents take several weeks to be effective (your acne may actually get worse during the first few weeks of treatment, then start to improve)

Do not use benzoyl peroxide with other topical acne products or retinoids

Avoid prolonged exposure to sunlight (UV)—use sunscreen and protective clothing; avoid drugs such as sulfas that make you more sensitive to the sun

Avoid multivitamins or nutritional supplements that contain vitamin A, tetracycline antibiotics, certain antacids (aluminum hydroxide), and certain birth control pills (progestin-only) while taking isotretinoin

Make sure you receive, read, and understand the *Isotretinoin Medication Guide* every time you get a prescription or refill

TABLE 12-3   **Medications for the Skin: Burn Medications and Acne Medications**

GENERIC NAME	BRAND NAME	AVAILABLE AS	COMMENTS
Burn Medications			
silver sulfadiazine	Silvadene, SSD	Cream	Watch for sulfa allergies
mafenide	Sulfamylon	Cream, powder for solution	Use with caution in sulfa-allergic patients
Acne Medications			
benzoyl peroxide	Panoxyl, others	Bar, cream, gel, liquid, lotion, foam	Antibacterial activity. Drying actions, for type 1 acne
isotretinoin	Claravis	10-, 20-, 30-, 40-mg caps	Absolutely contraindicated in pregnancy, for type 4 acne
salicylic acid	Clearasil, Neutrogena	Cream, liquid, gel, pads	mild acne
sulfur	Many combinations with other keratolytics	Cream, lotion, gel, pads, soap	mild acne
tretinoin	Retin-A	Cream, gel	Increases sensitivity to the sun

Note: Other preparations are available. This is a representative list.

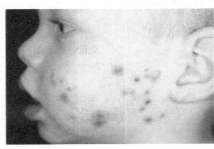 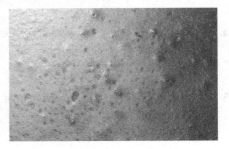

FIGURE 12-9 (A) Acne papules and nodules and (B) acne scarring. Courtesy of Robert A. Silverman, M.D., Clinical Associate Professor, Department of Pediatrics, Georgetown University.

A   **B**

CAUTIONS FOR TOPICAL MEDICATIONS

Skin medications by prescription or OTC are too numerous to mention. Many patients use products without adequate instruction in administration, side effects, or precautions. The health care professional has a responsibility to advise patients whenever possible to use great caution with self-medication to avoid ineffective or dangerous treatment. Both the health care professional and the layperson should *read instructions completely* before administration of any medication.

PATIENT EDUCATION

Patients using topical medications should be instructed regarding:

Even though these products are not in a pill form or may not require a prescription (in some cases), this does not mean they cannot cause harm if overused or misused

Never taking by mouth

Keeping out of reach of children

Being sure labels are not obscured and are read completely

Avoiding application to broken skin unless instructed otherwise

Discontinuing at once with any side effects and seeking medical advice

Not taking beyond the time limit listed on the medication container

Avoiding self-medication without medical advice

CASE STUDY A

Skin Medications

Anne Marie Reingardt noticed patches of irritated skin on her elbows, knees, and scalp. During an appointment with a dermatologist, she is diagnosed with psoriasis. The physician prescribed a keratolytic agent for treatment of the psoriasis. She would
benefit from the following information.

1. Keratolytic agents are used to control:
   a. Necrotic tissue
   b. Pruritus
   c. Scaling skin
   d. Fungal infections

2. A common side effect of a keratolytic agent is:
   a. Skin bruising
   b. Skin discoloration
   c. Glycosuria
   d. Severe skin irritation

3. Which instruction should Anne Marie receive about the keratolytic agent for her psoriasis?
   a. Treat irritated skin with the medication as needed.
   b. Avoid contact with the eyes.
   c. Discontinue use if the condition is no longer present or improves, even if midway through treatment.
   d. Use on surrounding tissues to ensure adequate coverage.

4. Which of the following is an example of a keratolytic agent?
   a. Collagenase
   b. Benzocaine
   c. Salicylic acid
   d. Ammonium lactate

5. Keratolytic agents can also be used to treat:
   a. Allergic contact dermatitis
   b. Fungal infections
   c. Eczema
   d. Warts

CASE STUDY B

Skin Medications

Mary Hanson, a 64-year-old female, is about to undergo a right total knee replacement. The nurse explains that an antiseptic
will be used preoperatively. She will find the following information helpful.

1. Antiseptics are substances that perform which of the following actions?
   a. They inhibit the growth of bacteria.
   b. They assist with the chemical debridement of tissue.
   c. They enhance the growth of healthy skin flora.
   d. They inhibit the replication of a virus.

2. The most preferred antiseptic for skin cleansing prior to surgery is:
   a. Povidone–iodine
   b. Terbinafine
   c. Mupirocin
   d. Chlorhexidine

3. Side effects of chlorhexidine can include:
   a. Petechiae
   b. Dermatitis
   c. Freckling of the skin
   d. Whitening of the skin

4. The nurse explains to Mary that she will need to perform the antiseptic scrub at home the night prior to the surgery. Mary should be instructed to:

a. Leave the medication on her skin after application

b. Apply the medication to her eyes and ears

c. Rinse her skin thoroughly after use

d. Apply the medication to all areas involving the dermis

5. The best surgical scrub for a patient with an allergy to iodine is:

a. Peridex

b. Betadine

c. Hibiclens

d. Bactroban

CHAPTER REVIEW QUIZ

Multiple Choice

1. What is the safest treatment of scabies in an extended care facility?

a. Lindane

b. Ketoconazole

c. Ivermectin

d. Nystatin

2. Which category of topical skin preparation is used to protect the skin and soothe irritation?

a. Antipruritic

b. Keratolytic agent

c. Enzymatic agent

d. Emollient

3. Oral antiviral medications are most effective if started within how many hours of the onset of symptoms?

a. 72

b. 96

c. 36

d. 48

4. Collagenase (Santyl) would be indicated to treat:

a. Hives

b. Scaly skin

c. Necrotic tissue

d. Psychiatric disorders

5. Which action should a patient take after using a nystatin oral preparation?

a. Spit out the excess.

b. Rinse the mouth.

c. Wipe off the excess.

d. Maintain NPO for at least 1h.

6. Which antipruritic would be most likely to cause a hypersensitivity reaction?

a. Synalar

b. Benzocaine

c. Cortaid

d. Desitin

7. Which preparation is used to prevent an infant from developing diaper rash?

a. Keratolytic

b. Protectant

c. Enzyme preparation

d. Antipruritics

8. A patient using a burn medication should be instructed to:

a. Allow the burn to be open to air

b. Disregard any signs of allergy

c. Use the aseptic technique to prevent infection

d. Use an enzymatic debriding agent to facilitate healing

9. Which of the following is an antibacterial cream used topically to treat impetigo?
   a. Lindane
   b. Bactroban
   c. Mycostatin
   d. Monistat

10. Patients with mild acne would most likely be treated with:
   a. Benzoyl peroxide
   b. Tetracycline
   c. Systemic hormones
   d. Isotretinoin

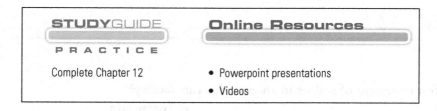

STUDYGUIDE

P R A C T I C E

Complete Chapter 12

Online Resources

- Powerpoint presentations
- Videos

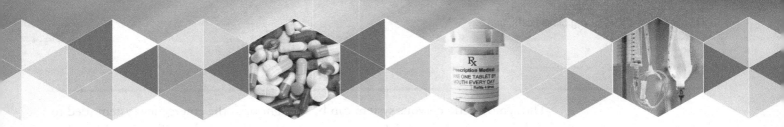

CHAPTER 13
AUTONOMIC NERVOUS SYSTEM DRUGS

KEY TERMS AND CONCEPTS

Adrenergic

Alpha-blockers

Anticholinergics

Autonomic

Beta-blockers

Cholinergic drugs

OBJECTIVES

Upon completion of this chapter, the learner should be able to

1. Compare and contrast characteristics of the four categories of autonomic nervous system drugs

2. List the most frequently used (key) drugs in each of the four categories and the purpose of their administration

3. Describe the possible side effects of each of the key drugs

4. Define the Key Terms and Concepts

The **autonomic** nervous system (ANS) can be thought of as being *automatic*, self-governing, or involuntary. That is to say, we have no conscious control over the action of the ANS. The autonomic system can be divided into the sympathetic and parasympathetic nervous system. The sympathetic system is your "alert system" that can quickly ready your body to face emergencies. The parasympathetic system can be thought of as your "resting and digesting" system and automatically helps to maintain the normal body functions again without your conscious effort. Chemical substances called *neurotransmitters* are released at the nerve endings within these systems to transmit the nerve impulses from nerve to nerve at the synapses or from nerve to smooth muscle or glands.

Drugs that affect the function of the ANS are divided into four categories based on whether they mimic or block the response of the sympathetic and parasympathetic nervous system:

1. Adrenergics (sympathomimetics = mimic sympathetic responses)
2. Adrenergic blockers (alpha- and beta-blockers = block sympathetic responses)
3. Cholinergics (parasympathomimetics = mimic parasympathetic responses)
4. Cholinergic blockers (anticholinergics = block parasympathetic responses)

ADRENERGICS

The sympathetic nervous system can be thought of as the emergency system used to mobilize the body for quick response and action. Key words to illustrate this action are *fright, fight,* and *flight.* If someone is startled in a dark place by a sudden motion, the sympathetic nerves are automatically mobilized to prepare the body to handle the fright by flight or a fight. The blood pressure, pulse, and respiration increase to supply more oxygen to the tissues. The peripheral blood vessels constrict, sending more blood inward to the vital organs and skeletal muscles needed for the fight or flight action. The bronchioles dilate to allow for a greater oxygen supply. The pupils dilate to allow more light to see the situation at hand.

The chemical substances (neurotransmitters) released at the sympathetic nerve endings are called catecholamines and include norepinephrine and dopamine. In addition, the hormone epinephrine is secreted by the adrenal glands in response to strong sympathetic stimulation. Drugs that mimic the action of the sympathetic nervous system are called sympathomimetic or **adrenergic.**

Actions of the adrenergics include:

Cardiac stimulation

Increased blood flow to skeletal muscles

Peripheral vasoconstriction

Bronchodilation

Dilation of the pupils (mydriatic action)

Uses of the adrenergics include:

Restoring rhythm in cardiac arrest

Elevating blood pressure in shock

Constricting capillaries (e.g., applied topically to relieve nosebleed or nasal congestion or combined with local anesthetics for minor surgery)

Dilating bronchioles in acute asthmatic attacks, bronchospasm, or anaphylactic reaction

Ophthalmic procedures (see Chapter 18, "Eye Medications")

Side effects of the adrenergics may include:

- ❗ Palpitations
- ❗ Nervousness or tremor
- ❗ Tachycardia
- ❗ Cardiac arrhythmias
- ❗ Anginal pain
- ❗ Hypertension
- ❗ Hyperglycemia

Tissue necrosis (when applied to laceration of periphery, e.g., nose, fingers, and toes because of blood flow restriction)

Headache and insomnia

Precautions/contraindications with adrenergics apply to those with:

Angina

Coronary insufficiency

Hypertension

Cardiac arrhythmias

Angle-closure glaucoma

Organic brain syndrome

Hyperthyroidism

Caution for adrenergics also with dose and route of administration; check dosage carefully (small amounts only). Give subcutaneous, intramuscular (IM; deltoid), or intravenous (IV).

Interactions of adrenergics may occur with:

Central Nervous System (CNS) drugs (e.g., certain general anesthetics, monoamine oxidase inhibitors [MAOIs], and antidepressants)

Propranolol (Inderal) or other beta-adrenergic blockers

Terazosin (Hytrin) or other alpha-adrenergic blockers

See Table 13-1 for a summary of the adrenergics.

Figure 13-1 shows an epinephrine syringe and epinephrine injector for administering epinephrine to treat or prevent anaphylactic shock.

TABLE 13-1 Adrenergics

GENERIC NAME	TRADE NAME	DOSAGE	COMMENTS
epinephrine	Adrenalin	0.1–0.5 mL 1:1,000 sol subcutaneously or IM[a] (deltoid) 5–10 mL 1:10,000 sol IV	For bronchospasm, asthma, cardiac arrest
	EpiPen, EpiPen Jr	0.3 mL (1:1,000 or 1:2,000) IM	anaphylaxis
ephedrine		25–50 mg IM, subcutaneously, or slow IV	To raise blood pressure
dopamine		2–5 mcg/kg per min IV initially; titrate to response	To raise blood pressure, cardiotonic
isoproterenol	Isuprel	0.02–0.2 mg IV or IM; 5 mcg/min infusion	For heart block or ventricular arrhythmias
norepinephrine	Levophed	2–30 mcg/min IV	For acute hypotension and severe shock
phenylephrine	Neo-Synephrine	40–80 mcg/min IV (severe); 2–5 mg IM/ subcutaneously or 0.1–0.5 mg IV (mild–moderate)	To raise blood pressure, ventricular arrhythmias

[a]Use caution with dosage (note concentrations).

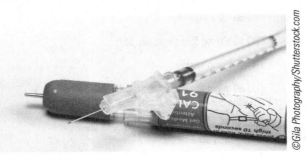

FIGURE 13-1 Epinephrine syringe and epinephrine injector (EpiPen).

©Gila Photography/Shutterstock.com

ADRENERGIC BLOCKERS

Drugs that block the action of the sympathetic nervous system are called adrenergic blockers. The most commonly used drugs in this category are the alpha- and beta-adrenergic blockers, or alpha-blockers and beta-blockers. Alpha-adrenergic blockers are discussed in Chapters 15 and 25. The prototype of the beta-adrenergic blockers is propranolol (Inderal) (Table 13-2).

Uses of the beta-blockers include treatment of the following:

Hypertension

Cardiac arrhythmias

Angina pectoris

Migraine headache

Tremor

TABLE 13-2   Adrenergic Blockers

GENERIC NAME	TRADE NAME	DOSAGE	COMMENTS
propranolol[a]	(Inderal)[b]	PO 40–160 mg daily in two to three divided doses initially	Begin with smaller dose and increase gradually to optimum dose for blood pressure control
	Inderal LA	PO 80–160 mg daily	Extended-release capsules
		PO 10–20 mg two to four times per day (initial dose)	For angina
		PO 80–320 mg daily	Extended-release dose
		PO 10–30 mg four times per day	For arrhythmias
		IV 0.5–3 mg slowly	Use extreme caution
		PO 80 mg initial dose, increase to 160–240 mg daily divided doses	For migraine

[a]A beta-adrenergic blocker or beta-blocker. Others are available and vary with condition (see Chapter 25).
[b]This brand name is no longer marketed, but the name is still commonly used.

Side effects of beta-blockers may include:

Hypotension

❗ Bradycardia

❗ Fatigue or lethargy

❗ Bronchospasm

❗ Nausea and vomiting

❗ Hypoglycemia

❗ Confusion

Precautions/contraindications apply to the use of beta-blockers with:

Abrupt discontinuation (decrease over several weeks)

Congestive heart failure or atrioventricular block

Hypotension

Asthma, chronic obstructive pulmonary disease (COPD)

Diabetes (can mask signs of hypoglycemia)

Interactions of beta-blockers may occur with:

Digoxin (frequently used together; monitor for bradycardia)

Insulin or oral antidiabetic agents

Theophylline

MAOIs and tricyclic antidepressants

Epinephrine (causes hypertensive response)

Phenothiazines (i.e., chlorpromazine, prochlorperazine)

PATIENT EDUCATION

Patients taking beta-blockers, frequently given for cardiovascular disease, should be instructed regarding:

Rising slowly from the reclining position to avoid postural hypotension

Reporting possible slow heartbeat and dizziness, difficulty breathing, or excessive weakness to the physician

If you have diabetes, checking with your health care professional before changing diet or the dose of your diabetic medication

Avoiding alcohol, antihistamines, muscle relaxants, tranquilizers, and sedatives because they potentiate CNS depression and sedation

Reporting sexual dysfunction or depression to the physician for possible dosage regulation or change to different medication

Not discontinuing the medication abruptly, except on advice of the physician

Consulting a physician or pharmacist before using over-the-counter (OTC) cold preparations

CLINICAL CONNECTION

Patient Compliance with Adrenergic Blockers

Patient compliance with adrenergic blockers, also called beta-blockers, when taken orally is poor. Beta-blockers are often discontinued or not taken regularly by patients because of various side effects. The most common is fatigue.

CHOLINERGICS

The parasympathetic nerve fibers synthesize and liberate *acetylcholine* as the mediator. Drugs that mimic the action of the parasympathetic nervous system are called parasympathomimetic or **cholinergic drugs** (e.g., bethanechol, neostigmine, pilocarpine, and pyridostigmine).

Actions of the cholinergics include:

Increased gastrointestinal (GI) peristalsis

Increased contraction of the urinary bladder

Increased secretions (sweat, saliva, and gastric juices)

Increased skeletal muscle strength

Lowered intraocular pressure

Constriction of the pupils

Slowing of the heart

Uses of the cholinergics include treatment of:

Nonobstructive urinary retention (bethanechol)

Neuromuscular blockade reversal (neostigmine)

Myasthenia gravis (pyridostigmine)

Xerostomia (dry mouth) (pilocarpine—Salagen)

Open-angle glaucoma (pilocarpine)

Side effects of the cholinergics may include:

❗ Nausea, vomiting, and diarrhea

❗ Muscle cramps and weakness

❗ Slowing of the heart and hypotension

❗ Sweating, excessive salivation, lacrimation (discharge of tears), and flushing

❗ Respiratory depression and bronchospasm

Acute toxicity or cholinergic crisis is treated with atropine sulfate IV. Atropine is a cholinergic blocker and therefore would block the effects of a cholinergic crisis.

Precautions/contraindications with the cholinergics apply to those with:

Benign prostatic hyperplasia (BPH)

GI disorders (e.g., ulcer and obstruction)

Asthma

Cardiac disorders

Hyperthyroidism

Interactions of cholinergics may occur with:

Procainamide and quinidine (have anticholinergic properties)

Local anesthetics (inhibit neuronal transmission in skeletal muscles)

See Table 13-3 for a summary of the cholinergics.

TABLE 13-3 **Cholinergics**

GENERIC NAME	TRADE NAME	DOSAGE	COMMENTS
bethanechol	Urecholine	10–50 mg PO – three to four times per day	For postpartum or postoperative urinary retention, *not* with benign prostatic hyperplasia (BPH)
neostigmine	Prostigmin	0.5–2.5 mg IM, subcutaneously or IV q1–3h	Primarily for neuromuscular blockade reversal
pilocarpine	Isopto Carpine	Ophthalmic drops; dose varies	To lower intraocular pressure in glaucoma
pyridostigmine	Salagen	5 mg PO three to four times per day	For the treatment of xerostomia (dry mouth)
	Mestinon	60–120 mg PO q3-8h	
	Mestinon Timespan	180–540 mg PO one to two times per day	Primarily for the treatment of myasthenia gravis
		(At least 6h between doses)	

PATIENT EDUCATION

Patients taking cholinergic drugs, or exposed to insecticides containing cholinergic agents (e.g., malathion), should be instructed regarding:

Reporting immediately to a physician or an emergency room any symptoms of prolonged GI distress (e.g., nausea, vomiting, and diarrhea), excessive perspiration, slow heartbeat, or depressed respiration

Avoiding combination of cholinergic medications with heart medications or cholinergic blockers

CHOLINERGIC BLOCKERS

Cholinergic blockers, or **anticholinergics**, are drugs that block the action of the parasympathetic nervous system. Therefore, they are also called parasympatholytic. Atropine is the classic example of a cholinergic blocker. A common use of anticholinergics is scopolamine transdermal patches to treat or prevent seasickness by decreasing gastric secretions and motility. Anticholinergic eye drops can be used to dilate the eyes by causing relaxation of the muscles of the iris (colored part of the eye), which is normally stimulated to constrict by acetylcholine, a parasympathetic response.

Anticholinergics most commonly used as preoperative medications include atropine and glycopyrrolate (Robinul). They reduce the secretions of the mouth, pharynx, bronchi, and GI tract and reduce gastric activity. Anticholinergics, as preoperative medication, are also used to prevent cholinergic effects during surgery, such as hypotension or bradycardia and some cardiac arrhythmias associated with general anesthetics or vagal stimulation. The vagus nerve is the major nerve of the parasympathetic nervous system and can be stimulated during intubation procedures and surgery. However, only *atropine* acts as a bronchodilator and reduces the incidence of laryngospasm that can occur during general anesthesia.

Actions of anticholinergics include:

Drying (all secretions decreased)

Decreased GI and genitourinary (GU) motility

Dilation of the pupils

CLINICAL CONNECTION

Ophthalmic Atropine

In practice, there are situations when it is necessary to dilate the pupils of the eyes, this means making the pupil bigger and wider. The most common eye drop used is atropine, which is an anticholinergic ophthalmic eye drop. When a patient goes to the eye doctor, often times it is easier to diagnose or treat diseases of the eye if the pupils are dilated because it is more open for the doctor to view to back of the eye. Additionally, dilating the pupils makes it easier to make some measurements for eye glasses. It is important to educate patients that after leaving their appointment, their eyes will be more sensitive to light, as atropine drops keep the eyes dilated for 4–24 h. This means patients should wear sunglasses in well-lit areas for the rest of the day. Atropine can also be used as a maintenance treatment for various eye conditions such as conjunctivitis. These patients should be instructed to wear eye protection and be cautious in well-lit areas.

Uses of the anticholinergics include:

Antispasmodic and antisecretory for GI or GU hypermotility

Preoperative and preanesthetic uses

Antidote for insecticide poisoning, cholinergic crisis, or mushroom poisoning

Emergency treatment of bradycardia and atrioventricular heart block with hypotension

Dilation of the pupils (mydriatic)

Prevention and treatment of bronchospasm (bronchodilator, e.g., Atrovent HFA [Hydrofluroalkane] inhaler)

Side effects of anticholinergics may include:

Fever or flushing

! Blurred vision and headache

! Dry mouth, constipation, and urinary retention

! Falls, delirium, and cognitive impairment, especially in older adults

! Palpitations and tachycardia (abnormally fast heartbeat)

Interactions with potentiation of sedation and drying occur with:

Antihistamines (e.g., diphenhydramine).

Precautions/contraindications apply to the use of atropine for those with:

Asthma and other COPD—atropine-type *inhalations of aerosols are recommended* rather than oral or parenteral administration, which can reduce and dry bronchial secretions and obstruct airflow. More on this in Chapter 26 concerning inhaled medications.

Angle-closure glaucoma

GI or GU obstruction

Cardiac arrhythmias

Hypertension

Hypothyroidism and hepatic or renal disease

See Table 13-4 for a summary of the anticholinergics.

TABLE 13-4 Cholinergic Blockers

GENERIC NAME	TRADE NAME	DOSAGE[a]	COMMENTS
atropine		0.4–0.6 mg IM, IV, subcu	Preoperative
		1–2 mg IM or IV q1h	For insecticide or mushroom poisoning
		0.5–1 mg IV	For bradycardia or atrioventricular block
		1% ophthalmic: 1–2 drops 1 h before needed	For pupil dilation
glycopyrrolate	Robinul	0.1–0.2 mg IM or IV	Preoperative
scopolamine	Transderm-Scop	72-h patch	Prevents motion sickness; reduces salivary flow
	Donnatal[c]	one to two tabs three to four times per day	For irritable bowel syndrome
homatropine	Isopto Homatropine	Dosage varies for ophthalmic drops[b]	Mydriatic

[a]Use caution to give correct dosage.
[b]Other anticholinergics used in ophthalmic conditions are discussed in Chapter 18.
[c]With atropine, hyoscyamine, and phenobarbital

PATIENT EDUCATION

Patients receiving cholinergic blockers should be instructed regarding:
- Dried secretions (e.g., dry mouth)
- Possible blurring of vision
- Reporting fast heartbeat or palpitations, feeling faint or falls, or trouble passing urine

Avoiding oral anticholinergics with chronic obstructive lung disease and asthma and using inhalants only as prescribed, never OTC

Sometimes it helps to have mnemonics or memory devices to sort out these similar-sounding drug categories. Therefore, see Figure 13-2 for a visual summary of the ANS drugs.

The Autonomic Nervous System

Sympathetic	Parasympathetic

A = Adrenergic Action

fright   fight   flight

 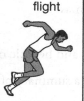

↑ BP, P, & R.

Fast

Bronchioles dilate
Pupils dilate

Peripheral blood vessels constrict

Adrenergic Drugs:

epinephrine (Adrenalin)
isoproterenol (Isuprel)
norepinephrine (Levophed)

Side effects: tachycardia, palpitations, hypertension, nervousness, hyperglycemia

C = Cholinergic Action

↑ Secretion = fluids flow

↑ Peristalsis and bladder contractions

↑ Increased muscle strength

↕ Respiration depressed

Slow

Pupils constrict ↓ intraocular pressure

Cholinergic Drugs:

bethanechol (Urecholine)
neostigmine (Prostigmin)
pilocarpine ophthalmic gtts

Side effects: nausea, vomiting, diarrhea, sweating, bradycardia, bronchospasm, respiratory depression.

B = β-adrenergic Blockers

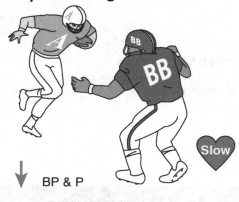

Slow

↓ BP & P

Beta-blocker:
propranolol (Inderal)

Side effects: hypotension, bradycardia, fatigue, depression, hypoglycemia

D = Cholinergic Blockers

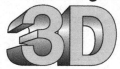 (3D effects)

Drying

Decreased motility G.I. and G.U.

Dilated pupils

↑ Heart rate **Fast**

Anticholinergic:
Atropine

Side effects: dry mouth, urinary retention, constipation, blurred vision, confusion, tachycardia

FIGURE 13-2 The ANS drugs can be as simple as A, B, C, and D.

CASE STUDY A

ANS Drugs

Lucy Westcott is a 47-year-old female who has a severe allergy to shrimp. Although at a cocktail party, she inadvertently ingests some shrimp from an hors d'oeuvre tray. She begins to experience signs of a severe reaction to the shrimp such as throat tightening and lip and eyelid swelling.

1. Which medication would be used as the first-line treatment for her symptoms?
  a. Levophed
  b. Neo-Synephrine
  c. Adrenalin
  d. Isuprel

2. When a patient is given an adrenergic medication, which action does the medication have on the ANS?
  a. It mimics a sympathetic response.
  b. It blocks a sympathetic response.
  c. It mimics a parasympathetic response.
  d. It blocks a parasympathetic response.

3. The EpiPen delivers an adrenergic medication, which has a primary effect of:
  a. The constriction of the pupils
  b. Bronchodilation
  c. Peripheral vasodilation
  d. Cardiac relaxation

4. A side effect that Suzanne may experience after the EpiPen injection is:
  a. Bradycardia
  b. Palpitations
  c. Migraine headache
  d. Hypotension

5. Which part of the ANS helps the body to be ready for emergencies?
  a. Parasympathetic
  b. Adrenal
  c. Cholinergic
  d. Sympathetic

CASE STUDY B

Cholinergic Blockers

Jeb Cranshaw is enjoying a Caribbean cruise on his honeymoon. However, on the second day of the cruise, he starts to feel queasy and seasick. His new wife suggests that he visit the ship's clinic for treatment.

1. Which type of drug will most likely be prescribed by the ship's physician?
  a. Beta-blocker
  b. Antihistamine
  c. Cholinergic
  d. Anticholinergic

2. Scopolamine is prescribed for Mr. Cranshaw. This medication will most likely be delivered by which route?
  a. IM
  b. IV
  c. patch
  d. PO

3. When educating Mr. Cranshaw about scopolamine, the ship's physician will tell him that he may experience:
  a. Nausea
  b. Dry mouth
  c. Sweating
  d. Slower heart rate

4. Mr. Cranshaw's wife is reading up on the general classification of the drug that he is taking and learns that one of these medications reduces the incidence of laryngospasm that can occur with general anesthesia. What is this medication?
  a. Glycopyrrolate
  b. Norepinephrine
  c. Ephedrine
  d. Atropine

5. Mr. Cranshaw's wife learns that which medication is often given preoperatively to reduce the secretions of the mouth and pharynx?

    a. Robinul   c. Levophed

    b. Isopto Homatropine   d. Urecholine

CHAPTER REVIEW QUIZ

Match the type of drug with the action. The type of drug may be used more than once.

Action	ANS drugs
1. _____ Increases muscle strength	**a.** Adrenergic
2. _____ Drying secretions	**b.** Adrenergic blocker
3. _____ Increases blood pressure	**c.** Cholinergic
4. _____ Increases peristalsis	**d.** Anticholinergic
5. _____ Lowers intraocular pressure	
6. _____ Antispasmodic	
7. _____ Bronchodilator	
8. _____ Lowers blood pressure	
9. _____ Constricts pupils	
10. _____ Antiarrhythmic	

Match the type of drug with possible side effects. The type of drug may be used more than once.

Side Effects	ANS Drugs
11. _____ Bronchospasm	**a.** Adrenergic
12. _____ Hyperglycemia	**b.** Adrenergic blocker
13. _____ Diarrhea	**c.** Cholinergic
14. _____ Flushing	**d.** Anticholinergic
15. _____ Lethargy	
16. _____ Hypoglycemia	
17. _____ Constipation	
18. _____ Nervousness	
19. _____ Cognitive impairment	

20. A cholinergic drug should be used with extreme caution in a patient with:

    a. Benign prostatic hyperplasia (BPH)   **c.** Hypothyroidism

    b. Hepatic disease   **d.** Renal disease

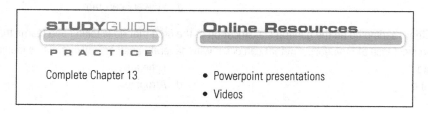

STUDYGUIDE   **Online Resources**

P R A C T I C E

Complete Chapter 13   • Powerpoint presentations

                                    • Videos

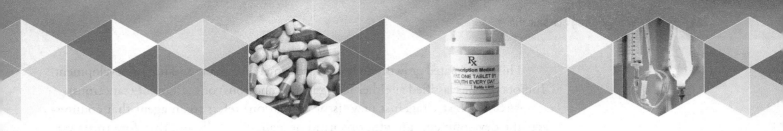

CHAPTER 14
ANTINEOPLASTIC DRUGS

KEY TERMS AND CONCEPTS

Antineoplastic

Benign

Chemotherapy

Cytotoxic

Immunosuppressive

Malignant

Palliative

Proliferating

OBJECTIVES

Upon completion of this chapter, the learner should be able to

1. Name three characteristics associated with the administration of antineoplastic drugs

2. Name and describe the major groups of antineoplastic agents

3. List the side effects common to most of the antineoplastic agents

4. Describe appropriate interventions in caring for patients receiving antineoplastic agents

5. Explain precautions in caring for those receiving radioactive isotopes

6. Describe the responsibilities of those caring for patients receiving chemotherapy

7. Explain appropriate education for the patient and family when antineoplastic agents are administered

8. List safety factors for those who care for patients receiving cytotoxic drugs

9. Define the Key Terms and Concepts

A healthy body needs cells to reproduce and grow in an orderly, regulated manner. However, sometimes conditions are altered in the body that trigger abnormal changes in the way the cells reproduce and grow. These triggers can cause cell growth to become uncontrolled, leading to overproduction or impaired cellular development (Figure 14-1).

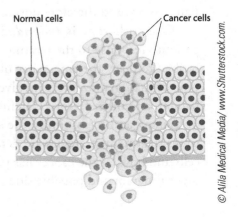

Normal cells   Cancer cells

© Alila Medical Media/ www.Shutterstock.com.

FIGURE 14-1 Cancer cells are identified by uncontrolled cell growth.

This unregulated growth can lead to abnormal cell, tissue, and tumor development. Tumors can be classified as either benign (noncancerous) or malignant (cancerous).

Antineoplastic (against new tissue formation) refers to an agent that counteracts the development, growth, or spread of malignant cells and therefore treats various types of cancers. Cancer therapy frequently includes a combination of surgery, radiation, and chemotherapy.

Chemotherapy is a constantly growing field in which many old and new drugs and drug combinations are used for palliative effects (alleviation of symptoms) or for long-term or complete remissions in the early treatment of cancer. Antineoplastic drugs are cytotoxic (destructive to cells), especially to cells that are proliferating (reproducing rapidly). Unfortunately, the toxic effects of the antineoplastic drugs are not confined to malignant cells alone; they also affect other proliferating tissues, such as the bone marrow, gastrointestinal (GI) epithelium, skin, hair follicles, white blood cells (WBCs), and epithelium of the gonads, resulting in numerous adverse side effects. It should be noted that all of these "normal" cell tissues affected by chemotherapy are ones that naturally grow and proliferate at a higher rate than other cells found in the body.

Significant developments continue in the use of targeted therapies that are designed to target only cancer cells, thereby sparing normal tissues. This therapy reduces host toxicity while simultaneously increasing toxicity to cancer cells and improving survival rates in patients with cancer. Many new drugs in the targeted therapy category called signal transduction inhibitors (STIs) are given by the *oral route*. The first cancer *treatment* vaccine for certain men with metastatic prostate cancer was recently approved, and many others are being tested in clinical trials.

Personalized oncology medicine, utilizing pharmacogenomic biomarkers (see Chapter 3), is a developing field where based on their genetic profile, individual patients and individual cancers that respond differently to oncology medications can be identified. This is the basis for the first-line treatment of metastatic breast cancer in patients with tumors that produce excess amounts of a protein called HER2, discussed later in this chapter.

Many antineoplastic agents also possess immunosuppressive properties, because they may decrease the production of WBCs and antibodies and reduce the inflammatory reaction. Suppression of the immune response results in increased susceptibility of the patient to infection.

Antineoplastic drugs are frequently administered in high doses on an *intermittent* schedule. Most normal tissues have a greater capacity for repair than do most malignant tissues, and therefore normal cells may recover during the drug-free period.

Chemotherapy is *individualized* and frequently modified according to the patient's response to the treatment. A *combination of several drugs* is frequently prescribed to delay the emergence of resistance, with the choice of agents based on the type of malignancy, areas involved, extent of the cancer, physical condition of the patient, and other factors. Careful planning is required to maximize the effectiveness of therapy and to minimize the side effects and discomfort for the patient. Often times treatment strategies are determined based on the aggressiveness of the cancer cells and how far the cancer has progressed upon diagnosis. Understanding the treatment program and possible side effects is essential for all concerned: the health care professional, the patient, and the family. Preplanning includes provision for symptomatic relief, such as antiemetics (drugs to prevent nausea), as well as reassurance and availability of support staff to answer questions, explore feelings, and allay fears.

The treatment of cancer is highly complex. Only health care professionals in oncology units, cancer treatment centers, or oncologist's offices would be expected to know the names of the numerous drugs. However, anyone who is in contact with patients on antineoplastic therapy should be aware of the frequent possible side effects and appropriate interventions for the comfort of the patient. Patient education and support are extremely important.

Antineoplastic agents can be generally classified into nine major groups: (1) antimetabolites; (2) alkylating agents; (3) mitotic inhibitors (plant alkaloids, taxanes); (4) antitumor antibiotics; (5) hormones and hormone modifiers (corticosteroids, antiestrogens, and antiandrogens); (6) biological therapies (interferons, colony-stimulating factors [CSFs], and monoclonal antibodies [MABs]); (7) targeted cancer therapies (STIs); (8) vaccines; and (9) radioactive isotopes.

About one-half of all cancer patients receive some type of radiation oncology therapy sometime during the course of their treatment. Radioactive substances are placed close to or implanted in the cancerous tissues (internal radiation therapy), or an external-beam radiation is passed in three dimensions, which is made possible with computer technology.

Only one or two examples of medications are presented for each category to identify the side effects specific to that group. It is not necessary to remember the names of these drugs as they are only representative of the many antineoplastic agents available. However, if you work extensively with cancer patients, knowing the drug names would become important, and the National Cancer Institute website would provide you with all the latest drugs and treatments available for the various types of cancers.

ANTIMETABOLITES

Antimetabolites work by interfering with DNA synthesis, repair, and cellular replication and are used in the treatment of various malignancies, especially those involving rapidly proliferating neoplasms (new growth). Some injectable antimetabolites include methotrexate and fluorouracil. Methotrexate is also available orally and has been used for severe, resistant cases of psoriasis, rheumatoid arthritis, and lupus. Fluorouracil is also available in a topical formulation (Efudex) to treat certain skin cancers.

Tissues that have a high rate of cellular metabolism such as neoplasms, hair follicles, buccal and GI tract lining, fetal cells, and bone marrow are most sensitive to the effects of the antimetabolites, which account for the side effects and cautions listed here.

Side effects of antimetabolites can include the following:

- ❗ Anorexia, nausea, vomiting, and diarrhea
- ❗ Ulceration and bleeding of the oral mucosa and GI tract

CLINICAL CONNECTION: METHOTREXATE DOSING

Many oral chemotherapy medications are administered on a daily basis, whereas methotrexate is ONLY dosed once weekly; it is generally given as multiple 2.5 mg tablets on the same day each week. This special dosing schedule is to allow the body to recover from the various side effects, and often times, folic acid is given on the days that the patient is not taking methotrexate to help as well. This is an important opportunity to educate patients that methotrexate is not taken like their other pills to ensure their treatment is successful and safe.

Note

Leucovorin (a reduced form of folic acid) is sometimes used as a "rescue agent" following methotrexate administration to reduce the side effects of methotrexate-induced hematological and GI toxicity.

- ! Bone marrow suppression, including leukopenia (abnormal decrease in WBC) with infection; anemia; and thrombocytopenia (abnormal decrease in blood platelets) with hemorrhage
- ! Rash, itching, photosensitivity, and scaling
- ! Alopecia (regrowth of hair may take several months)

Precautions/contraindications with antimetabolites apply to:

Renal and hepatic disorders

Pregnancy

GI ulcers

ALKYLATING AGENTS

Alkylating agents are used in the treatment of a wide range of cancers. Some alkylating agents include cisplatin and cyclophosphamide.

These agents prevent cell growth by damaging DNA needed for reproduction. They can cause long-term damage to the bone marrow. In a few rare cases, this damage can eventually lead to acute leukemia 5–10 years after treatment.

Side effects of alkylating agents can include the following:

- ! Nausea, vomiting, and diarrhea
- ! Mucosal ulceration; bone marrow suppression, including leukopenia with infection; anemia; and thrombocytopenia with hemorrhage
- ! Neurotoxicity, including headache, vertigo, and seizures
- ! Hemorrhagic cystitis with cyclophosphamide (mesna, a chemoprotectant, can be administered prior to chemotherapy to prevent this toxicity)

Rash and alopecia

Pulmonary fibrosis

Necrosis of tissue if intravenous (IV) drug solution infiltrates into tissues (for IV cannula placement, avoid areas of previous irradiation and extremities with poor venous circulation)

Precautions/contraindications with alkylating agents apply to:

Debilitated patients

Pregnancy

Renal disease (with cisplatin—major dose-limiting toxicity)

MITOTIC INHIBITORS

Mitosis refers to the process of cell division and reproduction. Mitotic inhibitors are often plant alkaloids and other compounds derived from natural products that block mitosis. They are used to treat many different types of cancer. These agents are also known for their potential to cause peripheral nerve damage and myelosuppression, which can be dose-limiting side effects.

Plant Alkaloids

Plant alkaloids, for example vinblastine or vincristine, which are derived from the periwinkle plant, are used in combination with other chemotherapeutic agents in the treatment of various malignancies. Vinorelbine (Navelbine), a semisynthetic agent derived from vinblastine, has been recommended as a treatment of choice for lung cancer in older patients.

Side effects of plant alkaloids can include the following:

- ❗ Neurotoxicity, including numbness; tingling; ataxia; foot drop; pain in the jaw, head, or extremities; and visual disturbances (less common with vinblastine and vinorelbine)
- ❗ Severe constipation or diarrhea, nausea, and vomiting
- ❗ Oral or GI ulceration
- ❗ Rash, phototoxicity (increased reaction to sunlight), and alopecia

Leukopenia with vinblastine (hematological effects less common with vincristine)

Necrosis of tissue if IV drug solution infiltrates into tissues (for IV cannula placement, avoid areas of previous irradiation and extremities with poor venous circulation)

Precautions/contraindications with plant alkaloids apply to:

Pregnancy

Hepatic dysfunction

Infection

Geriatric patients

Note

Intrathecal administration (into the spinal canal) of these agents is fatal. This route must not be used. Syringes containing these agents should be labeled, "Warning—For IV use only, fatal if given intrathecally."

CLINICAL CONNECTION

Extravasation

Extravasation occurs when a drug or liquid intended for IV administration leaks into the surrounding tissue (Figure 14-2). In particular, chemotherapy can cause painful irritation, and if left untreated can lead to necrosis of that tissue. In addition to treatment, patients can also get relief from this irritation from a cold or warm compress.

Different chemotherapy agents are relieved better by one or the other. Warm compresses work better for plant (vinca) alkaloids and taxanes, whereas cold compresses work better for anthracyclines, other alkylating agents, and antitumor antibiotics. Educating the patient on which to use could make a big difference for their relief.

(continued)

CLINICAL CONNECTION (*continued*)

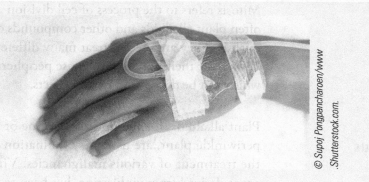

FIGURE 14-2 When a fluid leaks out of the vein and into the surrounding tissue, necrosis of that tissue can occur. The health care professional must be vigilant in monitoring the IV site to watch for swelling or pain as this site is showing early signs of swelling.

© Supoj Pongpancharoen/www .Shutterstock.com.

Taxanes

Paclitaxel, another plant alkaloid, was originally extracted from the bark of the Western (Pacific) yew. It is structurally different from other available antineoplastic agents. It is used as a second-line or subsequent therapy in patients with metastatic breast or ovarian carcinoma refractory to conventional chemotherapy.

Adverse side effects of paclitaxel are frequent and include:

- ❗ Bone marrow suppression—neutropenia, leukopenia, thrombocytopenia, and anemia
- ❗ Hypersensitivity reactions—can be severe, with flushing, rash, dyspnea, chest pain, hypotension, and bradycardia
- ❗ Peripheral neuropathy (occurs in up to 30% of patients)
- ❗ Nausea, vomiting, diarrhea, and mucositis (inflammation of the mucous membranes)
- ❗ Alopecia
- ❗ Necrosis of tissue if IV drug solution infiltrates into tissues

Precautions/contraindications with paclitaxel apply to:

Pregnancy

Hepatic dysfunction

Infection

Cardiac disease

Because of its severe adverse reactions, paclitaxel is administered only by IV under constant supervision of an oncologist, with frequent monitoring of vital signs and facilities available for emergency interventions if required.

Just to show the *Star Trek* quality of research in cancer medications, NAB-paclitaxel (Abraxane) is the first approved albumin nanoparticle drug. Paclitaxel is mixed with albumin nanoparticles (one billionth of a meter in size), which act as biological delivery agents to transport the drug to the needed site of action. See Figure 14-3 for a rendering of how nanoparticles work.

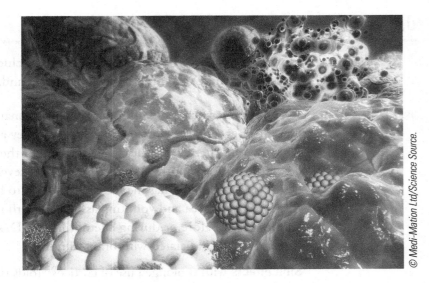

FIGURE 14-3 Illustration of nanoparticles (blue) containing cytotoxic drugs and targeting the tumor cells (purple). The orange cells represent dead and dying tumor cells.

© Medi-Mation Ltd/Science Source.

ANTITUMOR ANTIBIOTICS

Antitumor antibiotics are used to treat a wide variety of malignancies. Doxorubicin (Adriamycin) is considered the most active chemotherapy agent and is a critical component in the treatment protocols of breast, lung, gastric, and ovarian cancers and lymphoma, but it can permanently damage the heart if a maximum lifetime dose is reached. This means that regardless of the effectiveness these medications can only be used for a set period of time. Daunorubicin (Cerubidine), which is structurally related to doxorubicin, is primarily used for acute leukemias because of its lower incidence of cardiotoxicity. Other antitumor antibiotics include bleomycin and mitomycin. They are frequently used in combination with other drugs.

Side effects of antitumor antibiotics can include the following:

- **!** Anorexia, nausea, vomiting, and diarrhea
- **!** Bone marrow suppression (the acute dose-limiting toxicity with doxorubicin and daunorubicin)
- **!** Cardiotoxicity, including arrhythmias; congestive heart failure; and cardiomyopathy (cumulative dosing with most medications except bleomycin)
- **!** Pneumonitis and dyspnea; pulmonary fibrosis with bleomycin
- **!** Ulceration of the mouth or colon
- **!** Alopecia, rash, and scaling

  Tissue necrosis if IV solution infiltrates (with most meds)

Precautions/contraindications with antitumor antibiotics apply to:

Pregnancy

Liver disorders

Cardiac disease, especially congestive heart failure

> **Note**
>
> Side effects vary depending on specific medications. Always check side effects for each drug in this classification.

HORMONES AND HORMONE MODIFIERS

Hormones used in the treatment of cancer include the corticosteroids. Hormone modifiers include the antiestrogen and the antiandrogen agents.

Corticosteroids

Corticosteroids, such as prednisone, are used primarily for their suppressant effect on lymphocytes in leukemias and lymphomas. They are also frequently used in combination with other chemotherapeutic agents in the treatment of some types of cancer and before chemotherapy to help prevent severe allergic reactions. In addition, large doses of dexamethasone have been found to be effective in the prevention and treatment of nausea and vomiting associated with many antineoplastic agents, when administered before or during chemotherapy. Dexamethasone is also used to treat cerebral edema associated with brain tumors.

Side effects with prolonged use of corticosteroids (see Chapter 23 for a more detailed listing) include:

- ❗ Fluid retention, edema
- Cushingoid features (moon face)
- ❗ Nausea/vomiting, gastritis, and GI bleeding
- ❗ Osteoporosis with fractures

Antiestrogens

A *nonsteroidal* agent belonging to a class of drugs called selective estrogen-receptor modifiers (SERMs), tamoxifen, binds to estrogen receptors in various tissues. It can be used as a primary hormonal therapy both for metastatic estrogen receptor–positive breast cancer in both men and postmenopausal women and also for palliative treatment. Tamoxifen also stimulates estrogen receptors in bones and may help prevent osteoporosis.

Serious adverse side effects are rare and usually dose related. Nausea, vomiting, hot flashes, and night sweats can occur in up to 66% of cases but usually do not require discontinuation of the medication. Antidepressants may be prescribed to alleviate tamoxifen-associated hot flashes. Some antidepressants may reduce the potency of tamoxifen.

Anastrozole (Arimidex) and letrozole (Femara), which inhibit the final step in estrogen production, offer alternatives to tamoxifen in postmenopausal women with breast cancer. They can also cause nausea, vomiting, and hot flashes similar to tamoxifen but are more likely than tamoxifen to cause osteoporosis.

Antiandrogens

Antiandrogen drugs include leuprolide acetate, which suppresses testosterone production in the testes and is usually administered intramuscular (IM) (Lupron Depot) or subcutaneously (SC) (Eligard) on monthly regimens (every one, three, four, or six depending on the dosage) for prostate cancer. They are also used as hormonal therapy in the treatment of endometriosis. See Chapter 24 for more details.

Bicalutamide (Casodex) is an oral nonsteroidal antiandrogen, which interferes with the binding of testosterone to androgen receptors in the prostate and is used simultaneously with leuprolide in the treatment of metastatic prostate cancer.

Side effects of antiandrogens can include:

- ❗ Impotence
- ❗ Hot flashes, generalized pain, infection, constipation, and nausea

Sex hormones, including the estrogens, progestins, and androgens, are also used as antineoplastic agents in the treatment of malignancies involving the reproductive system (e.g., cancer of the breast, uterus, or prostate). These hormones are discussed in Chapter 24.

BIOLOGICAL THERAPIES

Biological therapy (also called immunotherapy, biotherapy, or biological response modifier therapy) is designed to repair, stimulate, or enhance cancer patients' natural immune systems to more effectively recognize and attack cancer cells. Some therapies are used to lessen the side effects caused by certain cancer treatments. There are different types of immunotherapy: The *active* or *direct* type (such as interferons) stimulates the body's own immune system to fight the disease. The *passive* or *indirect* type (such as MABs) uses immune system components created outside the body.

Interferons

Interferon alfa (Intron A), which is the type most widely used in cancer treatments, is a complex combination of many proteins that boost immune system response. Its antiviral action is described in Chapter 17. Interferons are used in the treatment of certain leukemias, melanoma, Kaposi's sarcoma, and non-Hodgkin's lymphoma. Interferons are also used to treat hepatitis B and C, multiple sclerosis, and other conditions.

Adverse side effects of interferons, sometimes severe, are experienced by almost all patients receiving interferon, varying with the dosage and condition. Most common side effects include:

- ! Flulike syndrome—fever, fatigue, chills, headache, muscle aches, and pains
- ! GI symptoms—anorexia, nausea, vomiting, diarrhea, and dry mouth
- ! Nervous system effects—sleep disturbances, depression, and neuropathy
- ! Hematological effects—especially leukopenia and anemia

    Dyspnea, cough, nasal congestion, and pneumonia

    Alopecia—transient

COLONY-STIMULATING FACTORS

CSFs such as erythropoietin (Epogen, Procrit) usually do not directly affect tumor cells. They encourage bone marrow stem cells to divide and develop into red blood cells (RBCs) and WBCs and platelets. Because anticancer drugs can damage the body's ability to make these cells, patients have an increased risk of developing infections, becoming anemic, and bleeding more easily. By using CSFs to stimulate blood cell production, oncologists can increase the doses of antineoplastics without increasing the risk of infection or the need for transfusions. CSFs are also used to increase the counts of RBCs and WBCs, so that chemotherapy can continue, as often times treatments are delayed if counts drop too low.

Refer to Chapter 25 for other uses of CSFs and their side effects.

MONOCLONAL ANTIBODIES

MABs are *exogenous* (*outside of body*) antibodies genetically engineered in the laboratory. MABs are designed to target only cancer cells, thereby sparing normal tissues (i.e., not *directly* cytotoxic). This reduces host toxicity while simultaneously increasing toxicity to cancer cells. One specific type of MAB is indicated where tumors have rich blood supplies, which can facilitate their growth and spread. Angiogenesis inhibitors (AIs) prevent the formation of new blood vessels that tumors need to grow and invade nearby tissue. Bevacizumab (Avastin), in combination with other agents, is indicated for the first-line treatment of patients with metastatic carcinoma of the highly vascularized colon, kidney, or lung. AIs may only stop or slow the growth of a cancer, not completely eradicate it.

Another MAB, trastuzumab (Herceptin), combined with paclitaxel, is indicated for first-line treatment of metastatic breast cancer in patients with tumors that produce excess amounts of a protein called HER2. *All MABs are administered intravenously.*

Side effects of MABs are common, especially with the first infusion, and can include:

- ❗ Fever and chills, headache, and dizziness
- ❗ Nausea and vomiting
- Itching, rash, and generalized pain

These reactions should occur less frequently with subsequent infusions.

Severe reactions can be minimized by *premedicating* with acetaminophen (Tylenol), diphenhydramine (Benadryl), and/or meperidine (Demerol). AIs (Avastin) may have side effects that are different from other MABs. Signs of severe reaction can include:

- ❗ Angioedema, hypotension, dyspnea, and bronchospasm (may be necessary to stop infusion)
- ❗ Hypersensitivity reactions (including anaphylaxis)
- ❗ Cardiac arrhythmias, angina, heart failure, cardiomyopathy; hypertensive crisis (with Avastin)
- ❗ Acute renal failure (not with Herceptin)
- ❗ Hematological toxicity (i.e., reduced WBCs); complete blood count and platelet count should be monitored frequently
- ❗ GI perforation, GI bleed; impaired wound healing (all with Avastin)

TARGETED THERAPIES

Targeted cancer therapies are drugs or other substances that block the growth and spread of cancer by interfering with specific molecules involved in tumor growth and progression. By focusing on molecular and cellular changes that are specific to cancer, targeted cancer therapies may be more effective than other types of treatment, including chemotherapy and radiotherapy, and are less harmful to normal cells.

Signal Transduction Inhibitors

One of the newer and largest grouping of targeted therapy drugs are called the STIs, which block specific enzymes and growth factor receptors that signal cancer cell proliferation. Imatinib (Gleevec) is one of the first clinically useful agents in this class and is approved for the treatment of chronic myelogenous leukemia and some rare types of cancers. The majority of STIs are given by the *oral* route. Side effects vary greatly depending on the indication, agent, and combination therapy used.

VACCINES

Vaccines are medicines that boost the immune system's natural ability to protect the body against "foreign invaders," mainly infectious agents that may cause disease. There are two broad types of cancer vaccines:

- *Preventive (or prophylactic),* which are intended to prevent cancer from developing in healthy people.
- *Treatment (or therapeutic),* which are intended to treat an existing cancer by strengthening the body's natural defenses against the cancer.

The FDA has approved two vaccines, Gardasil and Cervarix, that *protect* against infection by the two types of human papilloma virus (HPV) that cause approximately 70% of all cases of cervical cancer worldwide. Neither vaccine is indicated for the *treatment* of HPV infection nor will it protect against all HPV types not contained within the vaccine. Therefore, recipients of the vaccine should continue to undergo routine cervical and annual cancer screenings (Figure 14-4).

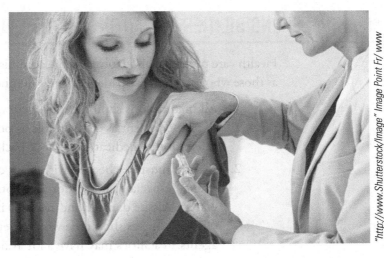

"http://www.Shutterstock/Image" Image Point Fr/ www.Shutterstock.com.

FIGURE 14-4 Young adults are encouraged to get Gardasil or Cervarix to help prevent the spread and incidence of these preventable types of cancer.

Patients who have latex hypersensitivity may be inappropriate candidates for the Cervarix prefilled syringe, as the tip cap and the rubber plunger of the needleless prefilled syringes contain dry, natural latex rubber.

The first cancer *treatment* vaccine, sipuleucel-T (Provenge), is approved for use in some men with metastatic prostate cancer. Sipuleucel-T is made from a patient's WBCs to stimulate the patient's immune system against the cancer and is manufactured for each patient individually.

See Chapter 17 for a discussion of traditional vaccines.

RADIOACTIVE ISOTOPES

Radioactive isotopes are also used in the treatment of certain types of cancer. Sometimes the radioactive material is injected into the affected site (e.g., radiogold, injected into the pleural or peritoneal cavity to treat the abnormal accumulation of fluid called ascites caused by the cancer). Radioactive sodium iodine is administered PO to treat thyroid cancer (thyroid cells naturally take up radioactive iodine). Radioactive material is sometimes implanted in the body in the form of capsules, needles, or seeds.

The newest targeted therapy provides the added benefit of radiation.

Radioimmunotherapy consists of MABs that have radioisotopes attached to them so that whatever the targeted antibody binds to can also be irradiated. Tositumomab (Bexxar) with iodine 131 is indicated for patients with refractory non-Hodgkin's lymphoma. The primary side effect after radioimmunotherapy is a decreased blood count occurring four to six weeks after treatment. The counts remain low for two to three weeks and then returns to normal. The distinct advantage of radioimmunotherapy is that it is usually given one time.

Health care professionals caring for patients receiving radioactive isotopes must observe special precautions to prevent unnecessary radiation exposure. Gowns and gloves should be worn when handling patient excreta such as feces, urine, and body secretions. Other isolation procedures, such as handling of linens, will be outlined in the facility's procedure manual. This protocol should be followed with great care by all those who come in contact with patients receiving radioactive materials, for the protection of patients as well as the health care professional.

CAUTIONS AND RESPONSIBILITIES FOR ANTINEOPLASTIC DRUGS

Health care professionals involved in the administration of antineoplastic agents, as well as those who care for these patients, have a number of very important responsibilities:

1. All medications should be given on time and exactly as prescribed to keep the patient as comfortable as possible and maximize the efficacy and safety of the medication. Check package inserts on all new drugs.

2. IV sites must be checked with great care because some antineoplastic agents (especially antitumor antibiotics and vinca alkaloids) can cause extreme tissue damage and necrosis if infiltration into surrounding tissues occurs. (Gloves should be worn when handling IVs with antineoplastic agents.) Facilities may have a kit available containing supplies and medications needed to treat extravasation.

3. IV fluids containing antineoplastic agents should not be allowed to get on the skin or into the eyes of the patient or the one administering the medication. Flush skin or eyes copiously if spills occur.

4. Antiemetics should be immediately available and administered as prescribed to minimize nausea and vomiting. Ondansetron (Zofran) and dolasetron (Anzemet) are examples of antiemetics used for this purpose (see Chapter 16).

5. Careful and frequent oral hygiene is essential to minimize discomfort and ulceration.

6. Soft foods and cool liquids should be available to the patient as required.

7. Accurate intake and output is important for the adequate assessment of hydration.

8. Careful observation and reporting of symptoms and side effects is an essential part of chemotherapy.

9. Aseptic technique is necessary to minimize the chance of infection in patients with reduced resistance to infection.

10. Careful assessment of vital signs is important to identify the signs of infection, cardiac irregularities, and dyspnea.

11. The health care professional and family must be informed about all aspects of chemotherapy and answer the patient's questions honestly. Awareness of verbal and nonverbal communication that gives clues to the patient's needs is absolutely necessary.

12. Careful attention to detail, astute observations, appropriate interventions, and compassion are an integral part of care when the patient is receiving chemotherapy.

13. The health care professional should reassure the patient that someone will be available to help at all times and should identify all resources available for both the patient and his or her family.

See Table 14-1 for a summary of antineoplastic agents' side effects.

PATIENT EDUCATION

Patients being treated with antineoplastic drugs and their families should be instructed regarding:

Side effects to expect, how long they can be expected to continue, and that they are frequently temporary

Comfort measures for coping with unpleasant side effects (e.g., antiemetics and antidiarrheal agents as prescribed)

Appropriate diet with foods that are more palatable and more likely to be tolerated (e.g., soft foods, bland foods, a variety of liquids, and especially cold foods in frequent, small quantities)

Careful aseptic technique to decrease the chance of infections and reporting any signs of infection (e.g., fever)

Careful oral hygiene with swabs to prevent further trauma to ulcerated mucosa

Observation for bleeding in stools, urine, and gums and for bruises, and reporting this to medical personnel

Reporting any persistent or unusual side effects, such as dizziness, severe headache, numbness, tingling, difficulty walking, or visual disturbances

Available community resources to assist and support the patient (e.g., Cancer Society, Hospice, or Home Health Services) as required and recommended by the physician

How to obtain information and answers to questions regarding treatment

The right of patients to terminate therapy if they wish

Cytotoxic Drug Dangers to Health Care Professionals

Most cytotoxic drugs are toxic substances known to be carcinogenic, mutagenic, or teratogenic. Anyone who prepares, administers, or cares for patients receiving cytotoxic drugs should be aware of the dangers involved. The American Society of Health-System Pharmacists (ASHP) has published a *Technical Assistance Bulletin*

TABLE 14-1   Side Effects of Antineoplastic Agents

POSSIBLE SIDE EFFECTS	DRUG CATEGORIES							
	ANTIMETABOLITES	ALKYLATING AGENTS	MITOTIC INHIBITORS (PLANT ALKALOIDS)	ANTITUMOR ANTIBIOTICS	HORMONE AND HORMONE MODIFIERS	INTERFERONS	MONOCLONAL ANTIBODIES	SIGNAL TRANSDUCTION INHIBITORS
GI effects: nausea, vomiting, diarrhea	X	X	X	X		X	X	X
Alopecia	X	X	X	X				
Suppressed bone marrow[a]	X	X	X	X		X (especially leukopenia)	X	
Ulcerated mucosa	X	X	X	X				
Photosensitivity	X							
Neurotoxicity	X	X	X			X		
Hypersensitivity			X	X			X	X
Cardiotoxicity	X	X		X		X	X	X
Respiratory dysfunction								
Hot flashes					X			
Impotence					X			
Flu-like syndrome						X	X	X
Renal toxicity		X					X	X
Extravasation		X	X	X				

[a]Includes leukopenia (low WBC count) and prone to infections, anemias, thrombocytopenia, and hemorrhage.

(TAB) that provides detailed advice on recommended policies, procedures, and equipment for the safe handling of cytotoxic drugs (see AHFS Drug Information). It is essential that policies and procedures be followed exactly as outlined on the labels provided by the drug company. Guidelines of the individual health care agency must also be followed to the letter for the safety of all concerned.

The danger to health care professionals from handling a hazardous drug stems from a combination of its inherent toxicity and the extent to which health care professionals are exposed in the course of carrying out their duties. This exposure may be from inadvertent ingestion of the drug on foodstuffs, inhalation of drug dust or droplets, or direct skin contact.

Recommended safe handling methods include four broad goals:

1. Protect and secure packages of hazardous drugs. Store them separately from nonhazardous drugs.

2. Inform and educate all involved personnel about hazardous drugs and train them in safe handling procedures.

3. Do not let the drugs escape from containers when they are manipulated (i.e., dissolved, transferred, administered, or discarded).

4. Eliminate the possibility of inadvertent ingestion or inhalation and direct skin or eye contact with the drugs.

Specific recommendations for cytotoxic drugs include the following:

1. When preparing these drugs, wear gloves, long-sleeved gowns, splash goggles, and disposable respirator masks.

2. For administration, wear long-sleeved gowns and gloves. Syringes and IV sets with Luer-Lock fittings should be used, and care should be taken that all fittings are secure.

3. Dispose of syringes, IV tubing and bags, gauze, or any other contaminated material such as linens in a leak proof, puncture-resistant container that is labeled "HAZARD."

4. Wear gloves and gown when handling excreta from patients receiving cytotoxic drugs.

5. Those who are pregnant, breast-feeding, or actively trying to conceive a child should not care for patients receiving cytotoxic drugs.

For more detailed instructions, see *ASHP Technical Assistance Bulletin on Handling Cytotoxic and Hazardous Drugs,* which is reproduced in the AHFS Drug Information book and updated based on information from Occupational Safety and Health Administration (OSHA), National Institutes of Health (NIH), National Study Commission on Cytotoxic Exposure, and the American Medical Association (AMA) Council on Scientific Affairs.

Antineoplastic therapy is complex and changes frequently with ongoing research. Therefore, you are not expected to remember the names of all of the antineoplastic agents. However, you need to know the *common side effects, interventions, cautions, and appropriate patient education.*

CASE STUDY A

Antineoplastic Drugs

The oncology infusion clinic's first patient of the day is Herman Johnson, a 72-year-old male with a new diagnosis of metastatic colon cancer. The oncologist has ordered a medication from a category of drugs as a first-line treatment that will *not* eradicate the cancer but *will* stop or slow the growth of cancer.

1. This category of drug is called a(n):
   a. Colony stimulating factor
   b. Vaccine
   c. Angiogenesis inhibitor
   d. Signal transduction inhibitor

2. Upon receiving his first dose, the nurse informs Mr. Johnson that he can expect which symptom(s)?
   a. Fever and chills
   b. Hot flashes
   c. Decreased platelet count
   d. Blood in his stools

3. Prior to a first dose, the nurse will administer which medication to minimize a potentially severe reaction?
   a. Morphine sulfate
   b. Motrin
   c. Mylanta
   d. Benadryl

4. During an infusion of Avastin, the nurse will be watching out for which possible side effect that may necessitate stopping the infusion?
   a. Nausea
   b. Bronchospasm
   c. Metallic taste in the mouth
   d. Headache

5. In the next several weeks, Mr. Johnson will be monitored for which side effect?
   a. Hypotension
   b. Low WBCs
   c. Constipation
   d. Excessive bruising

CASE STUDY B

Antineoplastic Drugs

During 39-year-old Geneva Moyet's annual physical, a physician palpates a swollen thyroid gland. A CT scan and biopsy determines that she has thyroid cancer. The physician refers her to an oncologist, who indicates that she should be treated with radioactive sodium iodide, a radioisotope.

1. With which route will this specific radioisotope be administered?
   a. IM injection
   b. Seed placement
   c. Orally
   d. Intravenously

2. What is a distinct advantage of radioimmunotherapy?
   a. It is usually given one time.
   b. It has no side effects.
   c. It is given once a month.
   d. No extra precautions need to be taken post-treatment.

3. Which of the following is the primary side effect of radioimmunotherapy?
   a. Diarrhea
   b. Nausea
   c. Fever
   d. Decreased blood count

4. Which should the nurse wear when handling patient excreta after radioimmunotherapy?
   a. Gloves only
   b. Gown and gloves
   c. Cap, gown, and gloves
   d. Cap, gown, gloves, and booties

5. Suppose that Geneva develops a low blood count. What category of drug would be given to her that would stimulate the bone marrow production of RBC and WBCs as well as platelets?
   a. Colony-stimulating factor
   b. Hormone modifiers
   c. Biological therapy (interferons)
   d. Antitumor antibiotics

CHAPTER REVIEW QUIZ

Match the term with the definition:

1. _____ Palliative
2. _____ Cytotoxic
3. _____ Antineoplastic
4. _____ Monoclonal antibodies
5. _____ Proliferating
6. _____ Exogenous antibodies
7. _____ Refractory
8. _____ Immunosuppressive
9. _____ Endogenous antibodies
10. _____ Clone

a. Target only cancer cells
b. Unresponsive to treatment
c. Within the cell
d. Produce a copy
e. Decreases antibody production
f. Alleviation of symptoms
g. Engineered in a laboratory
h. Reproducing rapidly
i. Destructive to cells
j. Counteracts malignant cell growth

Multiple Choice

11. Alkylating agents such as cisplatin and cyclophosphamide work by which method of action?
   a. They prevent growth by damaging DNA needed for reproduction.
   b. They assist in bone marrow depression.
   c. They block cell mitosis.
   d. They bind to estrogen receptors.

12. A tumor that is classified as benign is:
   a. Destructive to other cells
   b. Noncancerous
   c. Cancerous
   d. Resistant to radiation

13. A common side effect of an antimetabolite is:
   a. Numbness and tingling
   b. Phototoxicity
   c. Nausea and vomiting
   d. Visual disturbances

14. Which drug is used to treat cerebral edema associated with brain tumors?
   a. Leucovorin
   b. Anastrozole
   c. Letrozole
   d. Dexamethasone

15. Which antitumor antibiotic is known to be cardiotoxic and should not be used in patients with congestive heart failure unless no other options are possible?

a. Mitomycin

b. Daunorubicin

c. Adriamycin

d. Bleomycin

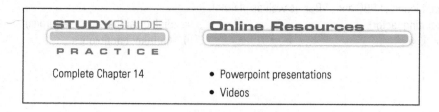

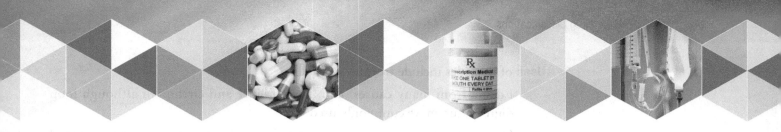

CHAPTER 15
URINARY SYSTEM DRUGS

OBJECTIVES

Upon completion of this chapter, the learner should be able to

1. Compare and contrast the four types of diuretics for uses, side effects, precautions and contraindications, and interactions and give examples of each type

2. Identify and describe medications given for acute and chronic gout to include side effects, precautions and contraindications, and drug interactions

3. Explain the role of certain antispasmodics used to reduce contractions of the urinary bladder

4. Identify the actions, uses, side effects, and precautions and contraindications for urinary analgesics to treat pain and cholinergic agents to stimulate bladder contraction

5. Describe the three different treatments for benign prostatic hyperplasia (BPH)

6. Describe appropriate patient education for all medications listed in this chapter

7. Define Key Terms and Concepts

DIURETICS

The most commonly used drugs influencing the function of the urinary tract are the **diuretics**, which increase urine excretion. Their main indication is to reduce the circulating fluid volume to help treat edema and hypertension. Diuretics are divided into five categories according to their action: thiazides, loop diuretics, potassium-sparing diuretics, osmotic agents, and carbonic anhydrase inhibitors. Carbonic anhydrase inhibitors such as acetazolamide (Diamox), which are used to lower intraocular pressure, are discussed in Chapter 18, "Eye Medications."

Thiazides and Related Diuretics

Thiazides are the most frequently used type of diuretic, increasing excretion of water, sodium, chloride, and potassium. An example is hydrochlorothiazide.

Uses of thiazides include treatment of:

Edema from many causes (e.g., heart failure and cirrhosis), although loop diuretics are more commonly used

Hypertension, either alone or combined with drugs from other classes (blood pressure is lowered by reducing peripheral vascular resistance as well as by decreasing fluid retention)

Prophylaxis of calculus (stone) formation in those with hypercalciuria (excess calcium in the urine)

Side effects of thiazides may include:

(!) Hypokalemia (potassium deficiency), may lead to cardiac arrhythmias; hyponatremia (low serum sodium level); hypercalcemia (abnormally high blood calcium level)

(!) Muscle weakness or spasm

Gastrointestinal (GI) reactions (e.g., anorexia, nausea, vomiting, diarrhea)

(!) Postural hypotension, vertigo, and headache

Fatigue, weakness, and lethargy

Skin conditions (e.g., rash and photosensitivity)

(!) Hyperglycemia and increased uric acid level

Precautions or contraindications with thiazides apply to:

Diabetes (may cause hyperglycemia and glycosuria)

History of gout (increased uric acid level)

Severe renal disease

Impaired liver function

Prolonged use (periodic serum electrolyte checks are indicated, and potassium supplements may be necessary to prevent hypokalemia)

Older adults because of greater sensitivity to thiazides (may cause low sodium level)

Patients with sulfonamide hypersensitivity

PATIENT EDUCATION

Patients being treated with thiazides should be instructed regarding:

Diet including potassium-rich foods (e.g., citrus fruits and bananas) or potassium supplements (check with the physician first)

A low-sodium diet prescribed by the physician if the diuretic is prescribed for hypertension

Notifying the physician of persistent or severe side effects

Administration with food (to reduce gastric irritation)

Administration in the morning to prevent disruption of sleep from frequent urination

Rising slowly from a reclining position to counteract postural hypotension

Limitation of alcohol consumption

Consulting the physician before adding other medications

Necessity for regular blood test to monitor electrolyte levels

Interactions of thiazides may occur with:

- Nonsteroidal anti-inflammatory agents (risk of renal insufficiency and reduced blood pressure control)
- Corticosteroids (increase potassium loss)
- Lithium (causes lithium intoxication)
- Hypotensive agents (potentiate blood pressure decrease)
- Digoxin (increased potential for digoxin toxicity)
- Probenecid (blocks uric acid retention)
- Antidiabetic agents (loss of diabetic control)

Loop Diuretics

These diuretics act directly on the loop of Henle in the kidney to inhibit sodium and chloride reabsorption, which in turn inhibits water reabsorption back into the bloodstream, leading to increased urine formation. Potent diuretics such as furosemide (Lasix), bumetanide (Bumex), and torsemide (Demadex) are not thiazides but act in a similar way to increase the excretion of water, sodium, chloride, and potassium. Their action is more rapid and effective than that of thiazides, with a greater *diuresis* (they do not lower blood pressure as well as the thiazides).

Uses of loop diuretics include treatment of:

- Edema associated with impaired renal function, heart failure, or hepatic disease
- Pulmonary edema
- Ascites caused by malignancy or cirrhosis
- Hypertension (if thiazides are ineffective, loop diuretics are sometimes combined with other antihypertensives, especially in patients with kidney disease)

Side effects of loop diuretics may include:

- ! Fluid and electrolyte imbalance with dehydration, circulatory collapse, and chest pain
- ! Hypokalemia with weakness (potassium supplements may be indicated especially for cardiac patients to prevent arrhythmias); hypocalcemia (abnormally low blood calcium level)
- ! Hypotension (close blood pressure checks are required)
- GI effects, including anorexia, nausea, vomiting, diarrhea, and abdominal pain
- ! Hyperglycemia and increased uric acid level
- Tinnitus, hearing impairment, and blurred vision
- Rash, urticaria, pruritus, and photosensitivity
- Headache, muscle cramps, mental confusion, and dizziness

Precautions or contraindications with loop diuretics apply to:

- Cirrhosis and other liver disease (careful monitoring is required)
- Kidney impairment

Alkalosis and dehydration

Patients on digoxin (cardiac arrhythmias are possible unless potassium is supplemented)

Those allergic to sulfonamides

Diabetes

History of gout

Pregnancy and lactation

Patients under 18 years of age (bumetanide and torsemide)

Interactions of loop diuretics are similar to those of thiazides:

Corticosteroids (potentiate potassium loss)

Lithium (toxicity risk is increased)

Hypotensive agents (potentiation of effects)

Digoxin (increased potential for digoxin toxicity and arrhythmias)

Additional interactions of loop diuretics may include:

Aminoglycosides increase the chance of deafness.

Indomethacin decreases the diuretic effect.

Salicylates with furosemide increase the chance of salicylate toxicity.

Anticonvulsants (e.g., phenytoin) reduce the diuretic effect of furosemide.

PATIENT EDUCATION

Patients being treated with loop diuretics should be instructed regarding the same information as patients taking thiazides:

Dietary or other potassium supplements as prescribed

Notifying the physician of side effects immediately

Taking with food before 6 p.m.

Rising slowly from a reclining position

Avoiding alcohol

Reporting sudden changes in urinary output, especially a decrease

Reporting abrupt or severe weight loss

Limiting exposure to sunlight while taking furosemide because of photosensitivity

Not taking any other prescribed or over-the-counter drugs without consulting the physician first

---

Potassium-Sparing Diuretics

Potassium-sparing diuretics such as spironolactone (Aldactone) and triamterene (Dyrenium) are sometimes administered under conditions in which potassium depletion can be dangerous. Potassium-sparing diuretics may also counteract the increased glucose and uric acid levels associated with thiazide diuretic therapy. Spironolactone is the diuretic of choice in patients with cirrhosis. It has also been shown to reduce deaths in patients with severe heart failure.

Potassium-sparing (saving) diuretics are seldom used alone but are usually combined with thiazide diuretics to increase the diuretic and hypotensive effects and to reduce the danger of **hyperkalemia** (excessive potassium retention). When combination products (e.g., Aldactazide or Dyazide) are given, supplemental potassium is usually *not* indicated, but this varies with individual circumstances and other medications taken concomitantly. *Periodic serum electrolyte checks are indicated.* Side effects of potassium-sparing diuretics are usually mild and respond to withdrawal of the drug, but may include:

- ❗ *Hyperkalemia* (especially with potassium supplements), which may lead to *cardiac arrhythmias*
- Dehydration or weakness
- GI symptoms, including nausea, vomiting, and diarrhea
- ❗ Fatigue, lethargy, and profound weight loss
- ❗ Hypotension
- ❗ Gynecomastia (enlargement of breast tissue in males) with spironolactone

Caution with potassium-sparing diuretics is indicated in patients with:

- Renal insufficiency
- Cirrhosis and other liver disease
- Pregnancy and lactation

Interactions may occur between potassium-sparing diuretics and:

- Potassium supplements, angiotensin-converting enzyme (ACE) inhibitors, angiotensin receptor blockers (ARBs), salicylates, and nonsteroidal anti-inflammatory drugs (NSAIDs), to cause hyperkalemia

PATIENT EDUCATION

Patients being treated with potassium-sparing diuretics should be instructed regarding:

- Avoiding potassium-rich foods and salt substitutes
- Reporting signs of excessive dehydration (e.g., dry mouth, drowsiness, lethargy, and fever)
- Reporting GI symptoms (e.g., nausea, vomiting, and diarrhea)
- Reporting persistent headache and mental confusion
- Reporting irregular heartbeat
- Monitoring weight and reporting sudden, excessive weight loss
- Rising slowly from a reclining position
- Taking medications after meals

Osmotic Agents

Osmotic agents (e.g., mannitol) are most frequently used to reduce intracranial or intraocular pressure. These agents are used mostly in emergency situations that involve cranial or spinal trauma and are used to reduce the risk of nervous system damage from swelling.

Side effects of osmotic agents can include:

- ❗ Fluid and electrolyte imbalance
- ❗ CNS symptoms, including headache, vertigo, and mental confusion
- ❗ GI symptoms, including nausea and vomiting
- ❗ Tachycardia, hypertension, and hypotension
- ❗ Allergic reactions
- ❗ Severe pulmonary edema

Extreme caution is indicated, and kidney and cardiovascular function should be evaluated before administration of osmotic agents to anyone with:

Kidney failure

Heart failure

Severe pulmonary edema

Pregnancy and lactation

PATIENT EDUCATION

Patients being treated with osmotic agents should be instructed regarding side effects to be reported to the physician immediately. The patient should be reassured that osmotic agents are always given under close medical supervision and serum electrolyte levels will be monitored frequently by blood tests to detect adverse reactions.

See Table 15-1 for a summary of drugs for diuresis.

TABLE 15-1   Drugs for Diuresis

GENERIC NAME	TRADE NAME	DOSAGE (VARIES WITH CONDITION)[a]
Thiazide and related diuretics (representative list—many others)		
hydrochlorothiazide	Microzide/HCTZ	12.5–100 mg daily
metolazone	Zaroxolyn	2.5–20 mg daily
Loop diuretics		
furosemide	Lasix	20–80 mg daily or BID[c], PO, IM, or IV
bumetanide	(Bumex)[b]	0.5–2 mg daily or BID[c], PO, IM, or IV
torsemide	Demadex	5–20 mg daily or BID[c], PO; slow IV dosage not to exceed 200 mg (*do not give IM*)
Potassium-sparing diuretics		
spironolactone	Aldactone	25–100 mg daily
triamterene	Dyrenium	50–100 mg bid pc
Combination potassium-sparing and thiazide diuretics		
spironolactone and hydrochlorothiazide	Aldactazide	25–50 mg daily (each component)
triamterene and hydrochlorothiazide	Dyazide, Maxzide	37.5 mg/25 mg, 50 mg/25 mg, 75 mg/50 mg 1 cap or tab daily
Osmotic agents		
mannitol	Osmitrol	Parenteral only; dose varies with condition

a. Dose may be higher for edema and heart failure.

b. This brand name is no longer marketed, but the name is still commonly used.

c. BID dosing is most often associated with the treatment of heart failure, patients should be instructed to take second dose in the middle of the day to avoid night time urination.

MEDICATIONS FOR GOUT

Gout is a form of arthritis and a metabolic disorder characterized by the accumulation of uric acid crystals in various joints (especially the big toe, ankle, knee, and elbow), tissues, and sometimes the kidneys, with resultant inflammation and pain. The management of gout includes treating acute attacks, uric acid–lowering therapy, and preventing recurrence of acute attacks. See Figure 15-1.

Acute gout is characterized by the sudden onset of pain, redness, warmth, and swelling in the affected joints. It occurs most commonly at night and in patients who are not well hydrated. Patients who are affected by gout can take nonpharmacological measures to help control their condition. Staying hydrated and avoiding or limiting fruit juices, seafood, red meats, and foods that are high in sugar and salt are dietary measures that help reduce the risk of acute gouty attacks. Smoking cessation and limiting alcohol consumption will also help.

Non-Steroidal Anti-inflammatory Drugs (NSAIDs) and Colchicine

NSAIDs such as naproxen, indomethacin, and ibuprofen, when started soon after the onset of symptoms, work quickly to relieve pain. NSAIDs should be used cautiously in patients with kidney disease, heart disease, or risk factors for GI bleeding (refer to Chapter 21 for more information on this class of drugs). Corticosteroids such as prednisone are useful in the treatment of acute gout in patients who cannot tolerate NSAIDs (see Chapter 23).

Colchicine is not an analgesic and does not affect uric acid clearance. It is used to relieve inflammation in acute gouty arthritis (must be given within 24h of the onset of symptoms for maximum effectiveness) and in the chronic management of gout. Colchicine can also be used prophylactically at low doses to prevent recurrent attacks.

Gout

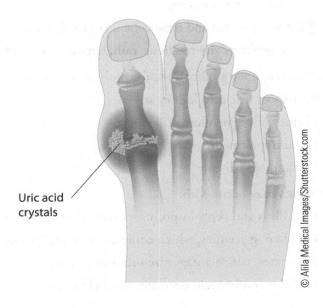

Uric acid
crystals

© Alila Medical Images/Shutterstock.com

FIGURE 15-1 Gout of the big toe due to uric acid formation.

Side effects of colchicine limit its use and can include:

Rash, alopecia

(!) GI upset, nausea, vomiting, and diarrhea (about 80% of patients cannot tolerate the frequent GI side effects)

Blood disorders and bone marrow suppression

PATIENT EDUCATION

Patients being treated with colchicine should be instructed regarding:
Large fluid intake to facilitate excretion of uric acid crystals.

Avoiding alcohol (increases the risk of adverse GI effects and increases serum urate [salt of uric acid] concentrations).

Medications used to treat gout chronically include the uricosuric agents and the xanthine oxidase inhibitors, which lower uric acid levels.

Uricosuric Agents

Uricosuric agents, such as probenecid, act on the kidneys by blocking reabsorption and thereby promoting urinary excretion of uric acid. This type of drug is used in the treatment of chronic cases of gout and frequent disabling attacks of gouty arthritis. However, the uricosuric agents have no analgesic or anti-inflammatory activity and are therefore not effective in the treatment of acute gout. During acute attacks of gout, the probenecid dosage is supplemented with colchicine, which has an anti-inflammatory action.

Probenecid is sometimes given with penicillin to potentiate the level of the antibiotic in the blood, for example with amoxicillin for some gonococcal infections. Probenecid is also given with cefoxitin to treat acute pelvic inflammatory disease.

Side effects of probenecid are rare but may include:

Headache

Nausea and vomiting

(!) Kidney stones and renal colic if large volume of fluids is not maintained

Hypersensitivity reactions, rash, hypotension, and anaphylaxis are rare

Precautions or contraindications for probenecid apply to patients with:

History of uric acid kidney stones

History of peptic ulcer

Renal impairment

Hematologic disease

Interactions may occur with:

Penicillins and cephalosporins, potentiating therapeutic effect of antibiotics

Oral hypoglycemics, which could cause hypoglycemia through potentiation

Salicylates, which antagonize uricosuric action

NSAIDs (probenecid decreases renal clearance)

PATIENT EDUCATION

Patients being treated with uricosuric agents should be instructed regarding:	Taking other medications at the same time only with the physician's order
Drinking large amounts of fluid	Taking medications with food
Avoiding taking large doses of aspirin products (aspirin doses of 325 mg per day or less are okay)	Reporting rash immediately

Xanthine Oxidase Inhibitors

Allopurinol (Zyloprim) is another medication used to treat chronic gout. This class of drugs also results in decreased serum and urinary levels of uric acid. It has no analgesic or anti-inflammatory activity and therefore is not effective in the treatment of acute gout.

Allopurinol is also used for the prevention of renal calculi in patients with a history of frequent stone formation and prevention of acute hyperuricemia during radiation of certain tumors or antineoplastic therapy.

Side effects of allopurinol can include:

> Rash
>
> ❗ Allergic reactions, also fever, chills, nausea, vomiting, diarrhea, drowsiness, and vertigo
>
> Severe hypersensitivity reactions are rare, but increase in older patients with renal impairment who receive allopurinol and thiazide diuretics in combination

Precautions or contraindications with allopurinol apply to:

> Impaired renal function
>
> History of hypersensitivity reactions
>
> Liver disease
>
> Pregnancy and lactation

Interactions of allopurinol may occur with:

> Antineoplastic drugs (potentiate side effects—azathioprine, mercaptopurine)
>
> Alcohol and diuretics (increase serum urate concentrations)

Febuxostat (Uloric) is the first new oral agent approved for gout since the early 1960s. It is more potent and has lower risk of hypersensitivity reactions compared to allopurinol. Febuxostat may have a higher risk of cardiovascular adverse events.

PATIENT EDUCATION

Patients being treated with allopurinol and febuxostat should be instructed regarding:	Avoiding alcohol, which increases uric acid
Drinking large quantities of fluid	Avoidance of purine-rich foods (liver, kidneys, shellfish, and red meat)
Taking medication after meals	
Stopping medication and reporting rash to the physician immediately	Avoiding other medications unless prescribed by the physician

BLADDER ANTISPASMODICS

Overactive bladder (OAB) is a condition characterized by two urinary symptoms: *frequency* and *urgency*. Frequency is defined as having to urinate more than eight times in 24h; urgency means the sudden need to urinate.

Antispasmodics, which are anticholinergic in action (blocking parasympathetic nerve impulses), are used to increase the capacity and decrease the urgency of the urinary bladder (see Chapter 13, "Cholinergic Blockers"). Antispasmodics, such as tolterodine (Detrol) and oxybutynin, are used to decrease bladder tone and suppress bladder contractions in patients with neurogenic bladder, resulting in decreased incontinence.

These drugs are used for the relief of symptoms such as urgency, frequency, nocturia, and incontinence. They have similar adverse side effects, especially in older adults.

Extended-release formulations (Ditropan XL, Detrol LA), patches (Oxytrol), and newer agents (Enablex, VESIcare) are less than or equally effective as oxybutynin IR (immediate release) but may cause fewer anticholinergic adverse effects. Recently the FDA approved an OTC patch called *Oxytrol for Women* (18 years or older); the Oxytrol patch remains prescription-only for men. Another anticholinergic, less commonly used as an antispasmodic, is hyoscyamine (Levsin), but adverse side effects are common in older adults.

Side effects of the **bladder antispasmodics** are ***anticholinergic*** in action and can include:

- **!** Drying of all secretions (especially in the eyes and mouth)
- **!** Drowsiness and dizziness—headache; fatigue
- **!** Urinary retention and constipation
- **!** Blurred vision
- **!** Mental confusion (especially with older adults)
- **!** Tachycardia, palpitations
- Nausea and vomiting
- Rash, urticaria, and allergic reactions

Precautions or contraindications with bladder antispasmodics apply for:

Older adults

Hepatic or renal disease and obstructive uropathy

Bladder or GI obstruction, or ulcerative colitis

Cardiovascular disease

Prostatic hyperplasia

Children—contraindicated for those under age 6 years. Ditropan XL is used effectively in children ≥6 years of age.

Pregnancy or lactation

Narrow-angle glaucoma

Interactions with bladder antispasmodics may include:

Other anticholinergic agents (can potentiate effects with possible toxicity)

Potassium salts (risk of GI irritation)

Mirabegron (Myrbetriq) is the newest bladder antispasmodic, which stimulates beta$_3$ receptors in the bladder to increase bladder capacity. It provides an alternative for patients who cannot tolerate the side effects of the anticholinergic antispasmodics. Common adverse effects of mirabegron include nausea, constipation, diarrhea, headache, dizziness, hypertension, and sinus tachycardia.

PATIENT EDUCATION

Patients being treated with bladder antispasmodics should be instructed regarding:

   Possible interactions with other drugs

   Reporting side effects that are troublesome for possible dosage adjustment

   Reporting effectiveness—inform patients that it may take several months to see effects

   Using caution driving or operating machinery

   Avoiding alcohol or other sedatives that potentiate drowsiness

   Seeking the advice of a health care professional before using over-the-counter *Oxytrol for Women*, to understand all of the FDA-required safe conditions for use

   Not crushing or chewing extended-release formulations (Enablex, Toviaz); not cutting or trimming patches (Oxytrol)

   Bladder retraining, toileting programs, and pelvic-floor exercises (Kegels), which may also be prescribed to improve bladder function

CHOLINERGICS

Bethanechol (Urecholine) is a **cholinergic** drug, stimulating parasympathetic nerves to bring about contraction of the urinary bladder in cases of nonobstructive urinary retention, usually postoperatively or postpartum. It has been called the "pharmacological catheterization." (See Chapter 13, "Cholinergics.")

Side effects of bethanechol are cholinergic in action and usually dose related, and can include:

   - ! GI cramping, diarrhea, nausea, and vomiting
   - ! Sweating and salivation
   - ! Headache and bronchial constriction
   - ! Slow heartbeat or reflex tachycardia and orthostatic hypotension
   - ! Urinary urgency

Precautions or contraindications of bethanechol include:

   Obstruction of the GI or urinary tract

   Hyperthyroidism

   Peptic ulcer and irritable bowel syndrome

   Asthma

   Cardiovascular disease—bradycardia

   Parkinsonism and seizure disorder

   Pregnancy and lactation

Interactions with bethanechol may occur with:

   Other cholinergic or anticholinesterase agents (e.g., neostigmine) administered concomitantly (can potentiate effects, with increased possibility of toxicity)

Quinidine or procainamide (antagonize cholinergic effect)

Atropine (antagonizes cholinergic effect—antidote in cases of cholinergic toxicity)

URINARY ANALGESICS

Phenazopyridine (AZO Standard) is an oral **urinary analgesic** or local anesthetic for urinary tract mucosa. It is used for a short time to relieve burning, pain, discomfort, and urgency associated with cystitis (bladder inflammation). It should not be taken for more than two days when used with an antibacterial agent.

Phenazopyridine is used *only for symptomatic* relief while waiting to see a physician and is not a substitute for the treatment of causative conditions. For treatment of urinary tract infections, anti-infective medication is required (see Chapter 17).

CLINICAL CONNECTION

Urinary Tract Infections

Urinary tract infections (UTI's) are characterized by symptoms that include increased frequency of urination or sudden urge to urinate, burning while urinating, cloudy or strong smelling urine, and possible pain in the lower abdominal area (Figure 15-2). UTI's are most common in women and the frequency of occurrence increases with age. In older adult patients, UTI's can often present with psychological symptoms that include confusion and delirium. Although UTI's are covered in depth in Chapter 17, some common antibiotics that are used for UTI treatment are Bactrim, Cipro, and Macrobid for a period of 7–14 days. Patients who have a history of UTI's should be educated to use proper hygiene and stay hydrated. As a health care professional, it is important to educate patients that although UTI's can resolve without treatment, it is important to seek treatment to avoid complications such as a kidney infection or damage to the urinary system.

Urinary Tract Infection

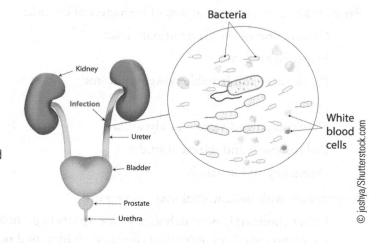

FIGURE 15-2 If left untreated, an uncomplicated UTI can travel up the ureter into the kidney and cause a more complicated infection called pyelonephritis.

© joshya/Shutterstock.com

Side effects of phenazopyridine are rare for the most part but can include:

Headache or vertigo

Mild GI disturbances

🚱 Discoloration of bodily fluids, including orange–red urine (common), which may stain fabric, and causes discoloration of contact lenses

Precautions or contraindications for urinary analgesics include:

Impaired kidney function, especially in older adults

Phenazopyridine may interfere with blood glucose measurements and urine ketone and protein kidney tests.

PATIENT EDUCATION

Patients being treated with phenazopyridine for urinary tract distress should be instructed regarding color change of urine to orange-red, which may stain fabric, and tears that may stain contact lenses.

Phenazopyridine is only temporarily effective against discomfort in the lower urinary tract and is not effective against infection. The cause of the discomfort must be determined and appropriate therapy, such as surgery or anti-infective medication, may be necessary to correct the condition.

TREATMENT OF BENIGN PROSTATIC HYPERPLASIA

Benign prostatic hyperplasia (BPH) is the most common benign tumor in men. BPH involves *hyperplasia* (an increase in the number of cells) leading to prostate enlargement, which interferes with urinary flow (Figure 15-3).

Benign Prostatic Hyperplasia

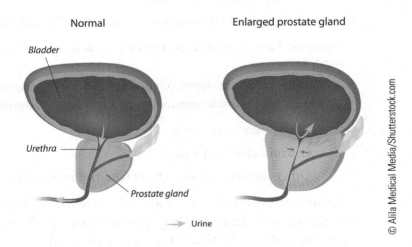

Normal

Enlarged prostate gland

Bladder

Urethra

Prostate gland

Urine

© Alila Medical Media/Shutterstock.com

FIGURE 15-3 Benign prostatic hyperplasia (BPH).

Drugs used to treat the symptoms of BPH include those that slow prostate growth (antiandrogens) and those that relax the bladder smooth muscle to make it easier for urine to flow from the bladder through the urethra (alpha-blockers).

Antiandrogens

Finasteride (Proscar) and dutasteride (Avodart) work by suppressing prostate growth and associated urinary obstruction and manifestations, for example urgency, nocturia, and urinary hesitancy. Proscar 5 mg, or Avodart 0.5 mg, is administered daily for a minimum of 6–12 months. This therapy appears to be suppressive rather than curative, and return of the hyperplasia is likely if the drug is withdrawn.

Side effects of **antiandrogens** include impotence, decreased libido, decreased ejaculate, and gynecomastia (including breast tenderness and enlargement). Side effects diminish after the first year of treatment.

Cautions: Patients should be screened first for cancer, infection, or other urinary dysfunctions. Antiandrogens can affect a blood test called PSA, used for the screening of prostate cancer (serum PSA concentrations may decrease even in the presence of prostate cancer). Liver function abnormalities may be exacerbated. Crushed tablets and soft gelatin capsules should *not be handled by pregnant women* (cause fetal damage).

Antiandrogens have not been associated with clinically important *drug interactions.*

Saw palmetto is a commonly used supplement for BPH, which might moderately reduce some BPH symptoms. The effects of co-use are not known at this time.

Alpha-Blockers

Tamsulosin (Flomax) blocks alpha-1 receptors found in smooth muscle in the bladder neck and prostate, causing them to relax. Consequently, the urine flow rate is improved and the symptoms of BPH are decreased. Alpha-blockers are considered to be the first-line therapy for the treatment of BPH. Other examples of **alpha-blockers** are doxazosin (Cardura) and terazosin (Hytrin), which are used in the treatment of hypertension, as well as for BPH (see Chapter 25, "Cardiovascular Drugs").

Side effects of alpha-blockers are infrequent but can include:

- ! Dizziness, headache, and nasal congestion
- ! Orthostatic hypotension
  - Palpitations (not Flomax)
  - Ejaculation dysfunction, decreased libido, and impotence

Cautions: Patients with a history of serious or life-threatening sulfonamide allergy (with Flomax):

Notify ophthalmologist of current or previous treatment with alpha-blockers—may be at risk for intraoperative floppy iris syndrome during cataract surgery.

Interactions may occur with:

Calcium channel blockers

Other antihypertensive agents (additive hypotensive effects)

Combination therapy with an antiandrogen (Proscar) and an alpha-blocker (Cardura) in patients with large prostates may significantly reduce the overall clinical progression of BPH and may reduce the need for invasive therapy compared to either agent alone (more data is needed, however).

Phosphodiesterase (PDE) Inhibitor

Tadalafil (Cialis), a PDE inhibitor approved for the treatment of erectile dysfunction, was recently approved to treat the signs and symptoms of BPH.

Caution: Important to read specific instructions on product label to reduce the risk of hypotension and fainting

See Table 15-2 for a summary of antigout medications, antispasmodics, cholinergic agents, analgesic agents, and agents for BPH.

TABLE 15-2   Other Drugs Affecting the Urinary Tract

GENERIC NAME	TRADE NAME	DOSAGE
Antigout medications		
colchicine	Colcrys	PO 0.6–1.2 mg daily in div. doses
Uricosuric agents		
probenecid		250–500 mg BID
probenecid w/colchicine		1 tab (500 mg/0.5 mg) BID
Xanthine oxidase inhibitors		
allopurinol	Zyloprim	100–600 mg daily
febuxostat	Uloric	40–80 mg daily
Bladder antispasmodics		
Anticholinergics		
tolterodine	Detrol	1–2 mg BID
	Detrol LA	2–4 mg daily
oxybutynin	(Ditropan)[a] Ditropan XL	2.5–5 mg two to four times per day
	Oxytrol patch (Rx)	5–30 mg daily
	Oxytrol for Women (OTC)	3.9 mg per day patch twice weekly
darifenacin	Enablex	7.5–15 mg daily
fesoterodine	Toviaz	4–8 mg daily
solifenacin	VESIcare	5–10 mg daily
hyoscyamine	Levsin	0.125–0.25 mg PO, SL, three to four times per day
Beta$_3$ agonist		
mirabegron	Myrbetriq	25–50 mg daily
Cholinergic[b]		
bethanechol	Urecholine	10–50 mg three to four times per day
Analgesic		
phenazopyridine	(Pyridium)[a] (Rx)	100–200 mg TID pc for 48 h only
	AZO Standard (OTC)	Dose varies depending on age range

(*continued*)

TABLE 15-2 **Other Drugs Affecting the Urinary Tract (*continued*)**

GENERIC NAME	TRADE NAME	DOSAGE
Agents for BPH		
Antiandrogens		
finasteride	Proscar	5 mg daily
dutasteride	Avodart	0.5 mg daily
Alpha-blockers		
doxazosin	Cardura	1–8 mg at bedtime
tamsulosin	Flomax	0.4–0.8 mg once daily 30 min after same meal or HS
terazosin	(Hytrin)[a]	1–10 mg at bedtime
Phosphodiesterase inhibitor		
tadalafil	Cialis	5 mg daily

a. This brand name is no longer marketed, but the name is still commonly used.
b. For bladder contraction.

CASE STUDY A

Urinary System Drugs

Ernesto Poligio, a 68-year-old male, is admitted to the hospital with shortness of breath, swollen ankles, and fatigue. His diagnosis is pulmonary edema.

1. Ernesto's physician prescribes a loop diuretic, which acts directly on what part of the kidney?
   a. Nephrons
   b. Bowman's capsule
   c. Renal pelvis
   d. Loop of Henle

2. The primary action of loop diuretics is to:
   a. Increase the excretion of water, sodium, chloride, and potassium
   b. Inhibit H_2O reabsorption back into the bloodstream
   c. Reduce peripheral vascular resistance
   d. Decrease fluid retention by promoting the excretion of uric acid

3. A potential side effect of a loop diuretic is:
   a. Hypokalemia
   b. Hypertension
   c. Hyperkalemia
   d. Renal colic

4. The nurse is preparing Mr. Ernesto for discharge and instructing him how to take his daily medication. One important point to include is to:
   a. Get 4h of sunshine a day
   b. Take medications at bedtime
   c. Avoid eating bananas
   d. Rise slowly from a reclining position

5. The nurse also makes sure that she reviews potential interactions with other medications and advises Mr. Ernesto to avoid:
   a. NSAIDs
   b. Diphenhydramine
   c. Digoxin
   d. Anticonvulsants

CASE STUDY B

Urinary System Drugs

Betty Weinstein is visiting her OB/GYN for her six-week postpartum checkup. She complains of burning, pain, and discomfort upon urination. Her physician prescribes a urinary analgesic to help relieve these symptoms.

1. The physician explains to Betty that urinary analgesics are given for a short time to alleviate symptoms associated with:
   a. Incontinence
   b. Nocturia
   c. Cystitis
   d. Prostatic hyperplasia

2. After giving Betty the prescription, the physician explains that the medication phenazopyridine can change the color of Betty's urine. What color will her urine be on this medication?
   a. Deep yellow
   b. Pink-tinged
   c. Pale yellow
   d. Orange-red

3. The physician also educates Betty on possible side effects of phenazopyridine, which include:
   a. Vertigo
   b. Fatigue
   c. Palpitations
   d. Nasal congestion

4. Prior to prescribing the medication, the physician reviews Betty's chart to make sure she does not have a cautionary condition. Patients with what condition would need to avoid phenazopyridine?
   a. Cardiovascular disease
   b. BPH
   c. Impaired kidney function
   d. Asthma

5. The physician also prescribes an antibiotic to be taken along with the phenazopyridine. Because of this, she explains to Betty that she should only take phenazopyridine for how many days?
   a. Two
   b. Four
   c. Six
   d. Eight

CHAPTER REVIEW QUIZ

Match the medication in the first column with the conditions in the second column that it is used to treat. Conditions may be used more than once.

Medication	Condition
1. ____ Proscar	**a.** Congestive heart failure
2. ____ Probenecid	**b.** Gout
3. ____ Hydrochlorothiazide	**c.** Benign prostatic hyperplasia (BPH)
4. ____ Ditropan XL	**d.** Incontinence
5. ____ Allopurinol	**e.** Edema
6. ____ Lasix	
7. ____ Cardura	
8. ____ Detrol	
9. ____ Demadex	
10. ____ Microzid	

Choose the correct answer.

11. Which medication is used prophylactically at low doses to prevent recurrent attacks of gout?
    a. Naprosyn
    b. Ibuprofen
    c. Indomethacin
    d. Colchicine

12. What type of intake is suggested for a patient on probenecid to prevent kidney stones and renal colic?
    a. Low sodium
    b. Large volume of fluids
    c. Low potassium
    d. Acidic fluids

13. Which instruction should be given to a patient taking allopurinol?
    a. Eat purine-rich foods.
    b. Avoid alcohol.
    c. Take medication with meals.
    d. Expect a slight rash.

14. In treating BPH, a patient taking Flomax might experience which side effect?
    a. Hypertension
    b. Dizziness
    c. Palpitations
    d. Hyperglycemia

15. What is a symptom or condition that is characterized by having to urinate more than eight times in 24 h?
    a. Nocturia
    b. Frequency
    c. Urgency
    d. Incontinence

16. Which of the following is the most uncommon medication used to treat a UTI?
    a. Macrobid
    b. Phenazopyridine
    c. Bactrim DS
    d. Oxybutynin

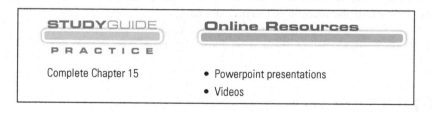

STUDYGUIDE
PRACTICE
Complete Chapter 15

Online Resources
- Powerpoint presentations
- Videos

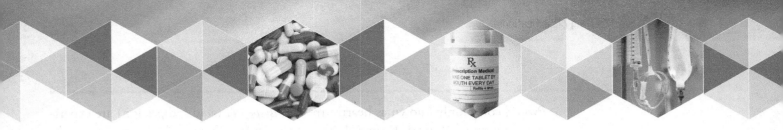

CHAPTER 16
GASTROINTESTINAL DRUGS

KEY TERMS AND CONCEPTS

Antacids

Antidiarrheal

Antiemetics

Antiflatulents

Antispasmodics

Antiulcer

Chemotherapy-induced nausea and vomiting (CINV)

Gastroesophageal reflux disease (GERD)

Histamine₂ blockers

Inflammatory bowel disease (IBD)

Laxatives

Postoperative nausea and vomiting (PONV)

Probiotics

Proton pump inhibitor (PPI)

OBJECTIVES

Upon completion of this chapter, the learner should be able to

1. Describe uses; side effects; precautions and contraindications; and interactions of antacids, antiulcer and agents for gastroesophageal reflux disease (GERD), agents for irritable bowel syndrome (IBS), antidiarrheal agents, antiflatulents, cathartics and laxatives, and antiemetics

2. Compare and contrast the seven types of laxatives according to use, side effects, precautions and contraindications, and interactions

3. Identify examples of drugs from each of the eight categories of gastrointestinal (GI) drugs

4. Explain important patient education for each category of GI drugs

5. Differentiate causes and treatment of *Helicobacter pylori* and *Clostridium difficile* infections

6. Define the Key Terms and Concepts

According to the National Institutes of Health, 60–70 million people suffer from digestive diseases. Gastrointestinal (GI) drugs covered in this chapter can be divided into the following eight categories based on their mechanism of action:

Antacids

Drugs for treatment of ulcers and gastroesophageal reflux disease (GERD)

GI antispasmodics

Agents for inflammatory bowel disease

Antidiarrheal agents

Antiflatulents

Laxatives and cathartics

Antiemetics

ANTACIDS

Pyrosis, commonly known as heartburn, and *dyspepsia* (acid indigestion) are experienced by up to 40% of the population in the United States at least once a month. Antacids act by partially neutralizing gastric hydrochloric acid and are widely available in many over-the-counter (OTC) preparations for the relief of indigestion, heartburn, and sour stomach. Other antiulcer agents are discussed later in this chapter. Antacids are also used at times as supplemental agents in the management of esophageal reflux.

Antacid products may contain aluminum, calcium carbonate, or magnesium, either individually or in combination. Most antacids also contain sodium. Sodium bicarbonate alone is not recommended because of flatulence, metabolic alkalosis, and electrolyte imbalance with prolonged use. Calcium carbonate, for example Tums, is rapid acting and possesses good neutralizing capacity but may cause constipation and kidney stones if overused.

The choice of a specific antacid preparation depends on palatability, cost, adverse effects, acid-neutralizing capacity, sodium content, and the patient's renal and cardiovascular function. Generally, antacids have a short duration of action, requiring frequent administration. Magnesium and/or aluminum antacids are the most commonly used. Magnesium can cause diarrhea, and aluminum causes constipation. Therefore, combinations, for example Maalox, Gelusil, and Mylanta, are frequently used to control the frequency and consistency of bowel movements.

Side effects with the frequent use of antacids may include:

- ❗ Constipation (with aluminum or calcium carbonate antacids)
- ❗ Diarrhea (with magnesium antacids)
- ❗ Electrolyte imbalance
- ❗ Urinary calculi (stone formation) and renal complications
- ❗ Osteoporosis (with aluminum antacids)
- ❗ Belching and flatulence (with calcium carbonate and sodium bicarbonate)

Precautions or contraindications with antacids apply to:

Heart failure

Chronic kidney disease or history of renal calculi

Cirrhosis of the liver or edema

Dehydration or electrolyte imbalance

Antacids may either increase or decrease the absorption of other medications. For many medications, this interaction does not result in patient harm. However, because they may decrease the effectiveness of the drug, antacids should not be taken within 2h of administering the following medications:

Anti-infectives, especially tetracyclines, quinolones, and isoniazid

Digoxin, indomethacin, and iron

Salicylates and thyroid hormones

Bisphosphonates (i.e., Actonel, Fosamax)

Antacids with the following drugs may increase action and precipitate side effects:

Diazepam, which increases sedation

Amphetamines and quinidine, which increase cardiac irregularities

Enteric-coated drugs may be released prematurely in the stomach (separate doses from antacids by 2h).

PATIENT EDUCATION

Patients using antacids should be instructed regarding:

Avoiding prolonged use (no longer than two weeks) of OTC antacids without medical supervision because of the danger of masking symptoms of GI bleeding or GI malignancy and causing the stomach to increase excess acid

Avoiding the use of antacids at the same time as any other medication because of many interactions (check with a pharmacist or physician concerning clinically important interactions)

Avoiding the use of antacids entirely or use with caution if the patient has cardiac, renal, or liver disease or fluid retention

Patients taking medicines for the management of esophageal reflux should also be instructed regarding avoidance of constrictive clothing, treatment of obesity (if appropriate), reducing meal size, avoiding lying down after meals, restriction of alcohol use, elimination of smoking, and elevating the head of the bed during sleep.

AGENTS FOR TREATMENT OF ULCERS AND GERD

H$_2$-Blockers

The histamine receptors found in the stomach are called H$_2$-receptors. H$_2$-receptor antagonists *reduce gastric acid secretion* by acting as **histamine$_2$ blockers**. They also reduce the amount of gastric acid released in response to stimuli such as food and caffeine. The drugs in this category, cimetidine, famotidine (Pepcid), and ranitidine (Zantac), are used *short term* for the relief of "acid indigestion and heartburn," **gastroesophageal reflux disease (GERD)**, esophagitis, and prevention of duodenal ulcer recurrence. Additionally, they are also used in the maintenance or long-term relief of the listed disease states but are dosed twice daily or at bedtime. Because they do not provide 24-h relief they are generally not considered first-line treatment unless proton pump inhibitors (PPIs) (discussed later in the chapter) are not able to be taken.

Side effects of H$_2$-blockers, usually transient and dose related, can include:

⚠ Diarrhea, dizziness, rash, and headache

⚠ Mild gynecomastia with cimetidine occurs infrequently and is reversible

⚠ Mental confusion (especially in older or debilitated adults; less with Pepcid)

Precautions or contraindications with H$_2$-blockers apply to:

Renal disease (may need to reduce dose and/or frequency)

Pregnancy

Lactation

Interactions with cimetidine may occur with increased blood concentrations of:

Warfarin (Coumadin) (also with high doses of Zantac)

Phenytoin

Beta-blockers

Benzodiazepines

Lidocaine

Theophylline (also with high doses of Zantac)

Tricyclic antidepressants

Note
There is less likelihood for drug interactions with Pepcid.

Proton pump inhibitors may interfere with the effectiveness of H_2-blockers; when given together the H_2-blocker is usually given at bedtime

All the H_2-blockers are available OTC for up to two weeks of self-treatment; beyond that time frame a physician should be consulted.

Proton Pump Inhibitors

GERD is caused by the excessive reflux of acidic gastric contents into the esophagus, resulting in irritation or injury to the esophageal mucosa characterized by heartburn and acid regurgitation. Serious complications include esophageal stricture, pulmonary aspiration, and esophageal cancer.

Omeprazole (Prilosec) is a gastric antisecretory agent (**proton pump inhibitor** or **PPI**), unrelated to the H_2-receptor antagonists. It is used for the *short-term* (four to eight weeks) symptomatic relief of GERD, for the *short-term* treatment of *confirmed* gastric and duodenal ulcers, and for erosive esophagitis and "heartburn." PPIs may be used *long-term* for severe GERD, preventing nonsteroidal anti-inflammatory drugs (NSAID)-induced ulcers, and hypersecretory conditions. Other drugs in this category include lansoprazole (Prevacid), rabeprazole (Aciphex), pantoprazole (Protonix), and esomeprazole (Nexium).

Side effects of PPIs can include:

- ❗ Diarrhea, constipation, nausea, vomiting, and abdominal pain
- ❗ Increased risk for pneumonia or intestinal (*Clostridium difficile*) infection

Long-term use on a regular basis of agents that reduce gastric acid can possibly result in vitamin B_{12} deficiency and low magnesium levels in the blood, especially in older adults.

In patients older than 50 years, long-term PPI therapy (at least one year), particularly at high doses, is also associated with an increased risk of hip, wrist, or spine fractures. A potential mechanism for this is PPIs' interference with calcium absorption.

Interactions of PPIs may occur with:

H_2-blockers (decrease PPI effectiveness)

Sucralfate (delays absorption of most PPIs)

Benzodiazepines, phenytoin, and warfarin (increased serum levels)

Ampicillin, ketoconazole, iron salts, vitamin B_{12}, bisphosphonates (results in poor bioavailability)

Food—Nexium, Prevacid, and Prilosec should be given on an empty stomach; Aciphex and Protonix can be given without regard to meals.

Note
PPIs available as slow-release (SR) tabs should *not* be chewed, broken, or crushed. PPIs available as SR caps may be opened and sprinkled on applesauce or yogurt, given with fruit juices, and swallowed immediately with water (do not chew or crush). Zegerid is an immediate-release product.

CLINICAL CONNECTION

Gastric and Duodenal Ulcer

Ulcers are a common condition that can affect any patient, although they increase with age, and are more common in those hospitalized and in women. The most common symptom of both gastric and duodenal ulcers is epigastric pain that is characterized by a dull or burning sensation. Gastric ulcers tend to exhibit this pain shortly after eating, whereas pain from duodenal ulcers tends to occur a few hours after eating as the food has now entered the small intestine area. If patients suspect they have an ulcer, it is important to determine if the likely cause is *Helicobacter pylori* or from chronic NSAID use. If the patient is a chronic NSAID user, then this is most likely the cause, if they are not chronically using NSAID's, *H. pylori* is most likely the cause. One can be tested noninvasively for *H. pylori* using a fecal antigen test, or invasively using an endoscope and a rapid urease test. Treatment of *H. pylori* ulcers is discussed in greater detail in Chapter 17 (Anti-Infective Drugs) but usually involves a PPI, two or more antibiotics, and a bismuth-based medication to coat the stomach. For NSAID-induced ulcers, it is important to discontinue the NSAID, or if this is not clinically possible, to initiate chronic PPI and/or H$_2$ antagonist therapy for at least one year. In either case, timely initiation of therapy is important to prevent further complications, which can include internal bleeding or the development of a gastric malignancy (cancerous tissue).

GASTRIC MUCOSAL AGENTS

Misoprostol (Cytotec)

Misoprostol (Cytotec), a synthetic form of prostaglandin E$_1$, inhibits gastric acid secretion and protects the mucosa from the irritant effect of certain drugs, for example NSAIDs (see Chapter 21), especially in those at risk, for example debilitated patients or older adults or those with a history of gastric ulcers. It is not Food and Drug Administration approved for the treatment of gastric or duodenal ulcers that are *unrelated* to NSAID use.

Side effects of Cytotec can include:

- ❗ Diarrhea, nausea, and abdominal pain (occurs early in the treatment and is usually self-limiting; take with food to minimize effects)

    Menstrual irregularities (begin therapy on the second or third day of the next normal menstrual period)

- ❗ Spontaneous abortion, possibly incomplete, with potentially dangerous uterine bleeding or maternal or fetal death

Precautions or contraindications for Cytotec include:

Women of childbearing age (unless the woman is capable of using effective contraceptives)

Pregnant women

Children under age 12

Interactions with antacids decrease the rate of absorption. Therefore, it is recommended that antacids should be given at least 2h away and should not be of a magnesium type (which exacerbates diarrhea).

Sucralfate (Carafate)

Sucralfate (Carafate), an inhibitor of pepsin, is another antiulcer agent that acts in a different way. Sucralfate is *administered on an empty stomach* and then reacts with hydrochloric acid in the stomach to form a paste that adheres to the mucosa, thus protecting the ulcer from irritation. The therapeutic effects of the drug result from local (i.e., at the ulcer site) rather than systemic activity.

Side effects of sucralfate are rare, with constipation occurring occasionally.

Interactions are possible with sucralfate altering absorption of certain drugs. Avoid giving other drugs within 2h of sucralfate, especially antibiotics and antacids.

Antacids may decrease binding of sucralfate to mucosa, decreasing effectiveness. Separate administration times by 30 min.

Helicobacter pylori Treatment

Helicobacter pylori bacterial infection plays a major role in the development of gastritis, gastric and duodenal ulceration, and gastric cancer (Figure 16-1).

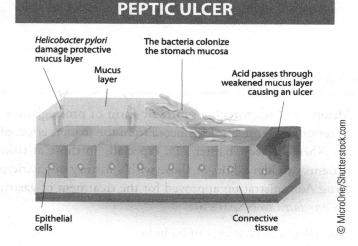

PEPTIC ULCER

Helicobacter pylori damage protective mucus layer

Mucus layer

The bacteria colonize the stomach mucosa

Acid passes through weakened mucus layer causing an ulcer

Epithelial cells

Connective tissue

© MicroOne/Shutterstock.com

FIGURE 16-1 The mechanism by which a *Helicobacter pylori*-induced ulcer is formed. In NSAID-induced ulcers it is the same, but NSAIDs inhibit the mucosal layer from forming around the stomach and can also irritate the gastric lining. Designua/www.Shutterstock.com.

PATIENT EDUCATION

Patients undergoing ulcer therapy should be instructed regarding:

Avoiding cigarette smoking, which seems to decrease the effectiveness of medicines in the healing of duodenal ulcers

Importance of close communication with the physician for possible dosage regulation of other medications taken at the same time

Structuring of environment to reduce stress factors and decrease tension to facilitate the healing of ulcers

Not taking antacids within 2h of any other drug

Taking medications on a regular basis and avoiding abrupt withdrawal, which could lead to rebound hypersecretion of gastric acid

Taking sucralfate (Carafate) 1h before meals, on an empty stomach, and not within 2h of any other medicine

Taking misoprostol (Cytotec) with meals and at bedtime with food, and avoiding magnesium products to lessen the incidence of diarrhea

Taking PPIs, esomeprazole (Nexium), lansoprazole (Prevacid), and omeprazole (Prilosec), on an empty stomach; rabeprazole (Aciphex) and pantoprazole (Protonix) can be given without regard to meals

That self-medication with OTC PPIs is not intended for *immediate relief* of heartburn

PPIs available as delayed-release dosage forms should *not* be chewed, broken, or crushed

Helicobacter pylori has been treated successfully with multiple-drug regimens (over 14 days). This treatment and possible side effects are discussed in Chapter 17, "Anti-Infective Drugs."

See Table 16-1 for a listing of the antacids, agents for ulcers and GERD, and protective gastric mucosal medications.

TABLE 16-1   Antacids, Antiulcer Agents, and Gastric Mucosal Agents

GENERIC NAME	TRADE NAME	DOSAGE
Antacids (only a sample, many other products are available)		
aluminum hydroxide gel		Suspension, 600 mg per 5 mL between meals & hs
calcium carbonate	Tums	Tabs, 500–2,000 mg orally in two to four divided doses daily
aluminum–magnesium combinations with simethicone	Maalox, Gelusil, Mylanta	Suspension, tabs; dose varies with product
Agents for ulcers and GERD		
H₂-blockers		
cimetidine		300 mg q6h PO
	Tagamet HB (OTC)	200 mg daily BID PO (two weeks max)
famotidine	Pepcid	20 mg BID or at bedtime–40 mg PO tabs at bedtime
		20 mg IV diluted q12h
	Pepcid AC (OTC)	20 mg daily or 10 mg BID (two weeks max)
with calcium carbonate and magnesium hydroxide	Pepcid Complete (OTC)	One to two tabs daily
ranitidine	Zantac	150 mg tabs BID or HS
		300 mg tabs BID or HS
		50 mg IV diluted or IM q6–8h
	Zantac 75, 150 (OTC)	150 mg daily or 75 mg BID (two weeks max)
Proton-pump inhibitors		
esomeprazole	Nexium	20–40 mg ac daily SR caps, susp, IV diluted
lansoprazole	Prevacid	15–30 mg ac daily SR caps,
		SoluTab; 30 mg daily IV diluted
	Prevacid 24 HR (OTC)	15 mg daily, SR caps (two weeks max)
omeprazole	Prilosec	20–40 mg qAM ac, SR caps, susp
	Prilosec OTC	20 mg daily ac SR tab (two weeks max)
with sodium bicarbonate	Zegerid	20–40 mg ac daily caps, susp
	Zegerid OTC	20 mg ac daily caps (two weeks max)
pantoprazole	Protonix	20–40 mg orally daily SR tabs, susp; 40 mg daily IV diluted
rabeprazole	Aciphex	20 mg daily SR tab

(*continued*)

TABLE 16-1   Antacids, Antiulcer Agents, and Gastric Mucosal Agents (*continued*)

GENERIC NAME	TRADE NAME	DOSAGE
Gastric mucosal agents		
misoprostol	Cytotec	100–200 mcg four times per day with meals and at bedtime with food
sucralfate	Carafate	1 g four times per day (1h ac and at bedtime), tabs, susp

Note: PPI's can be dosed BID in cases where daily dosing improves symptoms but does not last 24h.

GI ANTISPASMODICS OR ANTICHOLINERGICS

Dicyclomine

Antispasmodics or anticholinergics help to calm the bowel. Dicyclomine (Bentyl) is an anticholinergic and antimuscarinic agent used for the treatment of irritable bowel syndrome and other functional disturbances of GI motility. GI anticholinergics work by decreasing motility (smooth muscle tone) in the GI tract.

Side effects of dicyclomine, especially in older adults, can include:

- ❗ Dry mouth and constipation
- ❗ Blurred vision, dizziness, and drowsiness
- ❗ Urinary retention (decreases smooth muscle tone in the urinary tract)
  - Tachycardia, palpitations
- ❗ Confusion (especially in older adults)

Precautions or contraindications of dicyclomine include:

Glaucoma (narrow angle)

Unstable cardiac disease

Obstructive GI disease and ulcerative colitis

Obstructive uropathy (benign prostatic hyperplasia [BPH] and bladder obstruction)

Myasthenia gravis

Lactation

Interactions of dicyclomine include:

Phenothiazines (decreased antipsychotic effectiveness, increased anticholinergic side effects)

Tricyclic antidepressants (increased anticholinergic side effects)

Opiate agonists (additive depressive effects on GI motility or bladder function)

AGENTS FOR INFLAMMATORY BOWEL DISEASE

Inflammatory bowel disease (IBD) is a *chronic* condition that causes inflammation in the lining of the GI tract and includes Crohn's disease and ulcerative colitis. One of the main clinical features of this condition is abnormal defecation, which may be predominant constipation or diarrhea. There is no cure for IBD, and treatment strategies focus on symptom control and improvement in the quality of life.

Salicylates

Mesalamine (Asacol, Rowasa) and the prodrug sulfasalazine (Azulfidine) have chemical structures similar to those of aspirin and exhibit anti-inflammatory activity in the GI tract. They are used in the management of Crohn's disease and ulcerative colitis. These salicylates are all designed to reach the ileum and colon, bypassing the stomach and upper intestines. They are safe for long-term use and are well tolerated in most patients.

Side effects of salicylates (often more frequent and severe with sulfasalazine) can include:

- ! Anorexia, nausea, vomiting, diarrhea, and dyspepsia
- ! Abdominal pain, cramps, and bloating (with rectal administration)
- ! Headache, weakness, dizziness, and rash

Intolerance to sulfasalazine can be minimized by taking the enteric-coated product (Azulfidine EN-tabs).

Precautions and contraindications with sulfasalazine apply to those having:

- ! Allergy to salicylates
- ! Allergy to sulfonamides with sulfasalazine (can cause anaphylaxis or asthma attacks)
- ! Allergy to sulfites (Rowasa enema)

Renal impairment

Hepatic impairment (with sulfasalazine)

Interactions with sulfasalazine include:

Warfarin (increased risk of hemorrhage)

Methotrexate (increased bone marrow suppression)

Cyclosporine (decreased efficacy)

Oral diabetic agents (hypoglycemia)

Folic acid (absorption is inhibited)

Glucocorticoids

Glucocorticoids (prednisone, prednisolone, and hydrocortisone enema) are used to treat moderate to severe *active* forms of IBD in patients who are inadequately controlled with salicylates. The oral steroids do not require direct contact with the inflamed intestinal tissue to be effective. For a detailed discussion on these agents, see Chapter 23, "Endocrine System Drugs."

ANTIDIARRHEAL DRUGS

Antidiarrheal agents act in various ways to reduce the number of loose stools. Patients who are experiencing diarrhea should be instructed to stay hydrated with fluids such as water and electrolyte solutions such as Pedialyte. Sports drinks and sodas should not be used because of high sugar content, which can dehydrate the body further and worsen diarrhea.

Bismuth Subsalicylate

Bismuth subsalicylate (e.g., Kaopectate, Pepto-Bismol) has anti-infective and antisecretory properties, a direct mucosal protective effect, and weak antacid and anti-inflammatory effects. Kaopectate brand products have been reformulated several times over the years. Be aware that several formulations of "generic" Kaopectate are still available—check label contents and dosing carefully.

Side effects of bismuth subsalicylate are relatively uncommon at normal doses and include:

- ❗ Transient, occasional constipation
- ❗ Discoloration of tongue and stool (black color)
- Ringing in ears

Interactions with bismuth subsalicylate are possible, when these agents are administered concurrently with medications such as:

Warfarin (increases bleeding)

Aspirin and methotrexate (increases toxicity)

Quinolones and tetracyclines (decreases bioavailability)

Precautions or contraindications for bismuth subsalicylate include:

Salicylate (including aspirin) hypersensitivity

Children (<12 years old) or teenagers recovering from chickenpox or influenza (risk of Reye's syndrome)

Coagulation abnormalities and ulcers

Pregnancy and lactation

PATIENT EDUCATION

Patients treated with bismuth subsalicylate should be instructed regarding:

Avoiding self-medication for longer than 48h or if fever develops

Diet of a bland nature, excluding roughage and including foods containing natural pectin (e.g., apple *without* peelings and without sugar added)

Adequate fluid intake (especially tea *without* sugar for its astringent effect) or intake of oral electrolyte products (i.e., Gatorade, Pedialyte) to prevent dehydration

Contacting the physician immediately if complications develop or condition worsens and if observing blood in stool

Not using bismuth subsalicylate if allergic to salicylates (including aspirin) and in children or teenagers recovering from chickenpox or influenza

Considering all sources of salicylate if taking aspirin or other medications containing salicylate, so that toxic levels are not reached

Opiate Agonists: Diphenoxylate with Atropine and Loperamide

These products act by slowing *intestinal motility*, thus allowing for more reabsorption of fluid. Lomotil is a product combining diphenoxylate with atropine. It is a Schedule C-V controlled substance. Loperamide (Imodium) is available in various forms; all are OTC products, except for some capsule formulations, which remain prescription-only (see Table 16-2).

Side effects can include:

! Anticholinergic effects with Lomotil (e.g., drying of secretions, blurred vision, urinary retention, lethargy, confusion, or flushing)

! Abdominal distention, nausea, or vomiting with Lomotil or Imodium

Precautions or contraindications include:

Diarrhea caused by infection or poisoning

Fever over 101°F

Young children (under 3 years of age)

Pregnancy

Clostridium difficile colitis associated with antibiotics

Obstructive jaundice

Precautions or contraindications apply to older adults.

PATIENT EDUCATION

Patients taking antidiarrheal drugs should be instructed regarding:
  Not exceeding the recommended dosage; short-term (48 h) only
  Adequate fluid intake and bland diet

Reporting side effects or complications to the physician immediately, or if symptoms persist or worsen

Not taking these medications if diarrhea is caused by infection or food poisoning.

Probiotics

Probiotics are living microorganisms that can alter a patient's intestinal flora and may provide benefit in numerous GI diseases. The body's naturally occurring gut flora may fall out of balance in a wide range of circumstances, including the use of antibiotics or other drugs, excess alcohol, stress, certain diseases, or exposure to toxic substances.

Lactobacillus acidophilus is an acid-producing probiotic bacterium, available in several forms OTC. It is administered orally for the *treatment* of simple uncomplicated diarrhea caused by antibiotics, infection, irritable colon, colostomy, or amebiasis. *Lactobacillus* bacteria help to reestablish normal intestinal flora. The capsules, tablets, powder, or granules may be taken directly or mixed with cereal, food, milk, juice, or water.

Side effects tend to be mild and digestive (gas, bloating) in nature.

Precautions or contraindications for *Lactobacillus* apply to:

Anyone with a high fever; weakened immune system

Those sensitive to milk products or have a lactase deficiency

Long-term use, unless directed by the physician

Patients with prosthetic heart valves or valvular heart disease (risk of bacteremia)

Saccharomyces boulardii (Florastor) is a yeast used in dairy fermentation. It is derived from the intestinal microbiota of healthy humans. It is a probiotic often started within three days of antibiotic initiation and continued for three days after discontinuation to *prevent* diarrhea. Probiotic bacteria are also found in yogurt (Activia) and other dairy foods for the replacement of beneficial intestinal tract bacteria.

Clostridium difficile Infection

Clostridium difficile is one of the most common causes of infectious diarrhea in the United States. Symptoms of *C. difficile* diarrhea (CDD) may include watery diarrhea, nausea, and/or abdominal pain or tenderness. Complications may include sepsis, renal failure, toxic colitis, and death. CDD is caused primarily by the eradication of the native intestinal flora with broad-spectrum antimicrobials and overuse of PPI and H_2-blocker therapy. Please see Figure 16-2 for special considerations of patients with *C. difficile*.

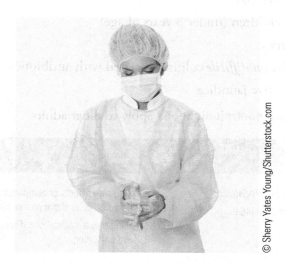

FIGURE 16-2 When a patient is hospitalized and diagnosed with *Clostridium difficile* they are moved to a contact isolation room to prevent the spread of infection. Barrier precautions such as this gown and thorough handwashing are very important. Alcohol-based hand sanitizers do not eliminate the *C. difficile* spores.

© Sherry Yates Young/Shutterstock.com

Oral medications include metronidazole (Flagyl) or vancomycin. See Chapter 17 for more information on these agents. Opiates and antidiarrheal medications may decrease GI motility, thereby increasing toxins in the intestine, so their use *should be avoided.*

ANTIFLATULENTS

Antiflatulents (e.g., simethicone) are used in the symptomatic treatment of gastric bloating and postoperative gas pains, by helping to break up gas bubbles in the GI tract.

No side effects, precautions and contraindications, or drug interactions have been reported.

PATIENT EDUCATION

Patients should be instructed to avoid gas-forming foods (e.g., onions, cabbage, and beans).

Precautions or contraindications apply only to infant colic because of limited information on safety in children.

See Table 16-2 for a summary of antispasmodic, IBD, antidiarrheal, and antiflatulent agents.

TABLE 16-2   GI Antispasmodic, IBD, Antidiarrheal, and Antiflatulent Agents

GENERIC NAME	TRADE NAME	DOSAGE
GI antispasmodics or anticholinergics		
dicyclomine	Bentyl	PO 20–40 mg four times per day caps, tabs; IM 20 mg q6h (two days max; switch to PO)
Agents for IBD		
Salicylates		
mesalamine	Asacol HD	2 × 800 mg PO TID (up to six weeks), DR tab
	Rowasa	4 g R at bedtime (retain 8 h; use three to six weeks), enema
	Canasa	1,000 mg R at bedtime (retain 1–3 h; use three to six weeks), suppository
sulfasalazine	Azulfidine	500 mg tab or DR tab
	Azulrfidine EN-tab	500 mg–1 g four times per day
Antidiarrheal agents		
Salicylates		
bismuth subsalicylate	Kaopectate, Pepto-Bismol	Susp, 30 mL or 2 tabs q30–60 min after each BM (max eight doses per day)
Opiate agonists		
diphenoxylate with atropine	Lomotil	Sol or tabs, 2.5–5 mg four times per day (max 20 mg per day)
loperamide	Imodium caps (Rx)	Sol, tabs, caps; 4 mg initially, 2 mg after each loose BM until stools are solid
	Imodium A-D (OTC)	(Rx maximum 16 mg per day; OTC maximum 8 mg per day × 2 days)
Probiotics		
lactobacillus acidophilus	Lactinex, Bacid	2 caps, 4 tabs, or 1 pkg granules three or four times per day
lactobacillus GG	Culturelle	1 cap PO BID (continue for one week after discontinuation of antibiotics)
saccharomyces boulardii	Florastor	2 caps PO BID (start within three days of antibiotic; continue for three days after discontinuation)
Antiflatulent		
simethicone	Mylicon	Liquid, tabs pc, and at bedtime 160–500 mg daily in divided doses

LAXATIVES AND CATHARTICS

Laxatives promote evacuation of the intestine and are used to treat constipation. Included in the laxative category are *cathartics,* or *purgatives,* which promote *rapid evacuation* of the intestine and alteration of stool consistency. Laxatives can be subdivided into seven categories according to their action: bulk-forming laxatives, stool softeners, emollients, saline laxatives, stimulant laxatives, osmotic laxatives, and chloride channel activator.

Many OTC laxatives are self-prescribed and overused by a large portion of the population. Prevention and relief of constipation is better achieved through natural methods (e.g., high-fiber diet, adequate fluid intake, good bowel habits, and exercise). Normal frequency of bowel movements varies from daily to several times weekly. When constipation occurs, the cause should be identified before laxatives are used.

Bulk-Forming Laxatives

Bulk-forming laxatives, also known as fiber supplements (e.g., psyllium, cellulose derivatives, polycarbophil, and bran), soften the stool by absorbing water and increase fecal mass to facilitate defecation. They are the treatment of choice for simple constipation unrelieved by natural methods. These products are available in powders, capsules, tablets, or wafers and *must be dissolved* or *diluted* according to manufacturers' directions (note label). The usual procedure is to take or dissolve the product in one *full glass* of water or juice to be taken orally and followed immediately with another glass of fluid. The proper dosage is administered one to three times per day. Laxative effect is usually apparent within 12–72 h.

Bulk-forming laxatives are the choice for older adults or laxative-dependent patients. They have been useful in maintaining regularity for patients with diverticulosis and in increasing the bulk of stools in patients with chronic watery diarrhea.

Precautions or contraindications for bulk-forming laxatives apply to patients with acute abdominal pain, partial bowel obstruction, dysphagia (difficulty in swallowing), or esophageal obstruction.

PATIENT EDUCATION

Patients should be instructed regarding:

Dissolving all bulk-forming products completely in one full glass of liquid and following that with another glass of fluid to prevent obstruction.

Administering immediately when dissolved, before thickening occurs.

Stool Softeners

Stool softeners (e.g., docusate) are surface-acting agents that moisten stool through a detergent action and are administered orally. Dosage required to soften stools varies widely depending on the condition and patient response. Stool softeners are the choice for pregnant or nursing women and children with hard, dry stools. The onset of action is usually 12–72 h.

Side effects are rare, with occasional mild, transitory GI cramping or rash.

Precautions or contraindications apply to acute abdominal pain or prolonged use (more than one week) without medical supervision

Caution to avoid stool softeners that also contain stimulant laxatives, for example Peri-Colace, Senokot-S.

PATIENT EDUCATION

Patients taking stool softeners should be instructed regarding:
  Discontinuance with any signs of diarrhea or abdominal pain
  Avoiding use for longer than one week without medical
    supervision

Interaction with mineral oil, which leads to mucosal irritation and
  systemic absorption of mineral oil
Taking large quantities of fluids to soften stool
Checking package label to be sure no cathartics are included

Emollients

Emollients promote stool movement through the intestines by softening and coating the stool. Mineral oil may be administered orally and is usually effective in 6–8 h. Mineral oil is sometimes administered rectally as an oil-retention enema (60–120 mL).

Side effects of emollients may include:

! Seepage of oil from rectum, causing anal irritation

! Malabsorption of vitamins A, D, E, and K only with prolonged oral use

Precautions or contraindications for oral mineral oil apply to:

Children under 5-years old

Bedridden, debilitated, or geriatric patients

Patients with dysphagia, gastric retention, or hiatal hernia

Pregnancy

Prolonged use

Concomitant use of stool softeners

PATIENT EDUCATION

Patients taking mineral oil should be instructed regarding:
  Avoiding frequent or prolonged use
  Using caution if having trouble swallowing or with aspiration of
    the oil (potential of lipoid pneumonitis if aspirated); never
    take mineral oil at bedtime

Interaction with docusate (stool softener), which can facilitate
  absorption of mineral oil, possibly increasing the risk of
  toxicity

Saline Laxatives

Saline laxatives (e.g., milk of magnesia (MOM) or citrate of magnesia) promote secretion of water into the intestinal lumen and should be taken only infrequently in single doses. Saline laxatives should not be taken on a regular or repeated basis unless directed by a physician. The onset of action is 0.5–3 h.

Side effects of saline laxatives used for prolonged periods or in overdoses can include:

! Electrolyte imbalance

! CNS symptoms, including weakness, sedation, and confusion

! Edema

! Cardiac, renal, and hepatic complications

Precautions or contraindications apply to:

Long-term use

Heart failure or other cardiac disease

Edema, cirrhosis, or renal disorders

Those taking diuretics

Acute abdominal pain

Colostomy

PATIENT EDUCATION

Patients taking saline laxatives should be instructed regarding:

Using caution as products of different strengths are available (MOM comes in 400, 800, and 1,200 mg per 5 mL concentrations)

Avoiding saline cathartics with certain medical conditions

Avoiding frequent or regular use of saline cathartics

Stimulant Laxatives

Stimulant laxatives (e.g., senna, castor oil, and bisacodyl) are cathartic in action, producing strong peristaltic activity, and may also alter intestinal secretions in several ways. Stimulant laxatives are habit forming, and long-term use may result in laxative dependence and the loss of normal bowel function. All stimulant laxatives produce some degree of abdominal discomfort. Their use should be confined to conditions in which rapid, thorough emptying of the bowel is required (e.g., before surgical, proctoscopic, sigmoidoscopic, or radiological examinations, or for emptying the bowel of barium following GI X-rays) or for patients on opioid therapy. Sometimes a combination of oral preparations, suppositories, and/or enemas may be ordered for these purposes. The onset of action is 0.25–8 h, depending on the preparation.

Side effects of stimulant laxatives are common, especially with frequent use, and can include:

(!) Abdominal cramps or discomfort and nausea (frequent)

Rectal and/or colonic irritation with suppositories

(!) Loss of normal bowel function with prolonged use

(!) Electrolyte disturbances and dehydration with prolonged use

Discoloration of urine with senna

Precautions or contraindications with stimulant laxatives apply to:

Acute abdominal pain or abdominal cramping—danger of ruptured appendix

Ulcerative colitis

Children and pregnant and lactating women

Long-term use

PATIENT EDUCATION

Patients taking stimulant laxatives should be given strong warnings against frequent or prolonged use because of the danger of laxative dependence and loss of normal bowel function.

Bisacodyl tablets should not be crushed or chewed or taken within 1h after milk or antacids because of gastric irritation.

Osmotic Laxatives

Osmotic laxatives such as glycerin, lactulose, polyethylene glycol (PEG), and sorbitol exert an action that draws water from the tissues into the feces and reflexively stimulates evacuation. Response and side effects vary with preparation. Lactulose response may take 24–48 h. Side effects include nausea, vomiting, flatulence, and abdominal cramps. Osmotic laxatives are also used to treat encephalopathy (brain and nervous system damage) in hepatic failure precipitated by GI bleeding and other conditions.

Glycerin rectal suppositories or enemas usually cause evacuation of the colon within 15–60 min. Glycerin may produce rectal irritation or cramping pain. Polyethylene glycol (Miralax) response can be seen in 0.5–3 h; however, two to four days of therapy may be required to produce a bowel movement. Side effects are similar to other drugs in this category; high doses of Miralax can cause electrolyte imbalances (hyponatremia, hypokalemia) with prolonged or excessive use.

Chloride Channel Activators

Lubiprostone (Amitiza) is a unique oral agent for the treatment of constipation. It increases intestinal fluid secretion by activating specific chloride channels in the intestinal epithelium. Lubiprostone alters stool consistency and promotes regular bowel movements without altering electrolyte balance or producing tolerance. Most patients experience a bowel movement within 24 h of the first dose.

Side effects of lubiprostone can include:

- Nausea and diarrhea
- Headache
- Abdominal bloating or pain and flatulence

Precautions or contraindications apply to:

- Severe diarrhea or bowel obstruction
- Renal or hepatic impairment
- Pregnancy and breast-feeding

PATIENT EDUCATION

Patients with constipation issues should be instructed regarding:

- High-fiber diet to prevent constipation, including roughage (e.g., bran, whole-grain cereals, and fresh fruits and vegetables)
- Adequate fluid intake
- Developing good bowel habits (e.g., regular, at an unrushed time of day)
- Regular exercise to develop muscle tone
- Avoiding any laxative with acute abdominal pain, nausea, vomiting, or fever
- Avoiding laxatives if any medical condition is present, unless prescribed by a physician. Bulk-forming laxatives are safest in the long term.
- Using only the mildest laxatives (e.g., stool softeners) on a short-term, infrequent basis
- Reporting any prolonged constipation, if above measures are ineffective, to a physician for investigation

Peripherally Acting Mu-opioid Receptor Antagonists

Naloxegol (Movantik) is a new oral agent specifically designed for the treatment of constipation caused by chronic or acute opioid use. It works by acting on the same mu-receptors that opioids do, but selectively inhibits the mu-receptors in the stomach. This action reduces or eliminates the opioid-induced delay in GI transit time cause by opioid stimulation that leads to constipation. It does not have action at other mu-receptors in the body, which means the analgesic properties of the opioid in use remain the same. Recently, this medication was a Drug Enforcement Administration (DEA) schedule II medication due to its structural relationship to opioids, but it has since been determined that there is no potential for abuse and therefore was removed from this schedule.

Side effects of peripherally acting mu-opioid receptor antagonists can include:

! Nausea and diarrhea

Flatulence

Precautions or contraindications with peripherally acting mu-opioid receptor antagonists apply to:

Severe GI obstruction

Patients with disruption to blood–brain barrier: may experience withdrawal-like symptoms

Severe hepatic impairment

Interactions may occur with:

CYP3A4 inhibitors will increase concentration of naloxegol

See Table 16-3 for a summary of laxatives.

PATIENT EDUCATION

Patients taking Movantik should be instructed to:

Take on an empty stomach 1 h before first meal of the day or 2h after

Avoid grapefruit or grapefruit juice

Swallow tablets whole, do not crush, split, or chew

Do not take other laxative medications while on this medication

Discontinue medication when or if opioid medication is discontinued

TABLE 16-3 Laxatives

GENERIC NAME	TRADE NAME	DOSAGE
Laxatives (only an example, many other products available)		
Bulk-forming		
psyllium	Metamucil, Konsyl-D, others	Powder, 1–3 tsp, dissolved in or 2–6 caps taken with full glass of fluid one to three times per day
Stool softener		
docusate	Colace, others	Oral caps, tabs, liquid 50–300 mg daily
Emollient		
mineral oil	Fleet mineral oil	15–45 mL PO daily; 60–120 mL R daily
Saline laxative		
magnesium hydroxide	Milk of magnesia	Susp, 15–60 mL daily

(continued)

TABLE 16-3 **Laxatives (*continued*)**

GENERIC NAME	TRADE NAME	DOSAGE
Stimulant laxatives		
senna	Senokot	8.6 mg tab, 1–4 BID or 10–15 mL syrup BID
with docusate	Peri-Colace, Senokot-S	1–2 tabs daily—BID
bisacodyl	Dulcolax	5–15 mg DR tabs, 10 mg suppository
	Fleet	10 mg/30 mL enema
Osmotic laxatives		
glycerine	Fleet suppository	1 suppository R PRN
lactulose	Enulose	15–60 mL PO daily (10 g/15 mL) (more frequently for hepatic encephalopathy)
polyethylene glycol	Miralax (OTC) GlycoLax (Rx)	17 g (1 capful) in 4–8 oz liquid daily (OTC—7 days max; Rx—14 days+)
sorbitol		30–150 mL PO of 70% solution
Chloride channel activator		
lubiprostone	Amitiza	8 mcg cap BID with food (IBD with constipation)
naloxegol	Movantik	24 mcg cap BID with food (constipation)
		12.5 to 25mg daily in the morning on an empty stomach (only use 12.5mg if patient unable to tolerate 25mg)

Note: This is only a representative sample. Others are available. Always read labels carefully, especially with OTC medications.

ANTIEMETICS

Antiemetics are used in the prevention or treatment of nausea, vomiting, vertigo, or motion sickness. Many different types of products are available, varying in their actions, the condition treated, and route of administration. Prevention is preferred over treatment of established nausea and vomiting.

Anticholinergics

Motion sickness is mediated by cholinergic and histaminic receptors in the inner ear. For prophylaxis of motion sickness, anticholinergic drugs such as dimen-hydrinate (Dramamine) or scopolamine are used. For greatest effectiveness, the Transderm-Scop patch is applied behind the ear 4h before anticipated exposure to motion (do not cut patch) and is effective up to 72h. Dramamine is administered orally 30 min before exposure to motion. Both of these drugs are also available for IM injection in patients who have already developed motion sickness.

Meclizine (Antivert) is an antihistamine used in the prevention and treatment of nausea, vomiting, and/or vertigo associated with motion sickness, and in the symptomatic treatment of vertigo associated with the vestibular system (e.g., Meniere's disease). The onset of action is about 1h and effects persist 8–24 h after a single oral dose. Although meclizine produces fewer adverse anticholinergic effects (dry mouth, confusion, urinary retention) than scopolamine, it can cause drowsiness, but to a lesser degree than dimenhydrinate (Dramamine). It is not recommended for children under age 12.

Antidopaminergics

Dopamine-receptor antagonists interfere with the stimulation of the chemoreceptor trigger zone (CTZ) in the brain, thereby blocking messages to the GI tract. The most frequently used agents to control nausea and vomiting in this class are prochlorperazine (brand name Compazine, which is no longer marketed) and promethazine (Phenergan), which are related to the phenothiazines, discussed in Chapters 20 and 26, respectively. These drugs are used for symptomatic relief, and their use must be supplemented by restoration of fluid and electrolyte balance, as well as determination of the cause of vomiting.

Antagonism of dopamine receptors in other areas of the brain, including those involved with movement, can lead to extrapyramidal reactions (tremors, difficulty walking, and muscular rigidity), which are common for drugs in this class at high doses. Prochlorperazine shows a high incidence of extrapyramidal reactions, especially in psychiatric patients receiving phenothiazines long term or in children. It is not recommended for children under age 12. *Caution with older adults. Not for long-term use.*

For *preoperative* preventive antiemetic effect or *postoperative* treatment for nausea and vomiting, promethazine is usually the drug of choice. Promethazine can be given *deep* IM (50 mg/mL concentration only) or via a central line (25 mg/mL concentration only), but *never* subcutaneously due to the risk of serious tissue injury that may occur. Metoclopramide (Reglan), a dopamine-receptor antagonist unrelated to other agents, is an antiemetic and a stimulant of upper GI motility. It accelerates gastric emptying and intestinal transit. It is used in a variety of GI motility disorders, especially gastric stasis, *short-term* (*up to 12 weeks*) treatment of GERD, and for the prevention (IM/IV only, not oral) of cancer chemotherapy–induced emesis. Extrapyramidal reactions can also occur with metoclopramide.

Serotonin-Receptor Antagonists

Serotonin is a major neurotransmitter involved in emesis located in the gut. Serotonin-receptor antagonists preferentially block serotonin receptors found centrally in the CTZ and peripherally in the intestines to control emesis. Ondansetron (Zofran) and dolasetron (Anzemet) are used for the prevention and treatment of **postoperative nausea and vomiting (PONV)** and for the control of **chemotherapy-induced nausea and vomiting (CINV)**.

These agents have fewer side effects (mainly headache, dizziness, drowsiness, and diarrhea) and are usually well tolerated.

Side effects of the antiemetics vary with the drug and dosage, but the most common include:

- ❗ Confusion, anxiety, restlessness (especially in older adults)
- ❗ Sedation, drowsiness, vertigo, weakness, and headache
- ❗ Diarrhea and depression (with Reglan)
- ❗ Dry mouth and blurred vision
- ❗ Extrapyramidal reactions (involuntary movements), especially in children and older adults with the antidopaminergics

  Cardiac arrhythmias, QT prolongation with high doses or too fast IV administration (see interactions)

Precautions or contraindications with antiemetics apply to:

Children and adolescents (increased risk of movement disorders) with antidopaminergics

Pregnancy and lactation

Debilitated, emaciated, or older adult patients (require reduced dose)

Angle-closure glaucoma

Prostatic hypertrophy

Cardiac arrhythmias or hypertension

Seizure disorders (seizure threshold lowered)

COPD and asthma (Phenergan suppresses cough reflex)

Interactions of antiemetics resulting in the potentiation of a sedative effect occur with:

CNS depressants, including tranquilizers, hypnotics, analgesics, antipsychotics, alcohol, muscle relaxants (potentiation of sedative effects)

Drugs that prolong QT interval (antiarrhythmics, tricyclic antidepressants, phenothiazines, atypical antipsychotics, "mycin" and quinolone antibiotics, and others)

Metoclopramide (other antiemetics also antagonize the stimulant effects of metoclopramide on the GI tract; promethazine can also increase the risk of extrapyramidal reactions if given with metoclopramide)

SSRI antidepressants (*serotonin syndrome* with promethazine and metoclopramide); serotonin syndrome is caused by excess serotonin release, leading to muscle rigidity, increased temperature, changes in blood pressure, confusion, and eventually death

See Table 16-4 for a summary of antiemetics.

TABLE 16-4 **Antiemetics**

GENERIC NAME	TRADE NAME	DOSAGE
Antiemetics		
Anticholinergics		
dimenhydrinate	Dramamine (po-OTC; inj-Rx)	50–100 mg PO or IM, IV q4h PRN for motion sickness (max 400 mg PO, 300 mg IM/IV)
meclizine	Dramamine Less Drowsy (OTC)	25–50 mg daily, 1 h before motion (repeat q24h PRN)
	Antivert (Rx)	25–100 mg in divided doses/Meniere's
scopolamine	Transderm-Scop	72-h patch for motion sickness
Antidopaminergics		
metoclopramide	Reglan	PO, IM, IV; dose varies with condition
prochlorperazine	(Compazine)[a]	5–10 mg PO, IM, IV, four times per day; 25 mg suppository BID
promethazine	Phenergan	Tabs, syrup, deep IM, IV, or suppository
		12.5–25 mg (never subcu; caution in older adults)

(continued)

TABLE 16-4 **Antiemetics (*continued*)**

GENERIC NAME	TRADE NAME	DOSAGE
Serotonin-receptor antagonists		
dolasetron	Anzemet	CINV[b]: 100 mg PO; PONV: 12.5 mg IV, 100 mg PO
ondansetron	Zofran	CINV: 0.15 mg/kg IV (over 15 min; max 16 mg), 24 mg PO; PONV: 4 mg IM, IV (over 2–5 min), 16 mg PO

Note: This is only a representative sample. Others are available. Always read labels carefully, especially with OTC medications.
a. This brand name is no longer marketed, but the name is still commonly used.
b. Dosage with PONV or CINV.

PATIENT EDUCATION

Patients taking antiemetics should be instructed regarding:

Taking these medications under medical supervision

Determining the cause of nausea and vomiting

Reporting effectiveness or complications

Administering only as directed

Not combining with any other CNS depressants, SSRI antidepressants, alcohol, or muscle relaxants unless prescribed by a physician (e.g., with cancer patients)

CASE STUDY A

Gastrointestinal Drugs

Derek Washington, a 42-year-old male, has called his physician's office to discuss an issue with the advice nurse. He has had diarrhea for the past 24h and would like a recommendation for a medication to relieve this condition.

1. The advice nurse suggests that Derek take some Pepto-Bismol, following the medication's label dosages. Which side effect may occur if he takes an amount over the recommended dosage?
   a. Dehydration
   b. Excessive thirst
   c. Hypoglycemia
   d. Black discoloration of the tongue and stool

2. The advice nurse also checks with Derek to see what other medications he is currently taking. The nurse explains that Derek should be cautious with which of the following when taking Pepto-Bismol?
   a. Iron
   b. Docusate sodium
   c. Warfarin
   d. Ibuprofen

3. Which type of diet will the nurse recommend for Derek while he is taking Pepto-Bismol?
   a. A full-liquid diet
   b. A diet high in roughage
   c. A bland diet
   d. A diet that avoids foods with natural pectin

4. The nurse also inquires about Derek's history of allergies to medication. Pepto-Bismol should be avoided in patients who are allergic to which drug?
   a. Penicillin
   b. Salicylates
   c. Naproxen sodium
   d. Glucocorticoids

5. The nurse recommends that Derek take Pepto-Bismol for no longer than:
   a. 48h
   b. 72h
   c. 96h
   d. 1 week

CASE STUDY B

Gastrointestinal Drugs

Helen Hoffmann is taking a bus trip to NYC with a group of friends. She is anxious about the trip because she often experiences motion sickness, so she consults with her physician.

1. Helen's physician suggests a medication to help prevent nausea and vomiting. Which medication will she be most likely to recommend?
a. Diphenhydramine
b. Meclizine
c. Promethazine
d. Prochlorperazine

2. After further discussion, the physician thinks that Helen would experience less motion sickness with a Transderm-Scop patch. To which area of the body is this patch applied?
a. On the inner wrist
b. On the upper arm
c. Behind the ear
d. On the anterior abdomen

3. How many hours prior to her bus trip should Helen apply the Transderm-Scop patch to prevent motion sickness?
a. 1h
b. 2h
c. 4h
d. 8h

4. The physician discusses other options for motion sickness treatment as well. Which medication can be given by IM injection to a patient who already has motion sickness?
a. Dimenhydrinate
b. Diphenhydramine
c. Nexium
d. Meclizine

5. Which additional instruction regarding the Transderm-Scop patch should the physician give to Helen prior to her bus trip?
a. The patch will be effective for 24 h.
b. The patch may cause excitability.
c. Do not cut the patch prior to application.
d. The patch will work only for motion sickness caused by bus travel.

CHAPTER REVIEW QUIZ

Match the medication in the first column with the condition in the second column that it is used to treat. Conditions may be used more than once.

Medication	Condition
1. ___ Nexium	**a.** Diarrhea
2. ___ Antivert	**b.** Flatulence
3. ___ Rowasa	**c.** GERD
4. ___ Lactinex	**d.** Meniere's disease
5. ___ Prevacid	**e.** Nausea and vomiting
6. ___ Transderm-Scop	**f.** Constipation
7. ___ Dulcolax	**g.** Inflammatory bowel disease
8. ___ Simethicone	**h.** Motion sickness
9. ___ Imodium	
10. ___ Phenergan	

Choose the correct answer.

11. With antacids, which of the following applies to administration?
    a. Before meals
    b. 2 h from other medications
    c. With Tagamet
    d. With milk

12. What is a frequent side effect of calcium carbonate antacids?
    a. Diarrhea
    b. Fluid retention
    c. Constipation
    d. Palpitations

13. A patient taking an antispasmodic may experience which side effect?
    a. Urinary retention
    b. Diarrhea
    c. Restlessness
    d. Excitability

14. *Clostridium difficile* infection is primarily caused by:
    a. Yeast overgrowth in colon
    b. Intermittent use of H_2 blocker therapy
    c. Eradication of native intestinal flora by antibiotics or another source
    d. Prolonged use of probiotics

15. When a patient complains of constipation, what is the first action that should be taken?
    a. Administer an osmotic laxative.
    b. Obtain an abdominal X-ray.
    c. Administer a bisacodyl tablet with milk.
    d. Identify the cause of the constipation.

16. An interaction of an antiemetic drug with another category of drug can result in a potentiation of a sedative effect. What is the second category of drug?
    a. Antiarrythmics
    b. Antidopaminergics
    c. Muscle relaxants
    d. Antacids

17. For patients who experience constipation directly resulting from opioid use, a new medication that may help them is?
    a. Movantik
    b. Scopalamine
    c. Amitiza
    d. Dulcolax

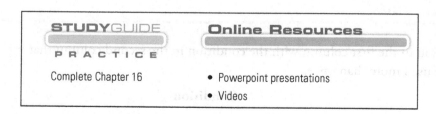

STUDYGUIDE

PRACTICE

Complete Chapter 16

Online Resources

• Powerpoint presentations
• Videos

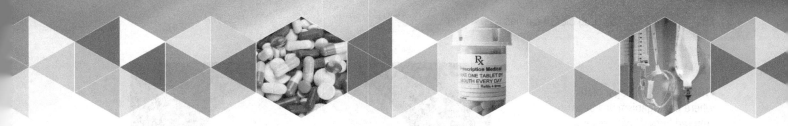

CHAPTER 17
ANTI-INFECTIVE DRUGS

KEY TERMS AND CONCEPTS

Adverse reactions

Aminoglycosides

Anaphylaxis

Antifungal

Antiretroviral (ARV)
  agents

Antituberculosis agents

Antiviral agent

Broad spectrum

Carbapenems

Cephalosporins

Culture and sensitivity
  (C&S) tests

Direct toxicity

Empiric

Macrolides

Opportunistic infections

Penicillins

Quinolones

Resistance

Sulfonamides

Superinfection

Tetracyclines

Urinary anti-infectives

Vaccines

OBJECTIVES

Upon completion of this chapter, the learner should be able to

1. Identify indications, side effects, precautions and contraindications, and interactions common to each category of anti-infectives

2. Explain the unique features of patient education appropriate for each category of anti-infectives

3. Describe the general instructions that should be given to every patient undergoing anti-infective therapy

4. Explain the mechanism for resistant organism development and its significance.

5. Define Key Terms and Concepts

According to the U.S. Centers for Disease Control and Prevention (CDC), over 28 million visits to office-based physicians and hospital outpatient departments are made annually for the treatment of infections and parasitic diseases. The first step in treatment is identifying the causative organism and the specific medication to which it is sensitive. **Culture and sensitivity (C&S) tests** will be ordered (e.g., wound, throat, urine, or blood), based on symptoms. See Figure 17-1. It is imperative to obtain the appropriate specimen before administering medication. Results of C&S tests will not be available for 24–48 h. In the meantime, depending on the clinical condition of the patient, the physician may order an empiric (best guess based on history) anti-infective regimen that would likely be active against the organisms encountered at the given site of infection (e.g., brain, lung, skin).

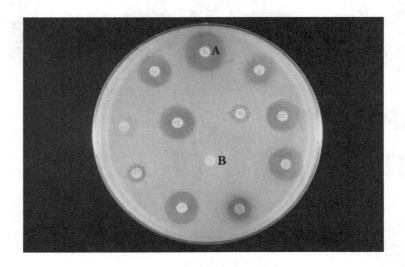

FIGURE 17-1 An agar plate where the organism has been cultured (grown) with several different antibiotic-containing paper disks placed on the "lawn" of organisms. Note the varying zones of inhibition or no growth. (A) A highly sensitive organism that is killed by the antibiotic. (B) A resistant organism that is not affected. Courtesy of the Centers for Disease Control and Prevention.

RESISTANCE

Sometimes organisms build up **resistance** to drugs that have been used too frequently or improperly, and then the drugs are no longer effective. According to the CDC, more than 70% of bacteria that cause hospital-acquired infections (HAIs; older term was nosocomial infections) are resistant to at least one of the drugs most commonly used to treat those infections. Also of concern, infections because of resistant organisms that were seen only in hospital settings are now increasingly being seen in the community. Antimicrobial resistance is rising not only in prevalence but also across all classes of antibiotics.

An example of an organism resistant to most antibiotics is methicillin-resistant *Staphylococcus aureus* (MRSA). Vancomycin IV is one of a small number of drugs effective against MRSA. The CDC also reports outbreaks of tuberculosis resistant to standard drug therapy (see "Antituberculosis Agents").

Some strains of enterococci have become resistant to most of the antibiotics, including vancomycin. Infections such as bacteremia, endocarditis, or urinary tract infections (UTIs), which are caused by vancomycin-resistant enterococci (VRE), can be very difficult to treat. Treatment options are limited, and mortality rates are high. Resistance to antiviral and antifungal agents is also an important clinical problem. Many strains of type A influenza are now resistant to oseltamivir (Tamiflu). Individuals infected with human immunodeficiency virus (HIV) wage a constant battle with resistance because the virus is only suppressed, not eradicated; that is, it is hidden in the patient's immune system by ongoing antiretroviral treatment. *Candida* species resistant to fluconazole are a growing problem in many health care institutions as well because of widespread use of this antifungal agent.

Anti-infective resistance is caused by many factors. Therefore, the strategies needed to combat the problem are also complex. Effective strategies include better patient and physician *education* on appropriate anti-infective use, accurate diagnosis, and targeted treatment of infections. Strict adherence to *preventive measures* such as routine handwashing or alcohol wiping between patient visits and rapid isolation of patients with resistant infections is also extremely important.

Selection of anti-infective drugs is based on several factors:

1. *Site of the infection.* This helps determine the initial empiric anti-infective regimen.

2. *Status of hepatic and/or renal function.* Lower doses or alternative drugs might be indicated with impairment.

3. *Age of the patient.* Some anti-infectives are more toxic to children or older patients. Lower doses or alternative drugs might be indicated.

4. *Pregnancy or lactation.* Some anti-infectives can cross the placenta and cause damage to the developing fetus, for example tetracycline or streptomycin. Others can be carried in breast milk and can cause toxicity to the infant.

5. *Likelihood of organisms developing resistance.* Sometimes a combination of drugs is used to decrease the chance of the organisms developing resistance to a single drug. Examples of combination therapy include sulfamethoxazole and trimethoprim combined to treat UTIs. Another example is the combination of three or more drugs to treat tuberculosis.

6. *Known allergy to the anti-infective drug.* In such cases, an alternative should be used.

ADVERSE REACTIONS

Adverse reactions to anti-infectives are divided into three categories:

1. *Allergic hypersensitivity.* This is an over-response of the body to a specific substance. A *mild* reaction with only rash, urticaria (hives), or mild fever is usually treated with corticosteroids or antihistamines, and the medication is *discontinued.* Sometimes severe reactions occur. *Severe* reactions may be manifested as anaphylaxis, a sudden onset of dyspnea, chest constriction, shock, and collapse. Unless treated promptly with epinephrine, corticosteroids, and CPR (cardiopulmonary resuscitation), death may result.

2. *Direct toxicity.* Results in tissue damage, such as ototoxicity (hearing difficulties or dizziness), nephrotoxicity (kidney problems), hepatotoxicity (liver damage), blood dyscrasias (abnormalities in blood components), phlebitis, or phototoxicity. Sometimes the damage can be permanent, or it may be reversible when the medication is discontinued. The health care professional's responsibility involves assessment of the physical condition and laboratory reports and potential *discontinuance* of the medication at the first sign of toxicity.

3. *Indirect toxicity, or superinfection.* Manifested as a new infection as a result of killing the normal flora in the intestines or mucous membranes, especially with broad-spectrum antibiotics and therefore allowing colonization of these areas with different resistant bacteria or fungi. Symptoms of superinfections can include diarrhea, vaginitis, stomatitis,

or glossitis. Treatment consists of antifungal medications, including buttermilk or yogurt in the diet, or administering probiotics (see Chapter 16) to help restore normal intestinal flora. Probiotics, available OTC, are also used prophylactically to prevent superinfections, especially in patients with severe colitis or in patients with a history of such infections.

VACCINES OR IMMUNIZATIONS

The CDC currently recommends routine vaccination to prevent 17 vaccine-preventable diseases that occur in infants, children, adolescents, or adults.

Information regarding vaccines and immunizations changes from time to time, and requirements may vary by state, territory, or country. The most up-to-date information regarding vaccines, immunization recommendations, and requirements can be obtained on the CDC website, http://www.cdc.gov/vaccines. You can also call the CDC Info Contact Center at 800-232-4636.

One recommendation of the CDC regarding influenza vaccine is relevant to your practice. The CDC now recommends that *all* individuals over 6 months old (including health care professionals) be given the influenza vaccine between August and November, annually. It is your responsibility to stress the importance of this prophylactic measure in helping to prevent serious, possibly fatal, complications from contracting virulent forms of influenza virus. There has been much controversy about whether vaccines and autism are linked. The first purported link was with the measles-mumps-rubella (MMR) vaccine. It has also been speculated that thimerosal, a mercury-containing preservative long used in vaccines, is linked to increased rates of autism. In both cases, after reviewing available data and studies, the Immunization Safety Review Committee (ISRC) of the Institute of Medicine (IOM) has determined that evidence is insufficient to demonstrate a causal relationship between vaccines and autism and therefore vaccinations should be recommended in all appropriate cases. A full immunization schedule for adults can be found in Figure 17-2.

ANTIBIOTICS

The term antibiotics refers to a large spectrum of medicines that are useful for treating and preventing infections caused by bacteria. These types of medications have no effect on viral, fungal, or other types of infections. Their improper use or use without proper indication can lead to resistance. This explains why antibiotics should not be used for treatment of the common cold, because it is a viral infection. Organisms can also become resistant if infections are treated incompletely or for a shorter duration than prescribed. Bacterial infections can vary greatly, therefore many different types of antibiotics have been developed that will be discussed in detail in the following section.

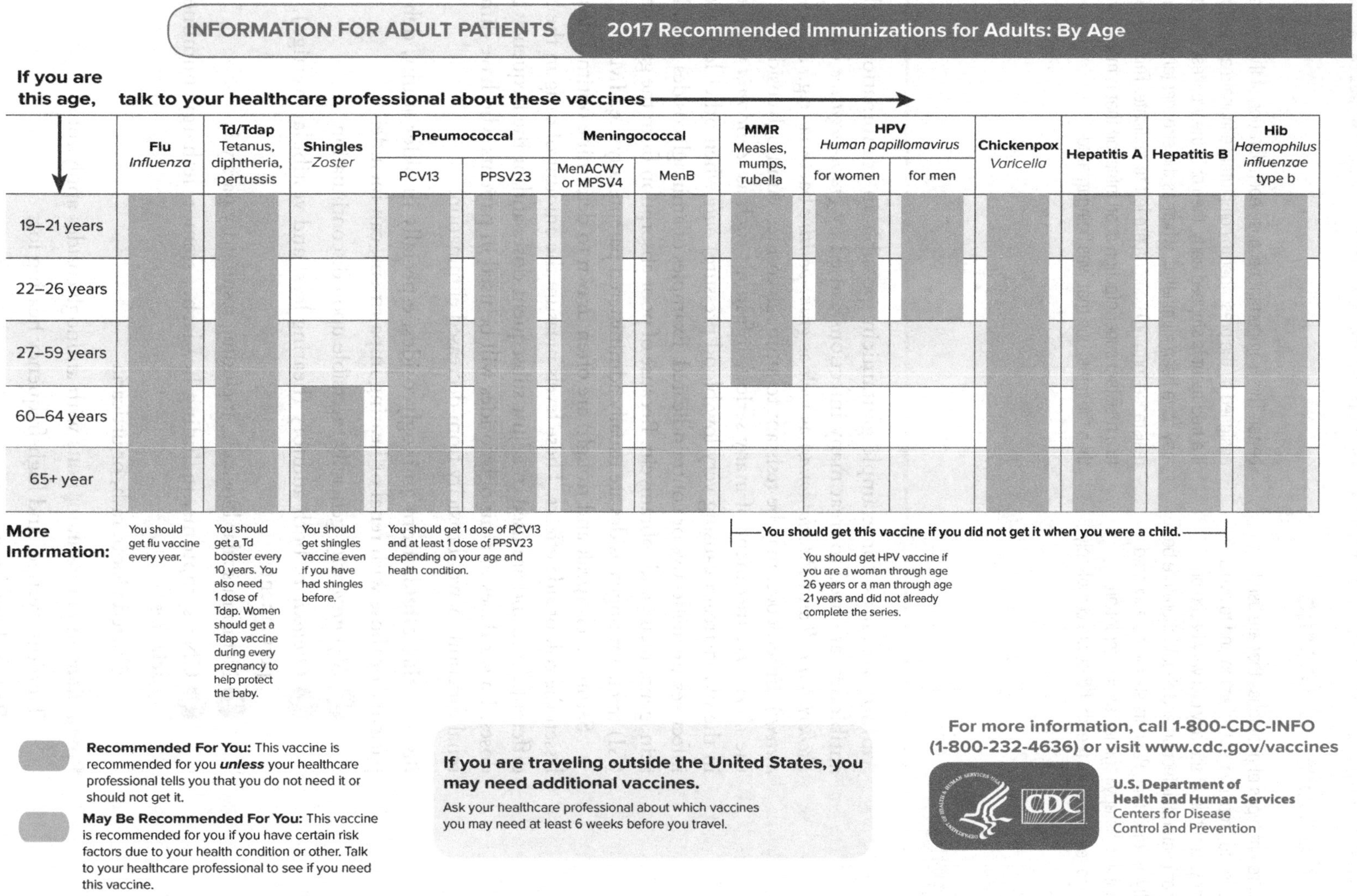

FIGURE 17-2 2017 Adult Recommended Immunization Schedule. *Courtesy U.S. Department of Health and Human Services and the Centers for Disease Control and Prevention.*

CLINICAL CONNECTION

Antibiotic Duration of Therapy

There are many different types of antibiotics that are used in different scenarios to properly treat infection and to avoid resistance. Similarly, duration of therapy can vary based on type and severity of bacterial infection and should therefore be considered equally as important. Patients should be educated to take every antibiotic therapy regimen until completion, even if they begin to feel better or feel that they are completely better. This is important because each duration of therapy is designed by the prescriber to completely eliminate all bacteria. If a treatment is stopped early, then only the weakest bacteria may have been eliminated, whereas the stronger (and possibly resistance-forming) bacteria are left to replicate. This can lead to a resistant superinfection or an infection that is more severe than the initial one that was being treated.

AMINOGLYCOSIDES

Aminoglycosides, for example gentamicin, possibly in combination with other antibiotics, are used to treat many infections caused by *gram-negative* bacteria (e.g., *Escherichia coli* and *Pseudomonas*) as well as *gram-positive* bacteria (e.g., *Staphylococcus aureus*). Enterococci may be resistant to aminoglycosides. Aminoglycosides are used in the *short-term* treatment of many serious infections such as *septicemia* (e.g., bacteria in the bloodstream causing very low blood pressure) *only* when other less toxic anti-infectives are ineffective or contraindicated. Examples of aminoglycosides include amikacin, gentamicin, and tobramycin. Because of poor absorption from the gastrointestinal (GI) tract, aminoglycosides are usually administered parenterally (i.e., IM or IV).

Serum levels (peak and trough) are often drawn to determine optimal dosing and lessen the risk of side effects. These levels measure the amount of drug in the blood at different times and are used to adjust subsequent doses and/or the frequency between doses. Lower doses of aminoglycosides will be used in patients who have diminished renal function to avoid toxicity from decreased elimination.

Serious side effects from aminoglycosides, especially in older adults, dehydrated patients, or those with renal or hearing impairment, can include:

- ❗ *Nephrotoxicity*, generally reversible upon discontinuation
- ❗ *Ototoxicity*, both auditory (hearing loss) and vestibular (vertigo), may be permanent
- ❗ Neuromuscular blockade, including respiratory paralysis
- ❗ CNS symptoms, including headache, tremor, lethargy, numbness, and seizures
- Blurred vision, rash, or urticaria

Precautions or contraindications with aminoglycosides apply to:

Tinnitus, vertigo, and high-frequency hearing loss

Reduced renal function

Dehydration

Pregnant or nursing women

Infants or older adults

Interactions of aminoglycosides may occur with:

Other ototoxic drugs (e.g., amphotericin B, polymixin B, bacitracin, and vancomycin)

General anesthetics or neuromuscular blocking agents (e.g., succinylcholine; can cause respiratory paralysis)

Antiemetics (may mask symptoms of ototoxicity)

PATIENT EDUCATION

Patients being treated with aminoglycosides should be instructed regarding:

Extreme importance of close medical supervision during therapy

Careful observation of intake and urinary output

Prompt reporting of any side effects, especially renal or hearing problems

CEPHALOSPORINS

Cephalosporins are semisynthetic beta-lactam antibiotic derivatives produced by a fungus. They are related to penicillins, and *some* patients allergic to penicillin are also allergic to cephalosporins. In general, cephalosporins are broad-spectrum antibiotics, active against many gram-positive and gram-negative bacteria. However, there are many different cephalosporins, and they vary widely in their activity against specific bacteria.

Cephalosporins are classified as first, second, third, fourth, or fifth generation, according to the organisms susceptible to their activity. First-generation drugs, for example cephalexin, are usually effective against gram-positive and some gram-negative organisms, such as those causing skin or soft tissue infections or UTIs.

Second-generation drugs, for example cefaclor, are usually effective against many gram-positive and gram-negative organisms, such as many strains causing bacterial pneumonia. Third-generation drugs, for example ceftriaxone, are usually effective against more gram-negative bacteria than the others and are sometimes used for the treatment of sexually transmitted infections (STIs) such as gonorrhea. Ceftazidime is extremely active against *Pseudomonas aeruginosa*. Cefepime (Maxipime), a parenteral cephalosporin with excellent activity against both gram-positive and gram-negative bacteria, is classified as a fourth-generation cephalosporin.

Ceftaroline (Teflaro) is an intravenous fifth-generation cephalosporin recently approved for the treatment of acute bacterial skin and skin structure infections and community-acquired bacterial pneumonia. It is the first cephalosporin that is active against resistant gram-positive pathogens including MRSA and vancomycin-resistant *S. aureus* (VRSA).

A C&S test may be helpful to determine which cephalosporin is appropriate depending on the organism(s) recovered. Different drugs are used to treat different infections of the respiratory tract, skin, urinary tract, bones, and joints; septicemias; some STIs; and endocarditis. They are also used prophylactically, especially in high-risk patients, for many types of surgery.

Side effects of cephalosporins can include:

- ⚠ Hypersensitivity, including rash, edema, or anaphylaxis (especially in those allergic to penicillin)
- ⚠ Blood dyscrasias (e.g., increased bleeding time or transient leukopenia)
- Renal toxicity, especially in older patients
- Mild hepatic dysfunction
- ⚠ Nausea, vomiting, and diarrhea
- ⚠ Phlebitis with IV administration and pain at the site of IM injection
- Respiratory distress
- Seizures

Precautions or contraindications with cephalosporins apply to:

- Known allergies, especially to penicillin (3%–7% cross-sensitivity; more so with first-generation cephalosporins)
- Prolonged use, possibly leading to superinfections or severe colitis (*Clostridium difficile*)

Interactions with cephalosporins can include:

- *Increased* effectiveness with probenecid
- Disulfiram-like reactions (flushing, tachycardia, shock) with alcohol ingestion and cefotetan

PATIENT EDUCATION

Patients being treated with cephalosporins should be instructed regarding:

Possible allergic reactions

Avoidance of alcohol

Reporting any side effects to the physician

Taking the medication without regard to meals but with food if stomach upset occurs

Attention to signs of abnormal bleeding (checking stools and urine for blood)

MACROLIDES

Macrolides, such as erythromycin, clarithromycin, and azithromycin, are used for the treatment of many infections of the respiratory tract, for skin conditions such as acne, or for some STIs when the patient is allergic to penicillin. Macrolides are considered among the least toxic antibiotics and are therefore preferred for treating susceptible organisms under conditions in which more toxic antibiotics might be dangerous (e.g., in patients with renal disease, pregnant women, or infants). Their most common use is seen with uncomplicated upper respiratory infections, where azithromycin will be used for a five-day regimen in the form of a Z-PAK (500 mg on the first day and then 250 mg for four days after) or a TRI-PAK (500 mg for three days).

Gram-negative bacilli are generally resistant to the macrolides, and resistant strains of Group A *Streptococci* and *Streptococcus pneumoniae* are increasing in number.

Clarithromycin, in combination with amoxicillin and lansoprazole (Prevpac Kit), is also used to treat *Helicobacter pylori* infection in patients with duodenal ulcer disease. See Chapter 16 for further discussion. Unrelated to its antibacterial effect, erythromycin in low doses stimulates gastric emptying. Therefore, it is used in the treatment of GI motility disorders.

Side effects from macrolides of a serious nature are rare, and mild side effects, usually dose related, can include:

- (!) Anorexia, nausea, vomiting, diarrhea, and cramps (take the medication with food or use smaller, more frequent doses)
- Urticaria and rash
- (!) Superinfections
- (!) Serious side effects can occur with some interactions. See the following discussion:

Precautions or contraindications with macrolides apply to patients with:

- Liver dysfunction and GI disease
- Electrolyte imbalances, certain cardiovascular diseases (can cause abnormal changes in the electrical activity of the heart that may lead to a potentially fatal irregular heart rhythm)

Interactions of macrolides (erythromycin and clarithromycin; potentially less with azithromycin) may occur with potentiation of the following drugs and possible toxicity:

- Carbamazepine (Tegretol) (ataxia, dizziness, and drowsiness)
- Cyclosporine (immunosuppressant with kidney or liver transplants)
- Theophylline
- Benzodiazepines (potentiation of sedative effects)
- Warfarin (may prolong prothrombin time and bleeding)
- Digoxin
- Statins (lead to myopathy)

- (!) **Warning.** Macrolides can cause abnormal, potentially fatal, cardiac arrhythmias when combined with the following drugs:
  - Calcium channel blockers—verapamil or diltiazem
  - Antiarrhythmic agents (i.e., sotalol; see Chapter 25)
  - *Azole* antifungals—fluconazole (Diflucan)
  - Quinolones

Always check the label, or ask a pharmacist, for any other dangerous interactions with macrolides. Interactions vary depending on the specific drug.

PENICILLINS

Penicillins are beta-lactam antibiotics produced from certain species of a fungus. They are used to treat many streptococcal and some staphylococcal and meningococcal infections, including respiratory and intestinal infections. Penicillin is the drug of choice for the treatment of syphilis and is also used prophylactically to prevent recurrences of rheumatic fever. Amoxicillin is the preferred drug of choice for infective endocarditis prophylaxis in dental procedures (2 g orally 1h prior to procedure) and is also used in combination with other drugs to treat *H. pylori* infection associated with *duodenal* ulcer disease (see discussion in the previous section and in Chapter 16). Amoxicillin is also considered first-line therapy for adolescents in the treatment of otitis media (ear infections).

Some semisynthetic penicillins have a wider spectrum of activity and are called extended-spectrum penicillins, for example piperacillin. These broad-spectrum penicillins are used in the treatment of infections caused by organisms such as *Pseudomonas*.

Some organisms, including both gram-positive and gram-negative bacteria, have become *resistant* to many forms of penicillin. To combat these organisms, amoxicillin is combined with clavulanic acid (Augmentin) and piperacillin with tazobactam (Zosyn), which are beta-lactamase inhibitors. They prevent beta-lactamase destruction of the penicillin with which they are combined, thus restoring or enhancing the intrinsic activity of the penicillin. C&S tests, when available, are essential to provide targeted therapy against the infecting organism.

Serious side effects of penicillins can include:

- ❗ Hypersensitivity reactions ranging from rash to fatal anaphylaxis
- ❗ Superinfections (especially with oral ampicillin) and pseudomembranous colitis (*C. difficile*)
- ❗ Nausea, vomiting, and diarrhea
- Blood dyscrasias, which are reversible with the discontinuance of the drug
- Renal and hepatic disorders (rare)
- CNS effects, for example confusion, anxiety, and seizures (especially with penicillin G)

Precautions or contraindications with penicillins apply to patients with:

History of serious allergy to penicillins or other beta-lactams (e.g., anaphylaxis, hives) (anaphylaxis has been reported with parenteral, oral, or intradermal skin testing)

Treatment for severe reactions includes discontinuance of the drug, immediate administration of appropriate medications (e.g., epinephrine and corticosteroids), and maintenance of a patent airway. Administration of antihistamines with penicillin will *not* prevent hypersensitivity reactions.

Interactions of penicillins include:

Potentiation of penicillin with probenecid (may be desirable)

Potentiation with anti-inflammatory drugs such as methotrexate and salicylates given concomitantly (at the same time; monitor for increased side effects)

Antagonistic effect (delayed absorption) of oral penicillins when given with antacids or with food

Antagonistic effect of some other anti-infectives on penicillin

Penicillin V or ampicillin may inhibit the action of estrogen-containing oral contraceptives.

PATIENT EDUCATION

Patients being treated with penicillins should be instructed regarding:

Discontinuance of the medication and *immediate* reporting of any hypersensitivity reactions (e.g., rash, swelling, or difficulty breathing)

Taking the medication on time as prescribed, for example on empty stomach, 1h before or 2h after meals, with full glass of water

Avoidance of antacids and alcohol

Possible decreased effectiveness of estrogen-containing oral contraceptives

CARBAPENEMS

Carbapenems such as meropenem (Merrem) belong to the beta-lactam class of antibiotics and have a very **broad spectrum** of activity against gram-negative and gram-positive organisms, including anaerobes and many multi-drug-resistant pathogens. They are primarily used to treat pneumonia, febrile neutropenia, intra-abdominal infections, diabetic foot infections, and significant polymicrobial infections. Carbapenems, similar to other beta-lactams, should be used cautiously in patients with documented penicillin allergies because of the potential for cross-reaction.

See Table 17-1 for a summary of the aminoglycosides, cephalosporins, macrolides, penicillins, and carbapenems.

QUINOLONES

Quinolones, such as ciprofloxacin (Cipro), levofloxacin (Levaquin) or moxifloxacin (Avelox) are used in adults for the treatment of some infections of the urinary tract, sinuses, lower respiratory tract, GI tract, skin, bones, and joints, and gonorrhea. Since these antibiotics are useful for treating many different infections, some organisms are showing increased resistance to the quinolones. Therefore, these agents should be reserved for infections that require therapy with a fluoroquinolone such as *Pseudomonas* infections or when a patient is allergic to other antibiotics.

TABLE 17-1 **Anti-infective Agents: Aminoglycosides, Cephalosporins, Macrolides, Penicillins, and Carbapenems**

GENERIC NAME	TRADE NAME	AVERAGE DOSAGE
Aminoglycosides		
amikacin		IM, IV 10–15 mg/kg per day in one to three divided doses
gentamycin		IM, IV 3–6 mg/kg per day in one to three divided doses
tobramycin		IM, IV 3–6 mg/kg per day in one to three divided doses
Cephalosporins		
First-generation		
cephalexin	Keflex	PO cap, liquid, tab 250–500 mg q6h
cefazolin		IM, IV 250 mg q8h to 2 g q8h
Second-generation		
cefaclor	(Ceclor)[a]	PO 250–500 mg q8h, cap, liq.
cefuroxime	Ceftin	PO tab, liq. 125–500 mg q12h
	Zinacef	IM, IV 750–1500 mg q8h–q6h
Third-generation		
cefdinir	(Omnicef)[a]	PO cap, susp. 300 mg q12h or 600 mg q24h
ceftazidime	Fortaz	IM, IV 1–2g q8–12h
ceftriaxone	Rocephin	IV, deep IM 250 mg–2 g daily
Fourth-generation		
cefepime	Maxipime	IV 500 mg–2 g q12h
		IM 500 mg–1 g q12h (UTI only)
Fifth-generation		
ceftaroline	Teflaro	IV 600 mg q12h
Macrolides		
erythromycin	Ery-Tab,	PO tab, cap 250 mg q6h–500 mg q12h
	E.E.S., EryPed	PO tab, susp. 400–800 mg q6–12h
	Erythrocin	IV 15–20 mg/kg per day divided q6h
clarithromycin	Biaxin	PO tab, liq. 250–500 mg q12h
	Biaxin XL	PO ER tab 1,000 mg daily
azithromycin	Zithromax Z-Pak	PO tab, IR susp. 500 mg one time, then 250 mg daily
	Zithromax Tri-Pak	PO tab 500 mg daily three times
	Zmax	PO ER susp 2 g one time
	Zithromax	IV 500 mg daily

(continued)

TABLE 17-1   Anti-infective Agents: Aminoglycosides, Cephalosporins, Macrolides, Penicillins, and Carbapenems (*continued*)

GENERIC NAME	TRADE NAME	AVERAGE DOSAGE
Penicillins		
penicillin G	Bicillin L-A	Deep IM 600,000–2.4 million units
penicillin VK	Pen VK	PO tab, liq. 250–500 mg q6h
amoxicillin	Amoxil	PO caps, liq. 250 mg–1 g q8h; 875 mg q12h
ampicillin		PO caps, liq. 250–500 mg q6h
		IM, IV 1–2 g q4–6h
Extended-Spectrum		
amoxicillin-clavulanate	Augmentin	PO tab, liq. 250–500 mg q8h, 875 mg q12h
	Augmentin ES	PO susp. 90 mg/kg in two divided doses (acute otitis media)
	Augmentin XR	PO tab 2,000 mg q12h
piperacillin-tazobactam	Zosyn	IV 2.25–4.5 g q6–8h
ampicillin-sulbactam	Unasyn	IV 1.5-3 g q6h
Carbapenems		
meropenem	Merrem	IV 500–1,000mg q8h

Note: Average dose ranges are listed. In severe infections, higher doses may be indicated. Many other anti-infectives are available. Only a few are represented here. Pediatric doses are computed according to the weight and condition of the child.

a. This brand name is no longer marketed, but the name is still commonly used.

Resistance has developed in strains of *P. aeruginosa* and *S. aureus*. Therefore, C&S tests should be performed to identify the causative organism *before initiating a quinolone treatment*, and therapy is adjusted if necessary.

Side effects of quinolones can include:

⚠ Nausea, vomiting, diarrhea, abdominal pain, and colitis (especially older adult patients)

⚠ CNS effects—headache, dizziness, confusion, irritability, seizures, and anxiety

Crystalluria (may require drinking liberal quantities of fluids)

⚠ Superinfection (treat infection appropriately, may need to stop the drug)

Hypersensitivity reactions or rash (rare)

⚠ Phototoxicity (exposure to sunlight can cause severe sunburn)

⚠ Possible cartilage or tendon damage (higher risk with older adults)

Precautions or contraindications with quinolones apply to:

Older adults, especially with GI disease or arteriosclerosis

Children or adolescents (*potential for cartilage damage*)

Those doing strenuous exercise during and several weeks after therapy (*potential for tendon rupture*)

Pregnancy and lactation

Seizure disorders

Cardiac disease (may cause or contribute to cardiac arrhythmias)

Interactions of quinolones may occur with:

Theophylline (ciprofloxacin can potentiate serious or fatal CNS effects, cardiac arrest, or respiratory failure)

Probenicid (increased blood levels of Cipro)

Warfarin (increased risk of bleeding)

Antacids and other preparations containing Fe, Mg, Zn, Ca (decrease absorption; do not give within 2h)

Sucralfate (Carafate) (contains aluminum ions, which decrease absorption)

PATIENT EDUCATION

Patients taking quinolones should be instructed regarding:

Not taking other medications without the physician's or pharmacist's approval

Drinking liberal quantities of fluids

Restricting caffeine intake—see CNS effects

Avoiding excessive exposure to the sun or use sunscreen with at least SPF 30

Avoiding strenuous exercise during and several weeks after therapy (potential for cartilage or tendon damage)

Reporting all side effects, especially rash or hypersensitivity signs

Geriatric patients should follow preceding instructions, especially reporting GI effects or CNS effects (see side effects list)

TETRACYCLINES

Tetracyclines are broad-spectrum antibiotics used in the treatment of infections caused by rickettsia, chlamydia, or some *uncommon* bacteria. Diseases such as Rocky Mountain spotted fever, atypical pneumonia, some STIs, and some severe cases of inflammatory acne are treated with tetracycline. Doxycycline can also be used to treat skin and skin structure infections caused by community-acquired MRSA, as well as upper respiratory infections and Lyme disease. Tetracycline in combination with bismuth salicylate and metronidazole (Helidac Therapy Kit) is also used to treat *H. pylori* infection associated with duodenal ulcer disease. See Chapter 16 for further discussion on this topic. However, some organisms are showing increasing resistance to the tetracyclines, and therefore they should be used only when other antibiotics are ineffective or contraindicated.

Side effects of tetracyclines can include:

⚠ Nausea, vomiting, and diarrhea (frequently dose related)

⚠ Superinfections such as vaginitis and stomatitis

⚠ Photosensitivity, with exaggerated sunburn

! Discolored teeth in fetus or young children

! Retarded bone growth in fetus or young children

Hepatic or renal toxicity (rare)

CNS symptoms such as vertigo and cerebral edema

Thrombophlebitis possible with IV therapy

Allergic hypersensitivity reactions (rare)

Precautions or contraindications with tetracyclines apply to:

Pregnancy and lactation

Children under age 8 years

Patients exposed to direct sunlight

Liver or GI disease

Renal disease (doxycycline preferred)

Interactions of tetracyclines may occur with the following antagonists (which decrease absorption):

Antacids, calcium supplements, or magnesium laxatives

Iron preparations and zinc

Antidiarrheal agents containing kaolin, pectin, or bismuth

Dairy products (doxycycline and minocycline not significantly affected)

Oral contraceptives (breakthrough bleeding or pregnancy may occur)

Tigecycline (Tygacil), a derivative of minocycline, is an IV antibiotic approved for the treatment of intra-abdominal and skin structure infections caused by several microorganisms, including MRSA; it also has significant activity against VRE. It should be reserved for more serious and resistant infections to maintain its full spectrum of activity.

PATIENT EDUCATION

Patients being treated with tetracyclines should be instructed regarding:

Avoiding exposure to sunlight

Avoiding this medication if pregnant or nursing or for a child under 8 years of age

Administering preferably on an empty stomach with full glass of water, 1h before or 2h after meals, unless there is gastric distress

Avoiding iron, calcium, magnesium, and antidiarrheal agents or dairy foods within 2h of taking tetracyclines

Not taking at bedtime to prevent irritation from esophageal reflux

Discarding any expired drug—nephrotoxicity can result from taking outdated drug

ANTIFUNGALS

Antifungal agents are used to treat specific susceptible fungal diseases. The medications are quite different in action and purpose and are therefore treated separately.

Amphotericin B

Amphotericin B is administered IV for the treatment of severe systemic, potentially fatal infections caused by susceptible fungi including *Candida*. It is sometimes considered the drug of choice to treat severe fungal infections resulting from immunosuppressive therapy (e.g., antineoplastic agents) or in patients with AIDS or those with severe illness (e.g., meningitis). *Severe side effects* are expected, and therefore close medical supervision (hospitalization) is usually required so that measures are available to provide symptomatic relief (e.g., antipyretics, antihistamines, and antiemetics).

Side effects of amphotericin B commonly include several of the following:

- ❗ Headache, chills, fever, hypotension, and tachypnea

  Infusion-related reactions

- ❗ Malaise, muscle and joint pain, and weakness

- ❗ Anorexia, nausea, vomiting, and cramps

- ❗ Nephrotoxicity (occurs to some degree in most patients, reversible in most cases upon completion of therapy)

  Anemia

- ❗ Hypokalemia and hypomagnesemia

Because of the many severe side effects and certain dose-limiting toxicities associated with conventional amphotericin B, other formulations have been developed. One example is a lipid-based product (Abelcet) that increases the tolerability of the drug without compromising its antifungal effects.

Fluconazole

Fluconazole (Diflucan) is one of the most widely prescribed antifungal agents. It acts against many fungal pathogens including most *Candida* without the serious toxicity of amphotericin B. Because of good patient tolerance and the convenience of both intravenous and oral dosage forms, this drug is appropriate for patients requiring prolonged antifungal therapy. It is used in the treatment of oropharyngeal (thrush) and esophageal candidiasis and serious systemic candidal infections (e.g., urinary tract and blood stream infections). Patients with recurrent candidiasis, especially those who are immunodeficient, may require maintenance therapy to prevent relapse. A single oral dose of fluconazole is effective in treating vaginal candidiasis, although it is now common practice to repeat the dose in 3–7 days to reduce the risk of recurrence or resistance.

Side effects of fluconazole can include:

- ❗ Moderate nausea, vomiting, abdominal pain, and diarrhea

  Rash

- ❗ Hepatic abnormalities

  Dizziness and headache

Precautions or contraindications with fluconazole apply to:

Pregnant or nursing women

Hepatic or renal disease

Interactions of fluconazole are common and may occur with:

Warfarin (increased prothrombin time could cause hemorrhage)

Oral antidiabetic agents (hypoglycemia can result)

Rifampin (can lead to clinical failure of fluconazole)

Statins (except pravastatin; increased risk of myopathy)

Benzodiazepines (increased CNS effects)

Micafungin

Micafungin (Mycamine) belongs to one of the newer classes of antifungals. Given IV, this drug provides new treatment options against *Candida* and *Aspergillus* species. Micafungin is indicated for the treatment of esophageal candidiasis and candidemia and for stem cell transplantation prophylaxis.

Side effects of Mycamine can include:

- (!) Headache and fever
- (!) Nausea, vomiting, and diarrhea
- (!) Infusion reactions
- (!) Neutropenia
- Hypokalemia and hypomagnesemia

Precautions or contraindications with Mycamine apply to:

Patients under age 18 years

Pregnancy and breast-feeding

Liver dysfunction

Renal disease

There are no major drug *interactions* with Mycamine.

Nystatin

Nystatin is structurally related to amphotericin B and is used orally to treat oral cavity candidiasis. It is also used as a fungicide in the topical treatment of skin and mucous membranes, for example the diaper area, mouth, or vagina (see Chapter 12, "Skin Medications").

Side effects of nystatin are rare but may occasionally include nausea, vomiting, and diarrhea with high oral doses.

Caution should be taken in the use of nystatin with pregnant or nursing women.

There are no significant drug *interactions* with nystatin because of its lack of absorption from the gut.

PATIENT EDUCATION

Patients on antifungal therapy should be instructed regarding:

Taking the medication for prolonged periods as prescribed, even after symptoms have subsided

Reporting relapses promptly to the physician

Reporting side effects immediately to the physician for possible dosage adjustment or symptomatic treatment

Not taking any other medications at the same time without physician approval (see Interactions)

ANTITUBERCULOSIS AGENTS

Tuberculosis (TB) is caused by a bacterium called *Mycobacterium tuberculosis*, which primarily attacks the lungs. According to the World Health Organization, approximately 8.5 million persons worldwide are infected with tuberculosis, and 1.5 million die from it annually. **Antituberculosis agents** are administered for two purposes: (1) to treat latent or asymptomatic infection (no evidence of clinical disease), for instance, after exposure to active tuberculosis and/or significantly positive PPD (purified protein derivative) skin test; and (2) to treat active clinical tuberculosis and prevent relapse.

For asymptomatic tuberculosis, the *treatment* consists of daily administration of isoniazid (INH) alone for 6–12 months to prevent development of the disease. For patients who are intolerant of INH or who are presumed to be infected with INH-resistant organisms, an alternative treatment of *rifampin with pyrazinamide* is given.

Treatment of clinical tuberculosis is challenging for two reasons:

1. Increasing incidence of tuberculosis is found particularly among certain high-risk populations (e.g., HIV-infected individuals, socioeconomically disadvantaged racial or ethnic minorities, homeless individuals).

2. Organisms have become resistant (multidrug and extensive drug resistant) because of patient noncompliance or failure to complete the 6- to 24-month conventional treatment.

Therefore, the CDC recommends the following treatment regimen:

1. The American Thoracic Society (ATS) and the CDC currently recommend *short-course regimens* (i.e., at least six months) for the treatment of uncomplicated pulmonary tuberculosis in adults. According to the ATS, CDC, and American Academy of Pediatrics (AAP), short-course regimens are also suitable for children. *Directly observed therapy (DOT)* should be used for all regimens administered two or three times per week whenever possible to ensure compliance.

2. The initial regimen for the treatment of tuberculosis should include INH given once daily for two months (in combination with rifampin, pyrazinamide, and ethambutol), followed by isoniazid and rifampin given daily, twice weekly, or three times per week for an additional four months (and at least three months beyond culture conversion). HIV-positive patients should always receive induction therapy with four drugs by DOT. When drug susceptibility results are available, the regimen should be altered as appropriate. In addition, treatment may be extended to nine months or longer in HIV-infected patients, dependent upon the clinical signs and symptoms or conversion of sputum cultures from positive to negative.

Although these drugs cross the placenta, they do not appear to have teratogenic effects. The CDC recommends that tuberculosis during pregnancy be treated initially with isoniazid, rifampin, and ethambutol for nine months. Streptomycin is not included because it may cause congenital ototoxicity. Since recommendations change because of resistant strains and newly developed information, consulting www.cdc.gov/mmwr for current CDC recommendations is advised.

Side effects of *INH* and *rifampin* are usually more pronounced in the first few weeks of therapy and can be treated symptomatically. Pyridoxine (vitamin B$_6$) is often given (25–50 mg PO daily) with INH to reduce the risk of CNS effects and peripheral neuropathy. Dosage changes are sometimes required in cases of acute toxicity, but the medication must *not* be discontinued. Side effects can include:

- ❗ Nausea, vomiting, and diarrhea
- ❗ Dizziness, blurred vision, headache, and fatigue
- Numbness and weakness of extremities
- ❗ Hepatic toxicity (especially those over 35 years and children; see precautions)
- ❗ Body fluids colored red-orange with rifampin
- ❗ Hypersensitivity reaction, with flu-like symptoms (sometimes with rifampin)

Precautions or contraindications with INH and rifampin apply to:

Chronic liver disease or alcoholics (periodic laboratory tests are required)

Impaired renal function

Children's doses of INH and rifampin should be limited to 10 and 15 mg/kg, respectively, to decrease the likelihood of hepatic toxicity.

Interactions with rifampin include:

Antagonism by oral hypoglycemics, corticosteroids, digitalis, anticoagulants, and *estrogen* (serum levels of these drugs are reduced when taking rifampin)

Decrease in the serum concentration of antiretroviral protease inhibitors (PIs) (may result in HIV treatment failure)

Interactions with INH include:

Potentiation by phenytoin (Dilantin); increased action (possible toxicity) when taken with isoniazid

Increase risk of hepatotoxicity with rifampin (versus each agent alone)

Alcohol (increases the possibility of liver toxicity with both INH and rifampin)

Antacids (avoid 2h before and after INH)

Side effects of ethambutol can include:

- ❗ Optic neuritis—with visual problems (reversible if discontinued early)
- ❗ Dermatitis, pruritus, headache, malaise, fever, confusion, joint pain, GI symptoms, and occasional peripheral neuritis

Precautions or contraindications with ethambutol include:

Visual testing before and during therapy

Impaired renal function (reduced doses indicated)

Diabetes, especially diabetic retinopathy

Ocular defects

Children under 13—and only in children whose visual acuity can accurately be determined and monitored

Pregnancy—caution

Patients with gout (ethambutol can cause hyperuricemia)

Side effects of pyrazinamide can include:

- ❗ Hepatic toxicity
- Gout (increased uric acid)
- ❗ Hypersensitivity
- GI disturbances

Precautions or contraindications with pyrazinamide apply to:

- People with a history of gout
- Diabetes
- Severe hepatic disease or alcoholism
- Children (potential toxicity)
- Pregnant or nursing women

Side effects of streptomycin, common to all aminoglycosides, include:

- ❗ Ototoxicity
- ❗ Nephrotoxicity

Streptomycin is administered by deep IM injection, alternating sites.

PATIENT EDUCATION

Patients taking antituberculosis agents should be instructed regarding:

- Taking rifampin on empty stomach for maximum absorption, or with food if nauseated
- Taking the prescribed medication for a *lengthy required period of time* even though asymptomatic
- Reporting side effects for possible dosage adjustment or prescription of other palliative medications to relieve discomfort
- Importance of frequent medical and laboratory checks

- Red-orange color of urine, feces, sputum, sweat, and tears with the use of rifampin
- Not wearing contact lens during rifampin treatment
- Interactions with other drugs (e.g., *birth control pills may be ineffective*)
- Avoidance of alcohol
- Importance of visual testing periodically during ethambutol treatment

See Table 17-2 for a summary of quinolones, tetracyclines, antifungal, and antituberculosis agents.

TABLE 17-2   **Anti-Infective Agents: Quinolones, Tetracyclines, Antifungals, and Antituberculosis Agents**

GENERIC NAME	TRADE NAME	AVERAGE DOSAGE	COMMENTS
Quinolones			
ciprofloxacin	Cipro	PO tab, susp. 250–750 mg q12h; IV 200–400 mg q8–12h	Do C&S before Rx, cartilage or tendon damage possible, phototoxicity
	Cipro XR	PO tab 500–1,000 mg per day (UTIs only)	
levofloxacin	Levaquin	PO tab, soln., IV 250–750 mg q24h	
moxifloxacin	Avelox	IV or PO 400 mg per day for 10–14 days	

(continued)

TABLE 17-2   Anti-Infective Agents: Quinolones, Tetracyclines, Antifungals, and Antituberculosis Agents (*continued*)

GENERIC NAME	TRADE NAME	AVERAGE DOSAGE	COMMENTS
Tetracyclines			
tetracycline		PO cap 250–500 mg q6–12h	Phototoxicity, discolored teeth in infants and children
doxycycline	Vibramycin	PO cap, tab, liquid, IV 100–200 mg daily. Can give double dose on day 1 as loading dose	Phototoxicity, discolored teeth in infants and children
tigecycline	Tygacil	IV 100 mg one time, 50 mg q12h	
minocycline	Minocin	PO 50–100 mg daily or BID	
Antifungals			
amphotericin B	Abelcet, AmBisome	IV dose varies with the condition and product formulation	Special IV precautions, protect from light
fluconazole	Diflucan	PO, tab, susp., or IV 50–400 mg daily	Prolonged or maintenance doses frequently
micafungin	Mycamine	IV 100–150 mg daily	Protect from light
nystatin		PO tab, susp. 500,000–1 million units three to four times per day, topical cream, oint., or powder	Continue treatment for 48 h after symptoms are resolved to prevent relapse
Antituberculosis agents			
ethambutol	Myambutol	PO tab 15–25 mg/kg per day (max 1,600 mg)	Always with other medications
isoniazid	INH	PO tab, liquid, IM 5 mg/kg per day (max 300 mg) or 15 mg/kg three times per week (up to 900 mg)	Preventive alone, or as treatment with other medications
pyrazinamide	PZA	PO tab 15–30 mg/kg per day (max 3 g) or 50–70 mg/kg two times per week	Always with other medications
rifampin	Rifadin	PO cap, IV 10 mg/kg per day (max 600 mg)	Initial phase with other drugs
streptomycin		IM (IV) 15 mg/kg per day (max 1 g)	Initial phase with other medications

Note: Other anti-infectives are available. Only a few are represented here. Pediatric doses are computed according to the weight and condition of the child.

MISCELLANEOUS ANTI-INFECTIVES

Clindamycin

Clindamycin has a wider spectrum of activity than lincomycin, from which it is derived. It is used in the treatment of serious respiratory tract infections, septicemia, osteomyelitis, serious infections of the female pelvis caused by susceptible bacteria, and for *Pneumocystis jirovecii* pneumonia associated with AIDS (see AIDS section in this chapter). It is also used in prophylactic regimen in dental procedures for penicillin-allergic patients. Clindamycin may be a viable therapeutic option for community-acquired MRSA.

Side effects of clindamycin that frequently occur can include:

⚠ Nausea, vomiting, diarrhea (drug should be discontinued if these symptoms develop), and colitis

⚠ Rash, pruritus, fever, and occasionally anaphylaxis

⚠ Local effects (minimize by deep IM or frequent IV catheter change)

Precautions or contraindications of clindamycin apply to:

History of GI, hepatic, or renal disease

Older adults

Children

Lactation (not recommended)

Metronidazole

Metronidazole (Flagyl) is a synthetic antibacterial and antiprotozoal agent that is effective against protozoa such as *Trichomonas vaginalis* and for the treatment of amebiasis and giardiasis. In addition, it is one of the most effective drugs available against anaerobic bacterial infections (intra-abdominal, skin, gynecological, septicemic, bone or joint, lower respiratory tract). Metronidazole is also useful in treating Crohn's disease, antibiotic-associated diarrhea, rosacea, and *H. pylori* infection (in combination with other drugs to avoid the development of resistance). It is available in oral, parenteral, and topical formulations. Because of its mechanism of action, metronidazole is a highly effective antimicrobial. Resistance to metronidazole is almost nonexistent.

Side effects of metronidazole include:

! Abdominal pain, nausea, and vomiting

Anorexia, metallic taste, and xerostomia (dry mouth)

! Headache, dizziness, and ataxia (defective muscle coordination)

! Flushing, rash, and urticaria

Peripheral neuropathy (rare) and seizures

! Dark urine (common but harmless)

Precautions or contraindications with metronidazole apply to:

History of blood dyscrasias

Lactation

Children (except for the treatment of amebiasis)

CNS and hepatic diseases

Avoid alcohol during and 48h after treatment

CLINICAL CONNECTION

Disulfuram-Like Reactions

Disulfuram-like reactions occur when a drug contains a structural feature that inhibits the proper breakdown of alcohol in the body. This causes the build-up of acetaldehyde, which leads to severe "hangover" effects felt severely and immediately. These symptoms include flushing, nausea, vomiting, thirst, chest pain, vertigo, and hypotension. Flagyl (metronidazole) is a commonly prescribed anti-infective medication that produces such a reaction if taken with alcohol. Patients who are taking metronidazole should be counselled to not only avoid alcoholic beverages, but also mouthwashes and elixirs that may contain alcohol. This type of reaction is sometimes desirable, in the case of alcohol abuse. The medication Antabuse is prescribed to deter chronic recovering alcoholics from relapsing and using alcohol (discussed further in Chapter 20).

Vancomycin

Vancomycin is structurally unrelated to other available antibiotics. IV vancomycin is used in the treatment of potentially life-threatening infections caused by susceptible organisms. It is the drug of choice for MRSA, treating gram-positive infections in penicillin-allergic patients, and some infections of the heart valves (endocarditis). The CDC reports that enterococci cause about one out of every eight infections in hospitals and that about 30% of these are caused by VRE.

Because vancomycin is poorly absorbed after oral administration, it is not used orally for widespread infections. It can be given orally to treat GI infections such as pseudomembranous colitis caused by the overgrowth of *C. difficile*. It is important to note that patients treated with IV vancomycin for systemic infections should not be switched to the oral form (a common practice with other antibiotics), because the oral form is not effective for treating systemic infections.

Side effects of vancomycin can include:

- ❗ Ototoxicity or nephrotoxicity (occurred primarily with older impure formulations) with IV use (discontinue with tinnitus, may precede deafness)
- ❗ *Local effects* (give only IV with care; can cause necrosis or thrombophlebitis)
- ❗ Rash ("Red Man's Syndrome"), anaphylaxis, and vascular collapse (hypersensitivity reactions reported in 5%–10% of patients)

    Pseudomembranous colitis caused by *C. difficile* infection (rare)

Precautions or contraindications with vancomycin apply to:

Older adults

Hearing impairment

Renal impairment (Serum drug levels are often drawn to determine the optimal dosing to maximize efficacy against MRSA. Kidney function is also monitored frequently by serum creatinine and blood urea nitrogen (BUN) to determine dosage adjustments.)

Pregnancy and lactation

AGENTS FOR VRE

Vancomycin has been used as "the last line of defense" against staphylococcal infections, as well as for certain streptococcal and enterococcal infections. However, in recent years, cases of VRSA and VRE have become more prevalent across the globe. Also, drug-resistant infections, particularly those by gram-positive pathogens, have spread from hospitals and nursing homes to communities, requiring the development of new drugs to combat these resistant strains.

Linezolid (Zyvox) is indicated for gram-positive infections and is approved for the treatment of bacterial pneumonia, skin and skin structure infections, and MRSA and VRE infections, including those infections caused by susceptible organisms that are complicated by bacteremia. Linezolid is effective in treating diabetic foot infections, which are among the most serious complications of diabetes (leading to amputation in severe cases) and are the leading cause of diabetes-related hospitalizations.

Linezolid administered by IV infusion or orally has implications for medication safety and drug interactions. Inappropriate use, leading to an increase in resistant organisms, is a concern, and treatment alternatives should be carefully considered before using linezolid in outpatient settings.

Side effects of linezolid can include:

! Nausea, headache, and diarrhea (stop medication and contact the physician if blood is present in the stool or abdominal pain occurs)

! Anemia and thrombocytopenia

Lactic acidosis

! Pseudomembranous colitis

Precautions or contraindications with linezolid apply to:

Blood dyscrasias

Cardiac disease and hypertension

GI disease and hyperthyroidism

Pregnancy and lactation

Infants

Interactions of linezolid may occur with:

Beta-blockers (worsen bradycardia)

Antidepressants (e.g., SSRIs can cause serotonin syndrome)

Migraine medications (triptans)

Sympathomimetics such as phenylephrine and pseudoephedrine (hypertensive reaction)

Foods or beverages with high tyramine content (see discussion in Chapter 20)

Daptomycin (Cubicin) is the first in a new class of antibiotics called lipopeptides with a spectrum of activity similar to vancomycin. It has greater activity against certain gram-positive bacteria. Daptomycin shows promise in treating VRE infections and endocarditis with associated bacteremia.

Side effects of daptomycin can include:

Constipation, nausea, injection-site reactions, and headache

! Elevated levels of creatinine phosphokinase (CPK), leading to myopathy (monitor CPK levels weekly)

Precautions or contraindications with daptomycin apply to:

Renal impairment (dosage adjustments required in severe diseases)

Pneumonia (daptomycin is inactivated by pulmonary surfactant and therefore is ineffective)

See Table 17-3 for miscellaneous anti-infectives and agents for VRE.

TABLE 17-3 Miscellaneous Anti-Infectives and Agents for VRE

GENERIC NAME	TRADE NAME	AVERAGE DOSAGE	COMMENTS
Miscellaneous anti-infectives			
clindamycin	Cleocin	PO cap, soln. 150–450 mg q6h, Peds 8–25 mg/kg per day divided doses, IM/IV 600 mg–2.7 g per day divided doses	
metronidazole	Flagyl	250–500 mg q8h–q6h IV, PO cap, tab (max. 4 g per 24 h)	Take without regard to meals; avoid all forms of alcohol
	Flagyl ER	PO ER tab 750 mg per day for seven days (for bacterial vaginosis)	Take on empty stomach
vancomycin	Vancocin	PO cap, soln.: 125–500 mg q6h for 7–10 days	For pseudomembranous colitis (IV route not effective)
		IV: 10–20 mg/kg IV q12–24h	IV dose varies according to age, weight, indication, renal function, and serum drug monitoring
Agents for VRE			
daptomycin	Cubicin	IV 4–6 mg/kg q24h	Adjust dosage with severe renal impairment
linezolid	Zyvox	PO tab, susp., IV 600 mg q12h	Watch for interactions with psychiatric meds

Note: Other anti-infectives are available. Only a few are represented here. Pediatric doses are computed according to the weight and condition of the child.

PATIENT EDUCATION

Patients taking antibiotics should be instructed regarding:

Never taking antibiotics for viral infections

Never taking antibiotics that were left over from the treatment of a previous infection or ones that were prescribed for someone else

Informing their physician *prior* to receiving any antibiotics of any allergies you have

Informing their physician if they are pregnant or breast-feeding

Unless directed otherwise, taking all antibiotics with a full glass of water on empty stomach, at least 1h before meals or 2h after meals

Not taking the medication with alcohol, antacids, or fruit juice

If side effects occur, notifying the physician or pharmacist

Reporting rash, swelling, or breathing difficulty to the physician *immediately*

Taking antibiotics at prescribed times to maintain blood levels; if you miss a dose, do not double the next dose—resume with the next scheduled dose

Taking entire prescription *completely*, *not* discontinuing when the symptoms of infection disappear

Not taking any other medications, prescriptions, or over-the-counter drugs at the same time as antibiotics without checking first with the physician or pharmacist regarding interactions

SULFONAMIDES

Sulfonamides are among the oldest anti-infectives. The increasing resistance of many bacteria has decreased the clinical usefulness of these agents. However, they are used most effectively in combination with other drugs, for example with trimethoprim (sulfamethoxazole and trimethoprim). In such combinations, resistance develops more slowly.

Sulfamethoxazole and trimethoprim (Bactrim) is used for the treatment of UTIs, especially acute, complicated UTIs; enteritis (e.g., travelers' diarrhea); and otitis media. In higher doses, it may also be considered as an oral alternative to vancomycin when treating certain MRSA infections. Sulfamethoxazole and trimethoprim is used in the treatment and prevention of *P. jirovecii* pneumonia in HIV-infected patients (see Treatment of Human Immunodeficiency Virus/AIDS Infections in this chapter). This combination drug is also used in the prevention of toxoplasmosis in HIV-infected patients.

Side effects of sulfonamides are numerous and sometimes serious, especially in AIDS patients, and can include:

- ❗ Rash, pruritus, dermatitis, and photosensitivity
- ❗ Nausea, vomiting, and diarrhea
- High fever, headache, stomatitis, and conjunctivitis
- Blood dyscrasias
- ❗ Hepatic toxicity with jaundice
- ❗ Renal damage with crystalluria and hematuria
- ❗ Hypersensitivity reactions (can be fatal)

Precautions or contraindications with sulfonamides apply to:

Impaired hepatic function

Impaired renal function or urinary obstruction

Blood dyscrasias

Severe allergies or asthma (some studies suggest approximately 3% of the population is allergic to sulfa drugs)

Pregnancy or lactation

Interactions with sulfonamides include:

Potentiation of anticoagulants and oral antidiabetics

Antagonism of local anesthetics (e.g., procaine may inhibit the antibacterial action of sulfa)

Potentiation of phenytoin (Dilantin) (e.g., increasing serum drug concentrations)

ACE inhibitors, potassium salts, and potassium-sparing diuretics (hyperkalemia)

PATIENT EDUCATION

Patients taking sulfonamides should be instructed regarding:

Importance of drinking large amounts of fluid to prevent crystalluria (crystals in the urine)

Discontinuance of sulfa at the first sign of rash

Reporting any side effects to the physician *immediately*

Avoiding exposure to sunlight

Ingestion of sulfa with food, which delays but does not reduce the absorption of the drug

URINARY ANTI-INFECTIVES

A UTI, defined as a symptomatic inflammatory response from the presence of microorganisms in the urinary tract, is one of the most common bacterial infections for which patients seek treatment. First-line **urinary anti-infectives** for empiric treatment of uncomplicated lower UTI are sulfamethoxazole–trimethoprim (discussed earlier) and nitrofurantoin.

Nitrofurantoin (Macrobid and Macrodantin) is most commonly used for initial or recurrent UTIs caused by susceptible organisms. This medication is a recommended oral treatment option for cystitis (bladder infection) in women but not men because tissue concentrations are generally lower, resulting in inadequate treatment of occult prostatitis. Because of the achievement of lower tissue concentrations, nitrofurantoin is never used to treat pyelonephritis in men or women. Treatment must continue for an adequate period of time to be effective and minimize recurrence of infection.

Side effects of nitrofurantoin can include:

- ⓘ Nausea and vomiting, which are less frequent if taken with milk or food
- Numbness and weakness of lower extremities
- Headache, dizziness, and weakness of muscles
- Cough; respiratory distress with prolonged use
- ⓘ Dark yellow or brown-colored urine
- Hemolytic anemia

Precautions or contraindications with nitrofurantoin apply to:

- Renal impairment (leads to loss of efficacy)
- Hepatic impairment
- Anemia
- Electrolyte abnormalities
- Asthma
- Pregnancy and lactation
- Children under 1 month of age

Interactions of nitrofurantoin include:

- Probenecid (increased risk of nitrofurantoin toxicity)
- Antacids containing magnesium (decreased effectiveness)
- Quinolones (antagonistic to each other if both are used for UTI)

PATIENT EDUCATION

Patients taking nitrofurantoin should be instructed regarding:
- Importance of taking the medication for required number of days
- Reporting side effects
- Taking medication with milk or food to reduce the incidence of nausea and vomiting
- Avoiding antacids
- Discoloration of the urine, which can stain underwear

See Table 17-4 for a summary of the sulfonamides and urinary anti-infectives.

TABLE 17-4 Sulfonamides and Urinary Anti-Infectives

GENERIC NAME	TRADE NAME	DOSAGE
Sulfonamides		
sulfamethoxazole (SMX) and trimethoprim (TMP)	Bactrim, Bactrim DS	Tab, suspension, IV 160 mg (TMP) q12h or 8–10 mg/kg per day in divided doses
Urinary anti-infectives		
nitrofurantoin	Macrodantin, Furadantin	Cap, suspension 50–100 mg four times per day for 5–7 days
	Macrobid	Cap, 100 mg bid for 5–7 days
		Tab, soln. 100 mg q12–24 h for 10–14 days

ANTIVIRALS

Acyclovir

The **antiviral agent** *acyclovir* is used predominantly in the treatment of herpes simplex, herpes zoster (shingles), and varicella zoster (chickenpox) infections. Acyclovir does not cure or prevent further occurrence of blister-like lesions. Topical application appears effective only with initial infections in relieving discomfort and shortening healing time of lesions (see Chapter 12, "Skin Medications"). Oral forms are most effective in the initial treatment of herpes to relieve pain and to speed healing of lesions and are also used to treat recurrent infections in some patients. In immunocompromised patients and children, parenteral treatment is recommended.

Herpes zoster (shingles) *is best treated within 24–72 h of onset* of rash (blister-like) or intense pain on the skin of one side of the trunk or head. Delayed treatment with an antiviral medication can lead to complications, such as intense pain and postherpetic neuralgia (PHN), lasting for weeks or months, especially in older adults. PHN is treated with tricyclic antidepressants (e.g., imipramine) or anticonvulsants (e.g., gabapentin). (See Chapter 19, section "Adjuvant Analgesics.")

Valacyclovir (Valtrex) is a prodrug that is converted to acyclovir as it is broken down within the body. The adverse reaction profile is the same as that for acyclovir but improved bioavailability means less frequent dosing for valacyclovir. Famciclovir (Famvir) has a similar spectrum of activity to acyclovir but has a longer duration of action and can be dosed less frequently.

Side effects of acyclovir are not common but can include:

Impaired renal function, especially with *rapid IV infusion*

⊘ Lethargy, tremors, confusion, and headache, especially with older adults

⊘ Rash, urticaria, pruritus, and photosensitivity

⊘ Nausea, vomiting, abdominal pain, and diarrhea

Precautions or contraindications with acyclovir apply to:

Children

Breast-feeding

Renal disease (adjust dosage)

Dehydration

Neurological abnormalities with high doses

Much work has been done in recent years to develop antiviral vaccines. Zostavax is a herpes zoster vaccine approved for the prevention of shingles in appropriate (no immunodeficiency, not pregnant, not allergic to latex) persons aged 50 years and older. The vaccine is administered in a single subcutaneous dose. It decreases the occurrence of herpes zoster by approximately 50%–70% and prevents the development of PHN by two-thirds. Additionally, if shingles does still develop after immunization it has been proven to be less severe. Zostavax can be given at the same time as the pneumococcal and the intramuscular flu vaccine.

PATIENT EDUCATION

Patients being treated with acyclovir should be instructed regarding:

The fact that acyclovir is usually effective only with *initial* infection in relieving pain and shortening healing of lesions but is *not* a cure, and there can be recurrences of lesions

Reporting side effects

Taking the medicine only as prescribed and not sharing the drug with others

Finishing full course as prescribed, even if feeling better

Avoidance of sexual intercourse when visible genital herpes lesions are present and using protection at other times

Neuraminidase Inhibitors

Oseltamivir (Tamiflu) and zanamivir (Relenza) belong to a class of antivirals called *neuraminidase inhibitors* and are indicated for the treatment of uncomplicated acute illness caused by influenza types A and B. Both are also indicated for prophylaxis but should not be considered a substitute for annual influenza virus vaccination, which remains the gold standard for reducing the impact of influenza. Instead, antiviral drugs are considered adjuncts to the prevention and control of influenza. Safety and efficacy for the prophylaxis of influenza infection in infants less than 1-year-old (for Tamiflu) and children less than 7 years old (for Relenza) are not yet established. Oseltamivir is given orally and zanamivir via inhalation; both will shorten the duration of illness about one day if taken *within 48h of the onset of symptoms.*

Because zanamivir is given via inhalation, its main side effect is airway irritation and bronchospasm, especially in patients with asthma and chronic obstructive pulmonary disease (COPD). In patients who are susceptible to bronchospasm, a bronchodilator can be concurrently administered (see Chapter 26 on respiratory drugs). Oseltamivir causes nausea, vomiting, and diarrhea in one out of four patients receiving it; these side effects can be lessened by taking the medication with food.

Ribavirin

A drug with the broadest spectrum of antiviral activity, *ribavirin* is used via nasal and oral inhalation for the treatment of infants and young children with respiratory syncytial virus (RSV) infections. It has also been used orally or parenterally (IV form available only through the CDC) in the treatment of other severe viral infections in adults, for example Lassa fever, Hantavirus, and hepatitis C (in combination with interferon alfa).

Side effects of ribavirin can include:

> ❗ Respiratory complications

> ❗ Hypotension and cardiac arrest

Anemia

Rash and conjunctivitis

Contraindicated during pregnancy or lactation. Health care professionals and visitors who are pregnant or lactating should be warned about the *serious risk of close contact with patients receiving ribavirin inhalation therapy.*

Interactions of ribavirin with NRTIs (agents for HIV), depending on the specific agent, can:

Antagonize antiviral action against HIV

Cause lactic acidosis

Cause hepatic failure

See Table 17-5 for a summary of the antiviral agents.

TABLE 17-5 **Antivirals**

GENERIC NAME	TRADE NAME	DOSAGE
Antivirals		Take entire Rx even if feeling better.
For herpes infections		
acyclovir	Zovirax	PO tab, cap, susp. 200–800 mg five times per day q4h, IV 5–10 mg/kg q8h
famciclovir	Famvir	PO tab 500 mg q8h
valacyclovir	Valtrex	PO tab 1,000 mg q8h
zoster vaccine	Zostavax	0.65 mL SC one time for prevention
For influenza		
oseltamivir	Tamiflu	PO cap, susp. 75 mg BID for five days
zanamivir	Relenza Diskhaler	Inhale 10 mg q12h for five days
For RSV		
ribavirin	Virazole	Powder/sol–inhalation
	Various	Oral, dose varies; primarily for hepatitis C

TREATMENT OF HUMAN IMMUNODEFICIENCY VIRUS/AIDS INFECTIONS

The CDC estimates that more than 1.2 million Americans are affected by HIV/AIDS, and approximately 18,000 people in the United States die each year from the disease. Treatment of HIV and AIDS infections is a highly specialized field. Those actively practicing in that field must be updated frequently on the many *new* medications and *frequently changing protocols*. If you are not actively practicing in this area, you would not be expected to be familiar with all of the many drugs for HIV (see Table 17-6). However, all health care professionals should be aware that there are numerous side effects and interactions specific to individualized medications. If you are caring for someone with HIV, it is imperative that you familiarize yourself with that particular individual's requirements by researching current information and consulting the pharmacist and/or infectious disease specialists. Additional resources are described following the section, which discusses drugs for HIV.

The treatment of HIV infection consists of highly active antiretroviral therapy (HAART) using combinations of three or more antiretroviral (ARV) agents and is one of several factors that has led to a decline in the U.S. mortality rate of AIDS. The primary approach to therapy is disruption of the virus at different stages in its reproduction. Eradication of HIV infection *cannot* be achieved with currently available ARV regimens. *The goals of HIV therapy are to achieve maximal and durable suppression of the viral load, restore and/or preserve immunological function, improve quality of life, reduce HIV-related morbidity, prolong survival, and prevent behavior-associated HIV transmission.*

The treatment of HIV-infected patients is complex because of the availability of numerous ARV agents and the rapid growth of new information. A patient's clinical condition, readiness for lifelong therapy, CD4 count, and plasma viral load are essential parameters to be used in decisions to initiate or change therapies. Current guidelines for the initial treatment of HIV infection recommend the use of two NRTIs with a protease inhibitor, a fusion inhibitor, or an NNRTI. Consult www.aidsinfo.nih.gov/guidelines for most current treatment information.

Antiretroviral Protease Inhibitors

Protease inhibitors (PIs) block the activity of the HIV enzyme essential for viral replication late in the viral life cycle. The first PI to be approved was saquinavir (Invirase), followed by more than eight other ARV protease inhibitors. (See Table 17-6 for names of other PIs.)

Side effects can include:

> All PIs are associated with GI intolerance, including nausea, vomiting, and diarrhea
>
> Taste alteration in patients receiving ritonavir, especially the liquid formulation
>
> Fat redistribution, hyperlipidemia, and insulin resistance
>
> Hyperglycemia, new-onset diabetes mellitus, diabetic ketoacidosis, and exacerbation of existing diabetes
>
> Increased spontaneous bleeding episodes in hemophilia patients (joints, soft tissues, intracranial, and GI bleeding)
>
> Indinavir may cause kidney stones (patients should drink at least 1.5 L per day of water to ensure adequate hydration and prevent kidney stones)

Interactions with PIs are many. Certain "statin" drugs are either contraindicated or require lower doses when given with PIs because of an increased risk of myopathy. Check with the pharmacist before administering PIs with other drugs.

Dietary considerations with PIs:

> Most PIs should be taken with food to reduce nausea and gastric irritation.
>
> Always check instructions regarding administration.

Nucleoside Reverse Transcriptase Inhibitors

NRTIs inhibit an enzyme responsible for viral replication early in the viral life cycle. Zidovudine (ZDV, Retrovir) was the first agent to be approved for the treatment of HIV, followed by more than six other NRTIs. (See Table 17-6 for names of other NRTIs.)

Because of the development of resistance, NRTIs must be used in combination with other ARVs. Combivir, a combination of zidovudine and lamivudine (there are currently six other combinations), allows patients to reduce the number of pills needed daily, which can be upward of 20 a day for certain drug combinations. Combivir plus Kaletra are a preferred regimen in pregnancy. Most NRTIs are dose adjusted in patients with renal dysfunction.

Side effects of NRTIs can include:

Lactic acidosis and liver dysfunction (infrequently, but with a high mortality rate)

Flare-up of chronic active hepatitis B with abrupt withdrawal of emtricitabine and lamivudine

Bone marrow suppression consisting of anemia and/or neutropenia with zidovudine

Pancreatitis with didanosine

Peripheral neuropathy and pancreatitis with didanosine and stavudine

Abacavir has been associated with hypersensitivity reactions that can be fatal. Prior to starting abacavir, it is recommended to obtain an HLA B5701 genetic test. If positive, abacavir should not be started because the patient will be at a higher risk of developing a life-threatening hypersensitivity reaction. Patients who develop signs or symptoms of abacavir hypersensitivity (which may include fever, rash, fatigue, nausea, vomiting, diarrhea, cough, and sore throat) should discontinue abacavir immediately.

Interactions of NRTIs include:

Alcohol

Antacids and iron preparations

Other drugs that are nephrotoxic

Non-Nucleoside Reverse Transcriptase Inhibitors

NNRTIs also inhibit an enzyme responsible for viral replication early in the viral life cycle. Nevirapine (Viramune) was the first NNRTI to be approved, followed by four others (see Table 17-6 for names of other NNRTIs). NNRTIs must be administered in combination with other ARVs due to development of resistance.

Adverse reactions with NNRTIs can include:

Hepatotoxicity and cutaneous reactions

Psychiatric adverse effects with efavirenz and rilpivirine

Side effects of NNRTIs can include:

CNS symptoms including dizziness, insomnia, abnormal dreams, and confusion

Interactions with NNRTIs are many. Check with the pharmacist before administering with other drugs.

Dietary considerations with NNRTIs:

Always check instructions regarding administration as some should be given ac and some pc.

Fusion Inhibitors

This class of ARV agents, called fusion inhibitors (FIs), has been shown to block entry of HIV into cells, which may keep the virus from reproducing. Enfuvirtide (Fuzeon) was the first FI approved for treatment-experienced patients with ongoing HIV replication despite current ARV use. It is administered by subcutaneous injection twice daily.

Almost all patients develop local site reactions to enfuvirtide, usually consisting of mild or moderate pain, erythema, itching, induration, nodules, and cysts. It is important to remember to rotate injection sites.

CCR5 Antagonists

CCR5 antagonists block a coreceptor required for HIV entry into human cells. Maraviroc (Selzentry) is the first oral CCR5 antagonist and is used in conjunction with other ARVs. Hepatotoxicity has been reported and may be accompanied by signs or symptoms of a systemic allergic reaction. Do not use maraviroc with St. John's wort as this combination can lead to treatment failure, and avoid certain ARV combinations.

TABLE 17-6 Drugs for HIV/AIDS

GENERIC NAME	TRADE NAME	CLASS ADVERSE EFFECTS
Antiretrovirals[a]		
Protease inhibitors (PIs)		
atazanavir	Reyataz	GI intolerance, hyperglycemia, dyslipidemia, many drug interactions
darunavir	Prezista	
lopinavir/ritonavir	Kaletra	
Nucleoside/nucleotide reverse transcriptase inhibitors (NRTIs)[b]		
abacavir	Ziagen	Lactic acidosis, liver dysfunction
lamivudine/zidovudine	Combivir	
tenofovir/emtricitabine	Truvada	
Non-nucleoside reverse transcriptase inhibitors (NNRTIs)		
efavirenz	Sustiva	Rash, hepatotoxicity, many drug interactions
rilpivirine	Edurant	
Fusion inhibitors (FIs)		
enfuvirtide	Fuzeon	Injection site reactions
CCR5 antagonists		
maraviroc	Selzentry	Hepatotoxicity
Integrase inhibitor		
raltegravir	Isentress	GI intolerance, CNS effects

a. Other drugs and combinations are being used investigationally in the treatment of HIV- and AIDS-related diseases. Dosage varies with condition. *Check dosage very carefully.*

b. *Other combination products available in this class are not listed.*

Integrase Inhibitor   Raltegravir (Isentress) is the first ARV in this class that is designed to slow the advancement of HIV infection by blocking the enzyme needed for viral replication. It is indicated for use in combination with other ARVs in treatment-experienced adults. Most common adverse effects are nausea, headache, diarrhea, and pyrexia. Rifampin can decrease plasma concentrations of raltegravir. Use caution with certain ARV combinations.

Although HAART is a significant advancement in the treatment of HIV, it is still not a cure. Other factors such as high cost, complicated regimens, patient adherence, and interactions with other therapies may limit the utility of these regimens.

HIV INFORMATION AND RESOURCES

Current recommendations for the clinical use of ARVs in the management of HIV-infected adults, adolescents, children, and infants may be found at:

National Institute of Health (NIH) Aids source
- https://aidsinfo.nih.gov/

Department of Health and Human Services
- http://aidsinfo.nih.gov/guidelines

Florida/Caribbean AIDS Education and Training Center
- www.FCAETC.org

AETC National Resource Center Drug Interactions
- www.aids-ed.org

Johns Hopkins HIV Guide
- www.hopkinsguides.com

National HIV Telephone Consultation Service
- www.nccc.ucsf.edu/about_nccc/warmline/

University of California, San Francisco
- http://hivinsite.ucsf.edu/

A card summarizing guidelines for the management of occupational and nonoccupational exposures to HIV, hepatitis B, and hepatitis C, including recommendations for postexposure prophylaxis (PEP), is available at www.FCAETC.org/Treatment. Pre-exposure prophylaxis (PrEP) for the prevention of HIV in men who have sex with men is also summarized. This card is intended to guide initial decisions about PEP/PrEP and should be used in conjunction with other guidance provided in the full reports. View the full reports at websites listed throughout card.

HIV/AIDS Education and Resource Center at 800-448-0440 or at www.aidsinfo. nih.gov. These guidelines are developed by the U.S. Department of Health and Human Services and the Henry J. Kaiser Family Foundation.

Once patients with HIV experience immunosuppression based on decreases in CD4 counts, they are at risk for many **opportunistic infections**. To learn about these infections and their respective treatments, please visit the Online Resources associated with this textbook.

In summary, note that many other anti-infective agents in all of the categories discussed in this chapter are available. This is a representative sample of drugs most commonly in use along with their indications, precautions or contraindications, side effects, and cautions.

PATIENT EDUCATION

Patients taking antiretrovirals should be instructed regarding:

    The fact that there is no cure for HIV, and opportunistic infections may develop

    Taking the drug in an upright position with full glass of water

    Taking the drug exactly as prescribed and not stopping abruptly

    Taking into account dietary considerations

Reporting any change in health status or side effects

Not exceeding the prescribed dosage

Not sharing the drug with others

Not taking any other drugs unless prescribed

CASE STUDY A

Anti-Infective Drugs

Thirty-seven-year old Constantine Karoulis suffered a torn Achilles tendon while playing flag football with some friends. He underwent an Achilles tendon repair, and 10 days postoperatively, he noticed green "pus" draining from his incision.

1. A culture of the wound revealed the gram-negative bacteria *Pseudomonas aeruginosa* as well as the gram-positive bacteria *Staphylococcus aureus*, growing in the wound. Which category of anti-infective drugs is best suited to treat this type of infection?

  a. Sulfonamides

  b. Quinolones

  c. Aminoglycosides

  d. Tetracyclines

2. Why are aminoglycosides most often administered either by IV or IM injection?

  a. Medications cause GI distress when given orally.

  b. A therapeutic dose cannot be reached when administered orally.

  c. Pills are difficult for the patient to swallow.

  d. The medication is poorly absorbed from the GI tract.

3. What method is used to determine optimal dosing for the aminoglycoside (gentamycin) that has been ordered for Constantine?

  a. Repeat C&S of wound drainage

  b. Serum peak and trough levels

  c. 24h urine analysis

  d. CBC with differential

4. What side effect can gentamycin IV cause?

  a. Syncope

  b. Nephrotoxicity

  c. Polyuria

  d. Lower extremity cramping

5. Constantine is taken back to the OR for a wound debridement, and gentamycin is ordered again for his wound infection. Postoperatively, an interaction may occur between gentamycin and which category of drug?

  a. Antiemetics

  b. Anti-inflammatories

  c. Analgesics

  d. Muscle relaxants

CASE STUDY B

Anti-Infective Drugs

Lillian Westcott is diagnosed with a UTI after complaining of burning upon urination. Her physician is preparing to write her a prescription for nitrofurantoin.

1. Prior to prescribing nitrofurantoin, the physician reviews Lillian's medical history because this medication should be used with caution in patients with:
   a. Diabetes
   b. Renal impairment
   c. Hypertension
   d. COPD

2. A common side effect of nitrofurantoin is:
   a. Tinnitus
   b. Numbness of hands
   c. Abdominal pain
   d. Brown-colored urine

3. The physician reviews Lillian's current medications because nitrofurantoin can interact with a certain drug that decreases its effectiveness. Which drug is this?
   a. Probenecid
   b. Warfarin
   c. An antacid containing magnesium
   d. Ibuprofen

4. Which of the following should the nurse make sure to include in Lillian's instructions for nitrofurantoin?
   a. Urine may become discolored.
   b. Take the medication with an antacid.
   c. Stop taking the medication when symptoms disappear.
   d. Take the medication with water.

5. The duration of drug therapy using nitrofurantoin for a UTI is how many days?
   a. Three
   b. Seven
   c. Ten
   d. Fourteen

CHAPTER REVIEW QUIZ

Match the medication in the first column with the condition in the second column that it treats. Conditions may be used more than once.

Medication	Condition
1. ___ nitrofurantoin (Macrodantin)	**a.** Herpes zoster and herpes simplex
2. ___ nystatin	**b.** MRSA and VRE
3. ___ fluconazole (Diflucan)	**c.** Urinary tract infections
4. ___ linezolid (Zyvox)	**d.** Tuberculosis
5. ___ ethambutol	**e.** Acne
6. ___ valacyclovir	**f.** Fungus
7. ___ erythromycin	**g.** Influenza A

Choose the correct answer.

8. What is the best method for preventing the spread of infection?
   a. Bleach patient care areas daily.
   b. Have patients wear a mask.
   c. Observe routine handwashing.
   d. Require masks and gloves for all health care personnel.

9. An over-response of the body to a specific substance is called:
   a. Hyperimmunity
   b. Superinfection
   c. Direct toxicity
   d. Allergic hypersensitivity

10. A sudden onset of dyspnea, chest congestion, shock, and collapse is called:
    a. Anaphylaxis
    b. Nephrotoxicity
    c. Dyscrasia
    d. Prophylaxis

11. When administering an anti-infective drug to an older patient, which of the following may be indicated for safe treatment?
    a. Alternate day dosing
    b. An increased dose
    c. A lower dose
    d. Once-a-day dosing

12. The best treatment for herpes zoster (shingles) will start within how many hours of the onset of the blister-like rash?
    a. 24
    b. 24–72
    c. 48
    d. 96

13. The physician orders an antibiotic to be given to a patient before surgery. What is this type of dosing called?
    a. Antiseptic
    b. Predetermined
    c. Prophylactic
    d. Proactive

14. Caution needs to be exercised when prescribing a cephalosporin to a patient with which known allergy?
    a. Seafood
    b. Penicillin
    c. Latex
    d. Peanuts

15. Which medication category may cause discolored teeth in young children?
    a. Tetracyclines
    b. Cephalosporins
    c. Aminoglycosides
    d. Carbapenems

16. What medication is used to treat oral cavity candidiasis?
    a. Nystatin
    b. Rifampin
    c. Isoniazid
    d. Amphotericin B

17. A patient receiving zanamivir might experience which side effect?
    a. Phlebitis
    b. Airway irritation
    c. Nausea
    d. Rash

18. The drug of choice for treating methicillin-resistant *Staphylococcus aureus* is:
    a. Metronidazole
    b. Ciprofloxacin
    c. Vancomycin
    d. Doxycycline

19. A patient taking an antiretroviral should be instructed that:
    a. OTC drugs are permitted in conjunction with an antiretroviral as long as dosing instructions on the label are followed.
    b. The drug should be taken in an upright position with a full glass of water.
    c. The drug reduces the risk of HIV transmission to other individuals.
    d. The medication may be stopped abruptly.

20. What side effect might protease inhibitors cause?
    a. Exacerbation of existing diabetes
    b. Constipation
    c. Dehydration
    d. Urinary tract infection

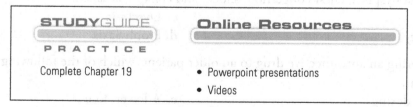

STUDYGUIDE

PRACTICE

Complete Chapter 19

Online Resources
• Powerpoint presentations
• Videos

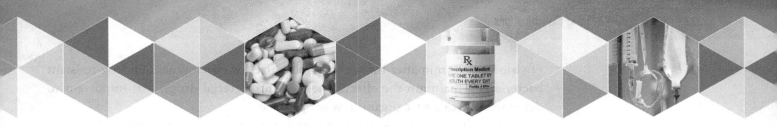

CHAPTER 18
EYE AND EAR MEDICATIONS

KEY TERMS AND CONCEPTS

Antiglaucoma agents

Anti-infective

Anti-inflammatory

Beta-adrenergic blocker

Carbonic anhydrase inhibitors

Cycloplegic

Intraocular pressure

Miotics

Mydriatics

Otic

Otitis media

OBJECTIVES

Upon completion of this chapter, the learner should be able to

1. Demonstrate the administration technique for instillation of ophthalmic medication to reduce systemic absorption

2. List and describe the five categories of ophthalmic medication

3. Identify side effects, precautions and contraindications, and interactions for each category of ophthalmic medication

4. Explain appropriate patient education necessary for each category of eye medication

5. Demonstrate the administration technique for instillation of otic medication

6. List and describe common uses for otic medications

7. Explain necessary patient education for otic medication administration

8. Define the Key Terms and Concepts

A ccording to the National Eye Institute, the most common eye diseases in Americans 40 years and older are age-related macular degeneration, glaucoma, cataracts, and diabetic retinopathy. Conjunctivitis, or inflammation of the conjunctiva (commonly referred to as "pink eye" or "red eye"), is one of the most frequent causes of patients seeking help. Allergens, irritants, mechanical abrasions, bacteria, and viruses all can cause conjunctivitis. Medications for the eye discussed in this chapter can be classified into five categories: anti-infectives, anti-inflammatory agents, antiglaucoma agents, mydriatics (pupil dilation), and local anesthetics.

ANTI-INFECTIVES

Many **anti-infective** ophthalmic topical ointments and solutions are available for the treatment of superficial infections of the eye caused by susceptible organisms. In general, ointments are preferable to drops in children and patients with poor adherence, whereas drops are preferred in adults because ointments will cause blurring of vision for 20 min after instillation. To reduce the development of drug-resistant bacteria and maintain the effectiveness of antibacterial drugs, it is important to determine the causative organism when possible.

Ophthalmic antibiotic preparations (singly and/or in combination) include macrolides, bacitracin, fluoroquinolones, sulfonamides, bacitracin–polymixin, and trimethoprim–polymyxin. Aminoglycosides are used less frequently owing to their toxicity to the corneal epithelium. When treating infections, if there is no improvement in two to three days, suspect microbial resistance, inappropriate choice of drug, or incorrect diagnosis. In these cases, the antibiotic can be switched to a different class, or the patient may have to return for a follow-up appointment.

In general, topical therapy is used for 7–10 days. Prolonged use may result in the overgrowth of nonsusceptible organisms including fungi. Always check the latest literature regarding resistant organisms and check the patient's history regarding allergies. See Chapter 17 for further details on anti-infective agents, resistance, and allergies.

PATIENT EDUCATION

Patients being treated with anti-infective ophthalmic preparations should be instructed regarding:

Using only as directed and checking dosage and frequency

Careful instillation into the lower conjunctival sac to avoid contamination of the tip of the dropper or ointment tube (see Figure 18-1)

Possible hypersensitivity reactions in patients with allergies of any kind

Discontinuance of the medication and reporting immediately to a physician any signs of sensitivity (e.g., burning and itching)

Careful handwashing to prevent the spread of infection to the other eye or other persons

Not using eye makeup or not wearing contact lenses while treating eye infections

Replacing contact eye makeup and contacts due to possible contamination by the causative organism

When using more than one ophthalmic product at the same time, space them at least 5 min apart (to ensure maximum absorption) and administer the more viscous preparation (i.e., ointment, suspension) *last*.

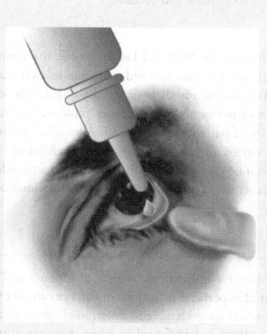

FIGURE 18-1 Instilling eye medication. Gently pull the lower lid down and have the patient look upward. Ophthalmic solution is dropped inside the lower lid.

Side effects of anti-infectives can include hypersensitivity reactions such as conjunctivitis, irritation, local burning, stinging, blurred vision, rash, and urticaria in persons with a history of allergy.

Precautions or contraindications for anti-infectives apply to:

Anyone allergic to the drug

Viral and fungal diseases of the ocular structure

Interactions may occur with prolonged use of corticosteroids, which can result in secondary ocular infections caused by suppression of immune response.

Antiviral ophthalmic preparations, used topically in the treatment of herpes simplex, keratitis (inflammation of the cornea), or conjunctivitis include trifluridine (Viroptic) ophthalmic solution. Dose is one drop to the lower conjunctival sac of the infected eye up to nine times daily at 2-h intervals while awake (maximum nine drops per eye per day or 21 days per episode).

MEDIALINK

See it in Action! Go to the Online Resources to view a video on Administering Eye Medications.

ANTI-INFLAMMATORY AGENTS

Anti-inflammatory ophthalmic agents are used to relieve inflammation of the eye or conjunctiva in allergic reactions, burns, irritation from foreign substances or postoperatively.

Corticosteroids

Various topical forms of the corticosteroids are also useful in the *acute* stages of eye injury to prevent scarring, for severe symptoms, or when the condition is unresponsive to other medications. However, corticosteroids should not be used for extended periods because of the danger of masking the symptoms of infection or slowing the healing process. In general, ophthalmic corticosteroids should be prescribed cautiously because they may cause sight-threatening complications when used inappropriately. Application of ophthalmic corticosteroids topically does not generally cause systemic effects. However, systemic absorption can be minimized by applying gentle pressure on the inner canthus of the eye following instillation of corticosteroid ophthalmic drops or ointment (see Figure 18-2).

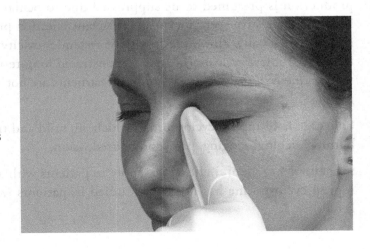

FIGURE 18-2 Apply gentle pressure on the inner canthus following administration of ophthalmic medications. Systemic absorption is thus minimized with medications such as corticosteroids, miotics, and mydriatics.

Side effects of corticosteroids can include:

- ⚠ Increased intraocular pressure (IOP; depends on the drug, dose, frequency, and length of treatment; less likely with fluorometholone)
- ⚠ Reduced resistance to bacteria, viruses, or fungi
- ⚠ Delayed healing of corneal wounds, thinning of cornea, and corneal ulceration
- ⚠ Stinging, burning, or ocular pain
- ⚠ Increased risk of developing cataracts

Precautions or contraindications with corticosteroids apply to:

Acute bacterial, viral, or fungal infections

Primary open-angle glaucoma

Pregnancy

Prolonged use

Ophthalmic corticosteroids are also available in combination with other antibiotics (i.e., Tobradex—tobramycin and dexamethasone; Blephamide—sulfacetamide and prednisolone). They are used to treat steroid-responsive inflammatory ocular conditions in which a corticosteroid is indicated and bacterial infection or risk of infection exists.

Nonsteroidal Anti-inflammatory Drugs

Nonsteroidal anti-inflammatory drug (NSAIDs) such as flurbiprofen (Ocufen) and ketorolac (Acular) ophthalmic drops are used to treat postoperative inflammation following cataract surgery. NSAIDs are not generally first-line agents for other eye conditions with inflammation but are an alternative to corticosteroids if a contraindication exists.

Caution applies to those who may be allergic to aspirin and other NSAIDs. Topical NSAIDs are relatively safe, with few local or systemic side effects. Ketorolac may sting or burn during application, but this may be alleviated by refrigerating the solution before use.

Ophthalmic Immunologic Agent

Topical cyclosporine (Restasis) increases tear production in patients whose tear production is presumed to be suppressed due to ocular inflammation. It is an immunosuppressive agent for organ transplant rejection prophylaxis when administered systemically. However, the risk of systemic toxicity is minimal when given topically. Topical cyclosporine has demonstrated long-term efficacy and safety in the treatment of dry eye disease (other treatments are not recommended for long-term use).

Side effects of topical cyclosporine, which are mild and transient, include ocular burning, itching, stinging, pain, and blurred vision.

Precautions or contraindications apply to patients with active ocular infections; topical cyclosporine has not been studied in patients with a history of herpes keratitis.

Antihistamines or Decongestants

Ophthalmic administration of antihistamines blocks histamine receptors in the conjunctiva, relieving ocular pruritis associated allergic conjunctivitis. Ophthalmic administration of decongestants causes vasoconstriction of blood vessels, thereby providing relief from minor eye irritation and redness. These two classes of drugs are also used in combination (i.e., Naphcon-A, Visine-A). See Chapter 26 on antihistamines for more information. The most common use for ophthalmic antihistamines is for seasonal allergies that precipitate symptoms such as redness, itchiness, or other irritation.

Many of these products contain the preservative benzalkonium chloride, which can accumulate in contact lenses, causing irritation. Manufacturers recommend that these products be used for no more than 72h. Patients should stop using a product and see a physician if they experience eye pain, changes in vision, continued redness or irritation of the eye, or persistent condition.

Ophthalmic Lubricants

Ocular lubricants such as artificial tear solutions provide a barrier function at the level of the conjunctival mucosa. They help to dilute and flush various allergens and inflammatory mediators that may be present on the ocular surface. Artificial tear products that contain preservatives may cause allergic reactions and should be stopped immediately. Ophthalmic lubricants are considered to be very safe and can be used as often as needed.

See Table 18-1 for a summary of anti-inflammatory ophthalmic drugs.

TABLE 18-1   Anti-Inflammatory Ophthalmic Drugs

GENERIC NAME	TRADE NAME	DOSAGE
Corticosteroids		
fluorometholone	FML	Oint, susp; varies with condition
prednisolone	Omnipred, Pred Forte	Sol, susp; varies with condition
	Many combinations with antibiotics	Oint, sol, susp; varies with condition
dexamethasone	Maxidex	Sol, susp, implant; varies with condition
	Many combinations with antibiotics	Oint, sol, susp; varies with condition
Nonsteroidal anti-inflammatory drugs		
flurbiprofen	Ocufen	Sol; varies with condition
ketorolac	Acular, Acular LS	Sol; varies with condition
Immunologic agent		
cyclosporine	Restasis	emulsion 0.05%; 1 drop q12h

Note: Percent and dose ordered *carefully!* Follow directions. Do not use for longer than prescribed.

This is a representative sample; many other products are available.

ANTIGLAUCOMA AGENTS

Glaucoma is a group of sight-threatening diseases of the eye in which there is increased intraocular pressure (IOP) due to obstruction of the outflow of aqueous humor. This causes deterioration of and damage to the optic nerve (which carries images on the retina to the brain), resulting in vision loss. According to the Glaucoma Research Foundation, of the 60 million people worldwide and the 2.2 million in the United States who have glaucoma, approximately half are unaware they have the disease. There are two main types of glaucoma:

1. ***Acute (angle-closure) glaucoma.*** Characterized by a sudden onset of pain, blurred vision, and a dilated pupil, this condition is considered a *medical emergency.* Although uncommon, if left untreated, blindness can result in a few hours or days. Treatment consists of miotics (e.g., pilocarpine), osmotic agents (e.g., mannitol) (see Chapter 15, "Diuretics"), carbonic anhydrase inhibitors (e.g., acetazolamide), and surgery to open a pathway for the release of aqueous humor.

2. ***Chronic (open-angle) glaucoma.*** Much more common and often bilateral, this condition develops slowly over a period of years with few symptoms except a gradual loss of peripheral vision and possibly blurred vision. Halos around lights and central blindness are late manifestations. Treatment consists of miotics, carbonic anhydrase inhibitors, and a local beta-adrenergic blocker, such as timolol (Timoptic) eye drops.

The first step in glaucoma therapy is early diagnosis via screening and ensuring the patient abstains from medications that may exacerbate glaucoma (i.e., potent corticosteroids, anticholinergics, and antihistamines). Antiglaucoma drugs, given to lower intraocular pressure, can be divided into five main categories based on their mode of action:

1. ***Carbonic anhydrase inhibitors,*** for example dorzolamide (Trusopt). Act by decreasing the formation of aqueous humor and have a diuretic effect.

Note

There is no cure for glaucoma, and any vision damage that has already occurred cannot be reversed. It is very important to continue treatment for a lifetime once diagnosed and to have regular eye exams to prevent further vision damage. This is especially important for diabetic patients who are predisposed to developing glaucoma.

2. *Miotics,* for example pilocarpine. Act by increasing the aqueous humor outflow.

3. *Beta-adrenergic blockers,* for example timolol. Act by decreasing the rate of aqueous humor production.

4. *Alpha-agonists,* for example brimonidine (Alphagan-P). Decrease the production of aqueous humor and increase outflow.

5. *Prostaglandin analogs,* for example latanoprost (Xalatan). Act by increasing aqueous outflow.

Currently, the beta-adrenergic blockers and prostaglandin analogs are the most frequently used topical medications. Drugs in different categories are sometimes given concomitantly. Combination products are available as well, for example timolol combined with dorzolamide (Cosopt) or with brimonidine (Combigan).

Carbonic Anhydrase Inhibitors

Carbonic anhydrase inhibitors (CAIs) such as acetazolamide reduce the formation of hydrogen and bicarbonate ions, which have a diuretic effect and reduce the production of aqueous humor. Oral acetazolamide (Diamox Sequels) has largely been replaced by topical preparations, which have fewer side effects, but is occasionally used in the adjunctive treatment of open-angle glaucoma or short-term preoperatively (IV or regular-release tabs) to reduce IOP in angle-closure glaucoma and is given with miotics.

Side effects of *oral and IV* CAIs, infrequent and usually dose related, can include:

- ❗ Nausea, vomiting, diarrhea, and constipation
- Thirst, taste alteration; frequent urination
- ❗ Drowsiness, fatigue, confusion, and seizures
- Numbness, muscular weakness, and tingling, with high doses
- Blood dyscrasias; electrolyte imbalance
- ❗ Hepatic and renal disorders (can lead to kidney stones)
- ❗ Photosensitivity (avoid excessive sunlight exposure)

Precautions or contraindications with CAIs apply to:

Chronic obstructive pulmonary disease (COPD)

Diabetes

Electrolyte, hematological, hepatic, pulmonary, and renal disorders

Sulfonamide hypersensitivity

Pregnancy and lactation

Interactions with CAIs are frequent because of increasing or decreasing excretion of other drugs and can include:

Decreased effects of lithium and oral antidiabetics

Increased effects of quinidine, amphetamines, and other diuretics

Hypokalemia with thiazides and corticosteroids

Dorzolamide (Trusopt) is a CAI that is applied *topically* to treat open-angle glaucoma. It is used as an adjunct to beta-blockers and is available as a combination product with timolol (Cosopt).

Side effects of dorzolamide can include:

- ! Burning or stinging and blurred vision

    Bitter taste

Caution applies to:

Those with sulfonamide hypersensitivity

Concurrent ophthalmic and oral CAIs

PATIENT EDUCATION

Patients being treated with CAIs should be instructed regarding:

Importance of follow-up with the physician

Reporting side effects and response to the physician for appropriate dosage regulation

---

Miotics, Direct-Acting

Miotics are medications that cause the pupil to contract. Miotics reduce IOP by increasing the aqueous humor outflow. They act by contracting the ciliary muscle; this mechanism also leads to blurred vision. Miotics (e.g., pilocarpine) are used in the treatment of open-angle glaucoma (considered third-line therapy due to side effects) or in the short-term treatment of angle-closure glaucoma before surgery.

Pilocarpine is also used after ophthalmic examinations in glaucoma patients to *constrict the pupil* and counteract the *mydriatic* (pupil-dilating) effects of other agents. Miotics are usually administered with acetazolamide and/or timolol. Because of its increased duration of effect and less frequent administration, pilocarpine hydrochloride gel (Pilopine HS) may provide some advantages over ophthalmic solutions, especially for long–term use with noncompliant patients.

Pilocarpine has cholinergic action and side effects. (See Chapter 13, "Cholinergics.")

Side effects of pilocarpine, usually dose related, can include:

- ! Blurred vision and myopia
- ! Twitching, stinging, and burning
- ! Ocular pain and headache
- ! Photophobia and poor vision in dim light

    Aggravation of inflammatory processes of the anterior chamber of the eye

    Cataracts and retinal detachment (due to ciliary muscle spasm)

Systemic effects with frequent or prolonged use or high doses of pilocarpine, especially in children, can include:

- ! Nausea, vomiting, and diarrhea
- ! Increased lacrimation, salivation, and sweating

  ❗ Hypotension and bradycardia

  ❗ Bronchospasm

Precautions or contraindications with pilocarpine apply to:

Angle-closure glaucoma *with acute inflammation*

History of retinal detachment or retinal degeneration

Acute inflammatory processes

Soft contact lenses in place

Corneal abrasion

Interactions of pilocarpine may occur with:

Topical atropine, which reduces effectiveness

PATIENT EDUCATION

Patients being treated with miotics should be instructed regarding:

Following directions carefully regarding time and amount

Administration by closing tear duct after instillation
(see Figure 18-2)

Reporting side effects to the physician for possible dosage adjustment

Administration at bedtime to reduce side effects

Not driving at night

Beta-Adrenergic Blockers

Timolol (Timoptic) is a *nonselective* **beta-adrenergic blocker** that is used topically to lower IOP in open-angle glaucoma by decreasing the rate of aqueous humor production.

Side effects of beta-blockers are infrequent and transient but may include:

Ocular irritation, tearing, conjunctivitis, or diplopia

Transient blurred vision with the gel formulation

  ❗ Aggravation of *preexisting* cardiovascular or pulmonary disorders, which may cause bradycardia, hypotension, dizziness, and bronchospasm

Precautions or contraindications with beta-blockers apply to:

Bradycardia, heart failure, and heart block

Patients receiving oral beta-blocker drugs

Asthma and chronic obstructive pulmonary disease (COPD)—betaxolol (Betoptic-S) can be used *with caution* in patients with bronchospastic pulmonary disease because it does not affect the pulmonary receptors

Pregnancy and lactation

Children

Diabetes and hyperthyroidism

Closed-angle glaucoma

Interactions of beta-blockers may occur with:

Other antiglaucoma drugs to help lower IOP

Oral beta-blockers to increase chances of hypotension, bradycardia, and heart block

PATIENT EDUCATION

Patients being treated with beta-adrenergic blockers should be instructed regarding:

Administration by closing tear duct after instillation to reduce systemic effects (see Figure 18-2); do not exceed the recommended number of drops

Caution in patients with cardiac or pulmonary disorders or who are taking oral beta-blockers

Importance of regular eye examinations

Continuous use of medications for glaucoma; *do not discontinue abruptly*

When administering more than one ophthalmic medication, allowing a time interval (at least 5 min) between medications; ophthalmic solutions should always be used before gels and suspensions to optimize the absorption of each medication

Alpha-Agonists

Brimonidine (Alphagan-P) is a selective alpha$_2$-agonist that decreases the formation and increases the outflow of aqueous humor. It does this without causing mydriasis and with minimal effects on cardiovascular or pulmonary hemodynamics. Brimonidine is an alternative for those for whom topical beta-blocker therapy is contraindicated.

Side effects of alpha-agonists can include:

Conjunctival redness, itchiness, stinging

Dizziness, drowsiness, dry mouth, and headache

Alpha-agonists have the potential to enhance the CNS depressant effects of ethanol, opiate agonists, anxiolytics, sedatives, and hypnotics.

PATIENT EDUCATION

Patients being treated with alpha-agonists should be instructed regarding reporting side effects to the physician immediately.

Because drugs in this class may cause fatigue or drowsiness in some patients, those who engage in hazardous activities should be cautioned of the potential for a decrease in mental alertness.

Prostaglandin Analogs

Regarded as first-line agents, latanoprost (Xalatan), travoprost (Travatan Z), and others are prostaglandin analogs that cause the greatest reduction in IOP by increasing the outflow of aqueous humor. They may be used concomitantly with other topical ophthalmic drugs to lower IOP (administer the drugs at least 5 min apart).

Side effects of prostaglandin analogs include:

Blurred vision, burning, macular edema, and stinging

Slow, gradual change in the color of the iris (resultant color change may be permanent)

Change in the length, thickness, and pigmentation of eyelashes (Latisse, a form of bimatoprost, is approved for the treatment of hypotrichosis, or inadequate eyelashes)

! Systemic effects rarely, including upper respiratory tract infection and muscle and joint pain

Precautions or contraindications with prostaglandin analogs apply to:

Active intraocular inflammation (may worsen condition)

Contact lens wearers

Hepatic and renal diseases

Pregnancy, lactation, and use in children

Drug interaction of prostaglandin analogs occurs with eye drops containing the preservative thimerosal (precipitation occurs). If such drugs are used, administer them with an interval of at least 5 min between applications. There are no other clinically significant drug interactions.

More frequent administration of prostaglandin analogs than the dosage indicated in Table 18-2 may actually decrease their IOP lowering effect. Refrigerate unopened bottle of Xalatan; once opened, the container may be stored at room temperature for six weeks. Travatan does not require refrigeration.

See Table 18-2 for a summary of antiglaucoma agents.

TABLE 18-2 Antiglaucoma Agents

GENERIC NAME	TRADE NAME	DOSAGE
Carbonic anhydrase inhibitors		
acetazolamide	(Diamox)[a]	Tab, IV, 125–250 mg two to four times per day (max 1 g per day)
	Diamox Sequels	ER cap 500 mg PO BID (max 1 g per day)
dorzolamide	Trusopt	Ophthalmic sol 1 drop TID
Miotics[b], direct-acting		
pilocarpine HCl	Isopto Carpine	Ophthalmic sol 1%, 2%, 4%[c], 1 drop up to four times per day
pilocarpine gel	Pilopine HS	Ophthalmic gel 4%c at bedtime
Beta-adrenergic blockers		
timolol	Timoptic	Ophthalmic sol 0.25–0.5%, 1 drop BID
	Timoptic-XE	Ophthalmic gel 0.25–0.5%, 1 drop daily
timolol 0.5% with dorzolamide 2%	Cosopt	Ophthalmic sol 1 drop BID
betaxolol	Betoptic-S	Ophthalmic susp 0.25%, 1 drop BID
Alpha-agonists		
brimonidine	Alphagan-P	Ophthalmic sol 0.1%, 0.15%, 0.2%; 1 drop TID (8 h apart)
brimonidine 0.2% with timolol 0.5%	Combigan	Ophthalmic sol 1 drop q12h

(*continued*)

TABLE 18-2   **Antiglaucoma Agents (*continued*)**

GENERIC NAME	TRADE NAME	DOSAGE
Prostaglandin analogs		
latanoprost	Xalatan	Ophthalmic sol 0.005%, 1 drop at bedtime
travoprost	Travatan-Z	Ophthalmic sol 0.004%, 1 drop at bedtime

a. This brand name is no longer marketed, but the name is still commonly used.
b. Constrict the pupil.
c. Wide variation in strengths available. Check carefully for correct percentage.
Note: Other antiglaucoma agents and combination drugs are available. This is a representative list.

PATIENT EDUCATION

Patients being treated with prostaglandin analogs should be instructed regarding:

Possibility of iris color change (increase of the brown pigment).

Contacting the physician immediately if ocular reactions develop.

Prostaglandin analogs contain a preservative that may be absorbed by contact lenses. Remove lenses prior to administration of the drug and wait 15 min before reinserting.

MYDRIATICS

Mydriatics (e.g., atropine) are used topically to *dilate the pupil* for ophthalmic examinations. Atropine also acts as a **cycloplegic** (paralyzes the muscles of accommodation). It is the drug of choice in eye examinations for children. However, other mydriatics, for example cyclopentolate, are more often used for adults because of faster action and faster recovery time.

Side effects of mydriatics, more likely in older adult patients, may include:

> (!) Increased IOP
>
> Local irritation, tearing, and burning sensation (transient)
>
> (!) Blurred vision (common)
>
> Flushing, dryness of skin, and fever
>
> Decreased salivation and sweating
>
> Confusion (caution in older adults)

Precautions or contraindications for mydriatics apply to:

> Angle-closure glaucoma
>
> Infants

Phenylephrine is an alpha-sympathomimetic that produces mydriasis without cycloplegia. Side effects and precautions or contraindications are similar to those of epinephrine (see Chapter 13, "Autonomic Nervous System Drugs").

LOCAL ANESTHETICS

Local ophthalmic anesthetics, such as tetracaine (*TetraVisc*), are applied topically to the eye for minor surgical and diagnostic procedures, removal of foreign bodies, or painful injury.

Side effects of local anesthetics are rare, except with prolonged use, but may include *hypersensitivity* (transient stinging) reactions such as *anaphylaxis in those allergic to the "-caine" local anesthetics* (ester type).

Contraindicated for prolonged use because of the danger of corneal erosions, delayed wound healing, and keratitis.

See Table 18-3 for a summary of the mydriatics and local anesthetics for the eye.

TABLE 18-3   Mydriatics and Local Anesthetics for the Eye

GENERIC NAME	TRADE NAME	DOSAGE	COMMENTS
Mydriatics[a]			
atropine	Isopto Atropine	Oint, sol 1%	Administered 60 min before exam
cyclopentolate	Cyclogyl	Ophthalmic sol, 0.5%, 1%, 2%[b]	Check carefully for percent
phenylephrine	Mydfrin	Ophthalmic sol, 2.5%, 10%	
Local anesthetics			
tetracaine	TetraVisc	Sol, 0.5%	Apply eye patch
proparacaine	Alcaine	Sol, 0.5%	Apply eye patch; store product in refrigerator

a. Dilate the pupil.
b. Wide variations in strengths are available. Check carefully for correct percentage.

PATIENT EDUCATION

Making certain the correct medication and correct percent solution are used as prescribed; there is a potential for certain eye drops to be prescribed for use in the ears, but ear drops should never be used in the eyes

Continuing glaucoma treatment for a lifetime and having regular eye exams to prevent future vision damage

Proper aseptic technique and handwashing to prevent contamination of the other eye, the dropper, or the ointment tube

Instillation of the *correct number of drops* or amount of ointment into the conjunctival sac in the proper order (see Figure 18-1); if the directions say to use two drops, wait for 5 min before putting another drop into the same eye

Closing the eye gently so as not to squeeze the medication out; gently blotting extra medication coming out of the eye with a tissue

Applying gentle pressure to inner canthus after instillation to minimize systemic effects (see Figure 18-2); do not rub your eyes

Avoiding use of an eyecup as an aid to administration due to the risk of contamination.

Monitoring storage requirements such as refrigeration and expiration dates closely (depending on the health care setting, eye medications may be assigned a shorter expiration date)—do not use outdated medication.

Keeping eye preparations out of the reach of children; most of these products are not originally provided in child-resistant packaging.

OTIC (EAR) MEDICATIONS

The ear is made up of three parts, the outer, middle and inner ear (Figure 18-3). Together these parts serve two main purposes, hearing and balance. When either one of these functions is disrupted, it is usually a sign that there is inflammation or blockage in one or more parts of the ear. There are two main categories of common ear conditions (1) ear infections and (2) earwax buildup. These two types of conditions generally involve only the outer and middle ear and will be the focus of this

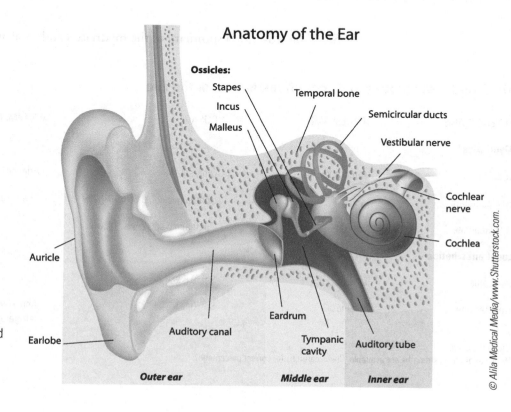

Anatomy of the Ear

Ossicles:
Stapes
Incus
Malleus
Temporal bone
Semicircular ducts
Vestibular nerve
Cochlear nerve
Cochlea
Auricle
Earlobe
Auditory canal
Eardrum
Tympanic cavity
Auditory tube
Outer ear
Middle ear
Inner ear

© Alila Medical Media/www.Shutterstock.com.

FIGURE 18-3 The ear contains many small structures that contribute to hearing and balance. Notice how inflammation or blockage would disrupt these functions.

section. Other, more serious conditions of the ear involve the inner ear. They are more difficult to treat and often require the care of an ear, nose, and throat specialist.

Otitis Media

Otitis Media (ear infections) occur most commonly in children, but can also occur in adults. They are caused most commonly by bacteria in the middle ear, which leads to inflammation (otitis media). In general, ear infections present with symptoms of pain (dull pulsing to sharp stabbing), tenderness, a feeling of "fullness" in the ear, fever, and difficulty hearing. It should be noted that infants or small children who cannot talk yet will often become fussy and cry while reaching toward the affected ear. This is an indicator that they may have an ear infection. Treatment for ear infections can be broken down into topical and systemic medications. Treatment always involves an antibiotic that can sometimes be paired with a steroid (topical) or NSAID (systemic) for inflammation and pain.

Topical Preparations for Ear Infections

Cipro (ciprofloxacin), Floxin (ofloxacin), and Cortisporin (polymixin B, neomycin, and hydrocortisone) are the most commonly used topical antibiotics. Cipro is also available in two combination formulations (Ciprodex and Cipro HC), which contain a steroid. Topical otic antibiotics are best suited for outer ear infections ("swimmers ear"). In general, ear drops are well tolerated, but minor side effects include irritation of the ear or burning and stinging when administering the drops. Treatment is usually prescribed for 7–14 days, and as always the patient should be instructed to continue to use the drops for the entire time period, even after symptoms have begun to improve or resolve.

There are also drops that are designed to just treat the pain and inflammation associated with an ear infection, these are always paired with an antibiotic (otic or systemic). These medications are Vosol HC (acetic acid and hydrocortisone) and Auralgan (benzocaine and antipyrine). Vosol HC does contain an antibacterial (acetic acid), but it is not an antibiotic and should not be used to eradicate an established infection. Proper administration of ear drops can be found at the end of Chapter 9. It should be noted that the technique is different between children and adults.

CLINICAL CONNECTION

Eye Drops for Ear Drops

Often times a patient will present to the pharmacy with a prescription for a topical **otic** (ear) antibiotic. Although it may seem incorrect, it is common practice to substitute an ophthalmic preparation (of the same active ingredient and concentration) if the pharmacy does not have the otic preparation in stock or it is not commercially available, if the otic preparation is not covered under the patient's insurance, or if the patient does not have insurance (ophthalmic preparations are generally less expensive). In these cases, the patient should be counselled that even though the bottle is labelled "ophthalmic," it is intended for otic use. Additionally, it should be noted that although you can use ophthalmic drops in the ears, you cannot use otic drops in the eyes. This is because all ophthalmic drops must be formulated with a pH that is acceptable for use in the eyes (around 7.4), whereas otic drops are not pH balanced or buffered. If an otic preparation were to be used in the eye extreme burning and irritation would occur.

Systemic Preparations for Ear Infections

When the inner ear is involved, or when patients' compliance or proper drop technique is a concern (in older adults or young children), systemic antibiotics and NSAIDs are preferable over topical preparations. Amoxicillin and Augmentin (discussed in Chapter 17) are the most commonly used antibiotics for otitis media. They are both available in a liquid suspension and an oral tablet. NSAIDs (discussed in Chapter 21) are usually paired with these systemic antibiotics to help alleviate pain and inflammation associated with the ear infection. They are also available as liquid suspensions or in oral tablet form.

Earwax Buildup and Blockage

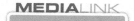

See it in Action! Go to the Online Resources to view a video on Administering Ear Drops.

When earwax accumulates in the ear canal, it can inhibit hearing and can cause pain. This type of condition is most commonly seen in older adults who are not able to properly groom themselves or in patients who are prone to produce more earwax than normal. Earwax buildup can directly lead to a blockage, but it is more common that a blockage occurs from the patient attempting to remove the earwax with a Q-tip or other object that results in the earwax being pushed deeper into the ear canal. Debrox (carbamide peroxide) is an OTC medication used to soften, loosen, and remove excessive earwax. If a patient is not successful after using this product, an ear nose and throat specialist may be needed for further assistance.

See Table 18-4 for a list of medications used for ear infections and earwax buildup.

TABLE 18-4   Otic Preparations and Medications for Earwax Buildup

GENERIC NAME	TRADE NAME	DOSAGE	COMMENTS
Topical antibiotics			
ciprofloxacin	Cipro	Otic sol, 0.2% ,3–4 drops BID for 7–14 days	Always use proper drop technique
ofloxacin	Floxin	Otic sol, 0.3%, 10 drops BID for 7–14 days	Often substituted with 0.3% ophthalmic drops
Combination topical antibiotics and steroids			
ciprofloxacin and dexamethasone	Ciprodex	Otic sol, 0.3%/0.1%, 4 drops BID for 7 days	Always use proper drop technique
ciprofloxacin and hydrocortisone	Cipro HC	Otic sol, 0.2%/0.1%, 3 drops BID for 7 days	
polymixin B, neomycin, and hydrocortisone	Cortisporin	Otic sol, 4 drops q6-8h	

(continued)

TABLE 18-4   Otic Preparations and Medications for Earwax Buildup (*continued*)

GENERIC NAME	TRADE NAME	DOSAGE	COMMENTS
Topical analgesics and anti-inflammatory agents			
acetic acid and hydrocortisone	Vosol HC	Otic sol, 1%/2%, 3–5 drops 4–6 times daily prn	Combination corticosteroid and antibacterial agent
benzocaine and antipyrine	Auralgan	Otic sol, 2–4 drops TID prn	Combination analgesic and anesthetic (currently not being manufactured)
Agents for earwax buildup			
carbamide peroxide	Debrox	Otic sol, 6.5% and 10%, 5–10 drops BID, max of 4 days (then consult ENT specialist)	Keep drops in ear for several minutes by tilting heading sideways and placing cotton in ear

CASE STUDY A

Eye Medications

Leena Shah is a 62-year-old female who has been experiencing a gradual loss of vision. She has recently been diagnosed with chronic (open-angle) glaucoma.

1. The ophthalmologist explains to Leena that glaucoma is a condition that results from:
   a. Bleeding into the aqueous humor space
   b. Obstruction of the outflow of the aqueous humor
   c. Hyperpigmentation of the aqueous humor
   d. Dehydration of the aqueous humor

2. The primary action of drugs for glaucoma is to:
   a. Increase intraocular pressure
   b. Decrease intraocular pressure
   c. Decrease external ocular pressure
   d. Increase external ocular pressure

3. The physician is preparing to write Leena a prescription for glaucoma treatment. She explains that the treatment will:
   a. Be short term (1–3 months)
   b. Be intermittent
   c. Continue for 6–12 months
   d. Continue for her lifetime

4. The physician determines that the best medication to treat Leena is a carbonic anhydrase inhibitor, which acts by:
   a. Decreasing the formation of aqueous humor
   b. Increasing blood flow to the aqueous humor space
   c. Reducing aqueous humor inflammation
   d. Decreasing blood flow to the aqueous humor space

5. Leena's physician starts her on acetazolamide at a low dose but explains that she may need to increase her dose. If her dose is increased, Leena may experience which side effect?
   a. Hyperactivity
   b. Urinary tract infection
   c. Taste alteration
   d. Urinary retention

CASE STUDY B

Eye Medications

Pia Ramirez is a 33-year-old female tennis player. She has been hit in the eye with a tennis ball and is experiencing severe pain.

1. Which medication would most likely be given to Pia to act as a local ophthalmic anesthetic?
a. Tetracaine
b. Atropine
c. Cyclopentolate
d. Phenylephrine

2. The physician applies a local ophthalmic anesthetic. What side effect may Pia experience?
a. Twitching of the eyelid
b. Anaphylaxis
c. Flushing of the eye's blood vessels
d. Profound itching

3. After being administered Alcaine, the nurse should instruct Pia to:
a. Store the medication at room temperature
b. Remain upright for 2h
c. Massage the eye every 4h
d. Wear an eye patch

4. What will the nurse instruct Pia to do after self-administering eye drops?
a. Blink rapidly.
b. Pull down her lower eye lid to let the excess medication drain out.
c. Apply pressure to the eyelid.
d. Close the eye gently so as not to squeeze the medication out.

5. Pia is cautioned to follow up with her physician if the pain continues. This is because prolonged use of an ophthalmic anesthetic can cause which complication?
a. Retinal detachment
b. Cataract formation
c. Corneal erosion
d. Conjunctival bleeding

CHAPTER REVIEW QUIZ

Match the medication in the first column with the condition in the second column that it is used to treat. Conditions may be used more than once.

Medication	Condition
1. ___ Cosopt	a. To dilate pupils
2. ___ Acular	b. Glaucoma
3. ___ tetracaine	c. Allergic reaction of eyes
4. ___ atropine	d. Postoperative inflammation
5. ___ prednisolone	e. Eye injury pain
6. ___ pilocarpine	
7. ___ Timoptic	
8. ___ Diamox Sequels	
9. ___ Travatan Z	
10. ___ phenylephrine	

Choose the correct answer.

11. The purpose of an ophthalmic decongestant medication is:
    a. To block histamine receptors
    b. Blood vessel vasoconstriction
    c. To block the tear duct
    d. Blood vessel vasodilation

12. What is the best form of ophthalmic medication for adults?
    a. Gel
    b. Ointment
    c. Drops
    d. Medicated patch

13. When administering more than one ophthalmic medication at a time, the minimum amount of time desired between the medications is:
    a. 5 min
    b. 15 min
    c. 30 min
    d. 1h

14. Which category of drug may exacerbate glaucoma?
    a. Anticoagulant
    b. Anti-inflammatory
    c. Antihypertensive
    d. Anticholinergic

15. Which medication is used at the end of an eye exam to constrict the pupil?
    a. Timolol
    b. Atropine
    c. Pilocarpine
    d. Brimondidine

16. Which medication would be the best choice for a patient who requires an antibiotic and steroid otic preparation?
    a. Ciprodex
    b. Ciprofloxaxin
    c. Auralgan
    d. Floxin

17. Patients who have earwax buildup should be instructed to:
    a. Do nothing, it will resolve on its own
    b. Attempt to remove with a Q-tip
    c. Use an antibiotic drop from a past ear infection
    d. Use Debrox OTC

18. You can use otic drops in the eyes but you cannot use ophthalmic drops in the ears? ____
    ____ True
    ____ False

STUDYGUIDE

Online Resources

P R A C T I C E

Complete Chapter 18

• Powerpoint presentations
• Videos

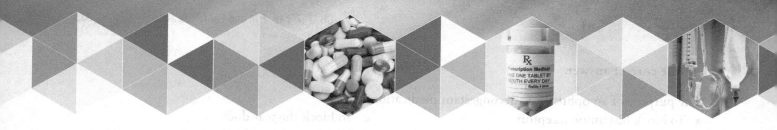

CHAPTER 19

ANALGESICS, SEDATIVES, AND HYPNOTICS

KEY TERMS AND CONCEPTS

Adjuvant

Analgesics

Antipyretic

Coanalgesic

Dependence

Endogenous

Endorphins

Hypnotics

Opioid agonists

Opioid antagonists

Paradoxical

Placebo effect

Sedatives

Subjective

Tinnitus

Tolerance

OBJECTIVES

Upon completion of this chapter, the learner should be able to

1. Compare and contrast the indications and actions of nonopioid, opioid, and adjuvant analgesics, sedatives, and hypnotics

2. List the side effects of the major analgesics, sedatives, and hypnotics

3. Describe the necessary information for patient education regarding interactions and cautions

4. Explain the precautions and contraindications to administration of the central nervous system (CNS) depressants mentioned in this chapter

5. Describe actions recently taken by the FDA and manufacturers and the associated impacts on the analgesic drug category

6. Define the Key Terms and Concepts

Analgesics, sedatives, and hypnotics depress central nervous system (CNS) action to varying degrees. Some drugs can be classified into more than one category, depending on the dosage. **Analgesics** are given to relieve pain. **Sedatives** are given to calm, soothe, or produce sedation. **Hypnotics** are given to produce sleep.

ANALGESICS

The most common reason patients seek out medical care is pain. The four most common types of pain reported by the National Center for Health Statistics are lower back, neck, migraine, and facial or jaw pain. Pain is **subjective** (i.e., it can be experienced or perceived only by the individual person). Health care professionals can assess a patient's pain by asking the patient to describe the pain and its location, and assess the pain's severity by using validated pain assessment scales. These scales are often based on a range of 1–10, or use symbolic facial expressions to show level of pain (Figure 19-1).

Pain has both psychological and physiological components. Some persons have a higher pain threshold than others because of conditioning, ethnic background, sensitivity, or physiological factors (e.g., endorphin release). **Endorphins** are **endogenous** analgesics produced within the body as a reaction to severe pain or intense exercise (e.g., "runner's high"). Endorphins block the transmission of pain. Endorphin release may be responsible for a **placebo effect**: relief from pain as the result of suggestion without the administration of an analgesic.

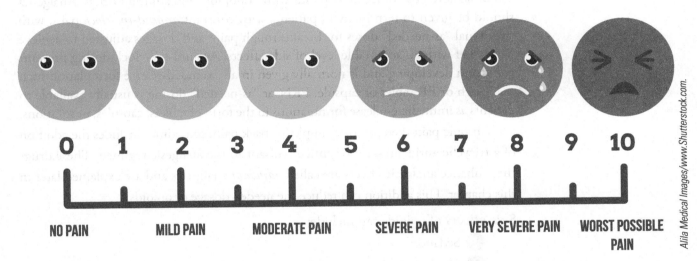

Alila Medical Images/www.Shutterstock.com.

FIGURE 19-1 Pain scales are used by health care professionals to assess pain at time of admission and to assess changes in pain levels.

Opioid Analgesics

Analgesics can be classified as opioid, nonopioid, and adjuvant. Opioids are classified as full or pure agonists, partial agonists, or mixed agonist–antagonists depending on the specific receptors they bind to and their activity at the receptor. Full agonists (e.g., morphine, hydromorphone, oxycodone, and fentanyl) are commonly used because their action is similar to that of opium in altering the perception of pain, and they do not have a ceiling to their analgesic effects. This means that there is no plateau to the amount of analgesic relief, the only limiting factor is side effects from higher doses. The pure agonist opioids will not reverse analgesia like the other classes (e.g., buprenorphine). Because of their potential for abuse and psychological dependence, **opioids** are classified as controlled substances in the United States and include both the natural opium alkaloids (e.g., morphine and codeine), the semisynthetics (e.g., hydromophone and oxycodone), and the synthetics (e.g., meperidine [Demerol] and fentanyl [Duragesic]). In November 2010, the Food and Drug Administration (FDA) requested a market withdrawal of all products containing propoxyphene (e.g., Darvon and Darvocet), which were linked to cardiac abnormalities and death from overdoses.

Opioids tend to cause tolerance (i.e., a larger dose of opioid is needed to achieve the same level of analgesia) and physiological dependence (i.e., physical adaptation of the body to the opioid and withdrawal symptoms after abrupt drug discontinuation) with chronic use. Addiction or psychological dependence is usually not a problem for patients who require opioids for acute pain management. The majority of people stop taking opioids when their pain resolves. Because of tolerance, the potential for developing dependence, and the potential for developing undesirable side effects, opioids are not used for extended periods except to relieve chronic pain, for example cancer pain, terminal illness, and nonmalignant pain in selected patients who do not benefit from other pain relief methods.

Adequate pain control is important for the terminally ill. Dependence is irrelevant for dying patients and should not be a consideration. More effective pain control can be achieved by combining opioids with nonopioid and adjuvant drugs. Analgesics should be given to terminally ill patients with constant *around-the-clock* pain, with additional "as-needed" doses for breakthrough pain, and dosages adjusted to achieve pain relief with an acceptable level of side effects. Around-the-clock dosing prevents pain from developing and is normally given in an extended-release formulation such as a patch or ER tablet or capsule. PRN or "as-needed" dosing is usually available to patients as immediate-release formulations in the form of tablets, capsules, or solutions.

Chronic pain therapy, for example for back pain, sometimes includes the addition of a tricyclic antidepressant or anticonvulsant to the analgesic regimen. These drugs that enhance analgesic effects are called *adjuvant* analgesics and are explained later in this chapter. This addition can reduce the needed dosage of opioids.

Side effects of opioids can include:

- ! Sedation
- ! Confusion, euphoria, restlessness, and agitation
- ! Headache and dizziness
- ! Hypotension and bradycardia
- Urinary retention; sexual dysfunction
- ! Nausea and vomiting (usually resolves within a few days) and constipation (occurs in more than 50% of patients and frequently requires treatment)
- ! Respiratory depression (appropriate dose titration reduces risk)
- ! Physical and/or emotional dependence; tolerance
- Blurred vision
- Seizures with large doses
- Flushing, rash, and pruritus (opiate agonists cause histamine release, especially codeine, morphine, and meperidine)

Precautions or contraindications with opioids apply to:

Head injury (i.e., conditions associated with increased intracranial pressure)

Cardiac disease (methadone has been associated with QT prolongation, which causes a cardiac arrhythmia that can be fatal in some patients) and hypotension

CNS depression

GI, hepatic, renal, and thyroid diseases

Chronic obstructive pulmonary disease (COPD) and asthma

Sleep apnea

Pregnancy and lactation

Children

Older adults and debilitated patients

Driving or operating machinery (may impair mental or physical abilities)

Addiction prone, suicidal, and alcoholic persons

Opiate agonist hypersensitivity (can try an opioid from a different chemical class, with close monitoring)

Abrupt drug discontinuation in patients taking opioids chronically

Interactions include potentiation of the effect of opioids with all CNS depressants, including:

Psychotropics

Alcohol

Sedatives and hypnotics

Muscle relaxants

Antihistamines

Antiemetics

Antiarrhythmics or antihypertensives

Preoperatively, an opioid like fentanyl is usually administered parenterally before the start of anesthesia, according to the directions of the anesthesiologist. Meperidine is not recommended for routine use owing to a metabolite that may accumulate and cause seizures in patients with kidney disease, although it is useful for the treatment

CLINICAL CONNECTION

Opioid-Induced Constipation

Although opioids are very effective for providing pain relief, they also have various dose-related side effects that can make taking them challenging. Of the previously discussed side effects, only constipation is not self-limiting. This means that all other side effects will improve over time as a patient continues therapy, but opioid-induced constipation (OIC) does not. OIC occurs because the digestive tract contains similar receptors (mu receptors) that are targeted in pain relief. When these receptors in the digestive tract are activated, transit time is slowed and constipation occurs. Often times an OTC stool softener or a stimulant laxative is sufficient but in more severe cases prescription strength medication is needed. Amitiza, Resistor, and Movantik are all medications used to treat severe OIC. Patients should also be instructed to stay hydrated and not remain stationary if possible. This is an important consideration for patients receiving opioid pain therapy, especially because it is often overlooked until OIC has already become an issue. Other laxative options and general constipation are discussed more in depth in Chapter 16.

Note

The **opioid antagonist** (reversal agent) naloxone (Narcan) is used in the treatment of opioid overdoses and in the operating room, delivery room, and newborn nursery for opiate-induced respiratory depression. Naltrexone (ReVia), a pure opioid antagonist, and sublingual buprenorphine, a partial opioid antagonist, are used separately and together (Suboxone) in the treatment of opioid dependence (see Chapter 20).

of post-op shivering. Morphine or hydromorphone are commonly used to manage moderate to severe pain due to their longer duration of effect and potency. Hydromorphone is four to eight times more potent than morphine, so caution is necessary to avoid medication errors.

Opioid agonists are available in various strengths, as concentrated oral solutions and in combination products. In January 2011, the FDA announced that drug manufacturers must begin to limit the strength of acetaminophen in *prescription* drug products, which are predominantly combinations of acetaminophen and opioids, to 325 mg per dosage form. This action will help reduce the risk of severe liver injury associated with acetaminophen. Carefully note the product and strength to be administered.

Hydrocodone-containing products, recently a Schedule III controlled substance, was the most commonly prescribed drug in the United States in 2011 (131 million prescriptions for 47 million patients). These products also consistently rank among the most-abused drugs (along with oxycodone) in the United States each year according to the DEA (see Chapter 20). These facts caused the DEA and the FDA to make hydrocodone-containing products a Schedule II controlled substance, limiting which kind of health care professionals can write for these products and eliminating the option for refills (see Chapter 1). Additionally, hydrocodone is now available in non–acetaminophen-containing formulations such as Zohydro ER and Hysinglia ER. Both are DEA Schedule II substances and are available in abuse deterrent formulations that are indicated for around the clock maintenance pain relief.

Tramadol

Tramadol (Ultram) is a centrally acting synthetic analog of codeine with a dual mechanism of action. It produces analgesia by weak inhibition of norepinephrine and serotonin reuptake and is an opioid receptor agonist. Tramadol has less potential for abuse or respiratory depression (although both may occur) and is currently a Schedule III controlled substance. However, doses above the normal therapeutic range produce several negative side effects.

Tapentadol (Nucynta) was developed in an attempt to take advantage of the positives associated with tramadol and fewer of its negatives. Tapentadol's mechanism of action does not involve serotonin reuptake, and clinical studies suggest a lower incidence of GI adverse effects. Tapentadol is classified as a Schedule II controlled substance.

Side effects and **precautions** of tramadol and tapentadol are similar to the opioids listed previously. It should also be noted that tramadol can lower the seizure threshold, so it may not be a good option in patients who have experienced a head trauma from an accident.

Interactions of tramadol and tapentadol occur with:

Monoamine oxidase inhibitors (MAOIs) or neuroleptics (may increase seizure risk)

Carbamazepine (Tegretol) antagonizes tramadol action

Selective serotonin reuptake inhibitors (SSRIs) (especially Paxil, Zoloft), tricyclic antidepressants, and triptans (may cause serotonin syndrome and increase seizure risk)

Note

By inhibiting reuptake, the substance (such as serotonin) will be around longer and therefore have a greater effect.

See Table 19-1 for a summary of the opioid analgesics.

TABLE 19-1   Opioid Analgesics[a]

GENERIC NAME	TRADE NAME	DOSAGE	USES/COMMENTS
butorphanol	(Stadol)[b]	1–4 mg IM, or 0.5–2 mg IV, or 1 mg (one spray) nasal spray q3–4 h PRN	Moderate to severe acute pain (e.g., migraine)
codeine		15–60 mg PO q4h PRN;	Mild to moderate acute, chronic, and cancer pain
		PO 10–20 mg q4–6h PRN (max 120 mg per day)	Antitussive dose
with acetaminophen[c]	Tylenol with Codeine	15–60 mg codeine PO q4–6h PRN	Max 360 mg codeine and 4 g acetaminophen per day from all sources
fentanyl citrate	Actiq (loz.) Fentora (buccal)	PO 200–400 mcg q4–6h PRN; or	Moderate to severe acute, chronic, or cancer pain
	(Sublimaze)[b]	25–100 mcg slow IV/IM	
hydrocodone with acetaminophen[d] hydrocodone	Lorcet Lortab Vicodin	PO 2.5–10 mg of hydrocodone (tab or liquid) q4–6h PRN	Moderate acute, chronic, or cancer pain, or antitussive; max 4 g acetaminophen per day
	Zohydro ER Hysinglia ER	10-50mg q12h 20-120mg q24h	Abuse deterrent formulations
hydromorphone	Dilaudid	PO 2–4 mg q4–6h PRN IM, IV, subcu 0.2–1 mg q2–4h PRN R 3 mg q6–8h PRN	Moderate to severe acute, chronic, or cancer pain
meperidine	Demerol	50–150 mg PO/IM/IV/subcu, q3–4h PRN	Short-term for moderate to severe *acute* pain
methadone	Dolophine Methadose	2.5–10 mg IM/IV/subcu/PO initially q8–12h PRN; maint. 5–20 mg PO q6–8h PRN	Severe chronic and cancer pain; also for narcotic withdrawal
morphine sulfate			
immediate release	morphine	PO 10–30 mg or PR 10–20 mg q3–4h PRN; IV (over 4–5 min); IM/subcu 2.5–15 mg q2–6h PRN	Moderate to severe acute, chronic, or cancer pain
extended release	MS Contin (tab) Avinza (cap) Kadian (cap)	PO, R 15–100 mg q8–12h PO 30 mg q24h (initially, titrate to response) PO 10 mg BID or 20 mg QD (initially, titrate to response)	Do not crush! OD can be fatal May open caps and sprinkle contents on applesauce; can give Kadian contents via a gastrostomy tube

(continued)

TABLE 19-1 Opioid Analgesics[a] (*continued*)

GENERIC NAME	TRADE NAME	DOSAGE	USES/COMMENTS
oxycodone			
controlled release	Oxycontin	PO 10–80 mg SR q8–12h	Serious abuse potential, overdose can be fatal; do not crush
immediate release	Roxicodone	PO 5–10 mg q6h PRN	Moderate to severe acute, chronic, or cancer pain
with aspirin[e]	Percodan	PO 1–2 tabs q4–6h PRN	Max 12 tabs per 24h
with acetaminophen[f]	Percocet	PO 1–2 tabs q4–6h PRN	Max 4 g acetaminophen per day
tramadol	Ultram	PO 50–100 mg q4–6h PRN, max 400 mg daily	Weak opioid analgesic for acute pain, not controlled federally
	Ultram ER	PO 100–300 mg daily	Do not crush; for chronic pain
with acetaminophen	Ultracet	PO 2 tabs q4–6h PRN	Max 8 tabs per day; for acute pain
tapentadol	Nucynta	PO 50–100 mg q4–6h PRN	For moderate to severe acute pain
	Nucynta ER	PO 50–250 mg SR q12h	For moderate to severe chronic pain; do not crush

a. Combination opioid products (check for allergies, especially aspirin combinations).
b. This brand name is no longer marketed, but the name may still be used.
c. Tylenol with Codeine tabs contain 300 mg acetaminophen plus codeine:
#2 tab 15 mg codeine, #3 tab 30 mg, #4 tab 60 mg (max acetaminophen dose 4 g/day).
acetaminophen with codeine elixir: 120 mg acetaminophen and 12 mg codeine per 5 mL.
d. Norco, Vicodin, Lortab: 325 mg acetaminophen and 5 mg, 7.5 mg, and 10 mg hydrocodone.
Vicodan tabs: 300 mg acetaminophen and 5 mg hydrocodone.
Vicodan ES tabs: 300 mg acetaminophen and 7.5 mg hydrocodone.
Vicodin HP tabs: 300 mg acetaminophen and 10 mg hydrocodone.
Lortab elixir: acetaminophen and hydrocodone concentrations vary depending on the manufacturer.
e. Percodan or Endodan tabs: 325 mg aspirin and 5 mg oxycodone.
f. Percocet, Roxicet, or Endocet: 325 mg acetaminophen and 5 mg oxycodone. (Other strengths are available.)

Nonopioid Analgesics

Nonopioid analgesics, many of which are available without prescription as over-the-counter (OTC) medications, are very popular. Therefore, it is extremely important that the health care professional be informed and responsible for patient education in this very important area of public health. The lay public needs to become aware of the dangers of self-medication, overdosage, side effects, and interactions, as well as the grave danger of poisoning to children and older adults by inappropriate use of these readily available drugs.

Nonopioids are given for the purposes of relieving mild to moderate pain, fever, and anti-inflammatory conditions, for example arthritis. This group of analgesics is also used as a coanalgesic in severe acute or chronic pain requiring opioids. The salicylates (aspirin) are most commonly used for their *analgesic* and antipyretic properties, as well as for their anti-inflammatory action. Other anti-inflammatory drugs, for example ibuprofen, are also used for their analgesic properties. The nonsteroidal anti-inflammatory drugs (NSAIDs) are discussed in Chapter 21.

Acetaminophen has analgesic and antipyretic properties but very little effect on inflammation. Aspirin and acetaminophen are frequently combined with opioids (see Table 19-1) or with other drugs for more effective analgesic action. See Table 19-2 for a representative sample of nonopioid analgesics and antipyretics. There are many other combination analgesic products available OTC. Patients should be instructed to check all ingredients in these combination products because of potentially serious adverse side effects, for example aspirin allergy or acetaminophen contraindications. When patients are taking acetaminophen, it is important to instruct them that other products (including OTC medications) containing acetaminophen should not be used without the knowledge and approval of their doctor or pharmacist.

TABLE 19-2 Nonopioid Analgesics and Antipyretics

GENERIC NAME	TRADE NAME	DOSAGE	COMMENTS
acetylsalicylic acid[a] (ASA, aspirin)	Ecotrin, Ascriptin, Bufferin	325–650 mg PO or rectal supp q4h PRN; larger doses for arthritis	Administer with milk or food; may cause Reye's syndrome in children and teenagers
acetaminophen	Tylenol (OTC)	325–650 mg PO or rectal supp q4h PRN (max 4 g/day)	No anti-inflammatory action; less effective than ASA for soft tissue pain
	Ofirmev (Rx)	1 g IV q6h PRN or 650 mg q4h PRN (>50 kg) weight based for less than 50 kg	For mild to moderate pain, fever; for moderate to severe pain with adjunctive opioid analgesics
combinations[b]			
ASA and caffeine	Anacin	2 tabs PO q6h PRN, max 8 per day	
ASA, acetaminophen, and caffeine	Excedrin	2 tabs/caps PO q6h PRN, max 8 per day	Also for the pain of migraine headaches
butalbital, caffeine, *with* *acetaminophen*	Esgic, Fioricet (Rx)	1–2 tabs/caps PO q4h PRN, max 6 per day	For tension headache or migraine
with aspirin	Fiorinal (C-III)		

a. Other nonsteroidal anti-inflammatory drugs with analgesic action are listed in Table 21-2.
b. Representative sample.

Salicylates and Other NSAIDs

Salicylate analgesic and anti-inflammatory actions are associated primarily with preventing the formation of prostaglandins and the subsequent inflammatory response prostaglandins help to induce. The salicylates, for example aspirin (ASA) and other NSAIDs, are also discussed in Chapter 21.

Side effects of salicylates and other NSAIDs, especially with prolonged use and/or high dosages, can include:

- ! Prolonged bleeding time
- ! Bleeding and frequent bruising
- ! Gastric distress, ulceration, and bleeding (which may be silent)

! Tinnitus (ringing or roaring in the ears) and hearing loss with overdose

Hepatic dysfunction

Renal insufficiency, decreased urine output with sodium and water retention, and renal failure

Drowsiness, dizziness, headache, sweating, euphoria, and depression

Rash

! Coma, respiratory failure, or anaphylaxis, which can result from hypersensitivity or overdosage, especially in children (watch for aspirin allergy)

! Gastrointestinal (GI) symptoms, which can be minimized by administration with food or milk or by using an aspirin buffered with antacids or in enteric-coated form

Poisoning (keep out of reach of children, especially flavored children's aspirin)

Precautions or contraindications for salicylates and other NSAIDs apply to:

GI ulcer and bleeding

Bleeding disorders in patients taking anticoagulants

Asthma

Children younger than 15 with influenza-like illness (because of the danger of Reye's syndrome)

Treatment of pain with NSAIDs after heart surgery

Pregnancy

Lactation

Vitamin K deficiency

Allergy to ASA (occurs in around 2% of the population)

Caution in use of salicylates and other NSAIDs must be taken with:

Anemia

Hepatic disease

Renal disease

Hodgkin's disease

Pre- or postoperative conditions (discontinue five to seven days before elective surgery)

Interactions of salicylates may also occur with NSAIDs and:

Alcohol (may increase potential for ulceration and bleeding)

Anticoagulants (potentiation)

Corticosteroids (gastric ulcer)

Antacids in high doses (decreased effects)

NSAIDs (decreased effects, increased GI side effects)

Do not give salicylates and NSAIDs together (unless approved by a physician)

Insulin or oral antidiabetic agents (increased effects; may interfere with certain urinary glucose tests)

Methotrexate (increased effects)

Probenecid (decreased effects)

Antihypertensives: angiotensin-converting enzyme (ACE) inhibitors, beta-blockers and diuretics (decreased effects)

Carbonic anhydrase inhibitors (toxic effects, e.g., Diamox)

Acetaminophen

Acetaminophen (Tylenol) is used extensively in the treatment of mild to moderate pain and fever. It has very little effect on inflammation. However, acetaminophen has fewer adverse side effects than the salicylates (e.g., does not cause gastric irritation or precipitate bleeding). Therefore, it is sometimes used only for its analgesic properties in treating the chronic pain of arthritis so that the salicylate dosage may be reduced to safer levels with fewer side effects in these patients.

Side effects of acetaminophen are rare, but large doses can cause:

- ! Severe liver toxicity
- ! Renal insufficiency (decreased urine output)
- Rash or urticaria
- Blood dyscrasia

Caution must be used with frequent acetaminophen use and alcohol ingestion because of potential liver damage. Caution must also be used with pregnancy and breast-feeding.

Contraindicated with hypersensitivity to acetaminophen or any component of the combination product.

Recently there have been major changes in acetaminophen liquid concentrations for pediatrics and lower dosing limits for adults. These *voluntary* changes are being implemented by manufacturers of acetaminophen and are designed to lower the risk of accidental overdoses when too much acetaminophen is ingested, resulting in liver toxicity. The traditional 80 mg/0.8 mL and 80 mg/1 mL concentrated infant drops are to be phased out, and all single-ingredient acetaminophen liquid products for pediatric patients are to be transitioned to a less concentrated children's formulation of 160 mg/5 mL and to include standardized dosing devices, such as oral syringes.

For adults, some manufacturers are lowering the maximum daily dose on single-ingredient acetaminophen products from 4,000 mg per day to 3,000 mg per day. Since these changes are voluntary, there is actually a greater potential for dosing confusion and errors during this transition period. It is imperative that parents, patients, and caregivers read the drug facts label for each specific product carefully to identify the concentration, recommended dosing, and directions for use of that particular product.

Note

Acetaminophen (Tylenol) is frequently combined with opioid analgesics when stronger pain relief is required. Some examples of such combinations include Tylenol #3, Lorcet, Lortab, Vicodin, Percocet, and Roxicet. For examples of other opioid combinations and for information regarding the proportion of the ingredients in each product, see Table 19-1 and the combination opioid products footnote below the table. Remember, all opioids are federally controlled substances.

Adjuvant Analgesics

These drugs were originally intended for the treatment of conditions other than pain. **Adjuvant** analgesics may enhance the analgesic effect with opioids and non-opioids, produce analgesia alone, or reduce the side effects of analgesics. Nerve pain (neuropathic pain) can be caused by certain disease states (diabetic neuropathy), infections (postherpetic neuralgia), and medications (certain chemotherapeutic agents and antiretrovirals). Fibromyalgia is a condition characterized by chronic, widespread musculoskeletal pain; muscle tenderness; sleep disturbances; and profound fatigue.

Both neuropathic pain and fibromyalgia may not be relieved by the pain medications discussed earlier. Two classes commonly used for analgesia in these conditions include anticonvulsants and specific classes of antidepressants. Another agent, lidocaine, is available topically in a patch (Lidoderm) and may be especially effective to treat nerve pain and other types of localized pain while avoiding the adverse effects of oral or parenterally administered medications.

Tricyclic Antidepressants

Tricyclic antidepressants are used in the treatment of fibromyalgia and nerve pain associated with herpes, arthritis, diabetes, and cancer; migraine or tension headaches; insomnia; and depression. Often, the patient will describe the pain as "burning." Tricyclic antidepressant actions are associated with increasing available norepinephrine and serotonin, which blocks pain transmission. Drugs in this class used commonly for pain include amitriptyline, desipramine, and nortriptyline. Allow two to three weeks to see therapeutic effects.

Side effects of tricyclic antidepressants (more so with amitriptyline) can include:

- **!** Dry mouth, urinary retention, delirium, and constipation
- **!** Sedation (take at bedtime)
- **!** Orthostatic hypotension
- **!** Tachyarrhythmias
- Heart block in cardiac patients

The degree of side effects varies with each antidepressant. Side effects may be additive with opioids (e.g., increased constipation, hypotension, and sedation).

Caution must be used with tricyclics if used with prostatic hypertrophy, urinary retention, increased intraocular pressure, and glaucoma.

Precautions or contraindications for tricyclics apply to hypersensitivity and recovery phase of myocardial infarction.

See Chapter 20 for more information on the tricyclic antidepressants.

Serotonin Norepinephrine Reuptake Inhibitors

Duloxetine (Cymbalta) and venlafaxine (Effexor XR) are antidepressants that inhibit the reuptake of both serotonin and norepinephrine. They do not affect histamine or muscarinic receptors like the tricyclics; therefore, anticholinergic side effects are not present. The SNRI antidepressants are used to treat diabetic neuropathy and fibromyalgia. Milnacipran (Savella), an SNRI with antidepressant activity, is indicated only for fibromyalgia.

Side effects of SNRIs include sleep disturbance, headache, nausea, stomach pain, diarrhea, constipation, dizziness, and sweating. Venlafaxine has the potential to increase blood pressure and heart rate.

Precautions or contraindications apply to narrow-angle glaucoma, hepatic (duloxetine, venlafaxine) or renal (milnacipran) impairment, abrupt discontinuation, patients with a history of suicidal ideation or behaviors, and substantial alcohol use.

Interactions with all SNRIs and serotonergics (such as MAOIs or SSRIs) may result in a serotonin syndrome that is characterized by a rapid development of hyperthermia, hypertension, rigidity, autonomic instability, and mental status changes that can include coma and delirium. Milnacipran has fewer interactions than the other SNRIs.

Anticonvulsants

Anticonvulsants (i.e., Neurontin and Tegretol), like tricyclic antidepressants, are commonly used for the management of nerve pain associated with neuralgia, herpes zoster (shingles), and cancer. Anticonvulsant therapy is implemented when the patient describes the pain as "sharp," "shooting," "shock-like pain," or "lightning-like."

Gabapentin (Neurontin) is generally considered a first-line *anticonvulsant* for neuropathic pain therapy, followed by carbamazepine (Tegretol) and lamotrigine (Lamictal). Carbamazepine is also indicated for trigeminal neuralgia (also known as tic douloureux), symptoms that include episodes of facial pain, often accompanied by painful spasms of facial muscles.

Pregabalin (Lyrica), a compound that is chemically and structurally similar to gabapentin, is a second-generation anticonvulsant approved by the FDA for use in fibromyalgia, diabetic neuropathy, and postherpetic neuralgia. Pregabalin has been designated as a Schedule V controlled substance because of its potential for abuse and dependence.

Side effects of anticonvulsants can include:

- ! Sedation, dizziness, and confusion
- ! Nausea, vomiting, constipation, and anorexia
- ! Ataxia and unsteadiness
- Hepatitis (not Lyrica)
- Rash, Stevens–Johnson syndrome (Lamictal—start low, slow titration upward)
- ! Bone marrow suppression
- Nystagmus, diplopia (double vision), and blurred vision
- Gingivitis (gabapentin)
- Weight gain and peripheral edema (pregabalin)

> **Caution**
> Do not confuse *Lamictal* (anticonvulsant) with Lamisil (antifungal).

Caution must be used with anticonvulsants if used with allergies, hepatitis, cardiac disease, and renal disease.

Precautions or contraindications with anticonvulsants include:

- Hypersensitivity
- Psychiatric conditions (increased risk of suicidal ideation and behavior)
- Pregnancy
- SA (sinoatrial) and AV (atrioventricular) block (Tegretol)
- Hemolytic disorders (Tegretol)
- Abrupt discontinuation

Interactions of anticonvulsants occur with:

Alcohol (decreased effects)

Antacids (decreased effects) (Neurontin)

Antineoplastics (decreased effects) (Tegretol)

CNS depressants (decreased effects) (Tegretol)

Folic acid (decreased effects) (Lamictal)

ACE inhibitors and the antidiabetic agents Actos and Avandia with Lyrica (increased risk of angioedema)

Antiretrovirals (increased or decreased effects) with Lamictal and Tegretol

LOCAL ANESTHETICS

The lidocaine patch (Lidoderm) is approved for the management of postherpetic neuralgia, although it can provide significant analgesia in other forms of neuropathic pain, including diabetic neuropathy and musculoskeletal pain such as osteoarthritis and lower back pain. Topical lidocaine provides pain relief through a peripheral effect and generally has little if any central action. The penetration of topical lidocaine into the intact skin is sufficient to produce an analgesic effect, but less than the amount necessary to produce anesthesia.

The lidocaine patch must be applied to the intact skin. Patches may be cut into smaller sizes with scissors before the removal of the release liner. To reduce the potential for serious adverse effects, patches are worn only once for up to 12-h within a 24-h period and then removed. If these patches are not removed for a 12-h period, tolerance can occur and the medication will be rendered ineffective. It may take up to two weeks to achieve the desired outcomes. It should be noted that although many patches cannot be cut, lidocaine patches are able to be cut into smaller or custom-sized pieces (Figure 19-2).

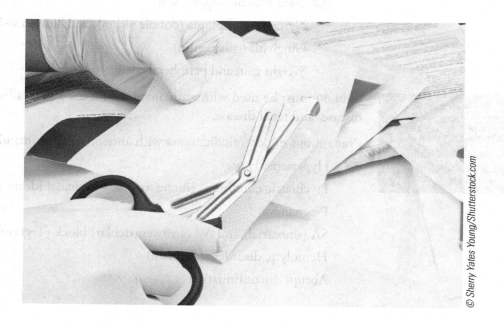

FIGURE 19-2 Lidocaine patches provide local pain relief, so it is convenient for patients to be able to cut them to cover exactly the area that they need treated.

© Sherry Yates Young/Shutterstock.com

Side effects of the lidocaine patch, local in nature, are generally mild and transient and include:

- ❗ Erythema, edema, and hives
- ❗ Allergic reactions

Precautions or contraindications for the lidocaine patch apply to:

Sensitivity to local anesthetics

Hepatic disease

Nonintact skin

Pregnancy, breast-feeding, and pediatric use

Handling and disposal to prevent access by children or pets

Drug interactions of the lidocaine patch occur with:

Antiarrhythmic drugs such as mexiletene

Local anesthetics

See Table 19-3 for a summary of adjuvant analgesics.

Note

Sometimes a local vasoconstricting agent such as epinephrine is given in conjunction with a local anesthetic injection such as lidocaine to further help localize the effect and thereby prolong the duration of the effect.

TABLE 19-3 **Adjuvant Analgesics and Local Anesthetic**

GENERIC NAME	TRADE NAME	DOSAGE[a]	COMMENTS
Antidepressants			
Tricyclics			
amitriptyline	(Elavil)[b]	PO 10–150 mg at bedtime	Use with caution in the older adults
nortriptyline	Pamelor	PO 10–150 mg at bedtime	Both of these are less likely to cause certain side effects vs. amitriptyline
desipramine	Norpramin	PO 10–150 mg at bedtime	
SNRIs[c]			
duloxetine	Cymbalta	PO 60–120 mg daily	
milnacipran	Savella	Titrate PO to 50–100 mg BID	For fibromyalgia only
venlafaxine	Effexor XR	PO 75–225 mg daily	
Anticonvulsants			
carbamazepine	Tegretol	PO 200–600 mg BID	Especially for trigeminal neuralgia; monitor serum levels periodically
gabapentin	Neurontin	PO 600–3,600 mg per day divided doses three to four times per day	For nerve pain, especially postherpetic neuralgia DEA considering adding schedule to gabapentin
lamotrigine	Lamictal	PO 25–200 mg BID	Slow titration to avoid rash
pregabalin	Lyrica	PO 150–600 mg per day in two to three divided doses	Slow titration to avoid rash (Stevens Johnson syndrome); for fibromyalgia, diabetic neuropathy, and postherpetic neuralgia

(continued)

TABLE 19-3 **Adjuvant Analgesics and Local Anesthetic (*continued*)**

GENERIC NAME	TRADE NAME	DOSAGE[a]	COMMENTS
Local Anesthetic			
lidocaine	Lidoderm	1–3 patches 5% daily (may be cut into smaller sizes)	For postherpetic neuralgia (on 12 h/off 12 h)

a. All adjuvants should be started at the lower end of the dosage range and titrated upward in small increments weekly according to the clinical response.
b. This brand name is no longer marketed, but the name is still commonly used.
c. Serotonin norepinephrine reuptake inhibitors.

ANTIMIGRAINE AGENTS

Migraine is the most common neurovascular headache and may include nausea, vomiting, and sensitivity to light or noise. Migraines (and most other forms of headache) respond best when treated early. Typically, patients who experience chronic migraines will have an aura before the migraine occurs that can help warn them a migraine is about to occur. Simple analgesics (see Table 19-2), NSAIDs (see Chapter 21), and opioid analgesics can be effective, especially if they are taken at the initial sign of migraine. Generally, opioids are reserved for refractory migraines that do not respond to other therapy options.

Serotonin Receptor Agonists (SRAs)

For those patients unresponsive to the aforementioned treatments, serotonin agonists were developed based on the observation that serotonin levels decrease, whereas vasodilation and inflammation of blood vessels in the brain increase, as the migraine symptoms worsen during an attack. SRAs are also effective in treating the nausea and vomiting associated with migraines because serotonin receptors are also found in the GI tract.

The first "triptan" approved was sumatriptan (Imitrex), followed by six others. SRAs are indicated for the acute treatment of migraines in adults and are not FDA approved for the prophylactic management of migraine headaches. Nasal spray formulations may be useful if the patient has nausea and vomiting or cannot swallow tablets. Individual responses to triptans vary; patients who do not respond to one triptan may respond to another. In general, these medications are taken at the onset of a headache (or first warning sign), and then repeated if needed in 2 h. Patients should be warned to not take more than two doses in a 24-h period unless directed to do so by their physician.

Side effects of SRAs include:

- ! Malaise, fatigue, dizziness, and drowsiness
- ! Nausea, vomiting, and diarrhea
- Asthenia, tingling, paresthesias, and flushing
- Pain or pressure in the chest, neck, or jaw
- ! Arrhythmias, angina, palpitations, myocardial infarction, and cardiac arrest

Precautions or contraindications with SRAs apply to:

Patients with cerebrovascular or cardiovascular disease

Uncontrolled hypertension

Peripheral vascular disease

Hepatic or renal disease (dose adjustments may be needed)

Older adults (who are more likely to have decreased hepatic function and more pronounced blood pressure increases and are at risk for coronary artery disease)

Pregnancy and lactation

Children

Drug interactions of SRAs occur with:

Ergot alkaloids (i.e., methylergonovine; additive vasospastic effects)

MAOIs elevate the plasma levels of *most* triptans (do not use within two weeks of discontinuing the use of the MAOI)

Most antidepressants potentiate the effects of serotonin (including SSRIs and tricyclics) and may result in serotonin syndrome (mental status changes, diaphoresis, tremor, hyperreflexia, and fever) when used in combination

Macrolide antibiotics, antiretroviral protease inhibitors, and "azole" antifungals with eletriptan (increased plasma levels) (do not use within at least 72 h of each other).

See Table 19-4 for information on antimigraine agents.

TABLE 19-4 Antimigraine Agents

GENERIC NAME	TRADE NAME	DOSAGE FORMS	INITIAL DOSE ADULT	REPEAT TIME (HOURS)	DAILY MAXIMUM DOSE (MG)
eletriptan	Relpax	Tablet	20–40 mg	2	40
frovatriptan	Frova	Tablet	2.5 mg	2	7.5
rizatriptan	Maxalt	Tablet	5–10 mg	2	30
	Maxalt-MLT	OD tablet	5–10 mg	2	30
sumatriptan	Imitrex	subcu	4 mg, 6 mg	1	12
		Nasal	5–20 mg	2	40
		Tablet	25–100 mg	2	200
zolmitriptan	Zomig	Tablet	2.5–5 mg	2	10
	Zomig-ZMT	OD tablet	2.5–5 mg	2	10
	Zomig	Nasal	5 mg	2	10

OD, orally disintegrating tablet.
Note: Representative sample; other products are available.

SEDATIVES AND HYPNOTICS

Sedatives and hypnotics are medications used to promote sedation in smaller doses and promote sleep in larger doses. Insomnia is one of the most prevalent sleep disorders, with symptoms occurring in approximately 33%–50% of the U.S. adult population. The prevalence of chronic insomnia is higher in women and older people. The sedative-hypnotics discussed in this section are classified as benzodiazepines (BZDs) and nonbenzodiazepines (non-BZDs). Some psychotropic drugs like trazodone and mirtazapine (see Chapter 22) and some antihistamines (see Chapter 26 and discussed next) are also used as sedative-hypnotics.

Antihistamines, for example diphenhydramine (Benadryl, Nytol, Sominex) and doxylamine (Unisom), have an extended half-life, remaining in the system longer. Because of slower metabolism and impaired circulation, the older or debilitated patient is particularly susceptible to *side effects*, such as blurred vision, dizziness, hypotension, confusion, and decreased coordination. These effects can continue for a longer time, resulting in "morning-after" problems. Tolerance can develop to sleep-inducing effect but not side effects. Therefore, antihistamines are not as effective as other available sedative-hypnotics.

None of these medications should be used for extended periods of time (>10 days) except under close medical supervision because of the potential for psychological and physical dependence. In addition, these medications depress the REM (rapid eye movement, or dream) phase of sleep, and withdrawal after prolonged use can result in a severe rebound effect with nightmares and hallucinations. Abrupt withdrawal of hypnotics, even after short-term therapy, for example one week, may result in rebound insomnia. Therefore, gradual reduction of dosage is indicated.

Before starting pharmacological treatment, patients should be encouraged to use nondrug interventions to combat insomnia. These include exercise during the day; avoiding daytime naps; avoiding heavy meals and activating medications near bedtime; and warm milk, back rubs, soft music, relaxation techniques, and other calming influences. In addition, avoidance of caffeine and alcohol should be stressed. Alcohol may help to initiate sleep but results in early awakening.

Barbiturates are rarely used now as sedative-hypnotics because of the many serious, potentially dangerous *side effects*, especially *CNS depression*. Phenobarbital is still used in the treatment of seizure disorders (see Chapter 22). However, there are many other safer and more effective hypnotics available. Therefore, the use of barbiturates for sedation is restricted to specific, limited circumstances in which the patient can be closely monitored (i.e., Brevital for general anesthesia induction and maintenance).

Benzodiazepines (BZDs) like temazepam (Restoril) and nonbenzodiazepines (non-BZDs) like zolpidem (Ambien) have supplanted barbiturates as sedative-hypnotics and have less potential for abuse. However, withdrawal effects are observed after long-term use, and *respiratory depression* (when taken with alcohol) can be potentially fatal. As mentioned earlier, the cause of insomnia should be established and underlying factors should be treated before a hypnotic is prescribed. Only short-term use (7–10 days) is recommended for most agents. Like BZDs, non-BZDs are classified as controlled substances because of the possibility of physical and psychological dependence.

Side effects of all the sedative-hypnotics can include:

- ❗ Daytime sedation, confusion, and headache—hangover
- ❗ Increased risk of falls (especially in older adults or with long-acting hypnotics)
- ❗ Dependence or withdrawal symptoms
- ❗ Amnesia, hallucinations, and bizarre behavior (may occur more often with triazolam [Halcion] than with other benzodiazepines)
- Metallic aftertaste with Lunesta
- ❗ Sleepwalking and engaging in complex tasks (i.e., "sleep eating," "sleep driving," and "sleep-sex")

Precautions or contraindications for all the sedative-hypnotics apply to:

- Hypersensitivity
- Severe liver impairment
- Coadministration of azole antifungals or protease inhibitors with triazolam
- Severe renal impairment
- Porphyria (with BZDs)
- Abrupt discontinuation
- Older adults
- Debilitated patients
- Addiction-prone patients
- Renal impairment
- Liver impairment
- Depressed and mentally unstable people
- Individuals who have suicidal ideation or behavior
- Pregnancy and lactation
- Children
- COPD and sleep apnea

Interactions of all the sedative-hypnotics with the following drugs can be dangerous and potentially fatal:

- Psychotropic drugs
- Alcohol
- Muscle relaxants
- Antiemetics
- Antihistamines
- Analgesics

Melatonin Receptor Agonist

Ramelteon (Rozerem) is the first FDA-approved prescription medication that acts on melatonin receptors, mimicking the actions of melatonin to trigger sleep onset. As a result of this mechanism of action, dependence and abuse potential are eliminated, and ramelteon is not classified as a controlled substance.

Ramelteon works quickly, generally inducing sleep in less than 1h (give within 30 min of going to bed with a high-fat meal or snack). There have been no studies comparing the effectiveness of ramelteon against other hypnotics or even against melatonin supplements (see Table 11-3 for information regarding melatonin). Dose reductions are not required in older adults; however, ramelteon should be used with caution in patients with hepatic impairment.

The use of ramelteon is contraindicated with fluvoxamine (Luvox), which inhibits the metabolism of ramelteon. Do not use ramelteon with melatonin because of the potential for additive sedative effects.

See Table 19-5 for a summary of the sedatives and hypnotics.

TABLE 19-5 Sedatives and Hypnotics (Use Hypnotics Short-Term Only)

GENERIC NAME	TRADE NAME	DOSAGE	COMMENTS
Benzodiazepines			
temazepam	Restoril	7.5–30 mg PO at bedtime	Intermediate onset, duration
triazolam	Halcion	0.125–0.25 mg PO at bedtime	Can cause amnesia, hallucinations, bizarre behavior, rapid onset, and short duration
Nonbenzodiazepines			
eszopiclone	Lunesta	PO 1–3 mg at bedtime	Rapid onset; not limited to short-term use
zolpidem	Ambien[a]	5–10 mg PO at bedtime	Rapid induction 30 min; short half-life (less than 3h); CR not limited to short-term use
	Ambien CR[a]	PO 6.25–12.5 mg at bedtime	
	Intermezzo	SL 1.75 or 3.5 mg one per night	For middle-of-the-night awakening with 4h left before planned wake time
zaleplon	Sonata	PO 5–10 mg at bedtime	Rapid onset, very short half-life
Melatonin receptor agonist			
ramelteon	Rozerem	PO 5–10 mg within 30 min of bedtime	Not limited to short-term use; not a controlled substance

Note: [a]Recent FDA warning suggests limiting dose in females to 5 mg regular release and 6.25 mg controlled release because of prolonged levels in blood and slower elimination than males.

Other Benzodiazepines will be discussed in Chapter 20, the ones included in this chart are specifically indicated for sleep.

MEDICAL MARIJUANA (CANNABIS)

Medical marijuana refers to the legal prescribed use of cannabis or its synthetic derivatives (cannabinoids) to treat a disease with symptoms of chronic pain, nausea, and severe decreased appetite. This type of treatment has not yet been well tested and is subject to the laws and regulations of each state where there is much variation. Medical marijuana treatments are considered as a treatment option most commonly in end of life situations where palliative care is a priority, or in severe diseases like cancer and HIV/AIDs. It is administered in various methods such as liquid tinctures, inhalation, and capsules by mouth (dronabinol) among others. Side effects include dizziness, feeling tired, increased appetite, and hallucinations. As a health care professional you will not be required to be fully knowledgeable on this topic but should be aware that this is a possible treatment option for some patients.

PATIENT EDUCATION

Patients taking analgesics, sedatives, or hypnotics should be instructed regarding:

Potential for physical and psychological dependence and tolerance with opioids, sedatives, and hypnotics

Taking only limited doses for short periods of time, *except* to relieve pain in terminal illness (in terminal cases, analgesics should be given on a regular basis around the clock to prevent or control pain)

Caution with interactions; *not* taking any medications (except under close medical supervision) that potentiate CNS depression (e.g., psychotropics, *alcohol*, muscle relaxants, antihistamines, antiemetics, cardiac medications, and antihypertensives)

Serious potential side effects with prolonged use or overdose of opioids, sedatives, and hypnotics (e.g., oversedation, dizziness, headache, confusion, agitation, nausea, constipation, urinary retention, and *potentially fatal* respiratory depression, bradycardia, or hypotension)

Tolerance with prolonged use, with increasingly larger doses required to achieve the same effect

Potential for overdose of sedatives or hypnotics and **paradoxical** reactions with older adults (e.g., confusion, agitation, hallucinations, and hyperexcitability)

Withdrawal after prolonged use of sedatives and hypnotics, possibly leading to rebound effects with nightmares, hallucinations, or insomnia

Mental alertness and physical coordination impairment, causing accidents or falls

Caution regarding OTC analgesic and sleep aid combinations and checking ingredients on the label; being aware of possible side effects with those containing aspirin (e.g., gastric distress or bleeding)

Not discontinuing abruptly

Proper storage and disposal of these medications

The website www.pain-topics.org is a very good noncommercial resource for health care professionals and their patients, providing open access to clinical news, information, research, and education for evidence-based pain-management practices.

CASE STUDY A

Analgesics

Seventy-two-year-old Maureen O'Malley is in the recovery room after just having undergone a right total hip replacement for severe arthritis.

1. The recovery room nurse will administer which category of medication *first* to relieve Maureen's pain?
   a. Hypnotic
   b. Sedative
   c. Analgesic
   d. Anti-inflammatory

2. After administering an opioid analgesic, the nurse should observe Maureen for which side effect?
   a. Constipation
   b. Respiratory depression
   c. Abdominal pain
   d. Hypoglycemia

3. The best method to assess Maureen's response to the analgesic is to observe:
   a. Her facial expression
   b. Her respiratory rate
   c. The rating of her pain on a pain scale
   d. The ability to open her eyes

4. While reviewing Maureen's medication orders, the nurse keeps in mind that which additional drug can cause potentiation of the opioid?
   a. Anti-inflammatory
   b. Stool softener
   c. Gastric ulcer medication
   d. Muscle relaxant

5. The nurse administering an opioid to Maureen will use extreme caution if she has a history of:
   a. Arthritis
   b. Allergy to penicillin
   c. COPD
   d. Cataracts

CASE STUDY B

Hypnotics

Sanjay Rudip has been experiencing insomnia for the past six weeks. At his annual physical, Sanjay reports to his physician that he saw a commercial for Lunesta (eszopiclone) and wants to know if this medication is right for him.

1. The physician explains to Sanjay that hypnotic medications should not be used for extended amounts of time except under close medical supervision. What is the primary reason for this?
   a. Loss of functioning due to an inability to stay awake during the day
   b. An increase in REM sleep as a withdrawal symptom
   c. Risk of cardiac arrest
   d. Physical and psychological dependence

2. Eszopiclone falls into which category of sedatives or hypnotics?
   a. Nonbenzodiazepine
   b. Benzodiazepine
   c. Melatonic receptor agonist
   d. Antihistamine

3. The physician discusses possible interactions of other drugs and hypnotic medications with Sanjay. Which category of drug may potentiate CNS depression when taken in conjunction with a hypnotic and should therefore be avoided?
   a. Anti-infective
   b. Antihistamine
   c. Anticoagulant
   d. Glaucoma

4. The physician warns Sanjay that when taking a hypnotic, he may develop tolerance. What does this mean?
   a. The body will release its own analgesia.
   b. A larger dose will be required over time to achieve the same effect.
   c. Sanjay will experience a lower pain threshold in the future.
   d. Relief from pain will be as a result of a suggestion without the actual administration of a medication.

5. A side effect of prolonged use of a hypnotic is
   a. Dizziness
   b. Tachycardia
   c. Urinary incontinence
   d. Asthma

CHAPTER REVIEW QUIZ

Match the medication in the first column with the classification in the second column. Classifications may be used more than once.

Medication

1. amitripytline
2. Vicodin
3. Imitrex
4. methadone
5. Percodan
6. Duragesic
7. fentanyl
8. codeine
9. Narcan
10. Tegretol

Condition

a. Antitussive
b. Opioid antagonist
c. Opioid analgesic with aspirin
d. Tricyclic antidepressant (adjuvant)
e. Opioid analgesic with acetaminophen
f. Nonopioid analgesic (not controlled)
g. Anticonvulsant (adjuvant analgesic)
h. Synthetic analgesic for acute pain
i. Opioid analgesic and narcotic withdrawal
j. Transdermal analgesic for chronic pain
k. Antimigraine

Choose the correct answer.

11. Which medication is used to treat opiate-induced respiratory depression?
    a. Butorphanol
    b. Naloxone
    c. ethadone
    d. Oxycodone

12. Nonopioid analgesics are commonly obtained by which method?
    a. From a pharmacist
    b. Over the counter
    c. With a prescription
    d. From a mail-order company

13. Salicylates are most commonly used for which properties?
    a. Analgesic or antipyretic
    b. Analgesic only
    c. Anti-inflammatory
    d. Antitussive

14. Which group of medications is used as a coanalgesic in severe or chronic pain?
    a. Opioids
    b. Nonopioids
    c. Hypnotics
    d. Sedatives

15. GI symptoms experienced from taking salicylates can be minimized by taking the medication by which of the following methods?
    a. With a small glass of water
    b. Divided doses
    c. Once-a-day dosing
    d. Enteric-coated pills

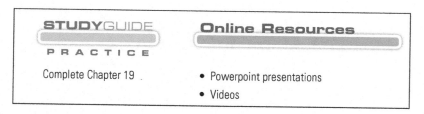

STUDYGUIDE

PRACTICE

Complete Chapter 19

Online Resources

- Powerpoint presentations
- Videos

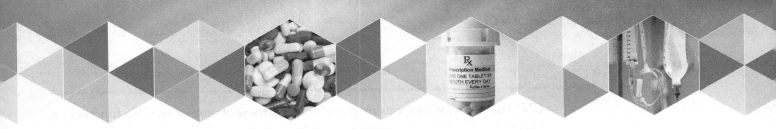

CHAPTER 20

PSYCHOTROPIC MEDICATIONS, ALCOHOL, AND DRUG ABUSE

KEY TERMS AND CONCEPTS

Addiction

Antidepressant

Antipsychotic

Anxiolytics

Ataxia

Atypical antipsychotics

Bipolar disorders

Chemical dependency

Extrapyramidal

Heterocyclic

Monoamine oxidase inhibitors (MAOIs)

Neurotransmitters

Psychotropic

Selective norepinephrine reuptake inhibitors (SNRIs)

Selective serotonin reuptake inhibitors (SSRIs)

Tardive dyskinesia

Tricyclics

OBJECTIVES

Upon completion of this chapter, the learner should be able to

1. Categorize the most commonly used psychotropic medications according to the following classifications: central nervous system (CNS) stimulants for promoting wakefulness and treating attention-deficit hyperactivity disorder (ADHD), antidepressants, antimanic agents for bipolar disorders, anxiolytics, and antipsychotic medications and tranquilizers

2. List the purposes, actions, side effects, interactions, and precautions and contraindications for psychotropic medications in common use

3. Describe the physiological effects of prolonged alcohol use

4. Explain the treatment of acute and chronic alcoholism

5. Compare and contrast drug addiction and habituation

6. Describe the effects of commonly used illegal drugs

7. List the responsibilities of a health care professional in combating drug abuse

8. Define the Key Terms and Concepts

Psychotropic refers to any substance that acts on the mind. Psychotropic medications are drugs that can exert a therapeutic effect on a person's mental processes, emotions, or behavior. Drugs used for other purposes can also have psychotropic effects. Examples of other medications that affect mental functioning are anesthetics, analgesics, sedatives, hypnotics, and antiemetics, which are discussed in other chapters.

Psychotropic medications can be classified according to the purpose of administration. The five classes are central nervous system (CNS) stimulants, antidepressants, anxiolytics, antimanic agents, and antipsychotic medications. Psychotropic medications are frequently prescribed concurrently with psychotherapy or professional counseling.

CNS STIMULANTS

CNS stimulant medications are given for the purpose of promoting CNS functioning. Drugs in this category include caffeine, amphetamine and methylphenidate preparations, and the wakefulness-promoting agents.

Caffeine

Fatigue and drowsiness are part of everyday life for millions of people. The only over-the-counter (OTC) drug proven safe and effective in helping fight fatigue and drowsiness is caffeine (at doses of 100–200 mg not more often than every 3–4 h), found in products like NoDoz and Vivarin. One prescription-only drug in this category, caffeine citrate (Cafcit), has been used in the treatment of neonatal apnea to stimulate the CNS's respiratory drive.

Prolonged, high intake of caffeine in any form may produce tolerance, habituation, and psychological dependence. Physical signs of withdrawal such as headaches, irritation, nervousness, anxiety, and dizziness may occur upon abrupt discontinuation of the stimulant. Excessive consumption of caffeine (especially when taken with alcohol or other drugs) can lead to life-threatening irregular heartbeats, heart attacks, and seizures. A rising number of patients, many of them young students, are being treated in emergency rooms for complications related to the consumption of highly caffeinated energy drinks.

Because caffeine crosses the placenta and is also distributed into the milk of nursing women, most clinicians recommend that those who are pregnant (because of a higher risk of miscarriage) or nursing avoid or limit their consumption of foods, beverages, and drugs containing caffeine, for example OTC analgesics or decongestants. All sources of caffeine should be included when calculating your daily intake.

Amphetamine and Methylphenidate Preparations

Other CNS stimulant drugs include the controlled substances (Schedule II) amphetamine/dextroamphetamine (e.g., Adderall) and methylphenidate (Ritalin), which are used to treat attention-deficit hyperactivity disorder (ADHD) in children over age 6 years and for narcolepsy. Amphetamine and methylphenidate preparations are the first-line therapy for ADHD. Ritalin is also occasionally used in the treatment of senile apathy and major depression refractory to other therapies. For ADHD, it is common practice for a patient to be on more than one stimulant preparation consisting of a long-acting delayed-release form and then an immediate-release formulation around midday.

Daytrana is a transdermal system that contains methylphenidate in a multi-polymeric adhesive matrix (making the drug difficult to extract) that is difficult to reapply once taken off. Vyvanse (lisdexamphetamine) is a prodrug that is converted to dextroamphetamine in the gastrointestinal (GI) tract and used to treat ADHD. Both products have the potential for a lower risk of abuse than other formulations.

The use of amphetamines to reduce appetite in the treatment of obesity is not recommended because tolerance develops rapidly and physical and/or psychological dependence may develop within a few weeks. *These drugs have a high potential for abuse and should be used only under medical supervision for diagnosed medical disorders.* However, when these drugs are used appropriately, as ordered by the physician, abuse potential (including other substances) and dependence appear to be minimal.

Side effects of the controlled CNS stimulants can include:

- ❗ Nervousness, insomnia, irritability, seizures, or psychosis from overdose
- ❗ Tachycardia, palpitations, hypertension, and cardiac arrhythmias
- Dizziness, headache, and blurred vision (dilated pupils with photophobia)
- ❗ GI disturbances, including anorexia, nausea, vomiting, abdominal pain, and dry mouth
- ❗ Habituation and dependence possible with prolonged use

A Food and Drug Administration (FDA) review of reports of serious cardiovascular adverse events in patients taking usual doses of ADHD products revealed reports of sudden death in patients with underlying serious heart problems or defects and reports of stroke and heart attack in adults with certain risk factors. FDA recommends that children, adolescents, or adults who are being considered for treatment with ADHD drug products work with their physician or other health care professionals to develop a treatment plan that includes a careful health history and evaluation of current status, particularly for cardiovascular and psychiatric problems (including an assessment for a family history of such problems).

Precautions or contraindications for the CNS stimulants apply to:

Treatment for obesity (never more than three to six weeks) without diet and exercise modifications (weight gain resumes after discontinuation of the medication)

Anxiety or agitation

History of drug dependence, alcoholism, or eating disorders

Hyperthyroidism

Cardiovascular disorders

Closed-angle glaucoma (not modafinil)

Pregnant or nursing women

Abrupt withdrawal (depression results)

Use with monoamine oxidase inhibitors (MAOIs) (may cause hypertensive crisis)

Caution must be used with sustained-release preparations differing in designations (CD, ER, LA, SR) and their respective dosing requirements (see Table 20-1).

Pediatric precautions: Prolonged administration of CNS stimulants to children with ADHD has been reported to cause at least a temporary suppression of normal weight and/or height patterns in some patients, and therefore close monitoring is required. Growth rebound has been observed after discontinuation, and attainment of normal adult weight and height does not appear to be compromised. CNS stimulants, including amphetamines, have been reported to exacerbate motor and vocal tics and Tourette's disorder, and clinical evaluation for these disorders in children and their families should precede use of the drugs. Children should also be observed carefully for the development of tics while receiving these drugs.

There is some evidence that medication use only during school days may be tried in children with controlled ADHD (in those children whose symptoms precipitate primarily in the school setting), but only if no significant behavior or social difficulties are noted. Once controlled, dosage reduction or interruption ("drug holidays") may be possible during weekends, holidays, or vacations.

Abuse of amphetamines: Signs and symptoms of chronic amphetamine abuse and acute toxicity are discussed later in this chapter in the section entitled "Drug Abuse." Treatment of acute toxicity is also described in that section.

Wakefulness-Promoting Agents

Modafinil (Provigil) and armodafinil (Nuvigil) are psychostimulant medications approved for narcolepsy, sleep apnea, and shift-work sleep disorder (resulting from night shift work) in adults and adolescents (>16 years old). The potential for abuse and dependence appears to be lower than that for the amphetamines and methylphenidate. These medications are effective in treating ADHD in children and adolescents (but not adults) but was not approved by the FDA, for this purpose, because of serious side effects that developed with the doses used in clinical trials. It has also not been demonstrated to promote weight loss.

Side effects of modafinil (Provigil) and armodafinil (Nuvigil) for approved indications are infrequent and include:

Mild headache, dizziness, nausea, and anorexia

Anxiety, insomnia, depression, and mood changes

Hypertension, palpitations, and tachyarrythmia

Cautions for the use of modafinil and armodafinil: Possible causes of fatigue and sleepiness should be determined before stimulant medicines are prescribed to increase wakefulness. Without adequate investigation, some common disorders, such as diabetes and sleep apnea, might go undiagnosed.

Reducing the necessary amount of restorative sleep for prolonged periods of time can result in mental and physical problems, especially neurological and cardio-vascular effects.

PATIENT EDUCATION

Patients receiving the controlled CNS stimulants should be warned regarding (utilize the Patient Medication Guide that is given out each time these products are dispensed):

Potential side effects

Potential for abuse and taking the medications only according to the physician's orders

Taking the medication early in the day to reduce insomnia

The fact that abrupt withdrawal may result in depression, irritability, fatigue, agitation, and disturbed sleep

Watching for signs of tics, gastric disturbance, insomnia, weight loss, or nervousness in children receiving amphetamines and methylphenidate and reporting them to the physician

Potential for dangerous cardiovascular side effects

Not chewing or crushing sustained-release products

For parents and caregivers, the potential for abuse with stimulants and signs of abuse such as running out of the medication early, rapid weight loss, and unusual changes in behavior.

Necessity for regular sleep in sufficient amounts to restore mental and physiological functioning to an optimal level while taking modafinil

SELECTIVE NOREPINEPHRINE REUPTAKE INHIBITOR (SNRI) FOR ADHD

Atomoxetine (Strattera) is a selective norepinephrine reuptake inhibitor (SNRI) and the first *nonstimulant, noncontrolled* drug approved for the treatment of ADHD. Atomoxetine, structurally related to fluoxetine, does not have a potential for abuse, has less insomnia and less effect on growth, and has been shown to be safe and effective in adolescents and children more than 6 years old and adults with ADHD. It has a longer onset to therapeutic benefit and reduced efficacy compared to the stimulants.

Side effects of SNRIs include:

- ! Dry mouth, reduced appetite, and fatigue
- ! Nausea, vomiting, constipation, and dyspepsia

  Urinary hesitation or retention

- ! Increased risk of suicidal tendencies in children and adolescents ("black box" warning)

Precautions or contraindications for SNRIs apply to:

Narrow-angle glaucoma

Cerebrovascular, heart, or hepatic disease

Possible growth disturbance during treatment

Interactions of SNRIs occur with:

Beta-agonists, vasopressor agents, and quinidine

Fluoxetine, paroxetine, venlafaxine, and MAOIs

See Table 20-1 for a summary of the CNS stimulants and nonstimulant medications for ADHD.

TABLE 20-1 Central Nervous System Stimulants and Nonstimulant Medications

GENERIC NAME	TRADE NAME	DOSAGE	COMMENTS
Stimulants			
caffeine citrate	Cafcit	PO 20–25 mg/kg one time and then 5–10 mg/kg per day	For neonatal apnea *Caution:* Do *not* use caffeine and sodium benzoate
amphetamine mixtures (amphetamine salts) (amphetamine/dextroamphetamine)	Adderall	PO 2.5–40 mg daily in one to three divided doses per day (4–6 h apart)	For narcolepsy, ADHD (attention-deficit hyperactivity disorder) (>3 years old)
	Adderall XR	PO 5–60 mg daily	For ADHD (>6 years old)
lisdexamfetamine	Vyvanse	PO 10–70 mg q A.M. (Starting dose is 30mg)	For ADHD (>6 years old)
methylphenidate	Ritalin, Methylin	PO 2.5–20 mg two to three times per day ac	For narcolepsy, ADHD (>6 years old)
	Ritalin SR, Metadate ER	10–60 mg divided doses (Note 8–h duration of action)	ER tabs, for ADHD, senile apathy, refractory depression
	Metadate CD, Ritalin LA	PO 10–60 mg q A.M.	ER (extended-release) caps for once-daily treatment of ADHD
	Concerta	PO 18–72 mg q A.M.	Tablet shell is excreted intact
	Daytrana Patch	10–30 mg daily to hip (Take 2 h before needed effect)	Remove patch after 9h
modafinil armodafinil	Provigil Nuvigil	PO 100–400 mg daily PO 150–250 mg daily	For narcolepsy, sleep apnea, and shift-work sleep disorder (>16 years old)
Nonstimulant			
atomoxetine	Strattera	PO 10–100 mg one to two times per day	Only noncontrolled, nonstimulant for ADHD (>6 years old)

ANTIDEPRESSANTS

Major depressive disorder (MDD) is a mental disorder characterized by an all-encompassing low mood accompanied by low self-esteem and loss of interest or pleasure in normally enjoyable activities. MDD is a significant health problem that affects about 15 million American adults annually. A national survey indicated that more than 16% of Americans will experience MDD in their lifetime.

The exact cause of depression is unknown, but it may result from a chemical imbalance in the brain. Chemicals in the brain, like dopamine, serotonin, and norepinephrine, are known as **neurotransmitters**. Substances that travel across the synapse (contact point of two neurons) transmit messages between nerve cells. If these neurotransmitters are reabsorbed by one nerve ending before they have had a chance to make contact with the next nerve cell, they cannot perform their function.

In depression, there may be a shortage of the neurotransmitters dopamine, serotonin, or norepinephrine.

Antidepressant medications, sometimes called mood elevators, are used primarily to treat patients with various types of depression. The five categories in general use are the tricyclic antidepressants, the **monoamine oxidase inhibitors (MAOIs)**, the **selective serotonin reuptake inhibitors (SSRIs)**, the **selective norepinephrine reuptake inhibitors (SNRIs)**, and the heterocyclic antidepressants. Although symptoms may be relieved in the first month, it is generally advisable to counsel patients to continue antidepressant therapy for six to twelve months or indefinitely to prevent relapse.

The FDA has directed manufacturers of *all* antidepressants to include a "black box" warning that antidepressants increased the risk of suicidal thinking and behavior (particularly during the first few months of therapy) in short-term studies in children and adolescents with manic depressive disorder and other psychiatric disorders. There were no occurrences of suicides in any of these studies. Anyone considering the use of antidepressants in a child, adolescent, or young adult must balance this risk with the clinical need. Patients should be observed closely for behaviors associated with these drugs (e.g., anxiety, agitation, panic attacks, insomnia, irritability, hostility, impulsivity, severe restlessness, hypomania, and mania) and communicate the same with the prescribing health care provider.

Tricyclics

Among the first antidepressants in clinical use, the mechanism of action of the **tricyclics** involves potentiation of norepinephrine and serotonin activity by blocking their reuptake. Their pharmacology also includes strong *anticholinergic* activity that is responsible for many of the side effects seen. Tricyclics may be lethal in overdose (cardiac conduction abnormalities or dysrhythmias).

The tricyclics have delayed action, elevating the mood and increasing alertness after two to four weeks. They are frequently given at bedtime because of a mild sedative effect. They should be used with caution (if at all) in older adults because of the strong sedative and anticholinergic properties of this drug class and the increased risk of falls. Tricyclics may be more effective than SSRIs in some cases of severe depression and are used as an adjunct in neuropathic pain control (see Chapter 19, "Analgesics, Sedatives, and Hypnotics").

Side effects of the tricyclics, such as imipramine (Tofranil), are anticholinergic in action and can include:

- ! Dryness of the mouth
- Increased appetite and weight gain
- ! Drowsiness and dizziness
- Blurred vision
- ! Constipation and urinary retention, especially with benign prostatic hyperplasia (BPH)
- Sexual dysfunction
- ! Postural hypotension, cardiac arrhythmias, and palpitation
- ! Confusion, especially in older adults

Precautions or contraindications for tricyclics apply to:

Cardiac, renal, GI, and liver disorders

Older adults

Glaucoma

Obesity

Seizure disorder

Pregnancy and lactation

Concomitant use with MAOIs

SSRIs (increase tricyclic blood levels)

Interactions of tricyclics occur with:

Certain antiarrhythmics and some quinolones (QT prolongation)

Clonidine (causing hypertensive crisis)

CNS drugs and alcohol

Monoamine Oxidase Inhibitors

The mechanism of antidepressant action of MAOIs involves increasing the concentrations of serotonin, norepinephrine, and dopamine in the neuronal synapse by inhibiting the MAO enzyme that degrades or breaks down these neurotransmitters.

The MAOIs, for example phenelzine (Nardil), are rarely used today because of potential serious side effects and numerous food, herbal, and drug interactions. They cannot be given until two weeks after tricyclics and other interacting drugs have been discontinued. These agents are typically reserved for refractory or atypical depression or those associated with panic disorders or phobias.

Side effects of MAO inhibitors are adrenergic in action and can include:

! Nervousness, agitation, and insomnia

! Headache

Stiff neck

! Hypertension or hypertensive crisis (can be fatal)

! Tachycardia, palpitation, and chest pain

Nausea, vomiting, and diarrhea

Blurred vision

Precautions or contraindications for MAOIs apply to:

Patients with cerebrovascular, heart, liver, and renal diseases

Children under 16 years

Pregnancy and lactation

Abrupt discontinuation

Interactions of the MAOIs with some drugs, foods, and herbal supplements can cause *hypertensive crisis*, manifested by severe headache, palpitation, sweating, chest pain, possible intracranial hemorrhage, and even death. Interactions may occur with:

Adrenergic drugs and levodopa

SSRIs and SNRIs (resulting in seizures, fever, hypertension, and confusion—"serotonin syndrome")

CNS depressants (resulting in circulatory collapse)

Foods containing tryamine, tryptamine, or tryptophan, such as yogurt, sour cream, all cheeses, liver (especially chicken), pickled herring, figs, raisins, bananas, pineapple, avocados, broad beans (Chinese pea pods), meat tenderizers, alcoholic beverages (especially red wine and beer), and all fermented or aged foods (e.g., corned beef, salami, and pepperoni)

Emsam (selegiline) is a selective MAOI (type B) administered as a transdermal patch indicated for the treatment of MDD in adults. Blockade of MAO enzyme reduces the metabolism of dopamine but not that of norepinephrine or serotonin. Transdermal administration allows for lower doses and direct absorption into the bloodstream, reducing the likelihood of a dietary tyramine–induced hypertensive crisis (see Chapter 22, "Anticonvulsants, Antiparkinsonian Drugs, and Agents for Alzheimer's Disease," for interactions and precautions or contraindications).

Selective Serotonin Reuptake Inhibitors

SSRIs are considered to be the first-line medications for the treatment of depression. They are preferred because of fewer side effects, greater safety in cases of overdose, and increased patient compliance.

The antidepressants in this category selectively block the reabsorption of the neurotransmitter serotonin, thus helping to restore the brain's chemical balance. Drugs in this class include fluoxetine (Prozac) and sertraline (Zoloft). Therapy may be required for several months or longer. Symptomatic relief may require one to four weeks, and there is prolonged elimination of the drug. SSRIs do not significantly affect cognition in older adults. Fluoxetine and escitalopram (Lexapro) are the only antidepressants recommended for the treatment of MDD in adolescents (aged 12–17 years), and fluoxetine is also approved for children aged 8 years and older.

Side effects of the SSRIs may include:

Sexual dysfunction

⚠ Nausea and other GI effects (the most common side effects during the first two weeks of therapy, but often transient)

Anorexia and sweating

⚠ Insomnia, anxiety, nervousness, tremor, drowsiness, fatigue, dizziness, and headache

Bleeding (because of impaired platelet aggregation)

Hyponatremia (low sodium levels)

QT prolongation with citalopram (Celexa) doses >40 mg per day that can lead to abnormal heart rhythm, which can be fatal

Caution with SSRIs applies to patients with the following conditions:

Liver or renal impairment

Suicide prone

Diabetes

Bipolar disorders (may precipitate manic attacks)

Underweight

Eating disorders

Pregnancy and lactation

Abrupt discontinuation

Interactions of SSRIs are possible with:

MAOIs (never take concurrently)

Amphetamines, most antidepressants, certain analgesics (fentanyl, tramadol), antiemetics (metoclopramide), antimigraines ("triptans"), antibiotics (linezolid), and OTC products (dextromethorphan, St. John's wort, tryptophan) (can result in serotonin syndrome—a potentially life-threatening reaction to excessive serotonin activity in the CNS.)

Anticoagulants, antiplatelet drugs, NSAIDs, and aspirin (increased risk of bleeding complications)

CLINICAL CONNECTION

Racemic Mixture of Drugs

Many medications are developed as racemic drugs. Racemic drugs consist of the active form of the drug combined with an inactive or a less active form. The inactive form of the drug does not contribute to the desired therapeutic effects but to the side effects associated with the medication. This becomes a problem at higher doses sometimes forcing the patient to discontinue the medication. To combat this side-effect problem, many drugs have been reformulated as purer forms containing only the active form of the drug or a greater percentage of the active form. This allows for prescribers to increase the dose without the severity of side effects. One example of this is the SSRI escitalopram (Lexapro), which is a purer form of the older drug citalopram (Celexa). Escitalopram contains only the active form of the drug, whereas citalopram (a racemic drug) contains a 50:50 mixture. In other words, 20 mg of escitalopram will give the same therapeutic benefits as 40 mg of citalopram, but with potentially less side effects. This strategy is used in other medications as well, but it should be noted that although this method is advantageous to therapy, it is more expensive to develop and produce the purer forms of drugs, which can sometimes limit availability to patients.

Selective Norepinephrine Reuptake Inhibitors

Duloxetine (Cymbalta) and venlafaxine (Effexor) are antidepressants that inhibit the reuptake of both serotonin and norepinephrine. They are also effective in patients with chronic pain (neuropathic pain, fibromyalgia, and musculoskeletal pain). Refer to Chapter 19 for details on these two agents.

Desvenlafaxine (Pristiq), also an SNRI, is the major metabolite of venlafaxine and is pharmacologically equiactive and equipotent to its parent compound. It is indicated for the treatment of MDD. The drug-related problems, warnings, and precautions associated with the use of desvenlafaxine are generally similar to those of other SNRIs.

Heterocyclic Antidepressants

The second-generation heterocyclic antidepressants are comparable in efficacy to the first-generation tricyclic antidepressants but have differing effects on dopamine, norepinephrine, and serotonin and distinctly different adverse effect profiles. Buproprion (Wellbutrin) is considered an *activating antidepressant* (like most SSRIs) and can be useful in cases of severe depression characterized by extreme fatigue, lethargy, and psychomotor retardation. It is also useful in helping to reduce relapse rates in persons who are quitting smoking (see Zyban in Chapter 26) and those patients who experience sexual dysfunction with other antidepressants. Buproprion has a risk of seizures, which increases with higher doses.

Mirtazapine (Remeron) is a *calming antidepressant* that can be useful in treating agitated depression, mixed anxiety and depression, and fibromyalgia. A common side effect of mitrazapine is weight gain, which can be helpful in patients with a poor appetite. Trazodone is highly sedating and is used in low doses as a hypnotic. It can be useful in higher doses in older adult patients for treating agitation secondary to dementia and treating activation side effects caused by the SSRIs.

Side effects of heterocyclic antidepressants can include:

- ❗ Drowsiness—common (except bupropion)
- ❗ Insomnia, restlessness, agitation, and anxiety (with bupropion)
- ❗ Dry mouth, nausea, dizziness, and confusion
- Priapism or impotence (trazodone; discontinue the drug)
- ❗ Weight gain (mirtazapine, trazodone)

Interactions of heterocyclics occur with:

Other CNS depressants, including alcohol, may potentiate sedation (mirtazapine, trazodone) or increase the risk of seizures (bupropion)

MAOIs (never take concurrently)

Food may decrease incidence of light-headedness

Caution with heterocyclics applies to:

Patients who are suicide prone

Patients with anorexia and bulimia (buproprion)

Seizure disorder

Cardiac or liver disorders

See Table 20-2 for a summary of the antidepressant agents.

TABLE 20-2 **Antidepressants**

GENERIC NAME	TRADE NAME	DOSAGE	COMMENTS
Tricyclics			
amitriptyline	(Elavil)[a]	PO 10–300 mg daily	All of these drugs interact with CNS drugs. Give at bedtime
desipramine	Norpramin	PO 100–200 mg HS or Q12H	Less sedation, anticholinergic S.E., and orthostatic hypotension
doxepin	(Sinequan)[a]	PO 50–300 mg daily	Also used topically for eczema (Prudoxin)
imipramine	Tofranil	PO 75–300 mg daily	Also effective for enuresis
nortriptyline	Pamelor	PO 25–150 mg daily	Older adults and adolescent patients need lower dose
MAOIs			
isocarboxazid	Marplan	PO 20–60 mg daily in divided doses	All of these drugs interact with many foods and other drugs, resulting in serious reactions
GENERIC NAME	TRADE NAME	DOSAGE	COMMENTS
phenelzine	Nardil	PO 45–90 mg daily in divided doses	
tranylcypromine	Parnate	PO 60 mg daily in divided doses	
SSRIs			
citalopram	Celexa	PO 10–40 mg daily	Doses >40 mg associated with QT prolongation
escitalopram	Lexapro	PO 5–20 mg daily	May be better tolerated than Celexa
fluoxetine	Prozac	PO 10–80 mg daily	Delayed response, long half-life; take in A.M.
paroxetine	Paxil	PO 10–60 mg daily	Older adults 1/2 dose; take in A.M.
	Paxil CR	PO 12.5–62.5 mg daily	Do not give with antacids
sertraline	Zoloft	PO 25–200 mg daily	Take in A.M.
SNRIs			
desvenlafaxine	Pristiq	PO 50–400 mg daily	Do not chew or crush
duloxetine	Cymbalta	PO 20–60 mg daily	Also used for neuropathy
venlafaxine	(Effexor)[a]	PO 75–375 mg divided doses	Take PC to lessen nausea
	Effexor-XR	PO 37.5–225 mg daily	Do not chew or crush; swallow whole
Heterocyclics			
bupropion	Wellbutrin	PO 100–150 mg two to three times per day	Take early in the day; space doses at least 6h apart to minimize seizure risk
	Wellbutrin SR	PO 150–200 mg daily–two times per day	Space doses at least 8h apart
	Wellbutrin XL	PO 150–400 mg	Give once daily in the A.M.

(continued)

TABLE 20-2   **Antidepressants (*continued*)**

GENERIC NAME	TRADE NAME	DOSAGE	COMMENTS
mirtazapine	Remeron	PO 15–45 mg daily	Take at bedtime; sedation is common
trazodone	Desyrel	PO 25–300 mg at bedtime for insomnia	Take pc to decrease dizziness and nausea; if drowsiness occurs, may give large portion of dose at bedtime
		PO 150–600 mg in divided doses for depression	

a. This brand name is no longer marketed, but the name is still commonly used.

ANTIMANIC AGENTS

Bipolar disorder, sometimes called manic depression, is a mental illness that is characterized by severe fluctuations in mood extremes (see Figure 20-1). Patients may experience high (mania) and low (depression) mood swings with a diminished capacity for daily functioning. The cause of bipolar disorder is most likely an imbalance in brain chemicals that affect mood. Without treatment, bipolar disorder is a debilitating condition that will not improve on its own.

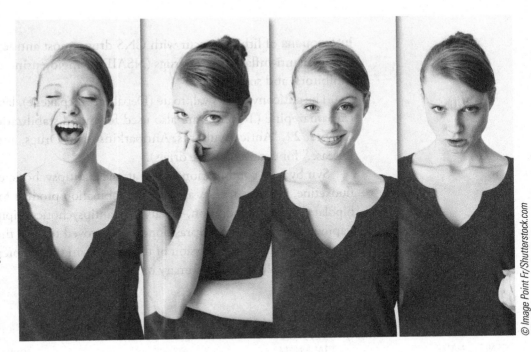

FIGURE 20-1 Bipolar disorder is often described as not being able to "settle" on one mood, often times going from extremely happy to upset or depressed and back again frequently and rapidly.

© Image Point Fr/Shutterstock.com

Lithium

Lithium salts are approved for the treatment of mania and the treatment and prophylaxis of bipolar disorder. They prevent more manic episodes compared with depressive episodes. Lithium is the only mood stabilizer that has lowered the suicide rate in bipolar patients. A maintenance dose is established by monitoring blood levels. Serum levels are checked seven days after starting or changing the lithium dose and every 6–12 months once a stable dose is established to maintain a level of 0.8–1.2 mEq/mL. Patients must be monitored and alerted for signs of toxicity.

Side effects of lithium can include:

- ❗ GI distress (usual initially and resolves—take medicine with meals)
- ❗ Cardiac arrhythmias and hypotension
- Thirst and polyuria (dehydration may cause acute toxicity)
- Weight gain
- ❗ Tremors (can be treated with propranolol)
- Thyroid problems—hypothyroidism, goiter

Signs of lithium toxicity can include:

- ❗ Drowsiness, confusion, blurred vision, and photophobia
- ❗ Tremors, muscle weakness, seizures, coma, and cardiovascular collapse

Caution with lithium when given to patients with the following conditions:

- Seizure disorders and parkinsonism
- Cardiovascular and kidney disorders
- Older adults and debilitated patients
- Thyroid disease

Interactions of lithium occur with CNS drugs, most antidepressants, diuretics, nonsteroidal anti-inflammatory drugs (NSAIDs), angiotensin-converting enzyme (ACE) inhibitors, and sodium salts.

The anticonvulsants valproate (Depakote, Depakene), lamotrigine (Lamictal), and carbamazepine (Tegretol) are also used for mood stabilization in bipolar illness (see Chapter 22, "Anticonvulsants, Antiparkinsonian Drugs, and Agents for Alzheimer's Disease," for details on these drugs).

Symbyax, a combination of the atypical antipsychotic olanzapine and the SSRI fluoxetine, is the first FDA-approved combination product for the depressive phase of bipolar disorder. In addition, the atypical antipsychotics aripiprazole, olanzapine, quetiapine, risperidone, and ziprasidone are approved to treat the manic phase of bipolar disorder. Refer to the discussion of these agents in this chapter for further details.

See Table 20-3 for a summary of antimanic agents.

TABLE 20-3 **Antimanic Agents**

GENERIC NAME	TRADE NAME	DOSAGE	COMMENTS
lithium	Lithobid	900–1,800 mg divided doses	0.8–1.2 mEq/mL (desired serum level)
carbamazepine	Tegretol, Tegretol XR	PO 600–1,600 mg in divided doses	4–12 mcg/mL (desired serum level)
lamotrigine	Lamictal	Titrate up to PO 200 mg daily	May be more effective than lithium for preventing depressive episodes

(continued)

TABLE 20-3   Antimanic Agents (*continued*)

GENERIC NAME	TRADE NAME	DOSAGE	COMMENTS
valproate	Depakote DR,	PO 750–2,500 mg per day (divided doses)	50–125 mcg/mL (desired serum level)
	Depakene		IR capsule, liquid
	Depakote ER	PO 250–1,000 mg per day	For migraine prophylaxis
olanzapine/fluoxetine	Symbyax	PO q p.m. (various strengths)	For bipolar depression

ANXIOLYTICS

Anxiety disorders are present in over 13% of individuals in the United States. Anxiety is the body's natural response to real or perceived danger. This natural response becomes a disorder when it is excessive and difficult to control and when it leads to significant distress and impairment. Types of anxiety disorders include social anxiety, post-traumatic stress disorder, panic attacks, and obsessive compulsive behavior.

Benzodiazepines

Benzodiazepines (BDZs) are sometimes referred to as anxiolytics or minor tranquilizers. They are useful for the short-term treatment of (1) anxiety disorders, (2) some psychosomatic disorders and insomnia, and (3) alcohol withdrawal. BDZs, such as diazepam (Valium), are also used as muscle relaxants, as anticonvulsants, in preprocedure testing, or preoperatively for sedation induction. Clonazepam (Klonopin), used primarily in the management of seizures (see Chapter 22), is also used in the treatment of panic disorder.

Anxiolytic BDZs, when given in small doses, can reduce anxiety and promote relaxation without causing sedation. Larger doses are sometimes prescribed at bedtime for their sedative effect. The role of BDZs in treating anxiety disorders is providing acute relief of anxiety symptoms while waiting for long-term treatment (e.g., SSRI or SNRI antidepressants) to take effect. BDZs do not treat the underlying cause of anxiety (abnormality of neurotransmitters) but rather only mask the symptoms.

Minor tranquilizers should not be taken for prolonged periods of time because *tolerance and physical and psychological dependence may develop*. Alprazolam (Xanax) is one of the most abused BDZs because of its quick onset of action, which leads to euphoria. All BDZs are classified as Schedule IV controlled substances. *Sudden withdrawal (missed doses/discontinuation) after prolonged use may result in seizures, agitation, psychosis, insomnia, and gastric distress.*

BDZs with a long half-life, such as clorazepate (Tranxene) and diazepam, should be avoided in older adults. Oxazepam (Serax), temazepam (Restoril) and lorazepam (Ativan) have medium to short half-lives and inactive metabolites and are less prone to accumulation in older adult patients or those with liver disease.

Side effects of the BDZs may include:

! Depression, hallucinations, confusion, agitation, bizarre behavior, and amnesia

! Drowsiness, lethargy, and headache

! **Ataxia** and tremor

! Increased risk of falls in older patients by ~50%

  Rash and itching

! Sensitivity to sunlight

Precautions or contraindications for BDZs apply to:

Mental depression

Suicidal tendencies; history of substance abuse

Depressed vital signs

Pulmonary disease and respiratory depression

Pregnancy and lactation

Children

Liver and kidney dysfunction

Older adults and debilitated patients (paradoxical reactions) and prolonged elimination time

Persons operating machinery

Interactions of BDZs with potentiation of effect may occur with:

CNS depressants (e.g., analgesics, anesthetics, sedative hypnotics, other muscle relaxants, antihistamines, and alcohol); NOTE: potentially lethal overdose when BDZs are mixed with alcohol or opioids

Antiretroviral protease inhibitors, macrolides (erythromycin), azole antifungals (ketoconazole, itraconazole), oral contraceptives, and calcium channel blockers (diltiazem, verapamil) all reduce the elimination of most BDZs, leading to increased and excessive sedation or impaired psychomotor function

Phenytoin (potentiation of phenytoin by raising serum concentration)

Grapefruit juice can potentiate the effects of orally administered alprazolam, midazolam, and diazepam, and should not be taken concurrently.

Midazolam (Versed) is a potent BDZ. It is used preoperatively to relieve anxiety and provide sedation, light anesthesia, and amnesia of operative events. Because of its more rapid onset of sedative effects and more pronounced amnesic effects during the first hour following administration, it is considered the drug of choice for short surgical procedures. Midazolam is usually administered IV, and the duration of amnesia is about 1h. It has also been used orally for preoperative sedation and to relieve anxiety with good results.

Midazolam may be used alone or in combination with an opioid such as fentanyl for painful procedures (e.g., endoscopy and cardiac catheterization with or without intervention). Midazolam is also used IV for the induction of general anesthesia, along with an opioid. This potent sedative requires individualized dosage with adjustment for age, weight, clinical condition, and procedure.

Side effects of midazolam can include:

! *Depressed respiration* with large doses, especially in older adults and those with COPD (chronic obstructive pulmonary disease)

> Paradoxical reactions (agitation or involuntary movements) occur occasionally
>
> Nausea and vomiting occasionally

Cautions with midazolam:

> Watch for apnea, hypoxia, and/or cardiac arrest
>
> Respiratory status should be monitored continuously during parenteral use
>
> Facilities and equipment for respiratory and cardiovascular support should be readily available; vital signs should be monitored carefully for changes in blood pressure or decrease in heart rate
>
> Patients with electrolyte imbalance, renal impairment, and congestive heart failure and children are at increased risk of complications

Contraindicated in pregnancy and those with acute narrow-angle glaucoma

Interactions of midazolam, which can potentiate the possibility of respiratory depression, occur with:

> Cimetidine (Tagamet) and ranitidine (Zantac)
>
> Same medications listed under BDZs

Other Anxiolytics

Other anxiolytics, not related to the BDZs, include buspirone (Buspar) and hydroxyzine (Vistaril). Unlike the BDZs, buspirone has no anticonvulsant or muscle relaxant activity, does not substantially impair psychomotor function, and has little sedative effect. It is indicated for the treatment of generalized anxiety disorder but not other anxiety disorders; it does not have activity against depression. Limited evidence suggests that buspirone may be more effective for cognitive and interpersonal problems, including anger and hostility associated with anxiety, whereas the BDZs may be more effective for somatic symptoms of anxiety.

Buspirone has a slower onset of action than most anxiolytics (two to four weeks for optimum effect). Therefore, it is ineffective on a PRN basis. It has little potential for tolerance or dependence and has been used without unusual adverse effects or decreased efficiency for as long as a year.

Side effects of buspirone (fewer and less severe) may include:

> Dizziness, drowsiness, and headache
>
> GI effects (e.g., nausea)

Caution with buspirone applies to renal and hepatic impairment.

Another short-term anxiolytic, chemically different from the BDZs, is hydroxyzine (Vistaril). It is an antihistamine (H_1-blocker) structurally related to meclizine (Antivert). Hydroxyzine is also used IM as a pre- and postoperative antiemetic and sedative.

Side effects of hydroxyzine, generally anticholinergic in nature, may include:

⚠ Drowsiness, ataxia, and dizziness

Urinary retention and mydriasis

Caution with hydroxyzine applies to:

GI, hepatic, respiratory, and urinary disorders

Closed-angle glaucoma

Older adults

Pregnancy (especially first trimester)

See Table 20-4 for a summary of antianxiety medications.

TABLE 20-4 Antianxiety Medications (Anxiolytics)

GENERIC NAME	TRADE NAME	DOSAGE	COMMENTS
Benzodiazepines (short-term use only)			
alprazolam	Xanax	PO 0.125–0.5 mg BID–TID	Abrupt withdrawal may cause severe side effects; one of the most abused BDZs
	Xanax XR	PO 0.5–6 mg q A.M.	For panic disorder
chlordiazepoxide	(Librium)[a]	PO 5–25 mg TID or four times per day	Larger doses needed for ethanol withdrawal
clorazepate	Tranxene	PO 7.5–60 mg daily in divided doses	If used in older adult patients no more than 15 mg daily
clonazepam	Klonopin	0.5–2mg daily or in divided doses	
diazepam	Valium	PO 2–10 mg TID, IV	Do not mix in syringe with other medications; also used as a muscle relaxant or IV in status epilepticus;
	Diastat	R 0.2 mg/kg	R for refractory seizures
lorazepam	Ativan	PO, IM, or IV 2–3 mg daily in divided doses	For older adults who are agitated
midazolam	(Versed)[a]	PO, IM, or IV dose varies with usage	Used preoperatively for short-term procedures
oxazepam	(Serax)[a]	PO 10–15 mg TID or four times per day	For older adults who are agitated
Other anxiolytics			
buspirone	Buspar	PO 15–60 mg daily in divided doses	Slow onset of action; may be used long term. Available in scored breakable tablets that can be broken for divided doses
hydroxyzine	Vistaril	PO 25–100 mg four times per day or 25–100 mg deep IM	Also used as an antiemetic and antipruritic or preoperatively

a. This brand name is no longer marketed, but the name is still commonly used.

ANTIPSYCHOTIC MEDICATIONS/MAJOR TRANQUILIZERS

Antipsychotic medications, or major tranquilizers, are sometimes called neuroleptics and consist of the traditional or *typical* (first-generation) and the newer or *atypical* (second-generation) agents. They are useful in two major areas:

- Relieving symptoms of psychoses, including delusion, hallucinations, agitation, and combativeness
- Relieving nausea and vomiting, for example prochlorperazine (Compazine) (see Chapter 16)

Most of the typical antipsychotics in use today are classified chemically as phenothiazines; for example, chlorpromazine (Thorazine) or butyrophenone derivatives such as haloperidol (Haldol). Dosage can be regulated to modify disturbed behavior and relieve severe anxiety in many cases without profound impairment of consciousness. These agents work primarily by blocking dopamine receptors, which accounts for their antiemetic effects but results in unbalanced cholinergic activity, which causes frequent extrapyramidal side effects (EPS) to include tardive dyskinesia (TD). The extrapyramidal system controls equilibrium and muscle tone, so EPS can include the muscle rigidity; tremors; difficulty walking; and involuntary, repetitive, and purposeless body movements called tardive dyskinesia. Despite their side effects, typical antipsychotics are still commonly used in the acute hospital setting because they are the only medications in this class available for IV administration.

The other class of antipsychotics, the atypical antipsychotics, for example risperidone, are chemically different from the phenothiazines, blocking both serotonin and transiently blocking dopamine receptors. This mechanism results in less potential for adverse effects, especially EPS and TD. The direct antagonism at the serotonin receptor (or the histamine-1 receptor), however, may account for the weight gain and other metabolic abnormalities seen with the atypical agents.

Although helpful in treating behavioral and psychological symptoms of dementia, typical or atypical antipsychotic drugs are *not* FDA-approved (black box warning) for the treatment of geriatric patients with dementia-related psychosis. Cerebrovascular adverse events (strokes, transient ischemic attacks, and cerebrovascular accidents), including fatalities (because of heart failure, sudden death, and infections), have been reported in older adults with dementia-related psychosis (Alzheimer's, vascular and mixed) being treated with antipsychotics.

Because there is no FDA-approved medication for the treatment of dementia-related psychosis, other management options (ruling out other causes, behavioral or environmental modifications, recreational activities, etc.) should be considered by health care providers. If antipsychotics must be utilized for dementia-related behaviors, they should be used at the lowest effective dose for the shortest duration necessary with appropriate documentation and justification of need.

Side effects of typical antipsychotics differ based upon the potency of the agent. Low-potency agents including chlorpromazine and thioridazine are more likely to produce sedation, hypotension, and anticholinergic effects. The remaining typical high-potency agents, including haloperidol, fluphenazine, and trifluoperazine, are more likely to produce EPS.

Side effects of all antipsychotics may include:
Postural hypotension, tachycardia, bradycardia, and vertigo

- ⚠ Anticholinergic effects (see Chapter 13 "Autonomic Nervous System Drugs"): dry mouth, constipation, urinary retention, blurred vision, fever, confusion, restlessness, agitation, and headache

- Jaundice, rash, photosensitivity, or hypersensitivity reactions

- Prolactin elevation with the typicals

- Agranulocytosis with clozapine (can be fatal)

- Metabolic effects (increased risk of hyperglycemia, insulin resistance, diabetes, weight gain, and elevated cholesterol) with the atypicals

Extrapyramidal side effects, severe CNS adverse effects, include:

- ⚠ Parkinsonian symptoms, for example tremors, drooling, dysphagia (more common in older adults)

- TD (involuntary and maybe irreversible, abnormal orofacial movements such as tics—more common in older adults, especially females)

- Dystonic reactions (spasms or abnormal muscle tone of the head, neck, or tongue—more frequent in children)

- Akathisia (uncontrollable motor restlessness—more common in children)

Treatment of parkinsonian symptoms includes concomitant administration of an anticholinergic antiparkinsonian agent, for example Artane or Cogentin (see Chapter 22). *Prophylactic administration of these drugs will not prevent extrapyramidal symptoms. These drugs will not alleviate symptoms of TD and can make them worse.* Dystonic reactions usually appear early in the therapy and usually subside rapidly when the antipsychotic drug is discontinued. Trihexyphenidyl (Artane), benztropine (Cogentin), or diphenhydramine (Benadryl) are used to treat dystonic reactions.

Precautions or contraindications for antipsychotics apply to:
Seizure disorders
Parkinsonian syndrome
Cerebrovascular disease
Severe depression
Pregnancy
Blood dyscrasias
Older adults and children
Hepatic, cardiovascular, and renal diseases
Prostatic hyperplasia and diabetes

Note
Tardive dyskinesia may become permanent and irreversible, and no treatment has been shown to be uniformly effective. Therefore, the best treatment is prevention. Patients receiving antipsychotic medication should be assessed for TD at the start of treatment and at least every six months with the Abnormal Involuntary Movement Scale (AIMS) (see Figures 20-2 and 20-3) or Dyskinesia Identification System: Condensed User Scale (DISCUS) available from www.med-pass.com and other websites. Dosage should not be terminated abruptly in those receiving high doses for prolonged periods of time.

INSTRUCTIONS: Complete Examination Procedure (reverse side) before making ratings.

Code: 0 = None, 1 = Minimal, may be extreme normal, 2 = Mild, 3 = Moderate, 4 = Severe

		(CIRCLE ONE)
FACIAL AND ORAL MOVEMENTS:	**1. Muscles of Facial Expression** e.g., movements of forehead, eyebrows, periorbital area, cheeks; include frowning, blinking, smiling, grimacing	0 1 2 3 4
	2. Lips and Perioral Areas e.g., puckering, pouting, smacking	0 1 2 3 4
	3. Jaw e.g., biting, clenching, mouth opening, lateral movement	0 1 2 3 4
	4. Tongue Rate only increase in movement both in and out of mouth, NOT inability to sustain movement	0 1 2 3 4
EXTREMITY MOVEMENTS:	**5. Upper (arms, wrists, hands, fingers)** Include choreic movements (i.e., rapid, objectively purposeless, irregular, spontaneous), athetoid movements (i.e., slow, irregular, complex, serpentine). Do NOT include tremor (i.e., repetitive, regular, rhythmic)	0 1 2 3 4
	6. Lower (legs, knees, ankles, toes) e.g., lateral knee movement, foot tapping, heel dropping, foot squirming, inversion and eversion of foot	0 1 2 3 4
TRUNK MOVEMENTS:	**7. Neck, shoulder, hips** e.g., rocking, twisting, squirming, pelvic gyrations	0 1 2 3 4
GLOBAL JUDGEMENTS:	**8. Severity of abnormal movements**	0 1 2 3 4
	9. Incapacitation due to abnormal movements	0 1 2 3 4
	10. Patient's awareness of abnormal movements Rate only patient's report	No awareness 0 Aware, no distress 1 Aware, mild distress 2 Aware, moderate distress 3 Aware, severe distress 4 No = 0 Yes = 1
DENTAL STATUS:	**11. Current problems with teeth and/or dentures**	No = 0 Yes = 1
	12. Does patient usually wear dentures?	

It is always preferable to perform the entire AIMS Examination. This establishes consistent testing conditions and allows test results to be compared. Nonambulatory residents may be observed informally for abnormal involuntary movements while in bed or in a wheelchair. Uncooperative residents should be observed during normal activities.

You must check one of these boxes: ☐ Full examination conducted and scored
☐ Scores from informal observations—Resident was:
   ☐ Not ambulatory—observed in   ☐ bed   ☐ wheelchair
   ☐ Not cooperative

RATER	DATE:	PATIENT	Resident #

FIGURE 20-2 Abnormal Involuntary Movement Scale (AIMS). This test, or a comparable one, is performed every three to six months with all patients receiving antipsychotic medication to identify any signs of tardive dyskinesia.

AIMS EXAMINATION PROCEDURE

Either before or after completing the examination procedure observe the patient unobtrusively, at rest (e.g., in waiting room).

The chair to be used in this examination should be a hard, firm one without arms.

1. Ask patient whether there is anything in his/her mouth (i.e., gum, candy, etc.) and if there is, to remove it.

2. Ask patient about the current condition of his/her teeth. Ask patient if he/she wears dentures. Do teeth or dentures bother patient now?

3. Ask patient whether he/she notices any movements in mouth, face, hands, or feet. If yes, ask to describe and to what extent they currently bother patient or interfere with his/her activities.

4. Have patient sit in chair with hands on knees, legs slightly apart, and feet flat on floor. (Look at entire body for movements while in this position.)

5. Ask patient to sit with hands hanging unsupported. If male, between legs, if female and wearing a dress, hanging over knees. (Observe hands and other body areas.)

6. Ask patient to open mouth. (Observe tongue at rest within mouth.) Do this twice.

7. Ask patient to protrude the tongue. (Observe abnormalities of tongue movement.)

◆ 8. Ask patient to tap thumb, with each finger, as rapidly as possible for 10–15 seconds; separately with right hand, then with left hand. (Observe facial and leg movements.)

9. Flex and extend patient's left and right arms (one at a time). (Note any rigidity and rate on DOTES.)

10. Ask patient to stand up. (Observe in profile. Observe all body areas again, hips included.)

◆ 11. Ask patient to extend both arms outstretched in front with palms down. (Observe trunk, legs, and mouth.)

◆ 12. Have patient walk a few paces, turn, and walk back to the chair. (Observe hands and gait.) Do this twice.

◆ Activated movement, some practitioners score these movements differently.

INTERPRETATION OF THE AIMS SCORE

- Individuals with no single score exceeding 1 are at very low risk of having a movement disorder.

- A score of 2 in only one of the seven body areas is borderline and the patient should be monitored closely.

- A patient with score of 2 in two or more of the seven body areas should be referred for a complete neurological examination.

- A score of 3 or 4 in only one body area warrants referring the patient for a complete neurological examination.

FIGURE 20-3 Abnormal Involuntary Movement Scale (AIMS). Examination procedure continued.

Interactions of the antipsychotics may include:

Potentiation with CNS depressants, anticholinergics, and antihypertensives

Drugs that prolong QT interval and increase the risk of life-threatening cardiac arrhythmias (antiarrhythmic agents, dolasetron, certain quinolones) with phenothiazines and ziprasidone

Dopamine antagonists (metoclopramide or promethazine), which increase the risk of TD and EPS

Antagonism with anticonvulsants (seizure activity may increase)

See Table 20-5 for a summary of the antipsychotic medications. See Figure 20-4 for a summary of the psychotropic drugs.

There is no "ideal" antipsychotic medication. Both conventional and atypical antipsychotic medications are associated with significant adverse drug reactions. However, research indicates a chemical component in many forms of mental illness. By altering abnormal levels of certain chemicals in the brain, such as serotonin, norepinephrine, or dopamine, many patients with mental or emotional illness have been helped. Psychiatric hospitalization has decreased since the advent of antipsychotic medications.

PATIENT EDUCATION

Patients taking antipsychotic medications should be instructed regarding (utilize Patient Medication Guides where available):

The importance of being compliant with medication and nonmedication therapy

Potential for psychological and/or physical dependence with prolonged use

Caution in taking the medication only in prescribed dosage and for a limited period of time under medical supervision to reduce the possibility of serious side effects from overdose or prolonged use

Reporting adverse side effects to the physician at once (e.g., dizziness, blurred vision, nervousness, palpitations and other cardiac symptoms, urinary retention, GI symptoms, adverse mental changes, and EPS

Avoiding chemical abuse (e.g., alcohol, nicotine, or drugs) and obtaining professional treatment when these conditions exist

Possible severe withdrawal reactions (e.g., seizures) after prolonged use of psychotropic medications (withdrawal should never be abrupt, and medical supervision is indicated for prolonged administration of any of the psychotropic drugs)

Caution with interactions; *not* taking any other medications (except under close medical supervision) that can potentiate CNS depression (e.g., analgesics, alcohol, muscle relaxants, antihistamines, antiemetics, cardiac medications, or antihypertensives)

Not taking grapefruit juice with the BDZs, especially alprazolam and diazepam

Older adult patients are more at risk for the side effects mentioned earlier because of slowed metabolism and cardiovascular, kidney, liver, and visual impairment. They should be issued the following cautions:

Rise slowly because of the potential for hypotension.

Avoid operating machinery or driving while taking these drugs until you know how they affect you. Report to the physician immediately any side effects, especially dizziness, confusion, sleep disturbances, or weakness.

Avoid taking any OTC drugs or herbal supplements without medical supervision.

Tell the prescribing physician about all other medicines you are taking, including eye drops.

TABLE 20-5   Antipsychotic Medications/Major Tranquilizers

GENERIC NAME	TRADE NAME	DOSAGE[a]	COMMENTS
Typical (*These drugs frequently cause EPS with long-term use. Monitor closely.*)			
Phenothiazines			
chlorpromazine	(Thorazine)[b]	PO 30–800 mg 1–4 doses daily, also deep IM, or IV	Primarily for agitation; also for nausea and vomiting and severe behavior problems
fluphenazine	(Prolixin)[b]	IM, PO 0.5–40 mg daily in divided doses	For older adults, reduce dose to ½ or ¼
perphenazine	(Trilafon)[b]	PO 4–64 mg daily in divided doses	For psychosis, nausea, and vomiting in adults
prochlorperazine	(Compazine)[b] Compro	PO, IM, or IV 5–10 mg PR 25 mg BID	For agitation; primarily for nausea and vomiting in adults
thioridazine	(Mellaril)[b]	PO 50–800 mg daily divided two to four times per day	For psychoneurosis, agitation, or combativeness
trifluoperazine	(Stelazine)[b]	PO 1–20 mg BID	For schizophrenia and short term for nonpsychotic disorders
Butyrophenone			
haloperidol	Haldol	PO, IV 0.5–30 mg daily divided two to three times	For agitation, especially with schizophrenia and delusions in older adults
	Haldol decanoate IM	IM 50–300 mg q4wk	
Atypical			
aripiprazole	Abilify	PO 2–30 mg daily IM 9.75 mg (for agitation)	For schizophrenia; adjunct treatment for depression
	Abilify Maintena	400 mg IM monthly	For schizophrenia maintenance
clozapine	Clozaril Fazaclo ODT	PO 12.5–900 mg (divided doses)	Monitor WBC, neutrophil count; agranulocytosis risk
olanzapine	Zyprexa	PO 5–20 mg daily	Reduce dose by ½ for older adults
	Zyprexa Zydis	IM 10 mg (maximum dose 30 mg per day)	For acute agitation Orally disintegrating tablet
paliperidone	Invega	PO 3–12 mg once daily	For schizophrenia; do not crush
	Invega Sustenna	IM 234 mg day 1, 156 mg in one week, and then 117 mg monthly	
quetiapine	Seroquel	PO 50–800 mg daily (divided doses)	Monitor for orthostatic hypotension
	Seroquel XR		Also for depression associated with bipolar
risperidone	Risperdal	PO 1–4 mg BID	Reduce dose by ½ for older adults
	Risperdal Consta	IM 25–50 mg q2wk	For schizophrenia or adjunct therapy for bipolar disorder
ziprasidone	Geodon	PO 20–80 mg BID with food	Greater risk of cardiac disorders

a. Varies with condition (divided doses).
b. This brand name is no longer marketed, but the name is still commonly used.

CENTRAL NERVOUS SYSTEM
Drugs that affect mental and emotional function and behavior

CNS STIMULANTS

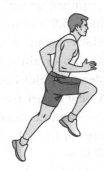

Indications
ADHD
Narcolepsy
Promote alertness
Neonatal sleep apnea

Example drugs
Ritalin
Adderall
Cafcit
Strattera

Antidepressants *(mood elevators)*

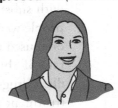

Indications: Treat Major Depressive Disorder (MDD)

Types of antidepressants
Tricyclics
MAOI's
SSRI's
SNRI's
Heterocyclics

Example drugs
Elavil
Marplan
Prozac
Cymbalta
Wellbutrin

Sedative-Hypnotics

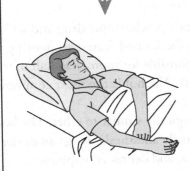

For SLEEP

Barbiturate and nonbarbiturates

phenobarbital (Luminal)
temazepam (Restoril)
zolpidem (Ambien)
zaleplon (Sonata)

Minor Tranquilizers
(antianxiety)

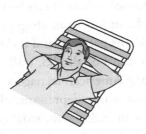

To CALM

Relieve anxiety

alprazolam (Xanax)
chlordiazepoxide (Librium)
diazepam (Valium)
buspirone (Buspar)
lorazepam (Ativan)

Major Tranquilizers
(antipsychotics)

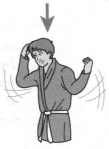

For DELUSIONS, HALLUCINATIONS

For VIOLENCE

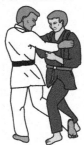

haloperidol (Haldol)
thioridazine (Mellaril)
risperidone (Risperdal)

FIGURE 20-4 Summary of psychotropic drugs.

DRUG ABUSE

Drug abuse can be defined as the use of a drug for other than therapeutic purposes. According to the Substance Abuse and Mental Health Services Administration (SAMHSA), an estimated 22.5 million individuals in the United States are diagnosed with substance abuse or dependence. Of this number, an estimated 15.4 million people were dependent on or abused alcohol alone, 3.9 million were dependent on or abused illicit drugs alone (marijuana, pain relievers, and cocaine had the highest rate of abuse), and 3.2 million were dependent on or abused both alcohol and illicit drugs. Drug abuse and addiction is considered a serious disease, which means treatment is paramount to recovery from it. A new report from SAMHSA stated that emergency department visits from the misuse and nonmedical use of ADHD stimulants more than doubled from 2005 to 2010, from 13,379 to 31,244; the greatest increase was among adults older than 18 years.

Drug **addiction** consists of the combination of all four of the following phenomena: tolerance, psychological dependence, physical dependence, and withdrawal syndrome with physiological effects. Habituation consists of psychological dependence only. **Chemical dependency** is the term used to describe a condition in which alcohol or drugs have taken control of an individual's life despite the problems related to their use and affect normal functioning.

ALCOHOL

Alcohol (ethyl alcohol, ethanol) can be classified as a psychotropic drug and a CNS depressant. It is the number one drug problem in the United States, accounting for nearly 100,000 deaths per year, and is directly responsible for more than half of traffic accidents (one-third of all U.S. traffic fatalities). Alcohol is the most commonly abused drug among American teenagers.

Alcohol is a fast-acting depressant, pharmacologically similar to ether. The body reacts to alcohol with excitement, sedation, and finally anesthesia. Large amounts of alcohol can result in alcoholic stupor, cerebral edema, and depressed respiration.

Alcohol is rapidly absorbed from the GI tract into the bloodstream. Alcohol depresses primitive areas of the cortex first and then decreases control over judgment, memory, and other intellectual and emotional functioning. Within a few hours, motor areas are affected, producing unsteady gait, slurred speech, and incoordination. Prolonged use can cause permanent CNS damage and result in peripheral neuritis, convulsive disorders, Wernicke's syndrome, and Korsakoff's psychosis with mental deterioration, memory loss, and ataxia.

Prolonged alcohol use affects almost all organs of the body. Chronic drinking causes liver damage and pancreatitis. Alcohol irritates the mucosa of the digestive system, leading to gastritis, ulceration, and hemorrhage. Alcohol can also lead to malabsorption of nutrients and malnutrition (see Figure 20-5).

Cardiovascular effects include peripheral vasodilation (producing the flushing and sweating seen with intoxication) and vasoconstriction of the coronary arteries. Alcohol increases the heart rate and, with chronic use, can cause cardiac myopathy, either directly or through metabolic and electrolyte imbalances. Potassium deficiency can cause cardiac arrhythmias.

Studies have shown an inverse association between the consumption of wine and coronary heart disease. In another study, it was determined that consumption of one or two drinks per day (five to six days each week) resulted in a reduced risk of myocardial infarction (MI) compared with nondrinkers. All this must be tempered with the deleterious effects of alcohol and the potential for abuse.

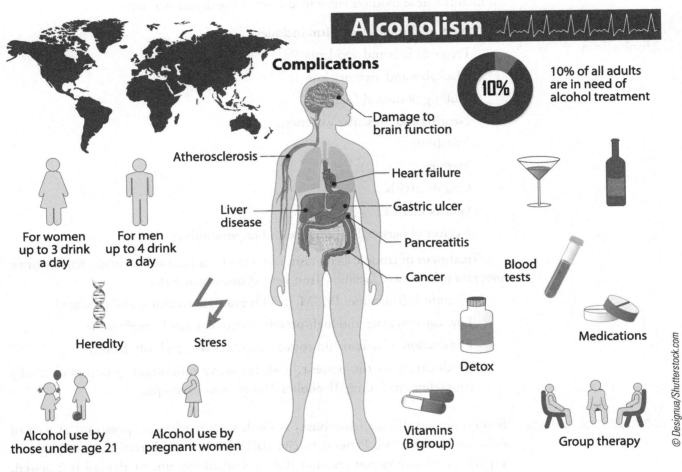

FIGURE 20-5 Alcohol abuse is common and can cause many long-term health issues.

ALCOHOL POISONING

Symptoms of acute alcoholic poisoning include cold, clammy skin; stupor; slow, noisy respirations; and alcoholic breath. Mortality associated with acute alcohol poisoning alone is uncommon but can be an important factor when mixed with recreational drugs.

Treatment includes close observation for:

Respiratory problems. Establish and maintain airway.

Vomiting. Prevent aspirations.

Seizures. Do not require treatment unless status epilepticus occurs.

Cerebral edema. Diuretics sometimes required (e.g., mannitol).

Electrolyte imbalance. IV fluids with thiamine, folic acid, magnesium sulfate, and vitamins added ("banana bag").

Alcohol withdrawal syndromes and delirium tremens. Treated with IV BDZs.

Fetal alcohol syndrome (FAS) is a teratogenic effect of ethanol. As few as two drinks early in pregnancy has been associated with FAS, although it is more commonly seen in infants whose mothers consumed four or five drinks per day.

Chronic Alcoholism

Symptoms of chronic alcoholism include:

Frequent falls and accidents

Blackouts and memory loss

Dulling of mental faculties

Neuritis and muscular weakness

Irritability

Tremors

Conjunctivitis

Gastroenteritis

Neglect of personal appearance and responsibilities

Treatment of chronic alcoholism can include an intensive in-house rehabilitation program in treatment facilities. Treatment frequently includes:

Vitamin B (thiamine) IV, IM, or PO; multiple vitamins; and folic acid

Low-carbohydrate and high-protein diet to combat hypoglycemia

Elimination of caffeine (in coffee, tea, chocolate, and soft drinks)

Reeducation of the patient, with intensive individual, group, and family counseling, including Alcoholics Anonymous techniques

Pharmacologic therapy

Sometimes disulfiram (Antabuse) is used, with patient cooperation, as part of *behavior modification.* Patients receive daily doses of disulfiram and are taught to expect a very unpleasant reaction if even a small amount of alcohol is ingested. There is some evidence that drinking frequency is reduced but minimal evidence that it facilitates abstinence. This treatment is used less frequently because of severe reaction potential and poor compliance.

Disulfiram–alcohol reactions can include:

Flushing and throbbing headache

Nausea and vomiting and metallic aftertaste

Sweating and dyspnea

Palpitation, tachycardia, and hypotension

Vertigo and blurred vision

Anxiety and confusion

PATIENT EDUCATION

Patients taking disulfiram should be instructed regarding:

Not taking within 12h of alcohol-containing preparations

Avoiding cough syrups, sauces, vinegars, elixirs, and other preparations containing alcohol

Caution with external applications of liniments, lotions, aftershave, or perfume

Signs of disulfiram–alcohol reaction

Reporting to emergency facility if effects do not subside or with severe reaction

Carrying identification card noting therapy

Avoiding other medications that may interact with disulfiram (e.g., metronidazole, anticoagulants, and phenytoin)

Another treatment for alcoholism includes the use of daily maintenance doses of naltrexone (ReVia), as part of counseling programs, to keep alcoholics sober after detoxification. Naltrexone is a long-acting opiate antagonist, which acts by blocking the pleasurable sensations associated with alcohol (and opiates) and therefore lessens the desire or craving to drink. Naltrexone reduces the frequency and risk of heavy drinking but does not necessarily enhance abstinence. It is better tolerated than disulfiram because it works to decrease the desire and rewards of drinking rather than elicit a punishment for consumption.

Side effects of naltrexone are usually minor and include:

GI side effects and decreased appetite

Headache, dizziness, and anxiety

Nausea and joint pains

Liver damage that can occur with doses larger than the recommended dose of 50 mg daily

Caution If naltrexone is given to someone currently dependent on opiates, it can send the addict instantly into severe, life-threatening withdrawal. Initiate therapy only if opiate free for 7–10 days.

Precautions or contraindications for the use of naltrexone include:

Patients with acute or severe liver problems

PRESCRIPTION DRUG ABUSE

According to the White House Office of National Drug Control Policy, prescription drug abuse is the nation's fastest growing drug problem. Prescription drugs are the second most abused category of drugs after marijuana, with nearly 22 million persons nationwide initiating the use of nonmedical pain relievers since 2002. It should be noted that all prescription drug abuse is illegal. This includes taking medication that is not prescribed to you by a doctor, taking medication prescribed to someone else, or taking medication more often or in higher doses than it was prescribed. According to the CDC, death rates from opioid overdoses have more than tripled since 1999 (in the United States in 2007, nearly 100 people died each day from a drug overdose).

Proper disposal and storage of prescription medication is important for deterring drug abuse. Keeping medications (especially those controlled by the Drug Enforcement Administration [DEA]) in a locked, secure space can help prevent theft, as well as not letting anyone but trusted caregivers and family members know their location. Additionally, disposal of controlled medications can be done in one of three ways. (1) Disposing in the normal trash but mixing with coffee grounds or pet litter in a way that makes them undesirable for consumption. This is the preferred method, but be sure to remove any personal information from bottles upon disposal. (2) Utilizing drop off days at local government facilities or locating a drop-box (usually at a police or fire station) where you can safely dispose of medication. (3) Flushing controlled medications down the toilet. Although this method is not preferred, controlled medications can be flushed if no other options are possible.

Although the majority of prescription drug abuse is conducted by the public, certain health care professionals have ready access to many prescription drugs, and, therefore, sometimes become involved in the illegal misuse of controlled substances. Prescription drugs most often abused by medical personnel are hydrocodone, oxycodone, and the BDZs. Counteractive measures include accurate recordkeeping of all controlled substances and recognition of the side effects and symptoms associated with drug abuse. (See Chapter 19 for a discussion of narcotic analgesics and see discussion earlier in this chapter of the anxiolytics.) Report suspected abuse to the person in authority; follow specific state agency reporting requirements.

Treatment of opiate addiction (fentanyl, oxycodone, hydrocodone, etc.) consists of a combination of counseling, behavioral therapy, and medications. Methadone, naltrexone, and buprenorphine are the medications approved for the treatment of opiate addiction. Methadone (an opioid agonist discussed in Chapter 19), sublingual buprenorphine (Subutex, a partial opioid antagonist), and buprenorphine with the opiate receptor antagonist naloxone (Suboxone) can be used during the detoxification process and for maintenance treatment. Naltrexone (ReVia), a pure opioid antagonist discussed earlier, is used in the maintenance therapy to block the pleasurable effects of opiates.

ILLEGAL DRUG ABUSE

This section describes four types of substances that can be produced illegally: the amphetamines, marijuana, cocaine, and the hallucinogens (LSD and PCP).

Amphetamines

Although amphetamines can be produced and prescribed legally, they are also produced in illegal labs. Two examples are methamphetamine ("crystal," "crank," "ice," "meth," "speed") and methylenedioxymethamphetamine (MDMA, "Ecstasy"). At normal dosage levels, administration of an amphetamine may produce tolerance within a few weeks. However, in hypersensitive individuals, psychotic syndrome may occur within 36–48 h of a single large dose of amphetamine. Some emotionally unstable individuals come to depend on the pleasant mental stimulation the drugs offer.

Symptoms of chronic abuse of amphetamines include:

- ❗ Emotional lability, irritability

  Anorexia

- ❗ Mental impairment, confusion, amnesia, and neurotoxicity

  Occupational deterioration and social withdrawal

  Continuous chewing or teeth grinding, resulting in trauma or ulcers of the tongue and lip

  Photophobia—frequently wearing sunglasses indoors

  Paranoid syndrome with hallucinations with prolonged use of high doses

  Tooth decay ("meth mouth")

Symptoms of acute toxicity from amphetamines can include:

- ❗ Strokes, cardiovascular symptoms including flushing or pallor, palpitation, tachypnea, tremor, extreme fluctuations of pulse and blood pressure, cardiac arrhythmias, chest pain, circulatory collapse

  Dilated pupils, diaphoresis, and hyperpyrexia

- ❗ Mental disturbances such as confusion, delirium, belligerence, combativeness, restlessness, paranoia, and suicidal or homicidal tendencies

- ❗ Fatigue and depression usually follow CNS stimulation

Treatment: There is no specific antidote for amphetamine overdosage. Treatment of an overdose is symptomatic and includes attention to airway, breathing, circulation, and administration of sedative drugs such as BDZs. General physiological supportive measures include treatment for shock or cardiac irregularities as appropriate. Administration of activated charcoal may help if it can be administered within 1–2 h after the substance was ingested. External cooling devices may be used to treat hyperthermia because antipyretics are not effective in this situation.

Abrupt withdrawal of amphetamines may unmask mental problems. Therefore, patients require careful supervision during withdrawal, and long-term follow-up may be required because some manifestations (e.g., depression) may persist for prolonged periods.

In an attempt to temper the meth epidemic, the Combat Methamphetamine Epidemic Act of 2005 (which took effect in 2006) banned OTC sales of ingredients commonly used to make methamphetamine. Pseudoephedrine (PSE), a popular and effective oral nasal decongestant, was the primary target of the act. PSE can now be stored and sold only under special conditions ("behind the counter") by pharmacies. Unfortunately, initial recordkeeping was store specific, and meth "smurfing" (the practice of going from one store to another to gain enough PSE to make meth) groups were formed to circumvent the law.

Chemically similar to methamphetamine as well as methylenediomethamphetamine (MDMA), the synthetic cathinones methylenedioxypyrovalerone (MDPV), mephedrone, and many others (collectively termed "bath salts") are an emerging family of highly addictive recreational drugs. "Bath salts" are designer stimulants not indicated for bathing but are falsely marketed as plant food, herbal incense, or more recently as jewelry or phone screen cleaner. The symptoms of abuse, toxicity, and treatment are similar to amphetamines, but the mental disturbances may be more prolonged, severe, and possibly permanent.

The DEA has classified MDPV, its salts, isomers, and salts of isomers as Schedule I substances (no accepted medical use) under the Controlled Substances Act. This regulation makes it illegal for anyone to sell or be in possession of these products. Unfortunately, chemists alter the chemical composition of the banned substance just enough that it still can be legally sold.

Marijuana

Tetrahydrocannabinol (THC) is the active ingredient in marijuana. Although classified technically as a CNS depressant, it also possesses properties of a euphoriant, sedative, and hallucinogen. Marinol (dronabinol—a synthetic form of THC) is approved for the prevention of chemotherapy-induced nausea and vomiting and is also used as an appetite stimulant in cachexia associated with AIDS or cancer.

The *Cannabis* plant grows over the entire world, especially in tropical areas. Potency varies considerably from place to place and time to time. Its composition varies widely, and the methods of administration do not provide a standardized and reproducible dose. This makes it difficult to evaluate the potential therapeutic effects of marijuana for certain disorders, and it is illegal under federal law. Nevertheless, 18 states and the District of Columbia currently have legalized "medical" marijuana for (1) severe nausea and vomiting associated with cancer chemotherapy, (2) weight loss associated with debilitating illnesses, (3) spasticity secondary to neurologic diseases, (4) pain syndromes, and (5) glaucoma.

THC, the active ingredient released when marijuana is smoked, is fat soluble and is stored in many fat cells, especially in the brain and reproductive organs. THC metabolizes slowly. A week after a person smokes one marijuana cigarette, 30%–50% of the THC remains in the body, and four to six weeks are required to eliminate all of the THC.

Side effects of marijuana include:

- ❗ Short-term memory loss, impaired learning, and slowed intellectual performance
- ❗ Perceptual inaccuracies and impaired reflex reaction (dangerous with driving)
- ❗ Apathy, lethargy, and decreased motivation
- Increased heart rate, anxiety, and panic attacks
- Lung irritation, chronic cough, frequent respiratory infections
- Reduced testosterone level and sperm count
- Reduced estrogen level, crossing of placental barrier, and transmission through mother's milk; miscarriage and stillbirth possible
- ❗ Delayed development of coping mechanisms in children and adolescents

Another newer illicit drug class coming on the scene is the synthetic cannabinoids, known as "spice," "K2," "skunk," fake weed, and other names. These products, which are abused by smoking, contain dried, shredded plant material and chemical additives that are responsible for their hallucinogenic effects. Spice users report experiences similar to those produced by marijuana, but in some cases these are stronger with unpredictable effects (rapid heart rate, hypertension, seizures, acute kidney injury, and myocardial ischemia, and in a few cases spice has been associated with heart attacks).

Because the chemicals used in spice have a high potential for abuse and no medical benefit, the DEA has designated it as a Scheduled I controlled substance, making it illegal to sell, buy, or possess it. Just like the "bath salts" mentioned earlier, however, makers of spice products evade these legal restrictions by substituting different chemicals in their mixtures.

Cocaine

Cocaine is a CNS stimulant and produces euphoria and increased expenditure of energy. The only approved medical use is as a local anesthetic, *applied topically only,* to mucous membranes of the laryngeal, nasal, and oral cavities.

Cocaine is highly addictive, causing dependence after even short-time use. It is abused by intranasal application (sniffing or snorting), intravenous injection, or inhalation (smoking "crack"). Nasal application can damage mucous membranes and/or the nasal septum. The effects of intravenous use are extremely rapid and dangerous and can be fatal. Smoking causes the most rapid addiction, sometimes after only one use. Cocaine crosses the placental barrier and has resulted in babies who are irritable, jittery, anorexic, and seizure prone. Cocaine use has caused numerous crimes and deaths. Severe depression can be associated with withdrawal, which is a lengthy and difficult process.

Side effects of cocaine, which are serious, include:

- Euphoria, agitation, and excitation
- Hypertension, chest pain, tachycardia, cardiac arrhythmias, or cardiac failure
  Anorexia, nausea, and vomiting
- Tremor and seizures
- Hallucinations, possible psychosis, and possible violent behavior
- Respiratory failure, strokes, and possible death from circulatory collapse
  Perforated nasal septum from prolonged nasal use

Hallucinogens

Lysergic acid (LSD) and phencyclidine (PCP), an animal tranquilizer, are hallucinogens. They produce bizarre mental reactions and distortion of physical senses. Hallucinations and delusions are common with confused perceptions of time and space (e.g., the user can walk out of windows because of the impression that he or she can fly). PCP is also an amnesic.

Side effects of hallucinogens include:

- Increased pulse and heart rate and rise in blood pressure and temperature
- Possible "flashbacks" months later
- Panic or paranoia (lack of control)
- Possible psychotic episodes; chronic mental disorders
  Possible physical injury to self or others

Dextromethorphan

Dextromethorphan (DXM), a semisynthetic morphine derivative, is a safe, effective, nonaddictive, OTC cough suppressant when used appropriately. Unfortunately, DXM (primarily the one found in Robitussin and Coricidin HBP products) is often abused by teens because of its phencyclidine-like euphoric effect, and the abuse of this agent may also be associated with psychosis and mania. The abuse of DXM can cause serious adverse events, such as brain damage, seizure, loss of consciousness, irregular heartbeat, and even death.

Flunitrazepam (Rohypnol)

Flunitrazepam (Rohypnol), an illegal drug of a different type, is a potent BDZ that is approved for use in Central and South America for ethanol withdrawal. Not approved in the United States, it is being used here as a recreational drug (sometimes snorted to offset cocaine withdrawal) and is known on the street as "roofies." It has also acquired the title "date-rape drug" because of its ability to induce amnesia, preventing the victim from recalling specific events while under the influence of the drug.

The Role of Medical Personnel

The role of the medical personnel in combating drug abuse includes:

Thorough knowledge of psychotropic drugs, action, and side effects

Willingness to participate in the education of the patient, the patient's family, and others in the community

Giving competent care to those under the influence of drugs in a nonjudgmental way

Recognizing drug abuse and making appropriate referrals without exception

Complete and accurate recordkeeping of controlled stocks of drugs that could be considered potential drugs of abuse

It is the responsibility of all medical personnel not only to recognize drug abuse but also to report any observed drug abuse to the proper person in authority. To look the other way not only enables the individual to continue to harm himself or herself but also endangers those in his or her care.

There are many services available to help medical personnel deal with drug abuse problems. Check with your state licensing agency or certification board for information about the programs in your area, such as the Impaired Nurse program. Local mental health clinics or psychiatric facilities can also provide assistance and information. Other agencies that can provide information include:

National Institute on Drug Abuse

www.nida.nih.gov

www.drugabuse.gov

www.clubdrugs.gov

National Institute on Alcohol Abuse and Alcoholism of the National Institutes of Health

ww.niaaa.nih.gov

Substance Abuse & Mental Health Services Administration

www.samhsa.gov

Alcoholics Anonymous, Narcotics Anonymous

www.aa.org, www.na.org

CASE STUDY A

Psychotropic Drugs

Kevin McClellan is a 19-year-old college student who, by his roommate's accounts, has been displaying "odd" behavior. The roommate convinces Kevin to visit the student health center with him and reports to the nurse that Kevin has had periods of "wild activity" alternating with periods of lying in bed for days at a time. The nurse reviews Kevin's records and finds that he has a history of bipolar disorder.

1. What is the drug of choice to treat patients with bipolar disorder?
   a. Buspirone
   b. Chlorpromazine
   c. Alprazolam
   d. Lithium

2. Patients on lithium should be monitored for correct dosing by which method?
   a. Observation of patient's behavior
   b. Serum lithium levels
   c. Patient reporting of his or her own behavior
   d. EKG every three months

3. Side effects of lithium can include:
   a. Hypotension
   b. Hypertension
   c. Weight loss
   d. Hyperthyroidism

4. While reviewing Kevin's chart, the nurse notes that he has been visiting the health center during the prior school year with complaints of photophobia. This indicates which complication?
   a. Retinal detachment
   b. Potential seizure activity
   c. Lithium toxicity
   d. Dehydration

5. All patients should be cautioned when taking lithium with which category of medications?
   a. Anticholesterol
   b. Angiotensin (ACE) inhibitors
   c. Anticoagulants
   d. Sulfonylureas

CASE STUDY B

Psychotropic Drugs

Jose Aquilar is a 33-year-old marine who has just completed a six-month tour of duty in Afghanistan. He has been home for over four weeks and is experiencing signs of post-traumatic stress disorder.

1. Jose has asked his personal physician for a medication to help him cope as he assimilates back into his daily life. What type of drug would the physician be most likely to prescribe to Jose for short-term use?
   a. Antipsychotic
   b. Anxiolytic
   c. Tranquilizer
   d. Antimanic

2. The physician warns Jose that when taking a minor anxiolytic, he may develop drug dependence. What does this likely mean for Jose?
   a. He will need larger doses over time to achieve the same effect.
   b. He will associate the drug with incidents from his tour of duty.
   c. He will find it difficult to make it through the day without the drug.
   d. He will rely on the drug during any emotional conflict.

(continued)

(*continued*)

3. The physician also explains that sudden withdrawal after prolonged use of an anxiolytic may result in which symptom?
   a. Development of tics
   b. Somnolence
   c. Insomnia
   d. Blurred vision

4. Side effects of benzodiazepines may include:
   a. Akathisia
   b. Neuritis
   c. Dystonia
   d. Ataxia

5. Physicians should use extreme caution when prescribing a benzodiazepine to a patient with a history of:
   a. Kidney disease
   b. Substance abuse
   c. Type II diabetes
   d. Reflex sympathetic dystrophy

CHAPTER REVIEW QUIZ

Match the medication in the first column with the classification in the second column. Classifications may be used more than once.

Medication

1. ___ Xanax

2. ___ lithium

3. ___ Risperdal

4. ___ amitriptyline

5. ___ Prozac

6. ___ Adderall

7. ___ Buspar

8. ___ Zyprexa

9. ___ Ativan

10. ___ Wellbutrin

Classification

a. Antipsychotic

b. Anxiolytic

c. Antidepressant

d. CNS stimulant

e. Antimanic

Choose the correct answer.

11. Close monitoring of a pediatric patient taking a CNS stimulant for ADHD is necessary to assess for:
    a. Temporary suppression of growth pattern
    b. Alopecia
    c. Weight gain
    d. Hypotension

12. A side effect of a selective norepinephrine reuptake inhibitor (SNRI) for ADHD is:
    a. Growth retardation
    b. Insomnia
    c. Increased potential for abuse
    d. Increased risk of suicidal tendencies in children and adolescents

13. With depression, there may be a shortage of what substance in the brain?
a. Glucose
b. Dopamine
c. Potassium
d. Monoamine oxidase

14. A common side effect of a tricyclic is:
a. Weight loss
b. Urinary frequency
c. Mouth dryness
d. Diarrhea

15. MAOIs can interact with some drugs and food and herbal supplements. These interactions can cause which side effect?
a. Hypoglycemia
b. Hypertensive crisis
c. Seizures
d. Hyponatremia

16. Tardive dyskinesia is characterized by which of the following?
a. Muscle laxity
b. Spasticity
c. Tremors
d. Involuntary, repetitive, and purposeless movements

17. Patients taking antipsychotic medications should be instructed:
a. To take medications with grapefruit juice for better absorption
b. To be aware that possible severe reactions may occur after short use
c. To be aware that there is a potential for psychological or physical dependence with prolonged use
d. To drink alcohol to calm the nerves if needed

18. A serious side effect of cocaine is:
a. Paranoia
b. Euphoria
c. Flashbacks
d. Panic attacks

19. The drug nicknamed the "date-rape drug," because of its ability to induce amnesia, is called:
a. Rohypnol
b. Lysergic acid
c. Fluticasone
d. Phencyclidine

20. Jared, a health care provider, suspects that another health care provider is abusing drugs. What is the first step that Jared should take?
a. Give the individual the benefit of the doubt and remain quiet.
b. Report any observed drug use to the proper person in authority.
c. Confront the individual and threaten to tell a person in authority.
d. Provide the individual with an 800 number for drug treatment and counseling.

STUDYGUIDE   **Online Resources**

PRACTICE

Complete Chapter 20

- Powerpoint presentations
- Videos

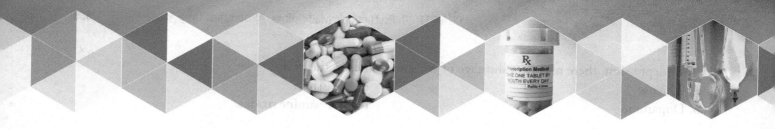

CHAPTER 21

MUSCULOSKELETAL AND ANTI-INFLAMMATORY DRUGS

KEY TERMS AND CONCEPTS

Anti-inflammatory

COX-2 inhibitor

Hormone replacement therapy (HRT)

Neuromuscular blocking agents (NMBAs)

NSAIDs

Osteoporosis therapy

Skeletal muscle relaxants

OBJECTIVES

Upon completion of this chapter, the learner should be able to

1. Identify the commonly used skeletal muscle relaxants
2. Describe the side effects to be expected with muscle relaxants
3. List the drugs that can interact with the muscle relaxants and cause serious potentiation of effect
4. Differentiate among the anti-inflammatory drugs and anti-rheumatic drugs
5. Explain the serious side effects of nonsteroidal anti-inflammatory drugs (NSAIDs)
6. List the drug interactions with NSAIDs
7. Explain appropriate patient education for those taking skeletal muscle relaxants and NSAIDs
8. Describe medications for osteoporosis prevention and treatment
9. Compare and contrast a cyclooxygenase-2 (COX-2) inhibitor and other NSAIDs
10. Define the Key Terms and Concepts

D isorders of the musculoskeletal system are rather common. Drugs used to treat such conditions may be classified into two broad categories: skeletal muscle relaxants and nonsteroidal anti-inflammatory drugs (NSAIDs). Corticosteroid therapy for inflammatory conditions is discussed in Chapter 23.

SKELETAL MUSCLE RELAXANTS

Some disorders of the musculoskeletal system can be attributed to structural defects (e.g., ruptured disks) that may require surgical intervention rather than medication. However, many disorders associated with pain, spasm, abnormal contraction, or impaired mobility do respond to medications classified as skeletal muscle relaxants. Acute, painful musculoskeletal conditions, such as backache or neck strain, are treated with a combination of muscle relaxants, rest, physical therapy, other nonpharmacological methods (e.g., hot or cold packs), and mild analgesics (e.g., nonsteroidal anti-inflammatory drugs [NSAIDs]). Muscle relaxants are given only on a short-term basis, and, after the acute pain subsides, exercises are usually prescribed by the physician to strengthen the weak muscles. Muscle relaxants can be used long term for certain conditions, but for acute injuries they should be used only until the problem is resolved.

Most muscle relaxant drugs affect the central nervous system (spinal cord and brain), with no direct effect on the skeletal muscle. The resulting action reduces muscle spasm, causes alterations in the perception of pain, and produces a sedative effect, promoting rest and relaxation of the affected part. Centrally acting drugs used to treat acute, painful musculoskeletal conditions include the benzodiazepines, such as diazepam (Valium) and methocarbamol (Robaxin). Refer to Chapter 20 for a discussion of the benzodiazepines.

A different type of muscle relaxant, dantrolene, causes a *direct* effect on skeletal muscles and is used in the management of spasticity resulting from upper motor neuron disorders such as multiple sclerosis or cerebral palsy. This medication is ineffective for amyotrophic lateral sclerosis (ALS) and is not indicated for the treatment of muscle spasms resulting from rheumatic disorders or musculoskeletal trauma (acute injuries).

Muscle relaxants also have moderate potential for abuse, as they can provide the patient with a feeling of euphoria. As discussed in Chapter 20, benzodiazepines are classified as Food and Drug Administration (FDA) schedule IV controlled substances. Additionally, Soma (carisoprodol) is also a schedule IV controlled substance. Although other muscle relaxants discussed throughout this chapter are not yet classified as controlled substances, health care professionals should still be aware that at high doses all muscle relaxants can exhibit the euphoric effects that can lead to abuse.

Side effects of skeletal muscle relaxants can include:

- ❗ Drowsiness, dizziness, or dry mouth
- ❗ Weakness, tremor, ataxia, and seizures
- Headache
- ❗ Confusion and nervousness
- Slurred speech
- Blurred vision
- ❗ Hypotension
- Gastrointestinal (GI) symptoms, including nausea, vomiting, diarrhea, or constipation
- Urinary problems, including enuresis, frequency, or retention
- ❗ Hypersensitivity reactions, including liver toxicity with dantrolene and tizanidine
- ❗ Respiratory depression

Precautions or contraindications for skeletal muscle relaxants apply to:

> Hypersensitivity to the muscle relaxant
> Pregnancy or lactation
> History of drug abuse
> Impaired kidney function
> Liver disorders
> Blood dyscrasias
> Chronic obstructive pulmonary disease
> Cardiac disorders
> Older adults
> Abrupt discontinuation
> Closed-angle glaucoma

Interactions with potentiation of effect occur between skeletal muscle relaxants and:

> Alcohol
> Analgesics
> Psychotropic medications
> Antihistamines

The MedlinePlus website www.nlm.nih.gov/medlineplus/backpain.html is a good resource for patient education and written materials on back pain.

See Table 21-1 for a summary of the skeletal muscle relaxants.

PATIENT EDUCATION

Skeletal Muscle Relaxants

Patients taking skeletal muscle relaxants should be instructed regarding:

Potential side effects (e.g., drowsiness, dizziness, weakness, tremor, blurred vision, hypotension, respiratory distress, or GI disorders); care with driving especially until effects are known

Avoidance of other CNS depressants at the same time (e.g., tranquilizers, antihistamines, or alcohol), which can cause serious CNS depression, and care with analgesics, only as prescribed by a physician

Importance of following the physician's orders regarding rest and physical therapy (e.g., heat and firm mattress or bed board

with back problems) and exercises as prescribed (after the acute pain subsides) to strengthen the weak muscles

The acronym RICE (rest, ice, compression [elastic bandage], elevation) represents appropriate care initially for musculoskeletal injuries to extremities. A recent addition has been the focus on prevention of the injury, so some modify the acronym to PRICE

Taking the medication only as long as absolutely necessary and observing caution regarding prolonged use, which could lead to physical or psychological dependence and withdrawal symptoms (e.g., seizures from abrupt baclofen or diazepam withdrawal after prolonged use)

TABLE 21-1   Skeletal Muscle Relaxants

GENERIC NAME	TRADE NAME	DOSAGE	COMMENTS
baclofen	Lioresal	PO 10–20 mg three to four times per day; intrathecal 300–800 mcg	For spasticity associated with spinal cord injury or spinal cord diseases
carisoprodol	Soma	PO 250–350 mg three to four times per day	Caution with asthma; watch for abuse potential (C-IV controlled substance)
cyclobenzaprine	Flexeril	PO 5–10 mg three times per day	Strongly anticholinergic side effects (structurally related to amitriptyline)
dantrolene	Dantrium	PO 25–100 mg two to four times per day (titrate to the lowest effective dose)	For multiple sclerosis and cerebral palsy, not for trauma or rheumatic disorders
methocarbamol	Robaxin	4–8 g PO daily in divided doses also IM and IV	For acute painful musculoskeletal conditions
tizanidine	Zanaflex	PO 2–8 mg one to three times per day (6–8 h intervals)	For increased muscle tone associated with spasticity, for example multiple sclerosis or spinal cord trauma

Note: This is a representative sample; other products are available.

Neuromuscular Blocking Agents

Another type of muscle relaxants that causes a direct effect on the muscles including the diaphragm are called **neuromuscular blocking agents (NMBAs)** such as succinylcholine and rocuronium (Zemuron), used during surgical, endoscopic, or orthopedic procedures. These drugs are potentially very dangerous and can result in respiratory arrest because of the potential to paralyze the major muscle of ventilation, the diaphragm.

NMBAs are *administered only* by anesthesiologists or specially trained personnel skilled in intubation, medically induced paralysis, and resuscitation. Since these agents paralyze the muscles, analgesics and sedatives are mandatory concurrent medications because the patient can still *feel* the pain but cannot react to it.

ANTI-INFLAMMATORY DRUGS

Anti-inflammatory drugs are used to treat disorders in which the musculoskeletal system is not functioning properly because of inflammation. Such conditions as arthritis, bursitis, spondylitis, gout, and muscle strains and sprains can cause swelling, redness, heat, pain, and limited muscle and joint mobility. Analgesics and corticosteroids are used at times for the acute stages of these disorders and are discussed in Chapters 19 and 23. The corticosteroids are not used for extended periods of time because of serious side effects. However, NSAIDs are frequently given for lengthy time periods in maintenance doses as low as possible for effectiveness.

Nonsteroidal Anti-inflammatory Drugs

NSAIDs, such as ibuprofen, inhibit the synthesis of prostaglandins, substances responsible for producing much of the inflammation and pain of rheumatic conditions, sprains, and menstrual cramps. No cure has been found for rheumatic disorders, but many medications are used to alleviate the pain and crippling effects.

Because of lower metabolic rates and other complications, older adults are particularly susceptible to side effects from NSAIDs and should be cautioned to report any undesirable signs or symptoms to their physician without delay.

The salicylates (e.g., aspirin) are the oldest drug in this category with analgesic, anti-inflammatory, and antipyretic effects (see Chapter 19). Many nonsalicylate NSAIDs are on the market, and some are tolerated better than aspirin by some patients, especially as short-term analgesics. However, with large doses and/or long term use, they all share many of the same side effects and interactions to some degree. Patients on prolonged therapy with any of the NSAIDs should be monitored carefully. Older adults or debilitated patients do not tolerate ulceration or bleeding (which can be "silent") as well as other individuals, and most reports of fatal GI events are found in these populations.

If chronic anti-inflammatory therapy must be continued despite GI ulceration, several options for the patient are available. Ideally after the ulcer heals, the patient could resume the NSAID with either misoprostol (Cytotec) or a proton pump inhibitor with close clinical monitoring for ulcer recurrence. Combination products are available, for example Arthrotec, which combines diclofenac (Voltaren) with misoprostol to protect the gastric mucosa. (See Chapter 16, "Gastrointestinal Drugs.")

Diclofenac is also available topically as 1% gel and a 1.3% patch (see Figure 21-1). Based on available data, topical NSAIDs seem unlikely to be associated with an increased risk of GI bleeding or renal failure. Serum concentrations of topical NSAIDs are much lower than those of oral NSAIDS; drug concentrations in meniscus, cartilage, and tendon sheath are much higher due to direct absorption of the drug through the skin into the tissues of the joints. However, until further evidence is available, the same oral NSAID warnings and precautions apply to the topical formulations as well.

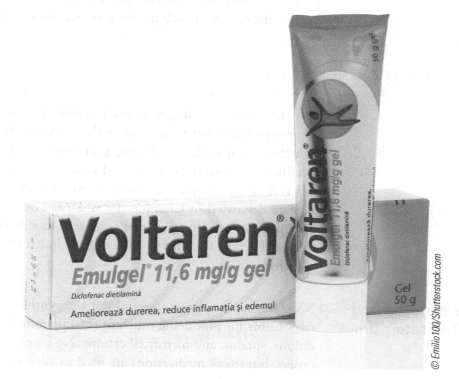

FIGURE 21-1 Voltaren Gel (now generic as diclofenac) is a unique topical NSAID that can be used for specific joint problems.

The FDA has issued a warning regarding the over-the-counter (OTC) non-selective NSAIDs: They should be used in strict accordance with label directions. Self-treatment with an OTC NSAID should not exceed 10 days, unless directed by a physician.

COX-2 Inhibitor

Celecoxib (Celebrex) is an NSAID that exhibits anti-inflammatory, analgesic, and antipyretic activities by *selectively* inhibiting cyclooxygenase-2 (COX-2) prostaglandin synthesis. However, it does not inhibit COX-1 and, therefore, does not inhibit platelet aggregation (clotting) or inhibit the production of mucosal-protective prostaglandins. Consequently, it does not pose the bleeding risks of the other *nonselective* NSAIDs described previously. Due to the specific action inhibiting COX-2 prostaglandin synthesis, Celebrex (and the partially selective NSAIDs) has the *potential* to cause fewer gastric problems and poses less risk of GI bleeding unless used concurrently with aspirin.

Earlier studies have suggested that there is a "good" and a "bad" prostaglandin as far as the heart is concerned. Suppressing both types in the way nonselective NSAIDs do would theoretically help the heart. If NSAIDs are prescribed, current evidence suggests that naproxen may have the best cardiovascular safety profile. The selective **COX-2 inhibitors** shut down only the "good" prostaglandin, raising the risk of high blood pressure, atherosclerosis, and clotting. However, both traditional NSAIDs and the COX-2 inhibitors can increase the risk of adverse events (recurrent MI or death) in patients who have a history of or who are at high risk for cardiovascular disease. Therefore, the benefits and risks in terms of pain relief and cardiovascular and GI safety must be weighed carefully for each individual.

The FDA has posted extensive NSAID (and acetaminophen) medication information at http://www.fda.gov/cder/drug/analgesics/default.htm. The health care professional has the responsibility to stay informed of the latest developments in this area.

Side effects of NSAIDs frequently include:

- ❗ GI ulceration and bleeding (may not be preceded by warning signs or symptoms)
- ❗ Epigastric pain, nausea, heartburn, and gastroesophageal reflux disease (GERD)
- Myocardial infarction (MI), thromboembolism, stroke, hypertension, and heart failure
- Fluid retention and peripheral edema
- Constipation
- Tinnitus and hearing loss
- Headache or dizziness
- Visual disturbances
- Hematuria and albuminuria (albumin in the urine)

! Rash, hypersensitivity reactions, and bronchospasm (especially with aspirin)

! Blood dyscrasias, especially prolonged bleeding time; anemia

Liver toxicity

Precautions or contraindications for NSAIDs apply to:

Asthma (may manifest aspirin sensitivity as bronchospasm)

Cardiovascular disorders (e.g., hypertension, heart failure; may cause fluid retention and edema)

Kidney disease

Liver dysfunction

History of GI ulcer or inflammatory bowel disease

Blood dyscrasias, especially clotting disorders or anemia

Children with viral infections (danger of Reye's syndrome with salicylates)

GERD

Older adults

Pregnancy and lactation

Those with aspirin and NSAID hypersensitivity

Those with sulfonamide hypersensitivity (should not take Celebrex)

These medications should be given with meals or milk to reduce GI side effects. Enteric-coated, timed-release capsules or buffered aspirin are sometimes also recommended to reduce gastric irritation.

Interactions of NSAIDs (especially salicylates) are many, but the most important clinically occur with:

Alcohol (potentiates the possibility of GI bleeding)

Anticoagulants (potentiate the possibility of bleeding; also true of vitamin E)

Corticosteroids (increase the chance of GI effects with prolonged administration of NSAIDs)

Aspirin (increases adverse GI effects and diminishes the risk-reducing effects of COX-2 inhibitors in the GI tract); nonselective NSAIDs may decrease the antiplatelet effects of aspirin (give the NSAID 30 min after or 8h prior to aspirin ingestion)

Antihypertensives (attenuated response)

Lithium (decreased clearance)

Methotrexate (potentiates and increases the risk of methotrexate toxicity)

Uricosurics (probenecid or sulfinpyrazone), whose action is antagonized by salicylates

See Table 21-2 for a summary of the NSAIDs.

CLINICAL CONNECTION

Medication Reconciliation

In an ideal world, each patient would only go to one doctor who treats all of their conditions and prescribes all of their medications, which are all filled at the same pharmacy. This would drastically cut down on gaps in care, duplications in therapy, and potentially dangerous drug interactions. As we know, this is not the case, therefore it is important to always take the time to get a complete list of medications that the patient is taking, including OTC medications. This practice is known as medication reconciliation and is a useful tool to identify potential problems in a medication regimen. Analgesics such as acetaminophen and NSAIDs are available both as prescriptions and OTC, so they are commonly involved in the aforementioned therapeutic duplications or interactions. NSAIDs are especially problematic because there is such a wide range of drugs and the names of these drugs are not similar. For example, a patient may be on Celebrex (celecoxib) for arthritis, and also be taking ibuprofen OTC for headaches. This patient is at an increased risk for stomach ulcers, kidney problems, and other side effects. Although there are many examples that could be given, proper medication reconciliation will help to avoid these types of situations, especially with medications like NSAIDs that are readily available and commonly prescribed, yet still have potential for serious adverse effects.

PATIENT EDUCATION

Patients taking NSAIDs should be instructed regarding:

Administering the medication with food to reduce gastric irritation

Caution with dosage (follow the physician's directions carefully regarding the amount of drug to reduce the chance of overdose)

Discontinuing drug and reporting to the physician any sign of abnormal bleeding (gums, stool, urine, and bruising), epigastric pain or nausea, ringing in the ears or hearing loss, visual disturbances, weight gain or edema, and skin rash

Avoiding taking any other drugs, either prescribed or OTC, without checking first with a physician or pharmacist

regarding possible interactions and duplication of the medication

Avoiding taking large amounts of aspirin or other NSAIDs with kidney, liver, or heart disease or with a history of GI ulcer (with these conditions, take only under medical supervision). Patients with asthma may manifest sensitivity to aspirin and other NSAIDs.

The danger that GI ulceration and bleeding can occur without previous warning signs or symptoms

Discontinuing NSAIDs before elective surgery or dental procedures to reduce the risk of serious bleeding (check with the physician or dentist)

Not taking Celebrex if allergic to sulfa

TABLE 21-2 Nonsteroidal Anti-inflammatory Drugs

GENERIC NAME	TRADE NAME	DOSAGE
Nonselective (traditional) NSAIDs		
diclofenac	(Voltaren DR)[a]	PO 150–225 mg daily in divided doses
	Voltaren XR	PO 100 mg one to two times per day
	Voltaren	Gel 2–4 g four times per day depending on the site (use supplied dosing cards)
	Flector	1 patch BID

(continued)

TABLE 21-2   Nonsteroidal Anti-inflammatory Drugs (*continued*)

GENERIC NAME	TRADE NAME	DOSAGE
Nonselective (traditional) NSAIDs (*continued*)		
ibuprofen	Motrin	PO 200–800 mg four times per day
	Motrin IB, Advil (OTC)	PO 200–400 mg q4–6h (max 1,200 mg per day, 10 days max)
	Caldolor	IV 400–800 mg q6h over 30 min (for hospitalized patients unable to take PO for pain or fever)
indomethacin	Indocin	PO, R up to 200 mg daily in divided doses
ketorolac	(Toradol)[a]	PO 20 mg one time, and then 10 mg q4–6 h (five days max)
		IM/IV 15–30 mg q6h (five days max)
naproxen	Naprosyn, Anaprox	PO 250–550 mg BID (q12 h)
	Aleve (OTC)	PO 220 mg q8–12h (max 660 mg per day, 10 days max)
oxaprozin	Daypro	PO 600–1,200 mg once daily
Partially selective NSAIDs		
etodolac	(Lodine)[a]	PO 600–1,200 mg daily in divided doses
meloxicam	Mobic	PO 7.5–15 mg daily or BID
nabumetone	(Relafen)[a]	PO 1,000–2,000 mg daily
Selective COX-2 inhibitor		
celecoxib	Celebrex	PO 100–200 mg daily or BID
Combinations		
diclofenac/misoprostol	Arthrotec 50, 75	PO 50 mg three to four times per day; 75 mg BID

a. This brand name is no longer marketed, but the name is still commonly used.
Note: Other NSAIDs are available. This is a representative list.

OSTEOPOROSIS THERAPY

Osteoporosis (porous bone) is defined as a systemic skeletal disease characterized by low bone mass and deterioration of bone tissue, leading to bone fragility and increased susceptibility to fracture, especially of the hip, spine, and wrist (Figure 21-2). It most commonly affects older populations, primarily postmenopausal women. The diagnosis of osteoporosis is determined by measuring one's bone mineral density (BMD), which serves as a predictor of future fracture risk. Osteoporosis therapy includes calcium and vitamin D supplementation and several prescription medications currently approved for the prevention and/or treatment of osteoporosis. Calcium and vitamin D supplementation should be started at the first sign of osteoporosis and in all patients who are considered to be at risk because of age, gender, or family history.

OSTEOPOROSIS

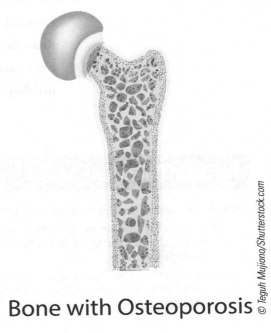

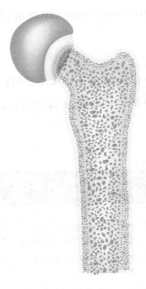

FIGURE 21-2 Osteoporosis is characterized by the breakdown of bone structure, this weakening can lead to fractures and other complications.

Normal Bone

Bone with Osteoporosis

© Teguh Mujiono/Shutterstock.com

Bisphosphonates

Bisphosphonates are nonhormonal agents that act directly to inhibit bone reabsorption, thereby increasing bone mineral density at the spine and hip, as well as decreasing the incidence of first and future fractures. Alendronate (Fosamax), ibandronate (Boniva), and risedronate (Actonel) have been approved for both the prevention and treatment of osteoporosis and are considered the first-line therapy. The bisphosphonates are also indicated for management of Paget's disease of the bone, a chronic disorder characterized by fractures, skeletal abnormalities, and significant bone pain.

Bisphosphonates bind strongly to and accumulate in bone, creating a reservoir of drug that is released back into systemic circulation gradually over a period of months or years after the treatment is stopped. Beneficial effects on BMD persist for some time, suggesting that a "drug holiday" could mitigate some of the risks associated with bisphosphonate therapy.

A new bisphosphonate, Reclast (zoledronic acid), is a once yearly infusion that has been shown to significantly decrease the risk of fractures and also to increase bone mass. It is the most potent bisphosphonate, but patients who are on it should be checked for proper renal function before starting it, and should be monitored throughout therapy. Other side effects and warnings are similar to other bisphosphonates.

Side effects of bisphosphonates can include:

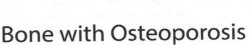 GI distress (nausea, dyspepsia, and esophagitis)

Abdominal and chest pain; bone and musculoskeletal pain

Caution with bisphosphonates applies to active upper GI problems, for example dysphagia, GERD, gastritis, or ulcers

Precautions or contraindications for bisphosphonates apply to:

Hypocalcemia

Renal failure

Drugs associated with gastric irritation (ASA, NSAIDs)

Inability to sit upright for 30–60 min after taking the drug

PATIENT EDUCATION

Patients taking bisphosphonates should be instructed regarding:

The importance of taking the medicine with a full glass of water (6–8 oz) at least 30 min before the first food, beverage, or medication of the day

Not lying down or eating or drinking anything else for at least 30–60 min to prevent reflux and avoid esophageal irritation

Contacting the health care provider if there is pain while swallowing, difficulty swallowing, worsening heartburn, or thigh or groin pain

Taking supplemental calcium and vitamin D if dietary intake is inadequate

Performing weight-bearing exercises

Modification of cigarette smoking and alcohol and caffeine consumption, if these factors exist

---

Hormones
Estrogens

Before menopause, estrogen helps to maintain a normal bone reabsorption rate in women. As will be discussed in Chapter 24, **hormone replacement therapy (HRT)**—estrogen with or without progestin—is recommended for postmenopausal osteoporosis prevention (secondary to estrogen deficiency) *only* when the patients are unable to take other agents and when the benefits outweigh risks. The FDA recommends prescribing the lowest possible dose for the shortest period of time. If HRT is started soon after menopause, estrogen prevents the accelerated phase of bone loss that occurs in the first five years after the onset of menopause.

Selective Estrogen Receptor Modifiers

Raloxifene (Evista) is a selective estrogen receptor modifier (SERM) with estrogen agonist activity on bone and lipids and estrogen antagonist activity on breast and uterine tissue. These properties result in increased bone mineral density, decreased bone reabsorption, and reduced fracture risk without promoting breast or endometrial cancer.

The incidence of vaginal bleeding and breast tenderness is lower with raloxifene than with HRT. However, in contrast to HRT, raloxifene can cause hot flashes and muscle cramps in the legs. Raloxifene is contraindicated in pregnancy and women with a history of thromboembolic disorders.

Calcitonin–Salmon

A synthetic form of the hormone calcitonin is available as a nasal spray (Miacalcin) or as a subcutaneous injection for the treatment of postmenopausal osteoporosis in women who are more than five years past menopause. Calcitonin is involved with calcium regulation, increases spinal bone density, and provides an analgesic effect in acute vertebral fractures. Calcitonin is reserved for women who refuse or cannot tolerate HRT or in whom HRT is contraindicated. Local nasal effects (e.g., irritation, redness, rhinitis, and epistaxis [nosebleed]) are the most common adverse effects from the nasal spray.

Store the unopened bottle of calcitonin in the refrigerator. Once the pump has been activated, store at room temperature in an upright position. Discard all unrefrigerated bottles after 30 days.

Parathyroid Hormone

Teriparatide (Forteo) is an injectable form of parathyroid hormone approved for postmenopausal women and men with osteoporosis who are at a high risk for having a fracture. It increases GI calcium absorption and renal tubular reabsorption of calcium, increasing the bone mineral density, bone mass, and strength. Common adverse effects include nausea, hypotension, dizziness, arthralgia (joint pain), and leg cramps. Safety and efficacy beyond two years has not been established and is not recommended.

Monoclonal Antibodies

Prolia (denosumab) is the newest treatment option for osteoporosis in both men and women. It works by inhibiting osteoclast (responsible for bone resorption) activity and is normally reserved for patients who are at a high risk of fracture or have proven to be intolerant to traditional therapy. Prolia is a subcutaneous injection and is given biannually. It is commonly used in combination with calcium and vitamin D supplementation and Forteo (teriparatide).

See Table 21-3 for a summary of osteoporosis therapy.

TABLE 21-3   Agents for Osteoporosis Prevention and Therapy

GENERIC NAME	TRADE NAME	PREVENTION DOSE	TREATMENT DOSE	COMMENTS
Hormones				
Selective estrogen Receptor modifier				
raloxifene	Evista	PO 60 mg daily	PO 60 mg daily	Can be given without regard to meals
Calcitonin–salmon				
calcitonin–salmon	Miacalcin	Not indicated	Intranasally 200 units (one activation) daily	Alternate nares
Parathyroid hormone				
teriparatide	Forteo	Not indicated	Subcu 20 mcg daily	For up to two years
Bisphosphonates				
alendronate	Fosamax	PO 5 mg daily ac	PO 10 mg daily ac	See Patient Education
		PO 35 mg qwk ac	PO 70 mg qwk ac	
			PO 40 mg daily ac for 6 months	For Paget's disease
ibandronate	Boniva	PO 2.5 mg daily ac	PO 2.5 mg daily ac	See Patient Education
		PO 150 mg qmo	PO 150 mg qmo	
			IV 3 mg bolus q3 months (over 15–30 sec)	
risedronate	Actonel	PO 5 mg daily ac	PO 5 mg daily ac	See Patient Education
		PO 35 mg qwk ac	PO 35 mg qwk ac	
		PO 150 mg qmo	PO 150 mg qmo	
zoledronic acid	Reclast	IV 5mg every 2 years	PO 30 mg daily ac for two months IV 5mg every 1 year	For Paget's disease Should be infused over at least 15 minutes
Monoclonal antibodies				
denosumab	Prolia	-	SC 60mg every 6 months	Supplement with calcium and vitamin D. Also used for certain cancers.

Note: Other dosing regimens are available.

CASE STUDY A

Musculoskeletal Drugs

Tavin Brown pulls a muscle in his back while helping his daughter move into her college dorm. He is now experiencing severe back spasms.

1. Tavin visits his primary care physician, who prescribes cyclobenzaprine, a skeletal muscle relaxant. He cautions Tavin that he might experience which side effect?
   a. Hypertension
   b. Dizziness
   c. Palpitations
   d. Insomnia

2. Tavin's physician also explains that this medication should be taken for which time frame?
   a. Intermittently as needed
   b. Short term
   c. Minimum of six months
   d. One year

3. The physician reviews Tavin's past medical history to determine if he has a condition that would require caution. What is an example of this?
   a. Past history of muscle strain
   b. Cataracts
   c. Impaired kidney function
   d. Past history of appendicitis

4. After prescribing the medication to Tavin, the physician cautions him to be careful in taking other medications with this muscle relaxant. What is one category of medications that may cause a potentiated effect?
   a. Antiemetics
   b. Anticoagulants
   c. Anticholinergics
   d. Antihistamines

5. Tavin has been taking cyclobenzeprine for two days. He has experienced some relief from his back spasms, but now is complaining of a dry mouth. What action would the physician take after hearing about this symptom?
   a. Advise him to discontinue the medication immediately.
   b. Advise him to take an antihistamine as he might be experiencing an allergic reaction.
   c. Explain that this is a common side effect.
   d. Inquire if he is experiencing urinary urgency.

CASE STUDY B

Anti-Inflammatory Drugs

Nahal Reddy has been experiencing pain in her right knee. After examination of the knee, her nurse practitioner (NP) recommends taking an NSAID drug.

1. The NP explains that the medication's action is to reduce inflammation by:
   a. Increasing the synthesis of prostaglandins
   b. Inhibiting the synthesis of prostaglandins
   c. Reducing white blood cells in the affected joint
   d. Increasing blood flow to the affected joint

2. Which age group is particularly susceptible to side effects from NSAIDs?
   a. Young children
   b. Young adults
   c. Postmenopausal women
   d. Older adults

3. A frequent side effect of NSAIDs is:
   a. Diarrhea
   b. Urinary frequency
   c. Hypotension
   d. GI ulceration and bleeding

4. In an effort to reduce the potential side effects while taking NSAIDs, the NP suggests that Nahal:
   a. Take the medication with a small sip of water
   b. Take the medication with meals
   c. Avoid enteric-coated capsules
   d. Take the medication on an empty stomach

5. Nahal expresses concern about taking medication, including the NSAID. What would be the most appropriate explanation from the NP regarding NSAIDs and the risk of cardiovascular disease?
   a. NSAIDs are not safe for heart patients.
   b. NSAIDs have a greater GI risk than cardiovascular risk.
   c. NSAIDs have no risk.
   d. NSAIDs can increase the risk of adverse events for individuals with a history of cardiovascular disease.

CHAPTER REVIEW QUIZ

Match the medication in the first column with the appropriate classification in the second column. Classifications may be used more than once.

Medication

1. ____ Dantrolene
2. ____ Arthrotec
3. ____ Mobic
4. ____ Actonel
5. ____ Voltaren
6. ____ Flexeril
7. ____ Nabumetone
8. ____ Evista
9. ____ Celebrex

Classifications

a. Combination NSAID
b. Osteoporosis therapy
c. Muscle relaxant for multiple sclerosis
d. Muscle relaxant for acute muscle strain
e. Partially selective NSAID
f. Nonselective NSAID
g. COX-2 inhibitor

Choose the correct answer.

10. Patients with which respiratory condition may manifest a sensitivity to aspirin and other NSAIDs?
    a. Allergies
    c. Cystic fibrosis
    b. Frequent upper respiratory infections
    d. Asthma

11. A patient taking an NSAID who develops ringing in the ears should be instructed to take which action?
    a. Discontinue the drug.
    c. Make an appointment with an audiologist.
    b. Go immediately to the ER.
    d. Reduce the dosage in half.

12. The mechanism of action of bisphosphonates is to:
    a. Increase bone development
    c. Inhibit bone resorption
    b. Increase bone resorption
    d. Increase calcium deposition into the bone

13. Which of the following is a selective estrogen receptor modifier?
    a. Alendronate
    b. Teriparatide
    c. Raloxifene
    d. Calcitonin-salmon

14. What is a key point to review with a patient taking a bisphosphonate?
    a. Take NSAIDs for discomfort
    b. Avoid weight-bearing exercise.
    c. Increase caffeine consumption.
    d. Sit upright for 30–60 min after taking the drug.

15. Combining salicylates and alcohol increases the risk for:
    a. Anemia
    b. The possibility of GI bleed
    c. Reye's syndrome
    d. The possibility of accelerated clotting time

16. Unless otherwise directed by a physician, what is the maximum number of days that an OTC NSAID should be taken?
    a. Three
    b. Seven
    c. Ten
    d. Fourteen

17. The muscle relaxant dantrolene is used to treat:
    a. Amyotrophic lateral sclerosis (ALS)
    b. Rheumatic disorders
    c. Poststroke contractures
    d. Spasticity associated with cerebral palsy

18. Suppose NSAIDs are suggested as a treatment for a lengthy time period. How will they most likely be prescribed?
    a. Variable doses on consecutive days
    b. Alternate day dosing
    c. A dose as low as possible for effectiveness
    d. A three-day drug holiday once a month

19. Which drug category may potentiate the possibility of bleeding when taking NSAIDs?
    a. Multivitamins
    b. Antianxiety drugs
    c. Antihistamines
    d. Anticoagulants

20. Which medication for osteoporosis would be a poor choice in a patient who has stage III renal failure?
    a. Calcium and vitamin D supplementation TID
    b. Actonel
    c. Prolia
    d. Reclast

STUDYGUIDE

Online Resources

P R A C T I C E

Complete Chapter 21

- Powerpoint presentations
- Videos

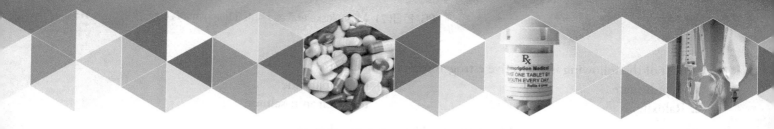

CHAPTER 22

ANTICONVULSANTS, ANTIPARKINSONIAN DRUGS, AND AGENTS FOR ALZHEIMER'S DISEASE

KEY TERMS AND CONCEPTS

Absence seizure

Alzheimer's disease

Anticholinergics

Anticonvulsants

Antiepileptic drug (AED) therapy

Antiparkinsonian drugs

Drug-induced parkinsonism (DIP)

Epilepsy

Febrile seizures

Mixed seizure

Neuroleptic malignant syndrome

Parkinson's disease

Partial seizures

Primary generalized seizure

Psychomotor epilepsy

Restless legs syndrome (RLS)

Status epilepticus

Temporal lobe seizures

Tonic-clonic seizures

Unilateral seizures

OBJECTIVES

Upon completion of this chapter, the learner should be able to

1. Compare and contrast different types of seizures
2. List the medications used for each type of epilepsy and common side effects
3. Describe the drug therapy for febrile seizures.
4. List the drugs used for parkinsonism and common side effects
5. Describe the patient education appropriate for those receiving anticonvulsants and antiparkinsonian drugs
6. Describe the drug therapy for the treatment of restless legs syndrome
7. Describe the drugs for the treatment of Alzheimer's disease
8. Define the Key Terms and Concepts

ANTICONVULSANTS

Seizures are brief, abnormal neuronal discharges in the brain that occur repeatedly and without warning. **Anticonvulsants** are used to reduce the number or severity of seizures in patients with epilepsy. **Epilepsy**, which is defined as two or more unprovoked seizures separated by 24h, is characterized by sudden attacks of altered consciousness, motor activity, or sensory impairment. Epilepsy is the fourth most common neurological disorder in the United States after migraine, stroke, and Alzheimer's disease.

Treatment is based on the type, severity, and cause of seizures. Although less than half of epileptic seizures have an identifiable cause, seizures may sometimes be associated with cerebrovascular disease, cerebral trauma, intracranial infection or fever, brain tumor, intoxication, or chemical imbalance. Sometimes the underlying disorder can be corrected, for example fever, hypoglycemia, or electrolyte imbalance, and anticonvulsive medicine is not indicated.

Seizures are described in two major groups that are differentiated by how and where they begin in the brain:

1. *Primary generalized seizures*—begin with widespread electrical discharge that involves both sides of the brain at once. The result is bilaterally symmetrical and without local onset; further classified as convulsive (tonic, clonic, and tonic-clonic) or nonconvulsive (absence, myoclonic, and atonic)

2. *Partial seizures* (also known as focal seizures)—begin with an electrical discharge in one limited area of the brain. If there is no loss of consciousness, it is classified as a simple partial seizure. If there is loss of consciousness, it is called a complex partial seizure. Less than 15% of all seizures are partial.

Treatment failure can be the result of inappropriate selection of an anticonvulsant for the specific type of seizure. For example, carbamazepine is used to treat many types of seizures; however, it is well known to aggravate myoclonic and absence seizures. Drug therapy is individualized, and the selection of the most appropriate drug is based on the seizure type and other patient factors. Once the treatment is started, approximately 50% of patients achieve adequate seizure control with monotherapy (one drug).

CLINICAL CONNECTION

Driving With Seizure-Related Conditions

Given the symptoms of seizures, it is understandable that it is not advisable for a person who has uncontrolled seizures to operate a vehicle in public to protect both themselves and others from potential harm. Even though this may seem logical, there are currently no definitive laws established to prohibit those affected with seizures from driving if they already have a valid driver's license. Instead, patients rely on the advice of their physician. In general, it is recommended that a person who has been diagnosed with an acute seizure disorder (from a car accident or other head trauma) should be symptom free for three to six months before resuming driving. For a person who suffers from a chronic seizure condition, it is recommended that the seizures are controlled one to two years before driving. Although these are recommendations and not laws, patients should be informed that they will be held liable for accidents that may occur if or when they drive against physician recommendations. Additionally, it should be noted that there are laws and regulations that vary by state that require new drivers to be seizure free for a period of time (similar to the above time frames) prior to being granted a license.

Primary Generalized Seizures

Generalized seizures include *tonic-clonic* (formerly called *grand mal*) and *absence* (formerly called *petit mal*) seizures and occur in about 40% of patients with epilepsy. Tonic pertains to tension or contraction, particularly muscle contraction. **Tonic-clonic seizures** are characterized by an abrupt loss of consciousness and falling, with tonic extension of trunk and extremities (tonic phase), followed by alternating contractions and relaxation of the muscles (clonic phase). The attack usually lasts 2–5 min, and urinary and fecal incontinence may occur. During the recovery period, patients are confused and sleepy and may complain of a headache.

Initial treatment consists *only* of preventing injury by removing any objects that could cause trauma, cushioning the head and turning it to the side, and loosening tight clothing, especially collars and belts. Do not try to open the mouth or force anything between the teeth, see Figure 22-1.

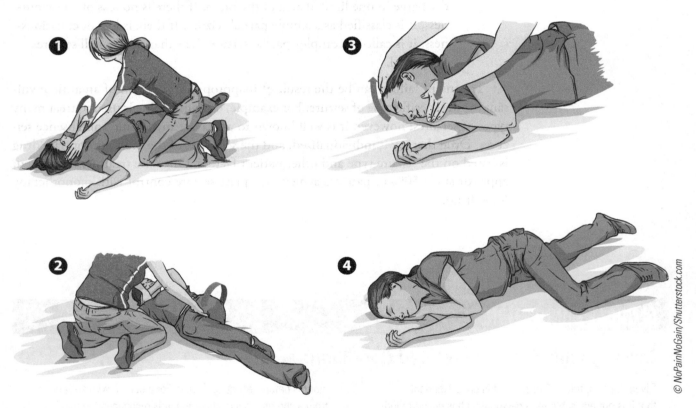

FIGURE 22-1 Bystanders should never attempt to inhibit the movement of a person who is having a seizure. The only action should be to safely assist them to the ground if needed, ensure the area is safe and to move them on their side.

If seizures are prolonged or so frequent that the patient does not regain consciousness between seizures, the condition is known as status epilepticus and is considered to be a true neurologic emergency. This condition has a reported fatality rate of up to 30%–40% after diagnosis. The treatment of choice is IV lorazepam (Ativan) administered slowly. Simultaneous loading with IV phenytoin or fosphenytoin is also recommended. In addition, if the cause of status epilepticus is known, reversal of the cause should be immediately addressed.

Absence seizures previously called petit mal, is so called because of the absence of convulsions. It is characterized by a sudden onset, a brief 10–20 sec loss of consciousness with no falling, and usually occurs initially in children. This can appear as staring into space. Absence seizures are not associated with postrecovery drowsiness. Patients with childhood absence epilepsy frequently achieve remission with increasing age or treatment.

Febrile seizures are the most common childhood seizure disorder, occurring in approximately 3% of children ages 6 months to 6 years. Its presence may signify a serious underlying acute infection such as sepsis or bacterial meningitis. Most febrile seizures are "simple"—single, brief (less than 15 min in duration), and generalized. Resolving the underlying condition is generally sufficient treatment for these types of seizures and daily medication is not necessary.

Partial Seizures

Partial seizures (also known as psychomotor epilepsy or temporal lobe seizures) account for up to 60% of new cases of epilepsy. They are caused by a lesion in the temporal lobe of the brain and limited to one cerebral hemisphere. Most seizures last from 10 sec. to 5 min. Complex symptoms can include confusion, impaired understanding and judgment, staggering, purposeless movements, bizarre behavior, and unintelligible sounds, but no convulsions. A partial seizure may be preceded by a subjective but recognizable sensation (an aura) that a seizure is going to occur.

Unilateral seizures affect only one side of the body. Some patients may have mixed seizure patterns combining more than one type. It is important to observe and report the type and length of seizures and general responsiveness to medications.

DRUG THERAPY FOR GENERALIZED AND PARTIAL SEIZURES

First-Generation Anticonvulsants

Prophylactic treatment of *generalized and partial seizures when indicated* should be started with a single drug such as valproate, lamotrigine, levetiracetam, carbamazepine, oxcarbazepine, or phenytoin. The dosage should be titrated to achieve seizure control or until the maximally tolerated dose is reached. The aim of this therapy is to prevent seizures without oversedation, and the dosage is adjusted according to the individual patient response and serum drug levels when available.

Side effects of phenytoin can include:

- ❗ Sedation, ataxia, dizziness, and headache
- ❗ Blurred vision, nystagmus, and diplopia
- ❗ Gingivitis (inflamed gums)

! GI distress, including nausea, vomiting, anorexia, constipation, or diarrhea

! Rash and dermatitis, Stevens–Johnson syndrome (a severe inflammatory disease affecting children and young adults), and lupus-like symptoms

Megaloblastic anemia (treated with folic acid)

Osteomalacia (bone softening, treated with vitamin D)

Syncope, arrhythmias, and hypotension with IV use

Precautions or contraindications with phenytoin apply to:

Kidney or liver disease

Diabetes

Heart failure, bradycardia, heart block, and hypotension

Pregnancy and lactation

Hematological disease

Abrupt discontinuation

There are many drug *interactions* and food or nutrient interactions with phenytoin, including:

Cimetidine, isoniazid, salicylates, SSRIs, sulfonamides, topiramate, and trimethoprim may increase the levels of phenytoin.

Phenytoin may decrease the effectiveness of "azole" antifungals, carbamazepine, estrogens, oral contraceptives, protease inhibitors, certain antidepressants and antipsychotics, valproic acid, and "statins."

Another medicine sometimes used for partial, generalized, or mixed seizures is carbamazepine (Tegretol). It has the advantage of minimal sedation and cognitive adverse effects.

Side effects of carbamazepine can include:

Ataxia, syncope (fainting), and visual difficulties

Risk for hyponatremia (decreased level of sodium in the blood)

! Cardiac, hematological, kidney, liver, and pancreas complications

Rash, for example Stevens–Johnson syndrome (see Glossary) (more likely to occur in Asian patients who test positive for an inherited variant of an immune system gene; FDA recommends genetic testing of patients of Asian descent prior to starting therapy)

Multiple *interactions* of carbamazepine occur with:

Phenytoin, phenobarbital, and rifampin (decrease levels of carbamazepine)

Calcium channel blockers, cimetidine, macrolides (e.g., erythromycin), azole antifungals, certain antipsychotics, protease inhibitors, valproic acid, and isoniazid (increase levels of carbamazepine)

Warfarin (increased metabolism, decreased effect)

Grapefruit juice potentiates action and can increase the risk of serious adverse effects. Do not take grapefruit juice with carbamazepine.

Note

The FDA has alerted health care professionals of an increased risk of suicidal ideation and behavior in patients receiving anticonvulsants to treat epilepsy, psychiatric disorders, or other conditions (e.g., migraine, neuropathic pain). All patients beginning treatment with anticonvulsants or currently receiving such treatment should be closely monitored for emerging or worsening suicidal thoughts and behavior, depression, and/or unusual changes in mood or behavior.

Oxcarbazepine (Trileptal), a second-generation oral anticonvulsant indicated for the treatment of partial seizures, is an analogue of carbamazepine. It is as effective as the first-generation agents and may be less likely than carbamazepine to cause CNS side effects and hematological abnormalities. Oxcarbazepine does not generally require drug level monitoring, and it appears to have less significant drug interactions.

Valproic acid (Depakene, Depakote) is considered a broad-spectrum anticonvulsant, useful for the management of many seizure types, including generalized tonic-clonic, absence, and myoclonic seizures. Dosage adjustments may be needed in hepatic diseases.

Side effects of valproic acid include:

- ! Weight gain and dyspepsia
- ! Alopecia, rash, and tremor
- ! Hepatotoxicity, life-threatening pancreatitis (black box warning), and blood dyscrasias

Multiple *interactions* of valproic acid occur with:

Carbamazepine, phenytoin, phenobarbital protease inhibitors, and rifampin (decrease valproic acid levels)

Chlorpromazine, felbamate, guanfacine, salicylates, and topiramate (increase valproic acid levels or effects)

DRUG THERAPY FOR FEBRILE SEIZURES

Routine treatment of febrile seizures involves searching for the cause of the fever and taking measures to control the fever (e.g., with the use of antipyretics). Most children with febrile seizures do not require anticonvulsant drugs. Those that do may be treated with rectal diazepam rectal gel if the seizure lasts longer than 5 min. The American Academy of Pediatrics Subcommittee on Febrile Seizures does not currently recommend continuous or intermittent antiepileptic drug (AED) therapy for children with one or more simple febrile seizures. A decision to use prophylactic AEDs for children with complex febrile seizures should be made on an individual basis taking into account the underlying risk factors for recurrence.

DRUG THERAPY FOR ABSENCE SEIZURES

The drug of choice for the management of absence epilepsy is often ethosuximide (Zarontin), which is effective only for this type of epilepsy and lacks the idiosyncratic hepatotoxicity of valproic acid. Other drugs sometimes used in the treatment of absence seizures, when Zarontin is ineffective, include clonazepam (Klonopin), valproic acid (Depakene), and lamotrigine (Lamictal).

Side effects of the drugs used for absence epilepsy can include:

- ! Sedation, dizziness, headaches, aggression, or irritability
- ! Gastrointestinal (GI) distress, including anorexia, nausea, vomiting, and diarrhea (take with food to minimize these effects)

Rash and blood dyscrasias

Precautions or contraindications with drugs used for absence epilepsy apply to:

Hepatic or renal disease

Pregnancy and lactation

Pancreatitis (with valproate)

Abrupt discontinuation

Interactions occur between ethosuximide and:

Carbamazepine, phenytoin, primidone, phenobarbital, valproic acid, rifampin, isoniazid, and antiretroviral protease inhibitors

Alternative formulations of traditional anticonvulsants have been developed, for example carbamazepine (Tegretol XR—extended release), diazepam (Diastat—rectal), fosphenytoin (Cerebyx—IM/IV), and valproate (Depacon—IV; Depakote ER—extended release). The primary advantage of these formulations may include improved adherence (fewer doses and/or better tolerability) or the availability of an injectable formulation (e.g., Depacon).

Second-Generation Anticonvulsants

The second-generation anticonvulsants include gabapentin (Neurontin), lamotrigine (Lamictal), levetiracetam (Keppra), oxcarbazepine, and topiramate (Topamax), which are used for the adjuvant treatment of partial (psychomotor) and generalized seizures. They are not currently considered superior in efficacy to the first-generation anticonvulsants in terms of seizure control. However, these agents usually do not require drug level monitoring, have fewer adverse effects (including effects on cognition), have fewer drug interactions than the first-generation anticonvulsants, and may improve adherence with once or twice daily dosing. All agents require a *slow titration period* to avoid central nervous system (CNS) adverse effects and to minimize the potential of a severe life-threatening rash with lamotrigine. The second-generation anticonvulsants should be used with caution in pregnant and lactating women and should not be abruptly discontinued.

See Table 22-1 for a summary of the anticonvulsants. (Refer to Chapter 19 for a discussion on phenobarbital, and Chapter 20 for a discussion on the benzodiazepines: lorazepam, clonazepam, and diazepam.)

TABLE 22-1 Anticonvulsants

GENERIC NAME	TRADE NAME	DOSAGE	COMMENTS
First Generation			
carbamazepine	Tegretol	PO 400 mg–1.2 g daily in three to four divided doses, susp, tabs	For partial or generalized seizures
	Tegretol XR	PO 200–600 mg BID, ERa caps, tabs	Extended release; do not crush or chew
fosphenytoin	(Cerebyx)[b]	IV, IM, dose varies	Caution—do not confuse with Celexa (antidepressant) or Celebrex (for arthritis)
phenytoin	Dilantin	PO 200–1,200 mg daily in divided doses, IV varies, no IM	For generalized or partial seizures and status epilepticus
ethosuximide	Zarontin	PO 250 mg–1.5 g daily in divided doses	For absence seizures only

(continued)

TABLE 22-1   **Anticonvulsants (*continued*)**

GENERIC NAME	TRADE NAME	DOSAGE	COMMENTS
First Generation			
valproic acid	Depakene[c], Depakote DR[d]	PO 15–60 mg/kg daily in two to three divided doses	For absence, partial, and generalized seizures
	Depakote ER[a]	8%–20% higher than the daily dose of Depakote given once daily	One dose per day; do not crush or chew
	Depacon	IV 15–60 mg/kg daily in divided doses	
Second Generation			
gabapentin	Neurontin	PO Initial dose of 300mg TID, titrate up to 600mg TID. Higher doses may be used if tolerated	Narrow spectrum agent with no drug interactions Max dose of 2400mg/day
			Decrease dose with renal dysfunction
lamotrigine	Lamictal	PO 100–250 mg BID (gradual titration to avoid the potential of severe skin rash)	Interactions with antiepileptic drugs mostly, hepatic and drug interaction dose adjustment needed
			Caution—do not confuse with Lamisil (antifungal)
levetiracetam	Keppra	PO, IV 500–3,000 mg daily divided BID	Broad-spectrum efficacy; no significant drug interactions
oxcarbazepine	Trileptal	PO 300–2,400 mg daily divided BID (renal dose adjustment may be needed)	Less significant drug interactions compared to carbamazepine; risk for hyponatremia
topiramate	Topamax	PO 50–200 mg daily BID (gradual titration; renal dose adjustment may be needed)	Interactions with antiepileptic drugs mostly; may affect cognitive function at high doses. Risk of metabolic acidosis, nephrolithiasis, and weight loss

a. Extended release.
b. This brand name is no longer marketed, but the name is still commonly used.
c. Regular release.
d. Delayed release.

PATIENT EDUCATION

Patients taking any anticonvulsant medication should be instructed regarding:

Reading the provided Medication Guide before they start taking an anticonvulsant and each time they get a refill

Caution with driving or operating machinery until they are regulated with the medication, because of drowsiness or dizziness

Reporting of any side effects, such as rash or eye problems, staggering, slurred speech, and any other symptoms

Careful oral hygiene until tenderness of the gums subsides as treatment progresses

Always taking the medication on time and *never* omitting dosage (abrupt withdrawal of the medication can lead to status epilepticus)

Wearing Medic-Alert tag or bracelet at all times in case of accident or injury

Taking the medication with food or milk to lessen stomach upset

Checking with the health care provider before initiating any new treatments, including OTC and herbal products. (Anticonvulsants are associated with numerous and potentially harmful drug–drug interactions.)

Not significantly altering the ingestion of grapefruit juice while on carbamazepine (Tegretol) because of potentiation of effect

Parents and teachers should be cautioned to observe and report changes in cognitive function, mood, and behavior in children receiving anticonvulsants

Some anticonvulsants cause an increased risk of birth defects if used during pregnancy; women of childbearing age taking anticonvulsants should be educated on using proper contraception

ANTIPARKINSONIAN DRUGS

Antiparkinsonian drugs are usually given for **Parkinson's disease (PD)**, a chronic neurological disorder characterized by fine, slowly spreading muscle tremors, rigidity, and generalized slowness of movement called bradykinesia (see Figure 22-2). PD is one of the most common neurodegenerative diseases in adults. As the disease advances, patients develop a tendency to fall, dementia, confusion, psychosis, sleep disturbances, and declining cognitive function. Most patients with PD progress to severe disability over 10–20 years. There is no cure for Parkinson's disease, and the goal of the treatment is to relieve symptoms and maintain mobility.

PARKINSON'S DISEASE

WHAT IS PARKINSON'S DISEASE?

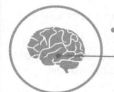
BRAIN
NEURON CELL

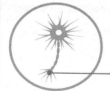
NEURON CELL
TERMINAL BRANCH

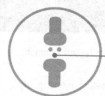
TERMINAL BRANCH
DOPAMINE

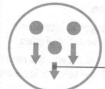
DOPAMINE
WEAK SIGNAL

PARKINSON'S DISEASE SYMPTOMS

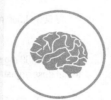
MEMORY LOSS, DEMENTIA
ANXIETY, DEPRESSION
HALLUCINATIONS

SLOW BLINKING
NO FACIAL EXPRESSION
DROOLING
DIFFICULTY SWALLOWING

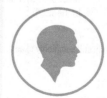
SHAKING, TREMORS
LOSS OF SMALL OR FINE
HAND MOVEMENTS

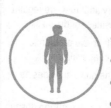
PROBLEM WITH BALANCE
OR WALKING
STOOPED POSTURE
ACHES AND PAINS
CONSTIPATION

FIGURE 22-2 Parkinson's disease overview.

The underlying pathology of PD is not completely understood, but normal dopamine activity as it relates to acetylcholine is diminished, and relative overactivity of cholinergic output results. This serves as the foundation of treatments for PD.

Before initiating treatment, it is important to rule out **drug-induced parkinsonism (DIP)** as a causative factor of PD. DIP is the most common form of *secondary* parkinsonism and is frequently unrecognized or misdiagnosed. Causes of DIP generally include dopamine receptor antagonists and other drugs that interfere with dopamine synthesis or release. Switching from, reducing, or discontinuing the offending agent (such as antipsychotics, calcium channel blockers, anticonvulsants, lithium, metoclopramide, and antidepressants) may be the most effective treatment option available.

Dopamine Replacement
Carbidopa–Levodopa

Levodopa crosses the blood–brain barrier, where it is converted to dopamine. Carbidopa enhances the effects of levodopa, thereby increasing the therapeutic effect of dopamine in the CNS and reducing its adverse reactions (e.g., nausea, vomiting, and low blood pressure upon standing). Sinemet (a combination of levodopa and carbidopa) is most often used for long-term treatment and is recommended as an initial drug treatment for patients with bradykinesia uncontrolled by other PD medications. As PD progresses, most patients will eventually require treatment with levodopa.

Side effects of Sinemet, which are numerous and frequent, can include:

- ❗ Dyskinesias (involuntary movements of many parts of the body)
- ❗ Nausea, vomiting, and anorexia (if given with food to prevent nausea, the protein load should be low to avoid competition for transport across the GI tract)
- ❗ Behavioral changes, anxiety, agitation, confusion, sleep disturbances, depression, hallucinations, and psychosis
- ❗ Hypotension, dizziness, and syncope

Precautions or contraindications for Sinemet apply to:

Abrupt discontinuation, which could lead to neuroleptic malignant syndrome (characterized by delirium, rigid muscles, fever, and autonomic nervous system instability)

Bronchial asthma or emphysema

Cardiac disease or hypotension

Active peptic ulcer

Diabetes and renal or hepatic disease

Glaucoma

Psychoses

Pregnant, postpartum, or nursing women

Interactions of Sinemet may occur with:

Antihypertensives (may potentiate hypotensive effect)

Antipsychotics (antagonistic by blocking the dopamine receptor)

Phenytoin (antagonizes levodopa)

Iron salts (reduce bioavailability)

Foods high in protein (reduce absorption)

Non-specific (type A) monoamine oxidase inhibitors (MAOIs) (may cause hypertensive crisis)

Patients receiving Sinemet for prolonged periods of time (two to five years) may develop a tolerance, resulting in ineffectiveness of the drug, called "wearing off." Sometimes, changing the timing of doses, adding an extra dose at the end of the day, or adding another agent from one of the drug classes listed below may bring the symptoms back under control.

Dopamine Agonists

The newer dopamine agonists (non-ergot derivatives) pramipexole (Mirapex) and ropinirole (Requip) are commonly used in conjunction with levodopa to delay the onset of levodopa-caused motor complications or used alone in early PD or in younger patients as a "levodopa-sparing" strategy. Dopamine agonists may reduce the required dose of levodopa for patients with advanced Parkinson's. The older dopamine agonists (ergot derivatives) such as bromocriptine (Parlodel) are used much less frequently now in PD because of serious adverse effects.

Some experts recommend dopamine agonists as initial monotherapy in patients less than 60 years old. These agents have a greater specificity for dopamine receptors and may have a neuroprotective effect, which leads to less dyskinesia, may delay the *wearing off* effect, and can postpone the need for Sinemet by several years.

Side effects of dopamine agonists are similar to those of Sinemet and can include:

⚠ Psychosis, hallucinations, obsessive behavior, impulsivity, confusion, and somnambulism or sleepwalking (higher risk compared to Sinemet)

⚠ Excessive sedation leading to "sleep attacks" during daily activities, including driving

⚠ Hypotension, syncope, and peripheral edema

⚠ Nausea and vomiting

Pulmonary, renal, and cardiac valve fibrosis with bromocriptine

Neuroleptic malignant syndrome with abrupt discontinuation

Interactions of dopamine agonists may occur with:

Antidopamine agents (i.e., antipsychotics, phenothiazines, metoclopramide) may decrease the efficacy of each agent

CNS depressants such as anxiolytics and hypnotic and sedative agents may increase the risk of somnolence

Rotigotine (Neupro patch) is a dopamine agonist applied topically with once daily dosing. The continuous transdermal delivery of drug may be advantageous for patients who have poorly controlled PD symptoms in the early morning, slowed GI motility associated with levodopa treatment, dysphagia, or have difficulty swallowing. Side effects of rotigotine are similar to other dopamine agonists, in addition to application site reactions (rotate the patch location).

MAO-B Inhibitors

Monoamine oxidase-B (MAO-B) is an enzyme responsible for breaking down dopamine and tyramine in the brain. In PD, MAO-B inhibitors will therefore increase the levels of dopamine.

Selegiline

Selegiline (*Eldepryl*) and *rasagiline* (*Azilect*) are selective MAO type-B inhibitors. Selegiline is sometimes prescribed as an adjunctive therapy for PD after levodopa has been used for several years and begins to "wear off," or become less effective. When Sinemet and selegiline or rasagiline are used *concurrently*, the Sinemet dosage is reduced by 10%–30% to lessen the chance of additive side effects.

Side effects of MAO B inhibitors include nausea, dizziness, confusion, abdominal pain, hallucinations, dry mouth, vivid dreams, dyskinesias, and headache. Selegiline is metabolized to amphetamine metabolites, which may contribute to its side effects (especially anxiety and sleeplessness); therefore the drug should be given no later than early afternoon.

Contraindicated with the following drugs that can interact with selegiline, resulting in rare but *severe* CNS toxicity, hyperpyrexia, hypertensive crisis, and even death. Do *not* use selegiline with:

   Meperidine (Demerol), methadone, and tramadol

   Tricyclic antidepressants

   Selective serotonin reuptake inhibitors (SSRIs) and selective norepinephrine reuptake inhibitors (SNRIs)

   Sympathomimetics (e.g., epinephrine, ephedrine, pseudoephedrine)

   Dextromethorphan and St. John's wort

   Abrupt discontinuation is contraindicated

When given at the recommended dosages, there is minimal danger of a hypertensive crisis associated with interactions of other MAOIs and certain foods (the "cheese reaction"). See Chapter 20 for a description of this reaction, which can occur if the recommended dosage is exceeded. No dietary restrictions are recommended for selegiline at the recommended dose.

An orally disintegrating tablet (ODT) formulation of selegilene (Zelapar) is available as an adjunct to levodopa. Selegilene ODT is absorbed through the buccal membrane, avoiding the first-pass hepatic metabolism. This results in a faster onset of action, the use of a lower dose, and fewer amphetamine metabolites.

Rasagiline

Rasagiline (Azilect) is currently the only MAO-B inhibitor approved as initial monotherapy for PD; it is also approved as an addition to levodopa later in the disease. Rasagiline is given only once daily, has no amphetamine metabolites, and is generally well tolerated. Side effects include headache, nausea, joint pain, hypotension, hallucinations, dyskinesias, depression, and dyspepsia. Contraindications are similar to selegiline.

Anticholinergic Agents

Drugs with anticholinergic and antihistaminic actions were the first to be used for tremors associated with PD and are still useful in the early stages of the disease in younger patients and for DIP. These agents restore the cholinergic–dopaminergic balance in PD. The anticholinergics include synthetic atropine-like drugs, such as benztropine (Cogentin) and trihexyphenidyl (Artane), which are used to treat parkinson-like tremors associated with the long-term use of antipsychotics or for other forms of parkinsonian syndromes. (See Chapter 13, "Autonomic Nervous System Drugs.")

Side effects of the anticholinergic agents are:

- ❗ Dry mouth
- ❗ Dizziness and drowsiness
- ❗ Blurred vision
- Constipation or urinary retention
- ❗ Confusion
- Depression
- Nausea
- ❗ Tachycardia

Precautions or contraindications for anticholinergics apply to:

Abrupt discontinuation (leads to rebound symptoms)

Closed-angle glaucoma

Use with caution in older patients because of the risk of cognitive impairment. Those with benign prostatic hyperplasia (BPH) are also at risk for urinary retention.

Amantadine

Another drug unrelated to the other antiparkinsonian agents is the antiviral agent amantadine. It alters dopamine release and has anticholinergic properties. Amantadine is used to treat parkinsonism (extrapyramidal reactions) associated with the prolonged use of phenothiazines, carbon monoxide poisoning, or cerebral arteriosclerosis in older adults. For PD, amantadine is generally used early in the disease as monotherapy, its efficacy may wane rather quickly (weeks or months), and it is of little benefit when added to levodopa.

Side effects of amantadine, usually dose related and reversible, can include:

- ❗ CNS disturbances, including depression, confusion, hallucinations, anxiety, depression, irritability, nervousness, and dizziness
- Headache, weakness, and insomnia
- ❗ Heart failure, edema, and hypotension
- ❗ GI distress, constipation, and urinary retention

Precautions or contraindications for amantadine apply to:

Abrupt discontinuation

Liver and kidney diseases (requires renal dose adjustment)

Cardiac disorders

Psychosis, neurosis, and mental depression

Epilepsy

Patients taking CNS drugs

COMT Inhibitors

Catechol-*O*-methyl-transferase (COMT) inhibitors, such as entacapone (Comtan) and tolcapone (Tasmar), block the enzyme responsible for metabolizing peripheral levodopa. COMT inhibitors increase the concentration of levodopa and dopamine. This allows the patient's dose of levodopa to be lowered and results in a decrease in the incidence or severity of the dose-related side effects of levodopa (e.g., dyskinesias, nausea).

Entacapone is also available in combination with carbidopa/levodopa (Stalevo), which provides the convenience of fewer pills, but dosing is less flexible for patients who need varying amounts of levodopa throughout the day. Because of the severe nature of adverse effects associated with tolcapone and extensive monitoring, it is reserved for patients who do not respond to other therapies.

Side effects of entacapone and tolcapone are similar and can include:

- ❗ Orthostatic hypotension
- ❗ Hallucinations
- ❗ Dyskinesia (levodopa dose may need to be decreased)

  Nausea and vomiting

- ❗ Diarrhea (can be severe) and abdominal pain

  Orange coloration of the urine

Hepatic injury with tolcapone (black box warning)—the treating physician is to obtain a patient-signed consent form acknowledging this risk; monitor hepatic enzymes throughout the treatment

Drug interactions: Patients taking entacapone or tolcapone should not receive *nonselective* MAOIs (phenelzine or tranylcypromine), but can take a *selective* MAOI such as selegiline. Concomitant use of CNS depressants should be avoided to prevent additive sedation.

PATIENT EDUCATION

Patients taking antiparkinsonian drugs should be instructed regarding:

Administration on a regular schedule as prescribed, with food to lessen GI distress; give carbidopa/levodopa with a low-protein meal if food is necessary to offset nausea

Avoiding abrupt withdrawal of the medication, which may greatly increase parkinsonian symptoms and the risk of neuroleptic malignant syndrome

Several weeks sometimes required before benefit is apparent

Caution with CNS drugs, alcohol, or antihypertensives (not taking other medicines, including vitamins, without physician approval)

Caution with driving or operation of machinery

The fact that drugs may cause drowsiness, dizziness, or lightheadedness; with pramipexole, there may be no warning signs before falling asleep while engaged in activities of daily living

Reporting adverse side effects to the physician (e.g., involuntary movements, blurred vision, constipation, urinary retention, GI symptoms, palpitations, and mental changes)

With dopamine agonists, there may be intense urges to gamble or spend money, increased sexual urges, bouts of binge eating, and other intense urges

Reporting any signs that the drug is no longer effective after prolonged use (sometimes after months or years the dosage may need to be increased or another drug may need to be substituted by the physician); avoiding any dosage changes without medical supervision

Maintaining physical activity, self-care, and social interaction, an essential part of therapy for Parkinson's disease

Rising slowly

See Table 22-2 for a summary of the antiparkinsonian drugs.

TABLE 22-2 Antiparkinsonian Drugs

GENERIC NAME	TRADE NAME	DOSAGE	COMMENTS
Dopamine replacement			
carbidopa and levodopa	Sinemet,	PO 10/100–200/2,000 mg in three to six divided doses pc	Immediate release tab
	Parcopa		Orally disintegrating tab
	Sinemet CR	PO 25/100–400/2,000 mg in two to four divided doses pc	Separate doses by at least 6h
Dopamine agonists			
bromocriptine	Parlodel	PO 1.25 mg BID with meals	Used with Sinemet; dosage gradually increased to optimum maintenance dose (up to 40 mg per day)
pramipexole	Mirapex	PO 0.125 mg TID (renal dose adjustments may be needed)	Increase to a max daily dose of 4.5 mg per day for desired effect balanced against side effects
ropinirole	Requip	PO 0.25 mg TID	Increase to a max daily dose of 24 mg per day for desired effect balanced against side effects
rotigotine	Neupro	2–8 mg/24h transdermally titrate upward by 2 mg per week; taper if discontinuing	Also for the treatment of restless legs syndrome
Anticholinergics			
benztropine	Cogentin	PO, IM, or IV 0.5–6 mg daily in one or divided doses	Not for the older adult
			For drug-induced parkinsonism and other forms of parkinsonian syndrome
trihexyphenidyl	(Artane)[a]	PO 1–15 mg daily in divided doses	For drug-induced parkinsonism and other forms of parkinsonian syndrome
COMT inhibitor			
entacapone	Comtan	200 mg with each dose of Sinemet (max 1,600 mg per day)	Use only with Sinemet
with carbidopa/levodopa	Stalevo	PO (various strengths) TID up to 6–8 tabs per day	Do not crush

(continued)

TABLE 22-2 Antiparkinsonian Drugs (*continued*)

GENERIC NAME	TRADE NAME	DOSAGE	COMMENTS
MAO B inhibitors			
rasagiline	Azilect	PO 0.5–1 mg daily	Reduce dose with hepatic impairment
selegiline	Eldepryl	PO 5 mg BID (second dose no later than 2 pm)	Used when levodopa wears off; levodopa dosage can be decreased
	Zelapar	PO 1.25–2.5 mg daily	Orally disintegrating tablet
Other agents			
amantadine	(Symmetrel)[a]	PO 100–400 mg in daily divided doses	Also for the treatment and prophylaxis of influenza A and drug-induced parkinsonism

a. This brand name is no longer marketed, but the name is still commonly used.

AGENTS FOR RESTLESS LEGS SYNDROME

Restless legs syndrome (RLS) is a sensorimotor neurologic disorder characterized by a distressing urge to move the legs, often accompanied by a marked sense of discomfort in the legs (aching, burning, pulling, itching, or tingling). RLS is triggered by rest or inactivity and is temporarily relieved by movement. It follows a circadian pattern, with symptoms being most intense in the evening and nighttime. It is usually disruptive to sleep, which is the primary reason patients seek treatment.

The etiology of RLS is either primary or secondary. Primary RLS involves the CNS and the dopaminergic pathway. The dopamine agonists pramipexole (Mirapex), ropinirole (Requip), and rotigotine (Neupro patch) used to treat PD (even though RLS is not related to PD) are FDA approved for RLS treatment as well. The dosages of the oral agents when used to treat RLS are typically only 10%–20% of those used to treat PD (50% for the transdermal patch) and are usually given 1–3 h before bedtime as a single daily dose. Apply the rotigotine patch at approximately the same time every day. The most worrisome side effects with the dopamine agonists in PD, such as dyskinesias, have not been observed in patients treated for RLS.

Gabapentin (Neurontin), benzodiazepines (such as clonazepam), and opioids (hydrocodone, oxycodone, tramadol) are second-line agents for RLS cases involving specific symptoms like continuous sleep disturbances or painful sensations in the extremities.

RLS may be secondary to other causes, including iron deficiency (with or without anemia), renal failure, diabetes, rheumatoid arthritis, fibromyalgia, vitamin deficiency (folate, B_{12}), hypothyroidism, and pregnancy. Treatment of secondary RLS focuses on identifying and treating the underlying cause. Medications that have the potential to aggravate RLS symptoms, such as metoclopramide, all neuroleptics, many antidepressants, and antihistamines, should be discontinued if possible.

AGENTS FOR ALZHEIMER'S DISEASE

Dementia is an umbrella term describing a variety of diseases and conditions that develop when nerve cells in the brain die or no longer function normally. **Alzheimer's disease (AD),** or dementia of the Alzheimer's type, is the most common type of dementia. It is characterized by a devastating, progressive decline in cognitive function, having a gradual onset, usually beginning between 60 and 90 years of age, followed by increasingly severe impairment in social and occupational functioning. AD is ultimately fatal.

Although the precise etiology of Alzheimer's disease is uncertain, cholinergic systems appear to be most clearly compromised and are frequently the target of current drug treatment. As AD progresses, behavioral and psychiatric symptoms are common. Nondrug interventions include trying to identify the problematic behaviors, understanding their triggers, and minimizing or eliminating those causes. These include maintaining a stable, low-stress environment; avoiding noise and glare; providing security objects; and daytime activity to improve nighttime sleep.

Cholinesterase Inhibitors

The first class of agents shown to be efficacious for the delay of symptoms in Alzheimer's disease is the cholinesterase inhibitors. These agents prevent the breakdown of acetylcholine in the synaptic cleft, thereby increasing acetylcholine levels and improving cognitive function, but do not treat the underlying pathology of the disease. They may slow the progression but do not cure the disease.

Tacrine (Cognex) was the first drug approved in this class but was associated with significant hepatotoxicity and a frequent dosing schedule and is no longer available. Donepezil (Aricept), galantamine (Razadyne), and rivastigmine (Exelon) are not associated with hepatotoxicity but do exhibit cholinergic side effects and dizziness. All drugs in this class cause GI upset (nausea, vomiting, diarrhea, abdominal cramps, anorexia, and weight loss), requiring slow dose titration to improve patient tolerance.

Interactions of cholinesterase inhibitors occur with:

Anticholinergics (may decrease effectiveness—avoid using together)

Cholinergics (bethanechol) and succinylcholine (may have a synergistic effect—monitor the patient closely)

Precautions or contraindications for cholinesterase inhibitors apply to:

GI bleeding and peptic ulcer disease

Cardiac disease (potential for bradycardia or syncope)

COPD (exacerbates the underlying disease)

Jaundice and renal disease

Pregnancy and lactation

Abrupt discontinuation (limit the sudden decline in cognitive function or increase in behavioral disturbances)

NMDA Receptor Antagonists

Memantine (Namenda) is the first *N*-methyl-*D*-aspartate (NMDA) antagonist approved for the treatment of moderate-to-severe dementia of the Alzheimer's type. Memantine is thought to selectively block the excitotoxic effects with abnormal transmission of the neurotransmitter glutamate. It can be used as monotherapy or in combination therapy with cholinesterase inhibitors. Memantine may be efficacious in the earlier stages of Alzheimer's disease as well, delaying the progression of symptoms, allowing patients to maintain certain daily functions for a little longer than they would without the drug.

Side effects of memantine involve the CNS, are dose-dependent, and include:

- (!) Confusion, cerebrovascular disorder, falls, and agitation
- (!) Dizziness, headache, constipation, and cough

Precautions or contraindications apply to pregnancy, lactation, use in children, and renal disease.

Drug interactions occur with other NMDA antagonists (amantadine, ketamine, and dextromethorphan) and certain antiarrythmics

Ultimately, the decision on whether to continue drug therapy in Alzheimer's patients is based on the quality of life, treatment goals, potential benefits, adverse effects, and costs. If the quality of life is poor, stabilizing or slowing further decline may not be an appropriate goal, and drug therapy should be discontinued.

See Table 22-3 for a summary of Alzheimer's drugs.

TABLE 22-3   Agents for Alzheimer's Disease (AD)

GENERIC NAME	TRADE NAME	DOSAGE	COMMENTS
Cholinesterase inhibitors			
donepezil	Aricept	PO 5 mg at bedtime, increase to 10 mg after four to six weeks, up to 23 mg	5 mg for mild to moderate AD 10 mg for mild, moderate, and severe AD
			23 mg for moderate to severe AD
	Aricept ODT		Orally disintegrating tablet
rivastigmine	Exelon	PO 1.5 mg BID with food	Increase to 3–6 mg BID (higher doses may be more beneficial)
		Patch 4.6 mg per 24 h titrate to 9.5 mg per 24 h after four weeks	Rotate application sites; can increase up to max effective dose of 13.3 mg per 24h
galantamine	Razadyne[a]	PO 4–12 mg BID with food	Caution with hepatic or renal disease
	Razadyne ER	PO 8 mg daily with food	Titrate to 16–24 mg once daily; do not crush

(continued)

TABLE 22-3   **Agents for Alzheimer's Disease (AD)** (*continued*)

GENERIC NAME	TRADE NAME	DOSAGE	COMMENTS
NMDA receptor antagonist			
memantine	Namenda	PO 5 mg per day initially titrate to 10 mg BID over four weeks	Can be used as monotherapy or in combination therapy with cholinesterase inhibitors
			CNS side effects, especially agitation
	Namenda XR	PO 7 mg per day initially, titrate to 28 mg once daily over four weeks	Do not crush or chew; may open capsule and sprinkle contents on applesauce before swallowing

a. Formerly Reminyl.

CASE STUDY A

Anticonvulsant Drugs

While standing in line with a friend at a local coffee shop, 22-year-old Danielle Miller abruptly loses consciousness and falls to the ground. For the next 2 min, she experiences alternating contraction and relaxation of her extremities. Her friend instructs the coffee shop cashier to call 911 to report that a customer is having a seizure.

1. What type of seizure is Danielle experiencing?
  a. Atypical
  b. Generalized
  c. Febrile
  d. Partial

2. After Danielle is treated in the ER and seen by a neurologist, she is prescribed carbamazepine. The nurse explains that she might experience what side effect from the drug?
  a. Hypernatremia
  b. Gingivitis
  c. Ataxia
  d. Headache

3. The nurse also cautions Danielle that carbamazepine has multiple interactions with other substances. Which of the following should she avoid because it can potentiate the effect of carbamazepine?
  a. Rifampin
  b. Phenobarbital
  c. Green tea
  d. Grapefruit juice

4. Which category of drug can increase the levels of carbamazepine?
  a. Calcium channel blockers
  b. Antidiarrheals
  c. Anticoagulants
  d. Antacids

5. Danielle is concerned about her quality of daily life while taking carbamazepine. What can the nurse explain as an advantage of taking carbamazepine for seizure control?
  a. No liver or kidney complications
  b. Minimal sedation and cognitive effects
  c. No cardiac complications
  d. Can be taken while pregnant

CASE STUDY B

Mitchell Grange is at the neurologist's office to receive the results of recent testing after Mitchell's complaints of muscle tremors, rigidity, and slow movement.

1. The physician explains that Mitchell has Parkinson's disease (PD), a chronic neurological disease characterized by:
   a. Akathesia
   b. Tardive dyskinesia
   c. Myocutaneous tightening
   d. Bradykinesia

2. The neurologist prescribes an antiparkinsonian drug, Sinemet, and instructs Mitchell on which of the following?
   a. The drug may cause increased wakefulness.
   b. Expect to see the benefits of the drug in three to five days.
   c. Take the drug with a small nonprotein snack to lessen GI distress.
   d. Stop taking the drug immediately if feeling side effects.

3. The physician also explains to Mitchell that caution should be exercised when he gets up to walk. This is because Sinemet can cause which side effect?
   a. Seizures
   b. Hypotension
   c. Blurred vision
   d. Muscular weakness

4. An abrupt discontinuation of Sinemet can lead to which complication?
   a. Myocardial infarction
   b. Severe shortness of breath
   c. Hypoglycemia
   d. Neuroleptic malignant syndrome

5. An interaction of Sinemet may occur with:
   a. Antihypertensives
   b. Multivitamins
   c. Antidepressants
   d. Foods high in carbohydrate

CHAPTER REVIEW QUIZ

Match the medication in the first column with the condition in the second column that it is used to treat. Conditions may be used more than once.

Medication	Condition
1. ____ Aricept	**a.** Seizures
2. ____ Entacapone	**b.** Absence seizure
3. ____ Neurontin	**c.** Parkinson's disease
4. ____ Lamictal	**d.** Extrapyramidal reactions
5. ____ Zarontin	**e.** Alzheimer's disease
6. ____ Amantadine	
7. ____ Depakote	
8. ____ Cogentin	
9. ____ Topamax	
10. ____ Razadyne	

Choose the correct answer.

11. A common side effect of phenytoin is:
   a. Hypertension
   b. Muscle cramps
   c. Sedation
   d. Dehydration

12. Health care professionals should closely monitor patients receiving anticonvulsants for which condition?
   a. Hyperactivity
   b. Mania
   c. Insomnia
   d. Suicidal ideation

13. Which of the following can interact with carbamazepine (Tegretol), potentiating the risk of side effects?
   a. Dairy products
   b. Grapefruit juice
   c. Aspirin
   d. Iron

14. Anticholinergics used to treat younger patients with PD may cause which side effect?
   a. Drooling
   b. Night sweats
   c. Dry mouth
   d. Bradycardia

15. Caution should be used when administering memantine to patients with Alzheimer's disease because there is an increased risk of:
   a. Diabetic ketoacidosis
   b. Falls
   c. Nausea and vomiting
   d. Decreased gag reflex

16. Patients taking any anticonvulsant medication should be instructed to
   a. Take the medication with food
   b. Expect slurred speech with the first dose
   c. Omit a dose if experiencing nausea
   d. Perform vigorous dental hygiene

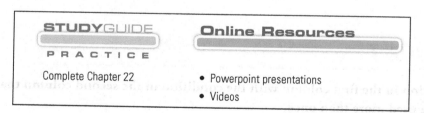

STUDYGUIDE

PRACTICE

Complete Chapter 22

Online Resources

- Powerpoint presentations
- Videos

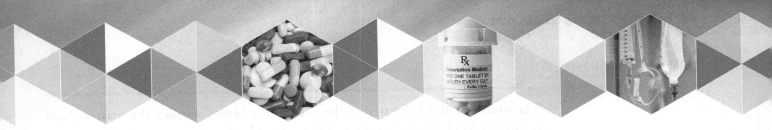

CHAPTER 23
ENDOCRINE SYSTEM DRUGS

KEY TERMS AND CONCEPTS

Antidiabetic

Antithyroid

Corticosteroids

Endocrine

Hormones

Hyperglycemia

Hypoglycemia

Hypothyroidism

Immunosuppressant

Sulfonylureas

OBJECTIVES

Upon completion of this chapter, the learner should be able to

1. Identify the hormones secreted by these four endocrine glands: pituitary, adrenals, thyroid, and pancreas

2. Describe at least five conditions that can be treated with corticosteroids

3. Explain the administration practice important to corticosteroid therapy

4. List at least four serious potential side effects of long-term steroid therapy

5. Compare and contrast medications given for hypothyroidism and hyperthyroidism

6. Describe the side effects of thyroid and antithyroid agents

7. Identify the symptoms of hypoglycemia and hyperglycemia and appropriate interventions

8. Explain the uses and side effects of oral and injectable noninsulin antidiabetics

9. Compare and contrast insulins according to their action (rapid, intermediate, and long-acting), naming the onset, peak, and duration of each category

10. Explain appropriate patient education for those receiving endocrine system drugs

11. Define the Key Terms and Concepts

The endocrine system, much like the nervous system, is a body control system. Unlike the nervous system, it often exerts its affects more slowly and over a longer period of time. *Endo* means *within* and endocrine refers to an internal secretion of *hormone*s produced by a ductless gland that secretes directly into the bloodstream. **Hormones** are chemical messengers that have specialized functions in regulating the activities of specific cells or organs as they travel though the bloodstream to their targets. Endocrine system drugs include natural hormones secreted by the ductless glands or synthetic substitutes. Hormones that affect the reproductive system are discussed in Chapter 24. This chapter covers four categories: pituitary hormones, adrenal corticosteroids, thyroid agents, and antidiabetic agents.

PITUITARY HORMONES

The pituitary gland, located at the base of the brain, is called the master gland because it regulates the function of the other glands. It secretes several hormones including somatotropin, adrenocorticotropic hormone (ACTH), thyroid-stimulating hormone (TSH), and gonadotropic hormones (FSH, LH, and LTH; see Chapter 24). The two pituitary hormones discussed in this chapter are somatotropin and ACTH.

The anterior pituitary lobe hormone, somatotropin, is called human growth hormone (HGH) because it regulates growth. Insufficient production of HGH will result in growth abnormalities, which should be treated only by an endocrinologist.

Adrenocorticotropic hormone (ACTH) is available only for parenteral use as corticotropin. Cosyntropin (Cortrosyn), a synthetic peptide of ACTH, is used mainly for the diagnosis of adrenocortical insufficiency. Treatment of associated disorders is usually reserved for the corticosteroids in which the dosage is more easily regulated and for which oral forms are available as well.

ADRENAL CORTICOSTEROIDS

The adrenal glands, located adjacent to the kidneys, secrete hormones called **corticosteroids**, which act on the immune system to *suppress the body's response to infection or trauma.* They *relieve inflammation, reduce swelling,* and *suppress symptoms* in acute conditions. Corticosteroid use primarily can be subdivided into two broad categories: (1) as replacement therapy when secretions of the pituitary or adrenal glands are deficient (e.g., for Addison's disease) and (2) as anti-inflammatory and **immunosuppressant** agents.

Corticosteroid therapy is *not curative* but is used as *supportive therapy with other medications.* Some conditions treated with corticosteroids include:

Allergic reactions (e.g., to insect bites, poison plants, chemicals, or other medications) in which there are symptoms of rash, hives, or anaphylaxis

Acute flare-ups of rheumatic or collagen disorders, especially where only a few inflamed joints can be injected with corticosteroids to decrease crippling or in life-threatening situations, such as rheumatic carditis or lupus

Acute flare-ups of severe skin conditions that do not respond to conservative therapy; topical applications are preferable to systemic therapy, when possible, to minimize side effects

Acute respiratory disorders such as status asthmaticus (persistent and intractable asthma) (intravenous preparations are preferable) and sarcoidosis or to prevent hyaline membrane disease in premature infants by administering IM to the mother at least 24h before delivery

Long-term prevention of symptoms in severe persistent asthma or chronic management of COPD (oral inhalations are preferable for both conditions) at the lowest possible effective dose

Malignancies (e.g., leukemia, lymphoma, and Hodgkin's disease), in which corticosteroids (e.g., prednisone) are used with other antineoplastic drugs as part of the chemotherapy regimen; treatment of nausea and vomiting associated with chemotherapy (e.g., dexamethasone)

Cerebral edema associated with brain tumor or neurosurgery

Organ transplant, in which corticosteroids are used with other immunosuppressive drugs to prevent the rejection of transplanted organs

Life-threatening shock owing to adrenocortical insufficiency; treatment of other forms of shock is controversial

Acute flare-ups of ulcerative colitis; short-term use only to avoid hemorrhage

Prolonged administration of corticosteroids can cause suppression of the pituitary gland with adrenocortical atrophy, in which the body no longer produces its own hormone. To minimize this effect, intermediate-acting corticosteroids (prednisone, methylprednisolone) can be given by alternate-day therapy when they are required for extended time periods. Withdrawal of corticosteroids following long-term therapy should always be gradual with step-down (i.e., tapering) dosage to allow the body's normal hormone production and regulation to return. This is especially important with patients whose therapy exceeds 14 consecutive days at a dose of 20 mg or prednisone (or equivalent) per day or more. Abrupt withdrawal can lead to acute adrenal insufficiency, shock, and even death.

Because of the potentially serious side effects, corticosteroids are administered for as short a time as possible and *locally if possible* to reduce systemic effects (e.g., in ointment, intra-articular injections, ophthalmic drops, and respiratory aerosol inhalants). Local administration reduces the dosage by avoiding the first-pass effect and going directly to the site of need. For *acute* episodes, some oral corticosteroids are available in *dose packs* (e.g., Medrol Dosepak, prednisone pak, DexPak TaperPak) to facilitate dose tapering.

Side effects of the corticosteroids used for longer than very brief periods can be quite serious and possibly include:

Adrenocortical insufficiency and adrenocortical atrophy

❗ Delayed wound healing and *increased susceptibility to infection*

Fluid and electrolyte imbalance, possibly resulting in edema, potassium loss, hypertension, and heart failure

❗ Muscle pain or weakness

❗ Osteoporosis with fractures, especially in older women

❗ Stunting of growth in children (premature closure of bone ends)

Increased intraocular pressure or cataracts

❗ Cushing's syndrome, including obesity of the trunk, "moon face," acne, hirsutism (see Glossary), amenorrhea, and *hyperglycemia*

Nausea, vomiting, diarrhea, or constipation

❗ *Gastric* or esophageal irritation, ulceration, or hemorrhage

⚠ CNS effects including headache, vertigo, insomnia, euphoria, psychosis, or anxiety

⚠ Petechiae, easy bruising, and skin thinning and tearing

⚠ Increased blood sugar or fluctuating blood sugar levels (counsel patients who test blood sugar regularly)

Precautions or contraindications apply to:

Long-term use (regulated carefully; avoid abrupt discontinuation)

Viral or bacterial infections (used only in life-threatening situations along with appropriate anti-infectives)

Fungal infections (only if specific therapy is concurrent)

Hypothyroidism or cirrhosis (exaggerated response to corticosteroids)

Hypertension or heart failure

Patients with psychosis or emotional instability

Diabetes (drugs increase hyperglycemia)

Glaucoma (drugs may increase intraocular pressure)

Cataracts (cause or worsening of cataracts)

History of gastric or esophageal irritation (may precipitate ulcers)

Children (drugs may retard growth)

Pregnancy and lactation

History of thromboembolic disorders or seizures

Interactions may occur with:

Barbiturates, phenytoin (Dilantin), and rifampin (may reduce the effectiveness of corticosteroids)

Estrogen and oral contraceptives (may potentiate corticosteroids)

Nonsteroidal anti-inflammatory agents or salicylates (e.g., aspirin may increase the risk of GI ulceration)

Diuretics (potentiate potassium depletion, e.g., thiazides and furosemide)

Live-virus vaccines and toxoids (long-term or high-dose corticosteroids inhibit the antibody response)

Bupropion (dose-related risk of seizures)

Haloperidol (increased risk of QT prolongation)

See Table 23-1 for a summary of the pituitary and adrenal corticosteroids.

TABLE 23-1 Pituitary and Adrenal Corticosteroid Drugs

GENERIC NAME	TRADE NAME	DOSAGE
Pituitary Drugs		
corticotropin (ACTH)	H. P. Acthar Gel	IM, subcu repository gel for injection
cosyntropin	Cortrosyn	IM and IV for adrenocortical insufficiency diagnosis

(continued)

TABLE 23-1 **Pituitary and Adrenal Corticosteroid Drugs (*continued*)**

GENERIC NAME	TRADE NAME	DOSAGE
Adrenal Corticosteroids[a]		
cortisone		PO for replacement
dexamethasone	(Decadron)[b]	PO, IV, IM
fludrocortisone	(Florinef)[b]	PO, for orthostatic hypotension
hydrocortisone	Cortef or Solu-Cortef	PO, IV, deep IM, subcu
methylprednisolone	Medrol, Depo-Medrol, or Solu-Medrol	PO, IV, deep IM, intra-articular
prednisone	Sterapred	PO (tab or liquid); do not confuse with prednisolone
triamcinolone	Kenalog	IM, intra-articular (never IV)

Note: Many other products are available. This is a representative list. Topical products are discussed in Chapter 12, and oral and nasal inhalation products are discussed in Chapter 26.
a. Dosage varies greatly depending on the condition treated; large doses may be given for acute conditions on a short-term basis; long-term therapy can be given on an alternate-day basis with intermediate-acting agents, and dosage is reduced gradually to lowest possible effective dose.
b. This brand name is no longer marketed, but the name is still commonly used.

PATIENT EDUCATION

Patients taking corticosteroids should be instructed regarding:

Following exact dosage and administration orders (never taking longer than indicated and never stopping medicine abruptly)

Notifying the physician of any signs of infection or trauma *while taking corticosteroids or within 12 months after long-term therapy is discontinued* and similarly notifying the surgeon, dentist, or anesthesiologist if required

Taking oral corticosteroids during or immediately after meals or with milk to decrease gastric irritation

Taking single daily or alternate-day doses prior to 9 A.M. Take multiple doses at evenly spaced intervals throughout the day but not near bedtime

Avoiding any other drugs at the same time (including OTC drugs, e.g., aspirin) without the physician's approval (antacids or other antiulcer drugs are sometimes prescribed)

Side effects to expect with the long-term therapy (e.g., fluid retention and edema)

Dangers of infection, delayed wound healing, osteoporosis, and mental disorders

Reporting any side effects to the physician immediately

THYROID DISORDERS

An estimated 20 million Americans will develop a thyroid disorder during their lifetime. The thyroid is an endocrine gland located in the front part of the neck and is responsible for regulating the rate of metabolism. When thyroid levels are low, the pituitary gland releases TSH. TSH promotes the biosynthesis and secretion of the two bioactive thyroid hormones thyroxine (T4) and triiodothyronine (T3, the active form of thyroid hormone). Thyroxine is the major product of the thyroid gland, and much of it is later converted in the body to the active T3 form.

Thyroid Agents

Thyroid agents can be natural (thyroid) or synthetic (e.g., Synthroid). Thyroid preparations are used in replacement therapy for **hypothyroidism**, the most common thyroid problem in the United States, which is caused by diminished or absent thyroid function. Synthetic agents, such as levothyroxine (Levoxyl), are generally preferred because T4 is a prohormone, and this allows the patient's own physiological mechanisms to control the production of T3. See Figure 23-1 for common symptoms of hypothyroidism.

Symptoms of HYPOTHYROIDISM

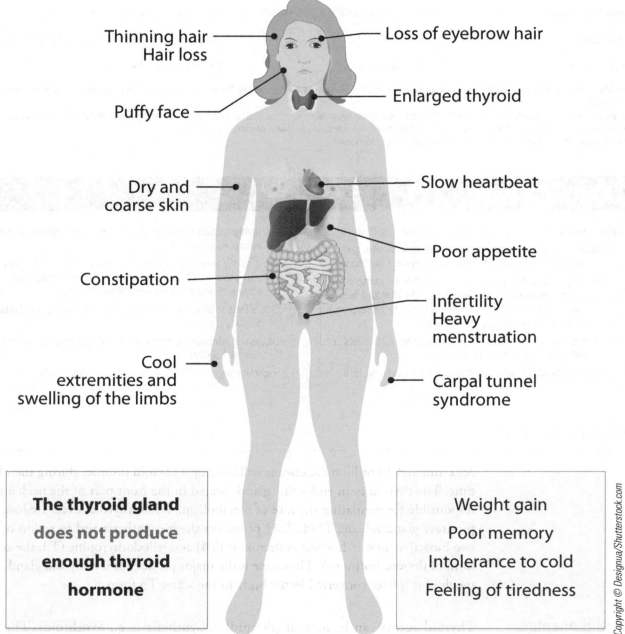

Thinning hair
Hair loss

Loss of eyebrow hair

Puffy face

Enlarged thyroid

Dry and coarse skin

Slow heartbeat

Poor appetite

Constipation

Infertility
Heavy
menstruation

Cool extremities and swelling of the limbs

Carpal tunnel syndrome

The thyroid gland does not produce enough thyroid hormone

Weight gain
Poor memory
Intolerance to cold
Feeling of tiredness

FIGURE 23-1 Hypothyroid disorders can present with symptoms that manifest throughout the body.

Hypothyroid conditions requiring replacement therapy include *cretinism* (congenital; requires immediate treatment to prevent mental retardation) and *myxedema* or adult hypothyroidism owing to simple goiter, Hashimoto's thyroiditis, pituitary disorders, medications (amiodarone, lithium), and thyroid destruction from surgery or radiation. Hypothyroidism causes slowed metabolism with symptoms ranging from fatigue, somnolence, dry skin, thinning hair, weight gain, constipation, sensitivity to cold, and irregular menses to mental deterioration (including depression) if untreated.

Transient hypothyroidism is rare, and thyroid replacement therapy for true hypothyroidism must be continued for life, although dosage adjustments may be required. Monitoring for toxic effects and periodic laboratory tests are recommended. Most patients are started on 100–125 mcg of levothyroxine as an initial dose. This starting value can vary based on severity of symptoms, TSH levels, and weight and body composition. Dosing adjustments are based off of patient reported symptoms for hyper or hypo thyroidism, as well as TSH levels that are generally drawn every four to six weeks until the dosage is stabilized.

Toxic effects are the result of overdosage of thyroid and are manifested in the signs of *hyperthyroidism*:

>   Palpitations, chest pain, tachycardia, cardiac arrhythmias, and increased blood pressure

>   Nervousness, difficulty concentrating, tremor, muscle weakness, headache, and insomnia

>   Weight loss (in spite of increased appetite), diarrhea, and abdominal cramps

>   Intolerance to heat, fever, and excessive sweating; easy fatigability

>   Menstrual irregularities; exophthalmos (bulging eyes)

Precautions or contraindications for thyroid apply to:

>   Cardiovascular disease, including angina pectoris, myocardial infarction and hypertension

>   Older adults (may precipitate dormant cardiac pathology)

>   Adrenal insufficiency (corticosteroids are required first)

>   Diabetes (close monitoring of blood glucose is required)

Interactions of thyroid may occur with:

>   Food (can diminish absorption by 50%)

>   Potentiation of oral anticoagulant effects if added after warfarin therapy is stabilized

>   Insulin and oral hypoglycemics (dosage adjustment is necessary)

>   Potentiation of adrenergic effect (e.g., epinephrine; watch closely!)

>   Estrogens and oral contraceptives (decreased thyroid response)

>   Amiodarone (contains about 37% iodine by weight but can cause either hypo- or hyperthyroidism; monitor for changes in thyroid function)

>   Aluminum/calcium/iron/magnesium salts, chromium, and sucralfate (decreased absorption; space several hours apart if possible)

>   Soy products (decreased response)

Note

The use of thyroid agents in weight reduction programs to increase metabolism when thyroid function is normal (euthyroid) is *contraindicated*, ineffective, and dangerous, leading to decrease in normal thyroid function and possibly life-threatening cardiac arrhythmias.

PATIENT EDUCATION

Patients being treated with thyroid medication should be instructed regarding:

Importance of taking the prescribed dosage of the thyroid medication consistently every day. It usually has to be taken for life. **Take on empty stomach 30–60 min prior to breakfast**

Importance of reporting any symptoms of overdose (e.g., palpitations, nervousness, excessive sweating, and unexplained weight loss)

Periodic laboratory tests to determine the effectiveness and proper dosage

Not changing from one brand to another or to a generic form without physician approval (if switched, TSH should be retested in six weeks)

CLINICAL CONNECTION

Narrow Therapeutic Index Drugs

Some medications are classified as narrow therapeutic index (NTI) drugs. This means that the range for therapeutic effect is very small, where a small increase in dosage could lead to an overdose (side effects) or a small decrease in dosage could lead to subtherapeutic effects. Because of this, these drugs are often dosed in micrograms rather than milligrams, which allows for more precise dosing for these often potent medications. NTI drugs often require laboratory monitoring to ensure that the desired drug levels are achieved. Levothyroxine (Synthroid) is one example of a NTI drug. Special care must be taken with NTI drugs, as an incorrect dose could have extreme effects. For example, patients are instructed to take levothyroxine on an empty stomach, if they do not do this regularly the absorption of the drug can vary greatly. Therefore, it is important to counsel patients to take exactly as prescribed, and to double check all doses upon dispensing NTI drugs.

Antithyroid Agents

Hyperthyroidism can be caused by Graves' disease (an autoimmune disorder where antibodies mistakenly attack the thyroid gland) and thyroiditis (inflammation of the thyroid gland). Orally administered radioactive iodine ablation (destruction) therapy is the most common treatment, and most patients are cured after a single dose. Surgery to remove all or part of the diseased thyroid is another permanent cure for hyperthyroidism but is seldom used now. The cure for hyperthyroidism is the destruction or removal of the gland resulting in hypothyroidism. This results in most people with hyperthyroidism needing lifelong hypothyroid treatment. See Figure 23-2.

Antithyroid agents (e.g., methimazole or Tapazole and propylthiouracil or PTU) are used *to relieve the symptoms of hyperthyroidism* in preparation for surgical or radioactive iodine therapy or for those who are not candidates for either procedure. Methimazole is generally considered the treatment of choice because it works faster and is less likely to cause liver injury than PTU. Antithyroid drugs are not helpful for the treatment of hyperthyroidism associated with thyroiditis, because this condition is due to the release, not the overproduction, of thyroid hormones.

Side effects of antithyroid agents are rare and may include:

Rash, urticaria, and pruritus (treat with antihistamines)

Abnormal sense of taste

Blood dyscrasias (especially agranulocytosis)

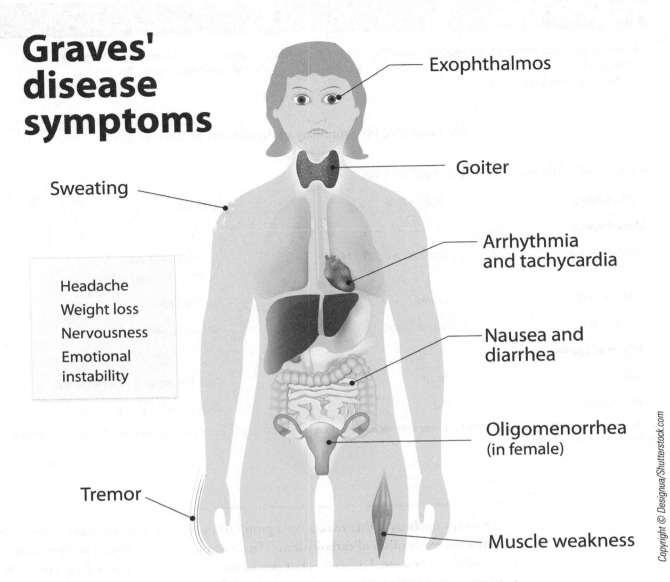

Graves' disease symptoms

- Exophthalmos
- Goiter
- Sweating
- Arrhythmia and tachycardia
- Nausea and diarrhea
- Oligomenorrhea (in female)
- Muscle weakness
- Tremor

Headache
Weight loss
Nervousness
Emotional instability

FIGURE 23-2 Graves' disease (hyperthyroid) can present with symptoms that manifest throughout the body.

Precautions or contraindications for antithyroid agents apply to:

Prolonged therapy (seldom used)

Patients older than 40 years old

Pregnancy and lactation

Hepatic disorders (black box warning with PTU)

Interactions occur with:

Other drugs causing agranulocytosis are potentiated

Excessive iodine intake or drugs containing iodine such as amiodarone (decreased efficacy)

PATIENT EDUCATION

Patients being treated with antithyroid medication should be instructed to:

Take doses at regular intervals

Notify the physician immediately of signs of illness (e.g., chills, fever, rash, sore throat, malaise, and jaundice).

See Table 23-2 for a summary of thyroid and antithyroid agents.

TABLE 23-2 **Thyroid and Antithyroid Agents**

GENERIC NAME	TRADE NAME	DOSAGE
Thyroid agents		
levothyroxine (T4)	Synthroid, Levothroid, Levoxyl	PO, 25–300 mcg daily[a] IV, 50% of PO dose initially
liothyronine (T3)	Cytomel	5–25 mcg daily
thyroid (T3 & T4)	Armour Thyroid	60–180 mg daily
Antithyroid agents		
methimazole	Tapazole	Tabs, 5–40 mg daily, in divided doses
propylthiouracil	PTU	Tabs, 100–400 mg daily in divided doses

a. When receiving orders for levothyroxine, caution is advised about decimal point placement (i.e., 0.025 mg vs. 0.25 mg) and dose conversions between mg and mcg, as medication errors have occurred.

ANTIDIABETIC AGENTS

Diabetes mellitus (DM) makes up a group of hormonal diseases characterized by impaired metabolism of carbohydrates, fats, and proteins that results in elevated levels of blood glucose. Diabetes is fast becoming one of the most prevalent and costly diseases in America, affecting almost 10% of the population, with many people not even knowing that they have the disease or at the prediabetic stage. Prediabetes is a condition where blood glucose levels are higher than normal but not high enough to be called diabetes.

DM is classified as insulin-dependent Type 1 (characterized by the destruction of pancreatic beta cells) or Type 2 (characterized by insulin resistance and deficiency). Type 1 diabetes was formerly described as juvenile diabetes because it was usually diagnosed in children and young adults. However, adults can also develop Type 1 diabetes and require insulin. Type 2 diabetes is the most common (90%–95%) form of diabetes. There is an increase in children and young adults with Type 2 because of an increase in the rate of obesity at an earlier age.

Type I diabetes results from a genetic or clinical destruction of pancreatic beta cells, whereas Type 2 results from a loss of sensitivity to insulin, which results from genetics or lifestyle (diet, exercise, etc.) or a combination of the two. Differences between the two disease states is outlined in chart Table 23-3.

TABLE 23-3   **Diabetes Type I vs. Type II**

CHARACTERISTIC	TYPE I	TYPE II
Age	Young (usually less than 35 years)	Older
Onset	Rapid (ketoacidosis)	Gradual with no symptoms in early stages
Body composition	Non-obese	Obese
Cause	Body cannot produce insulin	Insulin production is normal or altered to some degree. Body cells are resistant to insulin
Management	Insulin injections with diet and exercise	Oral /injectable non-insulin medications with insulin injections only if needed / diet and exercise

The result of long-term, poorly controlled diabetes is vascular injury, which is categorized as microvascular or macrovascular. Common microvascular complications include retinopathy, nephropathy, and neuropathy. Common macrovascular complications of diabetes include coronary artery disease (including myocardial infarction), cerebrovascular disease (including stroke), and peripheral vascular disease. DM is considered to be the seventh leading cause of death in the United States; about 70% of patients with diabetes die of heart disease or stroke. Health professionals of all disciplines have a responsibility to care for each patient in such a way that the risk of diabetic complications is minimized.

Medications that are administered to *lower blood glucose levels* include parenteral insulin and oral and injectable noninsulin antidiabetic agents.

Insulin

Insulin is required as replacement therapy for patients with Type 1 diabetes with insufficient production of insulin from the islets of Langerhans in the pancreas. Insulin is also required in patients with Type 2 diabetes who have failed to maintain satisfactory concentrations of blood glucose with therapy including dietary regulation and oral antidiabetic agents. Insulin is also indicated for patients with stable Type 2 diabetes at the time of surgery, fever, severe trauma, infection, serious renal or hepatic dysfunction, endocrine dysfunction, gangrene, or pregnancy. Insulin (regular) is used in the emergency treatment of diabetic ketoacidosis or coma.

Insulin must be administered parenterally because it is destroyed in the GI tract. Newer inhaled insulin preparations are currently being researched but are not yet used regularly in practice. All *injected* insulin products currently marketed are one of two types: biosynthetic human or analog. Biosynthetic insulins are referred to as "human" because their amino acid structure is identical to naturally occurring human insulin. Analog insulin (aspart, detemir, glargine, glulisine, and lispro) differs from human insulin only by substitution or position changes in the human insulin molecule, which mimics normal insulin secretion better than traditional insulins and reduces hypoglycemia. Biosynthetic and analog insulins are created using recombinant DNA technology.

Most of the insulin used today is U-100, which means that there are 100 units of insulin in each milliliter. The insulin syringe *must be marked U-100* to match the insulin used. Remember that on the 100-unit (1 mL) insulin syringe each line represents two units. If a smaller 50-unit (1/2 mL) syringe is used, each line represents one unit of insulin (see Chapters 4 and 9 for details). *Always have a clinician compare the insulin in the syringe with the dosage ordered to prevent errors*, which could have serious consequences. Another delivery option is prefilled insulin pens, which offer convenience and may help to avoid certain types of medication errors. In addition, implantable programmable insulin pumps are available that can administer insulin continuously through a catheter. Some pumps have internal glucose sensors to monitor levels. See Figure 23-3.

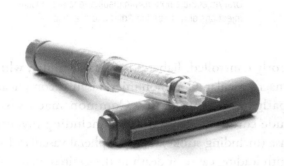

A

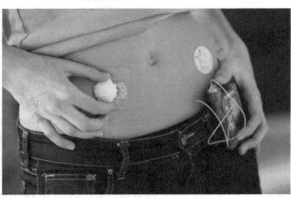

B

FIGURE 23-3 (A) Insulin pen: adjustable insulin dosage pen to regulate blood sugar levels. (B) Insulin pump: programmable implanted insulin pump administering continuous insulin subcutaneously to the fatty tissue layer. This pump has a glucose sensor to monitor glucose levels and adjust dosages. *Copyright © Rob Byron/www.Shutterstock.com. Garo/Phanie/Science Source.*

Insulin preparations differ mainly in their onset, peak, and duration of action (Table 23-4). Aspart, glulisine, and lispro insulins are ultra-*rapid acting* and have a *very short duration* of action. *Regular* insulin is *rapid acting* and has a *short duration*. *Regular* insulin may be given intravenously and intramuscularly as well as subcutaneously. Aspart, glulisine, and lispro are clear and rapid acting (onset in approximately 15 min). They peak in about 1h and last approximately 4h. They may be given subcutaneously or intravenously. *Isophane* (NPH) is intermediate acting; glargine and detemir are long acting, and they are administered subcutaneously.

TABLE 23-4　Insulins

ACTION	PREPARATION	TRADE NAME	ONSET	PEAK	DURATION
Rapid	aspart	Novolog	10–30 min	1–2 h	3–8 h
	glulisine	Apidra			
	lispro	Humalog			
Short	regular	Humulin R	30–60 min	1–5 h	6–10 h
		Novolin R			
Intermediate	isophane (NPH)	Humulin N	1–3 h	6–12 h	18–24 h
		Novolin N			
Long	glargine	Lantus	1–2 h	No pronounced peak	up to 24 h (dose dependent)

(continued)

TABLE 23-4   Insulins (*continued*)

ACTION	PREPARATION	TRADE NAME	ONSET	PEAK	DURATION
Ultra-long Acting	detemir	Levemir	1-2 h		
	degludec	Tresiba	1-2 h	No pronounced peak	Improved glycemic control
	glargine	Toujeo		No pronounced peak	Up to 24 h (more gradual release of insulin than Lantus)
Mixtures	NPH/reg	Humulin/Novolin 70/30, 50/50	30–60 min	1–4 h	16–24 h
	NPH/lispro	Humalog Mix 75/25, 50/50	15–30 min	1–6 h	12–24 h
	NPH/aspart	Novolog Mix 70/30	10–20 min	1–4 h	up to 24 h

Note: This is a representative list. Other insulin products are also available. Dosage varies. Because of limited use, beef- and pork-derived insulins and lente and ultralente insulins are no longer available in the United States. Before giving insulin, always check the expiration date on the vial and be sure that regular, as part, glulis-ine, and lispro insulins are clear and isophane insulins are cloudy. Isophane insulins are administered only subcutaneously, never IV. Rotate administration sites with each injection. Levemir, Novolin N, R, and 70/30 can be used for up to 42 days after opening when stored at room temperature. Opened vials of all other types of insulin may be stored at room temperature without loss of potency for 28 days. Stability of insulin pens and cartridges at room temperature vary depending on the product; they are never to be shared among patients as this may result in the transmission of blood-borne pathogens.

Rapid- or *short-acting* insulin is sometimes combined with isophane insulin in the same syringe. When two insulins are ordered at the same time, the *rapid-* or *short-acting insulin should be drawn into the syringe first.* Combinations of NPH and regular insulin are also available, for example Humulin 70/30 or Novolin 70/30. This combination provides rapid onset with a duration of up to 24 h. Insulin *glargine* and insulin mixtures should not be mixed with any of the other available types of insulin.

Diabetes therapy with insulin focuses initially on controlling fasting plasma glucose with the use of a long-acting insulin analog (Lantus or Levemir). If further glycemic control is needed, a mealtime (also known as bolus or prandial) rapid- or short-acting insulin may be added to reduce postmeal hyperglycemia. Regular insulin is best given 30–60 min before a meal. The rapid-acting insulins can generally be given 15 min before or immediately after a meal. Insulin mixtures should be given within 15 min before a meal.

Rapid- or *short-acting* insulin is sometimes ordered as *corrective dose insulin.* This means that the blood is tested for glucose and a specific amount of the insulin is administered subcutaneously based on the glucose level shown by the test. Doses are adjusted according to blood glucose response and insulin resistance (the amount of daily insulin required by patients in low-, medium-, and high-dose categories). For example, the physician might write an order to give rapid- or short-acting insulin subcutaneously with the following corrective dose scale according to the blood glucose levels:

Blood Glucose	Dosage of Rapid- or Short-acting Insulin		
	Low	Medium	High
>350	5 units	8 units	12 units & Call physician
301–350	4 units	7 units	10 units
251–300	3 units	5 units	7 units
201–250	2 units	3 units	4 units
151–200	1 unit	2 units	3 units
120–150	0 unit	1 unit	2 units
<120	No insulin		

Remember, this is only a *sample* corrective dose scale. It is now recommended that the traditional sliding scale coverage be reserved for patients who are newly diagnosed as diabetic to establish insulin requirements, started on enteral or parenteral nutrition, or started on glucocorticoids (e.g., prednisone). *Always check the physician's order carefully to determine the exact dosage of insulin, which varies with the individual.* Verification of insulin dosage with another caregiver is very important to prevent one of the most common and most dangerous of medication errors.

There are many different types of insulins available, and many have names or packages that look or sound alike. There has been confusion between "Lente" and "Lantus" and "Humulin" and "Humalog." Confusion is also possible with the premixed products "Humulin 70/30," "Humalog Mix 75/25," "Novolog Mix 70/30," and "Novolin 70/30." *Be extremely careful to give the right insulin and the right dose! If in doubt, consult the pharmacist.*

MEDIALINK

See it in Action! Go to the Online Resources to view a video on *blood glucose testing.*

Hyperglycemia

Hyperglycemia, or elevated blood glucose, may result from:

Undiagnosed diabetes

Insufficient insulin dose

Infections

Surgical or other trauma

Emotional stress

Other endocrine disorders

Medications (e.g., glucocorticoids such as prednisone)

Pregnancy

Symptoms of hyperglycemia may include:

Dehydration and excessive thirst

Anorexia and unexplained weight loss in persons under 40 years old

Polyuria (frequent urination)

Fruity breath

Lethargy, weakness, flu symptoms, and coma if untreated

Vision problems

Ketoacidosis (can be determined by testing urine for acetone)

Treatment of acute hyperglycemia includes:

IV fluids to correct electrolyte imbalance

Adding *regular* insulin to IV fluids

Interactions: Insulin action is antagonized by corticosteroids or epinephrine, necessitating increased insulin dosage. Atypical antipsychotics, protease inhibitors, thiazide diuretics, oral contraceptives, and estrogen may also increase insulin requirements. Beta-blockers (nonselective) with insulin pose risks of hypoglycemia or hyperglycemia and can mask the signs and symptoms (especially tachycardia) of hypoglycemia. Thiazolidinediones (Actos and Avandia) with insulin result in an increased risk of heart failure and edema.

Interactions of insulin with *potentiation of hypoglycemic effect* occur with:

Alcohol

Monoamine oxidase inhibitors (MAOIs)

Salicylates

Anabolic steroids

Hypoglycemia

It is estimated that 90% of all patients receiving insulin will experience a hypoglycemic event. **Hypoglycemia**, or lowered blood glucose, may result from:

Overdose of insulin and/or other antidiabetic medications

Delayed or insufficient food intake (e.g., dieting)

Excessive or unusual exercise

Change in the type of insulin, for example, from analog to human insulin

Symptoms of hypoglycemia may develop suddenly and are manifested usually at the peak of insulin action, including:

Increased perspiration, pallor, hunger, nausea, and vomiting

Irritability, confusion, or sudden unexplained bizarre moodiness or behavior change

Tremor, weakness, headache, hypothermia, or tingling of the fingers

Blurred or double vision

Tachycardia and shallow breathing

Loss of consciousness and convulsions if untreated

Hypoglycemic reactions in older diabetics may mimic a CVA (cerebrovascular accident)

Treatment of hypoglycemia includes:

If conscious, administration of 4 oz orange juice, candy, honey, or syrup (especially sublingual for faster absorption). After initial treatment, provide a protein snack, for example peanut butter, cheese, or a glass of milk. Then recheck blood glucose.

If comatose, administration of 10–30 mL of 50% dextrose solution IV or administration of 0.5–1 unit of glucagon (1 mg) SC, IM, or IV—follow with carbohydrate snack when the patient awakens to prevent secondary hypoglycemia.

Avoid giving excessive amounts of sugar or frequent overdoses of insulin, which can result in rebound hyperglycemia (Somogyi effect) from an accelerated release of glucagon. Treatment of rebound hyperglycemia involves reduction of insulin dosage with continuous monitoring of blood glucose.

Oral and Injectable Noninsulin Antidiabetic Agents

Type 2 diabetes results from insulin resistance (insulin produced but not used effectively by cells) combined with relative insulin deficiency. Type 2 diabetes is the leading cause of kidney failure, lower-limb amputations, and new cases of adult blindness. Patients may sometimes be treated with diet alone, that is, a low-calorie, low-fat diet;

avoiding simple sugars and alcohol; and substituting complex carbohydrates, such as whole-grain bread and cereals, brown rice, and vegetables high in fiber.

Frequently, however, it is necessary to combine diet and oral antidiabetic agents. Oral antidiabetic agents may be administered as a single daily dose before breakfast or two divided doses daily, before morning and evening meals. These medications are not a substitute for dietary management. Weight reduction, exercise, education, and modified diet are still considered the principal therapy for the management of Type 2 diabetes.

Symptoms of Type 2 diabetes may include:

Excessive weight gain after age 40

Excessive thirst (polydipsia)

Excessive urination (polyuria)

Excessive weakness, poor circulation, and slow healing

Visual problems

Oral and injectable noninsulin antidiabetic agents are available in several pharmacological classes with differing mechanisms of action, offering different avenues for reducing glucose levels. Because they work at different sites, they are often synergistic; some may be used in combination with one another or with insulin.

Biguanides

The biguanides, for example, metformin (Glucophage), work by decreasing hepatic glucose production and enhancing insulin uptake in muscle tissue. Metformin is the preferred initial first-line monotherapy or can be used in combination with sulfonylureas, alpha-glucosidase inhibitors, or insulin to treat Type 2 diabetics.

Side effects of biguanides may include:

⚠ GI effects (diarrhea, nausea, vomiting, bloating, flatulence, metallic taste, anorexia, and weight loss), which are generally mild and resolve during treatment; can take the medication with food to minimize epigastric discomfort

Lactic acidosis (a rare but serious metabolic complication) in patients with a history of ketoacidosis, severe dehydration, cardiorespiratory insufficiency, renal dysfunction, and chronic alcoholism with liver damage

Vitamin B_{12} deficiency (patients may present with peripheral neuropathy)

⚠ Hypoglycemia (rare when used without sulfonylureas or insulin)

Precautions or contraindications for biguanides apply to:

Impaired liver and kidney function

Patients with heart failure requiring pharmacologic treatment

Administration of radiocontrast dye (could result in acute alteration of renal function; withhold metformin just prior to tests with radioactive dye and for 48h after completion of the procedure)

Pregnancy and lactation

Children and older adults (especially those who are frail, anorexic, or underweight)

Drug interactions with biguanides include:

Increased metformin effect seen with alcohol, cephalexin, and cimetidine

Radiopaque contrast media (see contraindications)

Sulfonylureas

The oral hypoglycemic drugs known as **sulfonylureas** consist of first-generation agents (e.g., chlorpropamide, tolbutamide) and second-generation agents (e.g., glipizide, glyburide). The second-generation agents have mostly replaced the first-generation agents because of higher potency, shorter duration of action, better tolerance, and fewer drug interactions. The sulfonylureas work by increasing insulin production from the pancreas and by improving peripheral insulin activity. Although patients initially respond well to this class of drugs, glycemic control begins to wane after one to two years in most patients.

Side effects of sulfonylureas may include:

! GI distress (may subside with dosage regulation)

Dermatological effects, including pruritus, rash, urticaria, or photosensitivity

Hepatic dysfunction, including jaundice (rare)

! Weakness, fatigue, lethargy, vertigo, and headache

Blood dyscrasias, including anemia

! Hypoglycemia, especially in older adults

Possible increased risk of cardiovascular death (controversial)

Weight gain and water retention

Precautions or contraindications for sulfonylureas apply to:

Debilitated or malnourished patients

Impaired liver and kidney function

Unstable diabetes or Type 1 diabetes

Major surgery, severe infection, and severe trauma

Older adults (refer to Beers List in Chapter 27; chlorpropamide and glyburide, which have a longer half-life, greater chance of hypoglycemia, and also a risk of inappropriate antidiuretic hormone secretion [water intoxication])

Interactions of sulfonylureas with *potentiation* of hypoglycemic effect can occur with:

Beta-blockers, MAOIs, or probenecid

Alcohol with facial flushing (disulfiram-like reaction)

Cimetidine, miconazole, fluconazole, quinolones, or sulfonamides

Salicylates and other nonsteroidal anti-inflammatory drugs (NSAIDs)

Interactions *with antagonistic action* (larger dose may be required) can occur with:

Thyroid hormones

Thiazide and nonthiazide diuretics

Corticosteroids and phenothiazines

Estrogens and oral contraceptives

Calcium channel blockers

Rifampin and isoniazid

When these agents are administered or discontinued in patients receiving sulfonylureas, the patient should be observed closely for loss of diabetic control.

Alpha-Glucosidase Inhibitors

Alpha-glucosidase inhibitors such as acarbose (Precose) delay digestion of complex carbohydrates (e.g., starch) and subsequent absorption of glucose, resulting in a smaller rise in blood glucose concentrations following meals. Acarbose can be used as monotherapy or part of a combination regimen that includes insulin, metformin, or an oral sulfonylurea.

Side effects of alpha-glucosidase inhibitors may include:

⓵ High rate of GI effects (flatulence, abdominal distention/pain, loose stools), which tend to diminish with time or a reduction in dose; take at the start (with the first bite) of main meals

Elevated liver enzymes (dose-related, generally asymptomatic, and reversible)

Precautions or contraindications for alpha-glucosidase inhibitors apply to:

Impaired liver and kidney function

Patients with inflammatory bowel disease or intestinal obstruction

Pregnancy and lactation

Children

Drug interactions occur between alpha-glucosidase inhibitors and:

Digestive enzymes (effect of acarbose reduced)

Digoxin (reduced serum digoxin concentrations)

Estrogens and oral contraceptives (impaired glucose tolerance)

Incretin Therapies

Two naturally occurring hormones (incretins) called GIP and GLP-1 have been identified and are released by cells in the GI tract in response to food. Agents that mimic the actions of incretin hormones may be beneficial therapeutic options.

Exenatide (Byetta), a GLP-1 receptor agonist given *subcutaneously* twice daily, mimics the action of the incretin GLP-1. It also decreases glucagon secretion, delays gastric emptying time, and decreases food intake (increases satiety), resulting in weight loss. Bydureon is a long-acting form of the medication in Byetta and is given subcutaneously once weekly. Other drugs in this class are listed in Table 23-5.

Exenatide is indicated as adjunctive therapy for Type 2 patients who have not achieved glycemic control and are taking metformin, a sulfonylurea, or a glitazone.

Common *side effects* include nausea or vomiting, diarrhea, dyspepsia, gastroesophageal reflux, injection site reactions, and hypoglycemia (when given in combination with sulfonylureas). It is not recommended for use in patients with severe renal disease or a history of pancreatitis.

Sitagliptin (Januvia), saxagliptin (Onglyza), and linagliptin (Tradjenta), given *orally* once daily, are indicated for use as monotherapy in Type 2 patients or in combination with other agents when adequate glycemic control has not been achieved and may be preferred agents in older adults.

Common *side effects* include abdominal pain, diarrhea, nausea, vomiting, upper respiratory tract infection, and nasopharyngitis. Use these agents with caution (if at all) in patients with a history of pancreatitis. Dosage adjustments are required for renal disease (except for linagliptin).

Meglitinides

Nateglinide (Starlix) and repaglinide (Prandin) stimulate the beta cells of the pancreas to produce insulin. They can be used as monotherapy or in combination with metformin. Meglitinides have a rapid onset and short duration of action, and are to be taken before each meal.

Side effects of meglitinides may include:

- ! GI effects (nausea or vomiting, diarrhea, constipation, dyspepsia, and abdominal cramps)
- ! Hypoglycemia; initial weight gain
- ! Upper respiratory infection (URI), sinusitis, arthralgia, and headache

Precautions or contraindications for meglitinides apply to:

Diabetic ketoacidosis

Impaired liver function

Pregnancy and lactation

Children

Drug interactions with meglitinides include (refer to the listing under sulfonylureas):

Administer before meals to maximize absorption

Gemfibrozil (Lopid) may enhance or prolong effects

Thiazolidinediones

Pioglitazone (Actos) and rosiglitazone (Avandia) lower blood glucose by decreasing insulin resistance and improving sensitivity to insulin in muscle, liver, and adipose tissue. They can be used as monotherapy or concomitantly with other agents.

Product labeling for both pioglitazone and rosiglitazone includes black box warnings regarding the potential for these agents to cause or exacerbate congestive heart failure in some patients, and both are contraindicated with class III or IV heart failure. In addition, a black box warning for the potential increase in the risk of myocardial ischemia has been added to rosiglitazone's label, although the warning also states that the data concerning the increased risk of myocardial ischemia are inconclusive. Because of these precautions, only patients who are already established on this medication are normally given prescriptions for it. Additionally, physicians who wish to prescribe this medication must be registered with the Avandia-rosiglitazone Medicine Access Program.

Side effects of thiazolidinediones may include:

- ! Weight gain, fluid retention, and edema (Report weight gain over 6.6 lb, sudden onset of edema, or shortness of breath.)
- ! URI, sinusitis, pharyngitis, and headache

⚠️ Myalgia; atypical bone fractures (upper arm, hand, and foot)

Anemia

⚠️ Hypoglycemia (in combination with insulin or oral hypoglycemics)

Precautions or contraindications for thiazolidinediones apply to:

Impaired liver function

Heart failure (causes edema); pulmonary edema

May cause resumption of ovulation in premenopausal patients, increasing the risk for pregnancy

Pregnancy and lactation

Children

Drug interactions occur between thiazolidinediones and:

Insulins (increase the probability of weight gain, fluid retention, and CHF)

Pioglitazone with oral contraceptives (reduced effectiveness of the contraceptive)

Rosiglitazone with nitrates (increased risk of myocardial ischemia)

"Azole" antifungals (potentiation of hypoglycemic effect)

SGLT2 Inhibitor Therapy

Sodium-glucose co-transporter 2 inhibitors are the newest class of antidiabetic medications. Similar to other oral and injectable non-insulin medications they are only indicated for use in patients with type 2 diabetes. They can be used as monotherapy or in combination with oral medications. They work by decreasing the reabsorption of glucose in the kidney, essentially lowering available glucose to the body via excretion. Current drugs in this class include canagliflozin (Invokana), empagliflozin (Jardiance), and dapagliflozin (Farxiga). The most common side effects with these medications are vaginal yeast infections and urinary tract infections, along with increased desire to urinate. See Table 23-5 for a summary of the oral hypoglycemics.

TABLE 23-5 Oral and Injectable Noninsulin Antidiabetic Agents

GENERIC NAME	TRADE NAME	USUAL DOSAGE
First-generation sulfonylureas		
chlorpropamide	Diabinese	100–500 mg per day with meal (do not use for older adults)
tolbutamide	Orinase	250–3,000 mg per day or divided
Second-generation sulfonylureas		
glimepiride	Amaryl	1–8 mg per day with meal
glipizide	Glucotrol	2.5–40 mg per day ac or divided
	Glucotrol XL	5–20 mg per day with meal
glyburide	Diabeta	1.25–20 mg per day or divided with meal
	Glynase (micronized)	1.5–12 mg per day with meal

(continued)

TABLE 23-5 **Oral and Injectable Noninsulin Antidiabetic Agents (*continued*)**

GENERIC NAME	TRADE NAME	USUAL DOSAGE
Alpha-glucosidase inhibitors		
acarbose	Precose	25–100 mg TID, with first bite of meal
miglitol	Glyset	
Biguanides		
metformin	Glucophage	500–2,550 mg per day divided with meals
	Glucophage XR	500–2,000 mg per day with P.M. meal or divided
Incretin therapies		
GLP-1 receptor agonist		
exenatide	Byetta	*subcu* 5–10 mcg BID ac (A.M. & P.M. meal)
	Bydureon	*subcu* 2 mg weekly (any time of day)
liraglutide	Victoza	*subcu* 0.6–1.2 mg daily
dulaglutide	Trulicity	*subcu* 0.75–1.5 mg weekly
lixisenatide	Adlyxin	*subcu* starting at 10 mcg for 14 days and increasing to 20 mcg daily
DPP-4 inhibitors ("gliptins")		
linagliptin	Tradjenta	PO 5 mg daily
sitagliptin	Januvia	PO 50–100 mg daily
saxagliptin	Onglyza	PO 2.5–5 mg daily
Meglitinides		
nateglinide	Starlix	60–120 mg TID ac
repaglinide	Prandin	0.5–4 mg BID two to four times per day ac
Thiazolidinediones		
pioglitazone	Actos	15–45 mg per day
rosiglitazone	Avandia	4–8 mg per day or BID divided (restricted access/distribution)
SGLT2 inhibitors		
canagliflozin	Invokana	100-300 mg daily in the morning before first meal of day
empagliflozin	Jardiance	10-25 mg daily in the morning with or without food
dapagliflozin	Farxiga	5-10 mg daily in the morning with or without food
Combinations		
glyburide/metformin	Glucovance	1.25/250–20/2,000 mg per day or BID with meals
rosiglitazone/metformin	Avandamet	2/500–8/2,000 mg per day with meals or divided (restricted access/distribution)
sitagliptin/metformin	Janumet	50/500–50/1,000 mg BID with meals

Note: In older adults, start with the lowest dose possible and titrate upward to achieve desired glycemic control.

PATIENT EDUCATION

Patients with both Type 1 and Type 2 diabetes should be instructed regarding:

Prevention of hypoglycemia—the importance of control with proper drug and diet therapy and *never* skipping meals; do not consume alcohol on an empty stomach.

Early symptoms and treatment of hypoglycemia—carrying a ready source of carbohydrate (e.g., glucose tablets, lump sugar, or candy); orange juice, 4 oz, is also appropriate

Properly balanced diet (i.e., restricted calories); avoidance of simple sugars, alcohol, and foods high on the Glycemic Index (e.g., white bread, white potatoes, and white rice).

Substitute foods low on the Glycemic Index—complex carbohydrates, such as whole-grain breads and cereal and brown rice. Reduce fats, increase fiber, and be sure to have an adequate fluid intake.

Regular exercise and maintenance of proper body weight; weight reduction if obese

Importance of reporting to a physician *immediately* if nausea, vomiting, diarrhea, or infections occur (IV fluids may be required to prevent dehydration and acidosis)

Good foot care to reduce the chance of infections

Carrying identification card and wearing identification tag

Look-alike, sound-alike drugs: Actos/Actonel, glipizide/glyburide, insulin name pairs mentioned earlier

Taking the medication (oral or insulin) at approximately the same time each day and in proper relation to meals

Proper use of monitoring devices; check blood glucose as directed by the physician, especially with hypoglycemia or stress

For patients with Type 1 diabetes (those requiring insulin), the foregoing instructions are important, as well as these additional rules:

Rotate injection sites (Figure 23-4). Insulin is absorbed more rapidly in the arm or thigh, especially with exercise. Inject insulin into abdomen if possible for most consistent absorption.

Maintain aseptic technique with injections.

Have someone check the amount of insulin in the syringe or pen before injection, especially with older adults or those with vision impairment (retinal problems are common in diabetics).

Check all insulin for the expiration date.

Check regular insulin for clearness; do *not* give if cloudy or discolored.

Rotate isophane insulin vials to mix contents; do *not* give if solution is clear or clumped in appearance after rotation; do not shake the vial; rotate gently between hands (Figure 23-5).

If regular insulin is to be mixed with NPH, draw regular insulin into syringe first.

Unopened vials of insulin should be stored at 2–8°C and should not be subjected to freezing. The vial or pen in use may be stored at room temperature for a limited amount of time (depending on the product) without loss of potency.

Avoid exposure of insulin to extremes in temperature or direct sunlight. Do not put vial in glove compartment, trunk, or suitcase.

Regular insulin is sometimes administered as correction for elevated blood glucose readings as ordered by a physician.

Proper disposal of injectable products.

Notify the physician of illness, increased stress, or trauma. *More* insulin may be required under these circumstances.

Notify the physician if you increase your exercise significantly or if you are taking less than the usual amount of food. *Less* insulin may be required under these circumstances.

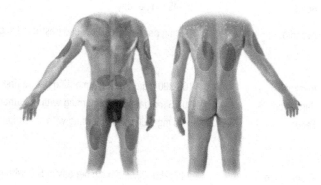

FIGURE 23-4 Common sites for insulin injection. Sites should be rotated and the site recorded each time on the medication record.

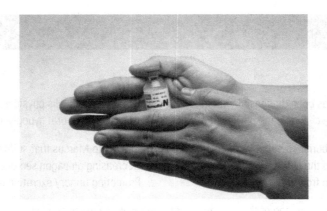

FIGURE 23-5 Rotate isophane and zinc insulin vials gently to mix contents. Do not shake.

CASE STUDY A

Endocrine System Drugs

After weeding in her garden, Marie Kilcline experiences a severe allergic reaction to poison ivy. She presents to her physician with a rash on her face, arms, and legs.

1. The physician prescribes a corticosteroid. How will this category of medication be most beneficial to Marie?
   a. As an antipruritic
   b. As an antineoplastic
   c. As an antidiabetic
   d. As an anti-inflammatory

2. The physician explains that side effects of the corticosteroid may include:
   a. Hypotension
   b. Hypoglycemia
   c. Increased susceptibility to infection
   d. Flushing of the hands and face

3. Prior to handing Marie her prescription, the physician reviews her medication history. He knows this is essential because of possible interactions with corticosteroids. Which drug may cause an interaction resulting in reduced effectiveness of the corticosteroid?
   a. Estrogen
   b. Salicylates
   c. Diuretics
   d. Phenytoin

4. When Marie picks up her corticosteroid medication at the pharmacy, she reads the label on the side of the bottle containing instructions on when to take her medication. Which of the following is most likely to be on this label?
   a. Take 1h before meals.
   b. Avoid taking with milk.
   c. Take 1h after meals
   d. Take 2h after meals.

5. Marie will be taking her medication for a prescribed amount of time. What will be the best method to discontinue her corticosteroid?
   a. Slowly taper the dosage.
   b. Stop the medication abruptly.
   c. Reduce the dose in alternating weeks.
   d. Administer an IV bolus and then discontinue the medication.

CASE STUDY B

Antidiabetic Agents

Forty-eight-year-old Marcus Wales has been diagnosed with new onset of Type 2 diabetes. His physician orders a low-fat, low-calorie diet. In addition to dietary changes, the physician would like to start him on an oral hypoglycemic drug.

1. The physician starts him on glyburide, a sulfonylurea medication. He explains to Marcus that sulfonylureas work by:

a. Blocking glucose uptake into the cell

b. Increasing insulin production from the pancreas

c. Decreasing glucagon secretion

d. Promoting urinary excretion of excess glucose

2. The physician explains to Marcus that one of the side effects of a sulfonylurea medication is:

a. Insomnia

b. Orthostatic hypotension

c. Excessive urination

d. Fatigue

3. Prior to prescribing the medication, the physician reviews Marcus's medical history. This is because sulfonylureas must be used with extreme caution in individuals who:

a. Are obese

b. Are asthmatic

c. Have impaired kidney and liver function

d. Have peripheral vascular disease

4. The physician cautions Marcus to call him prior to taking any other medication because of possible interactions. Which drug can potentiate the hypoglycemic effect of a sulfonylurea?

a. Quinolones

b. Penicillins

c. Antacids

d. Rifampin

5. What drug causes an interaction with sulfonylureas, resulting in an antagonistic action in which a larger dose may be required?

a. MAOIs

b. Testosterone

c. Corticosteroids

d. Narcotic analgesics

CHAPTER REVIEW QUIZ

Match the medication in the first column with the appropriate classification in the second column. Classifications may be used more than once.

Medication

1. ___ Glucophage

2. ___ prednisone

3. ___ Humulin R

4. ___ Synthroid

5. ___ Avandia

6. ___ Tapazole

7. ___ Isophane

8. ___ Prandin

9. ___ Lantus

10. ___ Humalog

Classification

a. Thyroid agent

b. Antithyroid

c. Oral antidiabetic agent

d. Corticosteroid

e. Insulin–rapid acting

f. Insulin–short acting

g. Insulin–intermediate acting

h. Insulin–long acting

Choose the correct answer.

11. The biguanide that decreases hepatic glucose production and enhances insulin uptake is which of the following?
    a. Glucophage
    b. Starlix
    c. Synthroid
    d. Cortrosyn

12. NTIs are characterized by which of the following?
    a. Very high doses are needed to show effects
    b. They have a small range for which they are safe and effective.
    c. They are administered with a narrow gauged needle
    d. They do not require laboratory monitoring upon initialization

13. A patient who is on a thyroid medication should be monitored for which potential side effect?
    a. Hyperglycemia
    b. Hypotension
    c. Muscle twitching
    d. Shortness of breath

14. Thyroid medication should be taken:
    a. At bedtime with a sip of water
    b. On an empty stomach 30–60 min prior to breakfast
    c. 30–60 min after breakfast
    d. With breakfast.

15. Insulin is administered parenterally because:
    a. It is easier to monitor dosage
    b. It is destroyed in the GI tract
    c. Insulin pills are difficult to swallow
    d. Parenteral dosing is tolerated better

16. To prevent a medication error, an insulin dose in a syringe:
    a. Should be color-coded for specific doses
    b. Should be drawn up with the nondominant hand for a better visualization of the dose
    c. Should only be verified by a pharmacist
    d. Should be verified by another clinician

17. What best describes the onset and duration of action of regular insulin?
    a. Delayed onset and short duration
    b. Extended onset and long duration
    c. Rapid onset and short duration
    d. Ultra-rapid onset and very short duration

18. The peak of rapid-acting insulins falls under which time frame postinjection?
    a. 1–2 h
    b. 1–5 h
    c. 6–12 h
    d. 12–24 h

19. What is one of the most likely symptoms of hyperglycemia?
    a. Weight gain
    b. Excitability
    c. Excessive thirst
    d. Urinary retention

20. Which of the following may potentiate the hypoglycemic effect of insulin?
    a. NSAIDs
    b. Corticosteroids
    c. Antidepressants
    d. Alcohol

21. Which preparation of insulin is used to correct elevated blood glucose?
    a. Lispro
    b. Regular
    c. Isophane (NPH)
    d. Glargine

22. Illness, increased stress, or trauma may have what effect on a prescribed dose of insulin?

    a. Less insulin may be required.

    b. The dose will need to be divided.

    c. More insulin may be required.

    d. No change in dosage will be required.

23. Which of the following is the main type of side effects observed with SGLT2 inhibitors?

    a. Urinary

    b. Respiratory

    c. Dermal

    d. Gastric

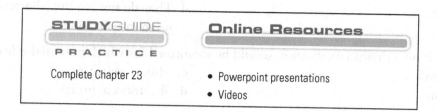

STUDYGUIDE

PRACTICE

Complete Chapter 23

Online Resources

- Powerpoint presentations
- Videos

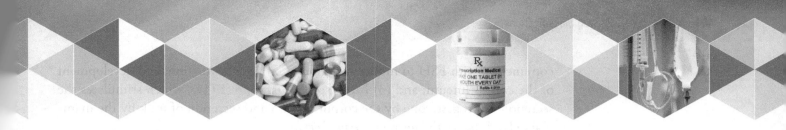

CHAPTER 24
REPRODUCTIVE SYSTEM DRUGS

KEY TERMS AND CONCEPTS

Androgens

Contraceptives

Erectile dysfunction (ED)

Estrogen therapy (ET)

Estrogen or progestin therapy (EPT)

Estrogens

Follicle-stimulating hormone (FSH)

Hormone therapy (HT)

Luteinizing hormone (LH)

Luteotropic hormone (LTH)

Oxytocin

Progesterone

Progestins

Testosterone

Tocolysis

OBJECTIVES

Upon completion of this chapter, the learner should be able to

1. Identify the uses, side effects, and precautions for the androgens

2. List the uses, side effects, and precautions or contraindications for the estrogens and progestins

3. Compare and contrast contraceptives

4. Describe the use of oxytocics and the precautions to be observed

5. Explain the uses of terbutaline, prostaglandins, and magnesium sulfate

6. Describe the uses of GnRH analogs

7. Explain drug therapy for erectile dysfunction

8. Present appropriate patient education for all drugs discussed in this chapter

9. Define the Key Terms and Concepts

H ormones that regulate the functions of the reproductive systems include *endogenous* chemical substances, which originate within different areas of the body. For the purpose of simplification, we will divide the reproductive hormones into four main categories: gonadotropic, androgens, estrogens, and progestins.

The pituitary gland is located at the base of the brain. The anterior lobe secretes four hormones. Those affecting growth, thyroid function, and adrenocorticosteroid production are discussed in Chapter 23. This chapter includes the gonadotropic hormones, which are secreted by the anterior and posterior pituitary lobes.

GONADOTROPICS

The gonadotropic hormones include (1) **follicle-stimulating hormone (FSH)**, which stimulates the development of ovarian follicles in the female and sperm production in the testes of the male; (2) **luteinizing hormone (LH)**, which works in conjunction with FSH to induce secretion of estrogen, ovulation, and development of the corpus luteum; and (3) **luteotropic hormone (LTH)**, which stimulates the secretion of progesterone by the corpus luteum and secretion of milk by the mammary gland, hence the term *lactogenic hormone*.

ANDROGENS

Androgens, the male sex hormones, are secreted mainly in the interstitial tissue of the testes in the male and secondarily in the adrenal glands of both sexes. Androgens, which stimulate the development of male characteristics (masculinization), include **testosterone** and androsterone.

Inadequate production of androgens in the male may be because of pituitary malfunction or to atrophy of, injury to, or removal of the testicles (castration), resulting in eunuchism or eunuchoidism. Eunuchoid characteristics include retarded development of sex organs, absence of beard and body hair, high-pitched voice, and lack of muscular development. Hypogonadism may also result in impotence or deficient sperm production (oligospermia).

Testosterone is absorbed from the gastrointestinal (GI) tract, but because of extensive metabolism by liver enzymes, oral bioavailability is poor. Replacement therapy is currently available in buccal, parenteral, and transdermal formulations. Synthetic androgens such as danazol and methyltestosterone are available for oral use but are used more often for conditions other than replacement therapy (see the following list) and have an increased potential for liver abnormalities.

Uses of androgens include:

Replacement in cases of diminished testicular hormone with testosterone (e.g., impotence, oligospermia, or andropause ["male menopause"])

Congenital hypogonadism (e.g., cryptorchidism or undescended testicles) or delayed puberty in the male

Acquired hypogonadism (e.g., orchitis, trauma, tumor, radiation, surgery of the testicles, or drug induced)

Palliative treatment of females with advanced metastatic carcinoma of the breast, for example, methyltestosterone (acting as an antiestrogen)

Treatment of endometriosis and fibrocystic breast disease, for example danazol, which is antiestrogenic and weakly androgenic

Treatment of cachexia with oxandrolone, an anabolic steroid with much greater anabolic effects than androgenic effects, thus promoting weight gain in patients with burns, trauma, AIDS, or chronic obstructive pulmonary disease (COPD)

Side effects of androgens can include:

⊘ Edema and hypertension (diuretics may be indicated)

⊘ Acne, increased oiliness of the skin and hair, or alopecia (male pattern baldness)

Oligospermia (deficient sperm production resulting in sterility)

Increased or decreased sexual stimulation or libido and impotence

Gynecomastia in males (enlarged breast tissue)

Hirsutism (excessive or unusual growth of hair), deepening of voice, and amenorrhea or other menstrual irregularities in females

⚠ Jaundice and hepatitis

Nausea and vomiting

⚠ Premature closure of bone ends in adolescents, with stunting of growth

⚠ Anxiety, depression, and headache

Increased low-density lipoprotein (LDL), decreased high-density lipoprotein (HDL), and insulin resistance

Precautions or contraindications for androgens apply to:

Cardiac, renal, and liver dysfunction (edema is common)

Men suspected of having carcinoma of the prostate or breast (stimulates growth of cancerous tissue)

Geriatric males (may increase the risk of or worsen prostatic hypertrophy and carcinoma or overstimulation sexually)

Prepubertal males who have not reached their full growth potential (may stunt growth by premature closure of bone ends)

Diabetes, obesity, or dyslipidemia (abnormal lipid profile)

Interactions of androgens may occur with:

Oral anticoagulants (potentiation may cause bleeding)

Decreased blood glucose and decreased insulin requirements in diabetics

Antiandrogens (dutasteride and finasteride)

Dangers of illegal use of anabolic steroids: Health care personnel have a responsibility to caution athletes, especially adolescents, regarding the hazards of taking illegal synthetic testosterone products to build muscle power, or physique. Besides the *potentially serious adverse side effects* just mentioned, another risk is *the development of psychosis* with delusions, paranoia, depression, mania, and aggression with violence.

All noncombination products in this class are classified as a controlled substance (C-III) by the DEA because of their abuse potential.

See Table 24-1 for a summary of the androgen agents.

TABLE 24-1 **Androgen Agents**

GENERIC NAME	TRADE NAME	DOSAGE	USES/COMMENTS
danazol	Danocrine	PO 100–400 mg BID	Endometriosis, fibrocystic breast disease
methyltestosterone	Android, Testred	PO, dose varies	Advanced breast cancer; replacement therapy
with estrogen	Covaryx, Covaryx H.S.	PO, dose varies (given cyclically)	Menopausal symptoms if estrogen alone is insufficient
oxandrolone	Oxandrin	PO 2.5–20 mg per day in divided doses	Treatment of cachexia associated with burns, trauma, AIDS, and COPD
testosterone	Depo-Testosterone Striant Androderm AndroGel Axiron	Deep IM, pellet implant, buccal; dose varies Transdermal patch Transdermal gel Transdermal solution (apply to axilla)	Hypogonadism, advanced breast cancer, replacement therapy

PATIENT EDUCATION

Patients on androgen therapy should be instructed regarding:

Taking only prescribed drugs according to directions

Skin irritation possible with transdermal formulations

Reporting side effects, especially edema, jaundice, nausea, or vomiting

Reporting sexual effects for males, such as decreased ejaculatory volume and excessive sexual stimulation, especially in geriatric patients beyond cardiovascular capacity

Sexual effects for females to expect (e.g., hirsutism and voice deepening)

Possibility of stunted growth when administered to adolescent boys before puberty

To avoid secondary exposure of children and partners, adults who use testosterone gels should target a discreet application site like the front and inner thighs or underarms (depending on the product used), wash their hands with soap and warm water after every application, and cover the application site with clothing once the gel has dried.

ERECTILE DYSFUNCTION MEDICATIONS

Erectile dysfunction (ED) is defined as the inability to achieve or maintain an erection sufficient for satisfactory performance. The incidence of ED increases with age, with an increased risk in those with diabetes, cancer, stroke, and cardiovascular disease. The principal mediator in attaining and maintaining an erection is nitric oxide, which ultimately causes smooth muscle relaxation in the corpus cavernosum of the penis, allowing the inflow of blood.

Phosphodiesterase (PDE) Inhibitors

Phosphodiesterase (PDE) inhibitors are a class of drugs given orally for the treatment of male ED, also referred to as impotence. Their introduction represented a significant advancement as other therapies required direct injection into the penis (Caverject) or insertion of a urethral suppository (Muse). The PDE inhibitors block PDE type 5, found in the corpus cavernosum, which is thought to impair the production of nitric oxide.

Sildenafil (Viagra) was the first PDE inhibitor approved to treat ED, followed by vardenafil (Levitra), tadalafil (Cialis), and avanafil (Stendra). These medications require sexual arousal for success. PDE is also found in various organs and tissues such as the prostate, pulmonary arteries, other blood vessels, retina, heart, liver, and brain. Sildenafil (as Revatio) and tadalafil (as Adcirca) are also approved to treat pulmonary hypertension; tadalafil (as Cialis) is approved for the treatment of signs and symptoms of benign prostatic hyperplasia (BPH).

Side effects of PDE inhibitors can include:

!! Headache, flushing, vision abnormalities, and dizziness

!! Hearing loss and tinnitus

   Dyspepsia, nasal congestion, rhinitis, diarrhea, rash, and back pain

!! Cardiovascular events (less than 2% of patients), including angina, syncope, tachycardia, palpitation, and hypotension

Precautions or contraindications for PDE inhibitors apply to:

Nitrates or alpha-blockers (e.g., Flomax, Cardura) (potentiates the hypotensive effects if used concurrently)

Older adults and patients with preexisting cardiovascular risk factors

Hepatic or renal function impairment

In the event of an erection persisting more than 4h, advise the patient to seek medical assistance immediately (tissue damage and permanent loss of potency may result)

Interactions occur between PDE inhibitors and:

Nitrates, antiarrhythmics, antiretroviral protease inhibitors, macrolides, quinolones, and some antifungals (potentiate/prolong hypotensive effect)

Grapefruit juice (use with caution; may potentiate hypotensive effect)

See Table 24-2 for a summary of the erectile dysfunction (ED) agents.

TABLE 24-2 Erectile Dysfunction (ED) Agents

GENERIC NAME	TRADE NAME	STARTING DOSE	USES/COMMENTS
sildenafil	Viagra	25–100 mg PO 1 h before sexual activity (max freq once daily)	Onset of action is 15–60 min; duration is up to 4 h
	Revatio	PO 20 mg TID IV 10 mg TID	For pulmonary hypertension
tadalafil	Cialis	5–20 mg PO 1–12 h before sexual activity (max freq once q24 h)	Onset of action is 15–45 min; duration is up to 36 h
		2.5 mg PO daily	Without regard to timing of sexual activity
		5 mg PO daily	For ED and BPH or BPH alone
	Adcirca	40 mg PO daily	For pulmonary hypertension
vardenafil	Levitra	10 mg PO 1 h before sexual activity (max freq once daily)	Onset of action is 25 min; duration is up to 4 h
avanafil	Stendra	50–200 mg 30 min before sexual activity (max freq once daily)	Onset of action is 30–45 min; duration is up to 6 h

Note: ED agents do not affect the libido and have no effects in the absence of sexual stimulation.

ESTROGENS

Estrogens, the female sex hormones, are produced mainly by the ovary and secondarily by the adrenal glands. Estrogens are responsible for the development of female secondary sexual characteristics, including breast enlargement, and during the menstrual cycle they act on the female genitalia to produce an environment suitable for fertilization, implantation, and nutrition of the early embryo. Estrogens also affect the secretion of the hormones FSH and LH from the anterior pituitary gland in a complex way. This results in the inhibition of lactation and ovulation, the latter process utilized in contraceptive therapy.

Menopause is a normal, natural life event that occurs in women as part of the aging process over a period of years but can be artificially induced by the surgical removal of the uterus and ovaries, chemotherapy, or other medical treatments. In menopause, levels of estrogen and progesterone are reduced, leading to the development of vasomotor symptoms (e.g., hot flashes and night sweats) and atrophic vaginitis (thinning, dryness, and inflammation of the vaginal walls; Figure 24-1).

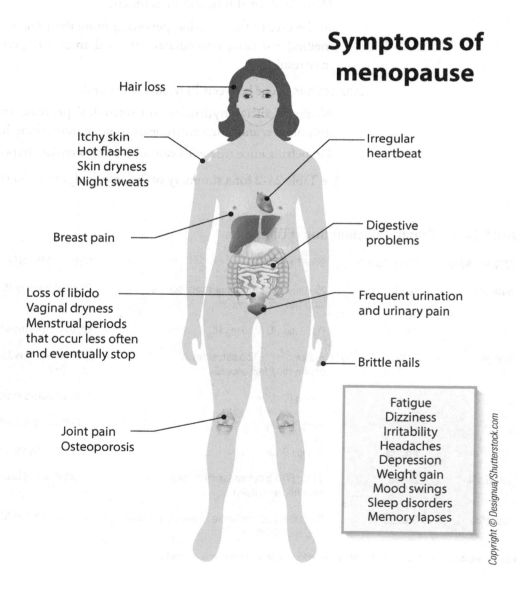

Symptoms of menopause

Hair loss

Itchy skin
Hot flashes
Skin dryness
Night sweats

Irregular heartbeat

Breast pain

Digestive problems

Loss of libido
Vaginal dryness
Menstrual periods that occur less often and eventually stop

Frequent urination and urinary pain

Brittle nails

Fatigue
Dizziness
Irritability
Headaches
Depression
Weight gain
Mood swings
Sleep disorders
Memory lapses

Joint pain
Osteoporosis

Copyright © Designua/Shutterstock.com

FIGURE 24-1 Menopause can present with various symptoms throughout the body and can change as menopause progresses.

Historically, estrogen replacement therapy was routinely used for relieving menopausal symptoms. Estrogen (in combination with progesterone if the woman has an intact uterus) is used in the management of severe menopausal symptoms.

Estrogen therapy (ET), that is, estrogen alone, has been associated with an *increased risk of endometrial carcinoma* in women with an intact uterus. When progestin is combined with estrogen (*combined hormone or* **estrogen and progestin therapy [EPT]**), the risk of endometrial cancer is substantially reduced.

In 2002, the results of the Women's Health Initiative (WHI) study were released. The main thrust of the WHI study was to determine the exact degree to which **hormone therapies (HTs)** presumably protected the heart and to investigate the degree to which some of the known and potential risks of HTs, such as breast cancer and blood clots, cancelled out any benefits. The WHI also explored whether HTs prevented fractures, colon cancer, and dementia, including Alzheimer's disease.

The authors of the WHI study announced not only that the risks of *combined HT* outweighed its benefits when used to prevent certain diseases, but the combined HT could actually *increase the risk* of certain conditions it was previously believed to prevent, such as heart attack. These findings and further research led to the establishment of the North American Menopause Society's (NAMS) new position statement on hormone therapy, which was published in 2012. This represents the most recent guidelines on HT use:

- HT remains the most effective treatment available for menopausal symptoms, including hot flashes and night sweats that can interrupt sleep and impair quality of life. Many women can take it safely.

- If you have had blood clots, heart disease, stroke, or breast cancer, it may not be in your best interest to take HT. Be sure to discuss your health conditions with your health care professional.

- How long you should take HT is different for EPT and ET. For EPT, the time is limited by the increased risk of breast cancer that is seen with more than three to five years of use. For ET, no sign of an increased risk of breast cancer was seen during an average of seven years of treatment, a finding that allows more choice in how long you choose to use ET.

- Most healthy women below age 60 will have no increase in the risk of heart disease with HT. The risks of stroke and blood clots in the lungs are increased, but in these younger age groups the risks are less than 1 in every 1,000 women per year taking HT.

- ET delivered through the skin (by patch, cream, gel, or spray) and low-dose oral estrogen may have lower risks of blood clots and stroke than standard doses of oral estrogen, but all the evidence is not yet available. Research will continue to bring valuable information to help women with their decision about HT.

For more information about menopause, visit the NAMS website: www.menopause.org.

Uses of estrogen therapy include:

Contraceptives (combined with progestin; these combination products are also used to treat menstrual irregularities and dysmenorrhea [painful menstruation])

Menopausal vasomotor symptom relief

Female hypogonadism owing to ovarian pathology or oophorectomy (ovary removal)

Postmenopausal prevention of osteoporosis (secondary to estrogen deficiency) *only* if unable to take other agents and if benefits outweigh the risks

Atrophic vaginitis from decreased secretions (low-dose vaginal cream biweekly)

Postcoital use after unprotected sexual intercourse (within 72h) of a single large dose to prevent, not terminate, pregnancy.

Palliative treatment for males with advanced, inoperable prostate cancer

Side effects of estrogen therapy, especially with high doses, can include:

(!) Increased risk of thromboembolic disorders, hypertension, myocardial infarction, and stroke

GI effects, including vomiting, abdominal cramps, bloating, diarrhea or constipation, and weight gain

Skin discolorations (acne may decrease or occasionally increase)

Fluid retention and edema

Increased serum triglyceride levels

Severe hypercalcemia in cancer patients with large doses

Folic acid deficiency (may require folic acid supplements)

Liver function abnormalities, including jaundice, anorexia, and pruritus

Breakthrough or irregular vaginal bleeding

Increased risk of cervical erosion and *Candida* vaginitis

(!) Headache, especially migraine, and depression

Visual disturbances

Breast tenderness, enlargement, and secretion

(!) Increased risk of gallbladder disease

(!) Cancer of the uterus with estrogen alone. Therefore, progesterone is recommended with estrogen. (See the WHI study and NAMS recommendations at the beginning of this section.)

Precautions or contraindications exist because the use of estrogens, especially in large doses, may be associated with the increased risk of several serious conditions. Before the estrogen therapy is begun, a complete history and physical examination are essential, and yearly physicals, including Pap test and mammogram, during therapy are important. Estrogens are contraindicated for anyone with a history of the following conditions, and estrogen therapy should be *discontinued with the signs of these conditions*:

> Hypertension, thromboembolic disorders (DVT, PE), stroke, and myocardial infarction
>
> Liver dysfunction
>
> Breast cancer (except for palliative treatment)
>
> Undiagnosed vaginal bleeding
>
> Visual disturbances, severe headaches, and migraine
>
> Shortness of breath and chest or calf pain
>
> Pregnancy

Other cautions for estrogens include the following:

> *Prolonged, continued* use of high-dose estrogens in postmenopausal women, which has shown an increased risk of endometrial cancer in some studies; therefore, cyclic administration at the *lowest* possible dose, is recommended with progesterone. Regular physical examinations, including a Pap test every year, are also recommended.
>
> Pregnancy, in which estrogens can cause serious fetal toxicity, congenital anomalies, and vaginal or cervical cancer for the offspring in later life. Estrogens should *never* be used to treat threatened abortions or if there is any possibility of pregnancy. A pregnancy test should be done before initiating therapy.
>
> Lactation
>
> Diabetes and heavy smokers

Interactions of estrogen include the following:

> Rifampin and isoniazid decrease estrogenic activity, and therefore other forms of contraception should be used with patients receiving rifampin or isoniazid.
>
> Corticosteroid effects are potentiated by estrogen.
>
> Laboratory test interference includes endocrine function tests, decreased glucose tolerance, and thyroid function tests.
>
> Oral anticoagulant, anticonvulsant, thyroid hormones, and hypoglycemic actions may be decreased with estrogen.
>
> Sunscreens with estradiol topical emulsion increases absorption.

PROGESTINS

Progesterone is a hormone secreted by the corpus luteum and adrenal glands. It is responsible for changes in uterine endometrium in the second half of the menstrual cycle in preparation for implantation of the fertilized ovum, development of maternal placenta after implantation, and development of mammary glands. Synthetic drugs that exert progesterone-like activity are called **progestins**.

Uses of synthetic progestins include:

Treatment of amenorrhea and abnormal uterine bleeding caused by hormonal imbalance

Contraception, either combined with estrogen or used alone

Postmenopausal—sometimes combined with estrogen in replacement cyclical therapy (note the risks)

Adjunctive and palliative therapy for advanced and metastatic endometrial or breast cancer (Megace—is also used for the anorexia, weight loss, and cachexia associated with acquired immunodeficiency syndrome [AIDS])

Management of paraphilia (sexual deviancy), especially pedophilia and sexual sadism (Depo-Provera, 100–500 mg IM weekly to monthly—the drug has been shown to decrease erotic cravings, but sexual deviance usually returns following discontinuance of the drug)

Side effects of continuous progestin use can include:

(!) Menstrual irregularity and amenorrhea, breakthrough bleeding, and spotting

(!) Edema and weight gain

Nausea

Breast tenderness, enlargement, and secretion

Jaundice, rash, and pruritus

Headache and migraine

Mental depression

(!) Thromboembolic disorders

Vision disorders

Possible decrease in bone density with prolonged use

Precautions or contraindications for progestins (similar to cautions with estrogen) apply to:

Any condition that might be aggravated by fluid retention (e.g., asthma, seizures, migraine, and cardiac or renal dysfunction)

History of mental depression

History of thromboembolic disorders, especially with tobacco smoking

History of cerebrovascular accident

Liver disorders

Undiagnosed vaginal bleeding

Pregnancy (progestins are no longer used to treat threatened abortion because of the potential adverse effects to the fetus)

Breast, cervical, uterine, and vaginal cancers (except for palliative treatment)

See Table 24-3 for a summary of the estrogens and progestins. Several different estrogen–progestin combinations are commercially available. Refer to the discussion of each individual agent.

TABLE 24-3   Estrogens and Progestins

GENERIC NAME	TRADE NAME[a]	DOSAGE	USES/COMMENTS
Estrogens			
estradiol	Estrace	PO, intravaginal, dose varies	Menopause, prostate cancer, breast cancer, dysfunctional uterine bleeding
	Vagifem	Vaginal tabs	Atrophic vaginitis
	Estrasorb EstroGel	Topical emulsion, Transdermal gel	Only for menopausal symptoms
	Climara, Vivelle	Transdermal patch, dose varies	
	Depo-Estradiol	IM, dose varies	Female hypogonadism, prostate cancer, menopausal symptoms
conjugated estrogens	Premarin	PO, vaginal cream, parenteral; dose varies with condition symptoms	Female hypogonadism, breast and prostate cancer, menopausal symptoms
esterified estrogens	Menest	PO, dose varies with condition	Female hypogonadism, breast and prostate cancer, menopausal symptoms
Progestins			
medroxyprogesterone	Provera Depo-Provera	PO tabs IM, dose varies	Abnormal uterine bleeding, menopausal symptoms, endometrial cancer, contraception
megestrol acetate	Megace, Megace ES (625 mg/5 mL daily)	PO 160–800 mg daily in divided doses	Endometrial and breast cancer, anorexia, and cachexia of AIDS
Estrogen–progestin combinations			
conjugated estrogens/ medroxyprogesterone	Premphase, Prempro	PO, dose varies	For menopausal symptoms
estradiol/norethindrone	CombiPatch	Transdermal, 1 patch two times per week (q3–4 days)	For female hypogonadism, menopausal symptoms
	Activella	PO, 1 tab daily	Osteoporosis prophylaxis; menopausal symptoms

Note: Because of adverse side effects, estrogen and progestin products should be administered at the lowest possible dose for effectiveness.

a. List of trade names is not all-inclusive as the products are too numerous to mention.

Contraceptive Agents

The use of combination *estrogen–progestin* contraceptives as a safe and an effective method of birth control has been well established. They act by suppressing the release of the pituitary hormones, FSH, and LH, thus resulting in the prevention of ovulation.

The *progestin-only* contraceptives prevent pregnancy by inhibiting ovulation, changing the amount or thickness of the cervical mucus, thus inhibiting sperm transport and creating a thin, atrophic endometrium not conducive to sustaining the fertilized ovum. The progestin-only preparations may be indicated for women who cannot tolerate estrogenic side effects or for whom estrogen is contraindicated. Examples would be estrogen-related headaches or hypertension. Other indications include breast-feeding women, because *progestin has no effect on lactation or nursing infants.* Young women who have a history of noncompliance on oral contraceptives might benefit from injections or intrauterine devices (IUDs). The failure rate for progestin-only preparations ranges from 0.5% for oral agents to 0.1%–0.3% for injections and implants and 0.2%–2% for IUDs.

Uses of combined or progestin-only contraceptives include:

> Prevention of pregnancy
>
> Treatment and/or improvement of other medical conditions, such as fibroids and endometriosis; premenstrual dysphoric disorder; painful, heavy periods; irregular cycles; and acne
>
> Other medical benefits of oral contraceptives include decreased incidence of ovarian cysts, ovarian or endometrial cancer, benign breast disease, and ectopic pregnancy and improved bone density during perimenopause; protective effect against pelvic inflammatory disease

Minor side effects of contraceptives include (most should resolve after a few months of use):

> Nausea
>
> Increased breast size and tenderness
>
> ❗ Fluid retention
>
> ❗ Weight gain or loss
>
> ❗ Bleeding between periods and breakthrough bleeding
>
> Scanty menstrual flow (considered a benefit)
>
> Changes in libido
>
> Mood changes
>
> Facial discoloration

Serious side effects of estrogen can include:

> ❗ Migraine headaches or headaches increasing in frequency and severity
>
> ❗ Severe depression
>
> Blurred vision or loss of vision

Precautions or contraindications for estrogen products apply to:

> Thrombophlebitis or thromboembolic disorder or history thereof
>
> History of cerebrovascular accident
>
> History of chest pain or MI
>
> Known or suspected history of breast cancer or other estrogen-dependent malignancy, or preexisting cervical cancer
>
> Pregnancy
>
> Major surgery with prolonged immobilization
>
> History of liver disease or impaired liver function

In addition to the preceding precautions or contraindications, estrogen–progestin contraceptives should be used **with caution** in the following conditions:

Women over 35 and currently smoking 15 or more cigarettes a day

Migraine headaches that start after initiating oral contraceptives

Perimenopausal women

Seizure disorder

Hypertension with resting diastolic above 90 or systolic above 140

High cholesterol; dyslipidemia

Obesity

Diabetes mellitus

Undiagnosed vaginal bleeding

Confirmed sickle cell disease

Lactation

Oral contraceptives may accelerate the development of gallbladder disease in women already susceptible

Interactions of estrogen products may include the following:

Many drugs may interact with oral contraceptives and alter the effectiveness, including pain relievers, alcohol, anticoagulants, antidepressants, tranquilizers or barbiturates, corticosteroids, rifampin, antiretrovirals, asthma drugs, beta-blockers, anticonvulsants, oral hypoglycemic drugs, St. John's wort, and vitamin C.

CLINICAL CONNECTION

Deep Vein Thrombosis Prevention

Although most side effects of oral contraceptives (OCs) are minor and manageable, deep vein thrombosis (DVT) is a serious risk consideration for women who chose this as a method of birth control. The highest risk patients are those over the age of 35, are obese, and who are smokers (especially those who smoke >15 cigarettes/day), but all women who are taking oral birth control should be informed of this risk and made aware of potential prevention strategies. OCs should be avoided in patients with a history of DVT (and related conditions like pulmonary embolism) and those patients requiring major surgery requiring prolonged immobilization. Additionally, patients who are deemed to have a higher risk of DVT/PE should be started on an OC with 30 mcg or less of estrogen and the progestin component levonorgestrel as these combinations show a lower DVT/PE risk than those with greater than 30 mcg of estrogen and the progestin component drospirenone. Finally, for those patients who are not considered to be at a higher risk of developing DVT/PE, they should be informed to stay active, especially during long car rides or plane flights, maintain a healthy BMI, monitor cholesterol and blood pressure, and to avoid smoking or consider smoking cessation if applicable. Compression socks and anticoagulation therapy can also be considered as preventative options.

PATIENT EDUCATION

Women taking oral contraceptives should be instructed regarding:

Using backup contraception for the first month on oral contraceptives and for the first two weeks with Depo-Provera

Taking the contraceptive at the same time every day (Every product comes with specific directions to follow if an oral contraceptive dose is missed. The general instruction is that the pill should be doubled up until the patient has caught up, using a backup method until the period begins. If three pills or more are missed, the patient is instructed to throw away the pack until she starts her period and then begin a new pack of pills. Stop oral contraceptives if pregnancy is suspected and stop smoking.)

Using backup contraception when taking other medicines that may alter effectiveness (see Interactions)

Reporting the following symptoms to the health care professional should they occur while on oral contraceptives: chest pain, shortness of breath, severe headache, dizziness, weakness, numbness, eye problems, breast lumps, or severe leg pains in the calf or thigh

The fact that oral contraceptives do not protect against HIV, AIDS, or other sexually transmitted diseases

CHOICE OF CONTRACEPTIVES

This section discusses the choice of contraceptive methods by women with various characteristics and medical conditions. Health care professionals should always consider the individual clinical circumstances of each person seeking family planning services.

Estrogen–Progestin Contraceptives

Estrogen–progestin oral contraceptives are available in several formulations and varieties of chemical preparations. They are usually classified according to their estrogen content and formulation as follows:

1. Monophasic preparations contain the same proportion of estrogen and progestin in each tablet.

2. Biphasic preparations contain two sequences of progestin doses and less than 50 mcg estrogen.

3. Triphasic preparations contain three sequences of progestin doses and less than 50 mcg estrogen. (See Figure 24-2.)

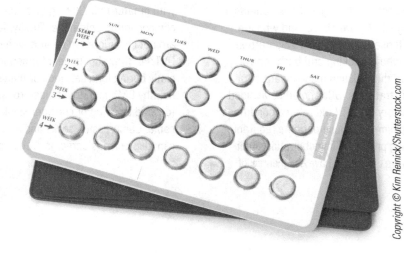

FIGURE 24-2 A triphasic 21/7 oral contraceptive. It is designed to mimic natural hormonal release in the body and has three different doses of oral contraception (1 week each) and a fourth week that is a hormone free interval.

4. Four-phasic preparations contain four sequences of estradiol valerate, a synthetic estrogen, and two (middle) sequences of the progestin dienogest.

The biphasic and triphasic formulations are intended to deliver the hormones in a manner similar to physiological processes.

Extended- or continuous-cycle oral contraceptives differ from traditional 21/7 products by decreasing or eliminating the hormone-free interval (HFI). Consecutive days of HT may extend to 84 or 365 days, with the HFI shortened to zero, two, or four days instead of the typical seven-day interval. Reasons for considering an extended- or continuous-cycle product include decreasing the typical menstrual symptoms (especially headaches) experienced during the HFI; improving efficacy in women who forget to restart the pill; and patient preference to decrease the frequency of menstrual-like bleeding, although breakthrough bleeding is more likely.

Choice of a particular contraceptive will be made after considering the patient's history, hormone-related side effects, prior use, and desired effect. In general, whenever possible, start on monophasic regimens with the smallest dose of estrogen (20 mcg for most women) and progestin (levonorgestrel or norethindrone) that is compatible with a low failure rate and meets the individual needs of the woman.

Broad categories are listed in Table 24-2. Individual oral contraceptives are too numerous to mention in their entirety; however, a few examples in each category are included.

Progestin-Only Contraceptives

These preparations are recommended for patients who do not tolerate estrogen or in whom it is contraindicated. The choice of the method of delivery (i.e., oral tablets, injection, or IUD) should be made to appropriately accommodate the patient's needs and compliance. It should be noted that use of Depo-Provera injections may be considered among the risk factors for development of osteoporosis (partially reversible upon discontinuation).

Progestin-Containing Intrauterine Device (IUD)

Mirena contains a reservoir of levonorgestrel, a synthetic progestin. It releases small amounts of progesterone daily, providing five years of continuous contraception protection. The mechanism of action of the IUD is not fully understood but is generally thought to have an inhibitory effect on sperm migration, change in the ovum transport, and alteration of the endometrium. The progestin in the IUD is thought to offer support to all of these actions.

There are many considerations, precautions or contraindications, and side effects that must be addressed when considering the IUD as a method of contraception, but are too numerous to mention here. The purpose of including the IUD here is to inform the reader that it is one of several delivery systems in the use of progestin as a contraceptive drug.

Postcoital Contraception

Although the use of combined estrogen–progestin contraceptive pills as a means of emergency or postcoital contraception is not without risk, it is an available option to women who are exposed to an unintentional risk of pregnancy. This includes such circumstances as a broken condom, rape, defective barrier methods, lost or forgotten oral contraceptives, or any other method that is not available at the time that it is needed. Emergency contraception options in the United States include estrogen and progestin combinations, progestin-only products, and progesterone agonist/antagonist.

When using postcoital or morning-after contraception, it is essential that the woman's history is reviewed, that she is informed of the risks and benefits of postcoital contraception, and that she gives informed consent. There is no medical condition for which the risks of emergency contraception use outweigh the benefits; therefore, emergency contraception *can be taken* by women with contraindications to conventional oral contraceptives. Emergency contraception should *not* be used as a regular method of birth control and is not as effective as other forms of contraception.

Women already on certain estrogen–progestin combination oral contraceptives can take a higher dose of their regular pill for use as emergency contraception if administered within 72h of unprotected intercourse. Typical dosages for oral contraceptives in this instance would be Lo/Ovral, Seasonale, or Triphasil, four tablets taken in two doses, 12h apart, for a total of eight tablets. For more information on birth control pills that can be used for emergency contraception, refer to the Princeton University website www.not-2-late.com. Side effects, which include nausea and vomiting, headache, and breast tenderness, usually subside within one or two days after treatment. Again, it must be noted that postcoital contraception must be administered within 72h of unprotected intercourse and is more effective the sooner it is taken after having unprotected sex.

Next Choice is an emergency contraceptive formulation containing two tablets of the progestin levonorgestrel; Plan B One-Step contains one tablet. Progestin-only emergency contraception is more effective and causes less nausea and vomiting than the oral contraceptive combinations. The first tablet should be taken as soon as possible but within 72h after having unprotected intercourse. For Next Choice only, the second tablet must be taken 12h after the first. Taken within three days of sexual intercourse, these progestin-only medications prevent ovulation or, if ovulation has already occurred, *block implantation of the fertilized egg*. Both are available to be purchased over-the-counter (OTC) without a prescription or proof of age.

Ulipristal acetate (Ella) is a progesterone agonist/antagonist, which is effective for the prevention of pregnancy when taken up to five days after the event. It most likely works by delaying or inhibiting ovulation. Ulipristal is available by prescription only and is not intended for more than one episode of unprotected intercourse in a menstrual cycle. The recommended dose is one tablet as soon as possible within five days; if vomiting occurs within 3h of taking the tablet, consider repeating the dose. Side effects include headache, vomiting, abdominal pain, and dysmenorrhea.

See Table 24-4 for a summary of contraceptive agents.

TABLE 24-4 **Contraceptive Agents**

GENERIC NAME	TRADE NAME[a]	DOSAGE	USES/COMMENTS
Monophasic preparations			
50 mcg estrogen	Necon 1/50 Ovcon-50	PO	Contain the same proportion of estrogen and progesterone in each tablet
35 mcg estrogen	Norinyl 1/35 Ortho-Novum 1/35 Brevicon	PO	
30 mcg estrogen	Lo/Ovral	PO	
	Seasonale		Extended-cycle regimen
	Yasmin		
20 mcg estrogen	YAZ	PO	Extended-cycle regimen
	Lybrel		Continuous-cycle regimen
	Ortho Evra	Transdermal	1 patch q7days for three weeks per cycle
Biphasic preparation—2 sequences progestin/1 part estrogen			
	Seasonique	PO	Extended-cycle regimen
	Mircette		
Triphasic preparation—3 sequences progestin/one part estrogen			
	Trivora	PO, dose varies	
	Ortho-Novum 7/7/7		
	Ortho-Tri-Cyclen		
Four-phasic preparation—four sequences estrogen/two sequences progestin			
	Natazia	PO, dose varies	Effective for heavy menstrual bleeding
Progestin-only preparations			
	Ortho Micronor	PO	"Mini-pill"
	Depo-Provera	IM, 150 mg q3m	
	Mirena	Intrauterine device (IUD)	
Postcoital contraception			
levonorgestrel	Lo/Ovral, Seasonale	PO, 4 tabs q12h for total of 8 tabs (must be administered within 72 h)	With norgestrel- and levonorgestrel-containing combination products (dose varies with other products)
	Next Choice	PO, 1 tab q12h for a total of 2 tabs (within 72 h)	Available OTC for 17+ years; Rx only for ≤16 years old
	Plan B One-Step	PO, 1 tab single dose (within 72 h)	Now available OTC with no age restrictions
ulipristal	Ella	PO, 1 tab single dose (within 120 h)	Rx only

Note: Because of adverse side effects, estrogen and progestin products should be administered at the lowest possible dose for effectiveness.

a. List of trade names is not all-inclusive as the available oral contraceptives are too numerous to mention.

PATIENT EDUCATION

Patients taking estrogen, progesterone, or combinations of the two should be instructed regarding:

Importance of following the prescribed schedule with contraceptives

Taking with or after evening meal or at bedtime, same time every day

The fact that these products do not protect against HIV infection or other STDs

Minor adverse effects of contraceptives, for example edema, weight gain, and nausea

Possible serious side effects and the importance of reporting any signs of cardiovascular or kidney disorders, liver or gallbladder dysfunction, rash, jaundice, GI symptoms, visual disturbance, severe headache, breast lumps, irregular vaginal bleeding, shortness of breath, and chest or calf pain

Increased risk of stroke or myocardial infarction (MI) for smokers

Regular breast self-examination

Complete physical examination including Pap test at least yearly

Avoidance of all estrogen or progestin products if pregnant (however, note that the American Academy of Pediatrics considers both estrogens and progestins to be generally compatible with breast feeding)

DRUGS FOR LABOR AND DELIVERY

In addition to the hormones secreted by the anterior pituitary gland, there is also a hormone secreted by the posterior pituitary lobe: **oxytocin**. This hormone stimulates the uterus to contract, thus inducing childbirth. Oxytocin also acts on the mammary gland to stimulate the release of milk. Synthetic chemicals used to stimulate uterine contractions are called *oxytocics* and include *oxytocin* and prostaglandin E_1 and E_2.

The goal of labor induction at term is to facilitate the vaginal delivery of a healthy infant. Induction of labor may be required for pregnancies that go beyond term, those in which premature rupture of the membranes occurs, or pregnancies in which there are maternal or fetal indications for early delivery.

Oxytocin

Uses of oxytocin (IV infusion of dilute solutions slowly and at a carefully monitored rate) include:

Induction of labor with at-term or near-term pregnancies associated with hypertension (e.g., preeclampsia, eclampsia, or cardiovascular or renal disease), maternal diabetes, or uterine fetal death at term

Stimulating uterine contractions during the first or second stages of labor if labor is prolonged or if dysfunctional uterine inertia occurs

Pelvic adequacy and other maternal and fetal conditions must be evaluated carefully prior to the induction of labor. Cesarean section may be preferable and safer in some instances.

Side effects of oxytocin are dose related and can be serious, resulting even in maternal or fetal death. *Extreme caution* with administration and *constant maternal* and *fetal monitoring* are required to prevent dangerous side effects such as:

❗ Tetanic contractions with the risk of uterine rupture

Cervical lacerations

❗ Abruptio placenta

Impaired uterine blood flow

Amniotic fluid embolism

❗ Fetal trauma, including intracranial hemorrhage or brain damage

❗ Fetal cardiac arrhythmias, including bradycardia, tachycardia, and premature ventricular contractions

❗ Fetal death because of asphyxia

With large amounts of oxytocin, watch for:

❗ Severe hypotension

❗ Tachycardia and arrhythmias

❗ Postpartum hemorrhage

Subarachnoid hemorrhage

Hypertensive episodes

Precautions or contraindications for oxytocin apply to:

Elective induction of labor merely for physician or patient convenience, which is *not* a valid indication for oxytocin use

Cephalopelvic disproportion and unfavorable fetal position or presentation

Uterine or cervical scarring from major cervical or uterine surgery

Fetal distress when delivery is not imminent

Placenta previa, prolapsed cord, and multiparity

Prolonged use with eclampsia

Prostaglandins

Prostaglandins are released as a natural part of the cervical ripening process. Prostaglandins causing the contraction of the myometrial muscle include dinoprostone or prostaglandin E_2 (Prostin E_2, Cervidil, Prepidil), the oral synthetic prostaglandin E_1 analog, misoprostol (Cytotec), and the prostaglandin F2-alpha analog carboprost (Hemabate). All prostaglandins stimulate smooth muscle in the GI tract, accounting for the GI side effects seen.

Uses of dinoprostone intravaginal gel or vaginal insert include:

Cervical ripening

Uses of dinoprostone vaginal suppositories or carboprost injection include:

Therapeutic abortion in the second trimester (beyond the 12th week)

Uterine evacuation in cases of intrauterine fetal death in late pregnancy; benign hydatidiform mole; or fetuses with acephaly, erythroblastosis fetalis, or other congenital abnormalities *incompatible with life*

Uses of carboprost injection include:

Treatment of postpartum bleeding because of uterine atony that is unresponsive to conventional management including oxytocin IV, uterine massage, uterine manipulation, and injectable ergot preparations

Side effects of prostaglandins can be minimized by the administration of a prior test dose and symptomatic treatment of such effects as:

- ❗ GI hypermotility, including nausea, vomiting, and diarrhea (decreased by premedication with antiemetics and antidiarrheal agents)
- ❗ Bradycardia, hypotension, hypertension, and arrhythmias
- ❗ Dizziness, syncope, flushing, and fever
- ❗ Bronchospasm, including wheezing, dyspnea, chest constriction, and chest pain
- Cervical laceration or uterine rupture (less common)
- Retained placenta (less common)

Precautions or contraindications for prostaglandins include:

Use only by trained physicians in a hospital where intensive care and surgical facilities are available

Contraindicated with a history of pelvic surgery, uterine fibroids, cervical stenosis, and acute pelvic inflammatory disease

Caution with asthma, hypertension, and cardiovascular or renal disease

Previous history of C-section

Mifepristone (RU-486)

Mifepristone (Mifeprex) is an antiprogesterone drug that is used to terminate an unwanted pregnancy (in conjunction with misoprostol). There are detailed requirements (including informed consent) to ensure that women fully understand the process. The drug is sold directly to trained physicians and is not available in pharmacies. Patient education (*Mifepristone Medication Guide*) is very important for the proper administration of this drug.

Mifepristone is for use only very early in pregnancy—within 49 days from the beginning of a woman's last menstrual period. Mifepristone blocks the action of progesterone, a hormone essential for maintaining pregnancy. Without progesterone, the uterine lining thins, so the embryo cannot remain implanted and grow. It requires three visits to a qualified physician to complete the treatment:

1. At the first visit, the physician will determine the gestational status. If the woman qualifies for the procedure, she must sign an informed consent agreeing to the necessary visits. She will then receive three mifepristone pills to be taken by mouth.

2. The second step requires the woman to swallow a second drug two days later to fully detach the embryo from the uterus and expel it. Misoprostol (Cytotec) causes uterine contractions with miscarriage-like cramping and bleeding.

3. The third step requires a follow-up visit to the physician within two weeks to make sure the abortion is complete. In case of hemorrhage, it might be necessary to consult the physician sooner. Studies have shown that mifepristone is 77%–92% effective in terminating pregnancy. However, in some cases, a curettage of the uterine cavity is required to remove any remaining products of conception.

Side effects of mifepristone can include:

> ⚠ Diarrhea and nausea

> ⚠ Uterine hemorrhage in about 5% of patients

> Infection if the embryo is not completely expelled

> A malformed child if the second and third steps are not completed

Precautions or contraindications of mifepristone apply to:

> Ectopic pregnancy

> Any time after 49 days from the beginning of a woman's last menstrual period

> Current long-term corticosteroid therapy

> Bleeding disorders

> Current anticoagulant therapy

The FDA recently approved mifepristone (Korlym) for the treatment of hyperglycemia in patients with Cushing's Syndrome who have Type 2 diabetes and are not candidates for or responding to prior surgery. Korlym is contraindicated in pregnancy.

Methylergonovine

The semisynthetic ergot alkaloid methylergonovine is used for the prevention and treatment of postpartum and postabortion hemorrhage.

Side effects of methylergonovine occur most commonly when administered IV undiluted or too rapidly, or in conjunction with regional anesthesia or vasoconstrictors, and can include:

> ⚠ Nausea and vomiting

> ⚠ Dizziness, headache, diaphoresis, palpitation, dyspnea, and arrhythmias

> Hypertension (more common) or hypotension

> Numbness and coldness of extremities with overdose (peripheral vasoconstriction)

> Seizures with overdose

Precautions or contraindications for methylergonovine include:

> When administered during the third stage of labor, may lead to retained placenta

> Contraindicated with cardiovascular disease, especially hypertension, and with hepatic and renal impairment

> Patients with preeclampsia or eclampsia

Terbutaline

Terbutaline, although classified as a bronchodilator drug primarily used for pulmonary disorders, is also used with careful monitoring in the management of preterm labor. Its sympathomimetic action inhibits uterine contractions (tocolysis) by smooth muscle relaxation. Although the manufacturer does not recommend its use for preterm labor, it is used off-label for this purpose in urgent situations with careful monitoring in the hospital setting. It is available for oral, IV, or subcutaneous administration but is only used subcutaneously or intravenously for this problem.

Side effects of terbutaline include:

> ❗ *Maternal* nervousness, tremors, increased heart rate, headache, nausea, vomiting, hypotension, heart palpitations, cardiac arrhythmias, myocardial ischemia, and metabolic abnormalities (hyperglycemia and hypokalemia)
>
> *Fetal* tachycardia, hypotension, hyperbilirubinemia, hypoglycemia, hypocalcemia, and intraventricular hemorrhage

Caution with terbutaline applies to:

> Watching the patient closely for signs of pulmonary edema. Should not be used in patients with hypertension, cardiac disease, hyperthyroidism, diabetes, or history of seizures.

Precautions or contraindications for terbutaline (black box warning) apply to:

> *Prolonged tocolysis* (use beyond 48–72 h), for terbutaline administered by injection or by continuous infusion pump because of the potential for serious maternal cardiovascular events and death

Magnesium Sulfate

Preeclampsia is characterized by new-onset hypertension, edema, and proteinuria during pregnancy. Patients become eclamptic when they develop new-onset grand mal seizures in the presence of preeclampsia and require immediate medical intervention. Treatment of severe preeclampsia or eclampsia consists of controlling elevated blood pressure (see Chapter 25) and utilizing magnesium sulfate injection for the prevention and control of seizures.

Magnesium sulfate acts by depressing the CNS, blocking neuromuscular transmission, and causing cerebral vasodilation, thus producing anticonvulsant effects. It has also been used in the management of uterine tetany associated with the use of oxytocic agents. Magnesium sulfate also acts peripherally, producing vasodilation and lowering the blood pressure. Patients receiving this drug must be monitored closely for vital signs and reflexes.

Side effects of magnesium sulfate, which can be serious and even fatal, can include:

> ❗ Flaccid paralysis and CNS depression
> ❗ Circulatory collapse, cardiac depression, and cardiac arrest
> ❗ Pulmonary edema and fatal respiratory paralysis
>
> Flushing and sweating and hypotension
>
> Fetal toxicity at high doses (rare with proper use and monitoring)
>
> The antidote for overdose of magnesium sulfate (e.g., respiratory depression or heart block) is IV administration of calcium gluconate.

Precautions or contraindications when using magnesium sulfate apply to:

> Impaired renal function
>
> Heart block or myocardial damage
>
> Prolonged use because of potential respiratory depression in the neonate

See Table 24-5 for a summary of drugs for labor and delivery.

TABLE 24-5 Drugs for Labor and Delivery

GENERIC NAME	TRADE NAME	DOSAGE	COMMENTS
Oxytocics[a]			
methylergonovine	(Methergine)[b]	PO, IM; dosage varies	For postpartum hemorrhage
oxytocin	Pitocin	IV, IM	For the induction of labor and for postpartum hemorrhage
Prostaglandins			
dinoprostone	Prostin E2	Vaginal supp., 20 mg	For therapeutic abortion
	Cervidil	Vaginal insert, 10 mg	For cervical ripening
	Prepidil	Intravaginal gel, 0.5 mg	For cervical ripening
misoprostol	Cytotec	Tablets	For pregnancy termination (used with mifepristone)
carboprost	Hemabate	IM, dose varies	For refractory postpartum bleeding, pregnancy termination
Tocolytic[c]			
terbutaline		IV, subcu, dose varies	Short-term for premature labor (PO now contraindicated for this use)
Treatment for preeclampsia or eclampsia			
magnesium sulfate		IM, IV; dosage varies	Watch for respiratory complications

a. Stimulate uterine contractions.
b. This brand name is no longer marketed, but the name may still be commonly used.
c. Inhibit uterine contractions in preterm labor.

OTHER GONADOTROPIC DRUGS

Drugs classified as analogs of *gonadotropin-releasing hormones* (GnRH) act in the pituitary to suppress ovarian and testicular hormone production and inhibit estrogen and androgen synthesis. Leuprolide (Lupron) has been used as an antineoplastic agent to inhibit the growth of hormone-dependent tumors. It has been used to reduce the size of the prostate and inhibit prostatic tumor growth. Lupron has also been used following other therapies, for example mastectomy, radiation, and/or other antineoplastic drugs to treat breast cancer. It is sometimes combined with the antiestrogen drug tamoxifen in the treatment of breast cancer (see Chapter 14 for dosage and side effects).

GnRH analogs that inhibit gonadotropin secretion, for example Lupron and Synarel, are used in the management of endometriosis. Endometriosis is a condition where endometrial tissue develops outside the uterus, causing pelvic or lower back pain. GnRH analogs inhibit ovulation and stop menstruation (similar to what occurs in menopause), thereby providing pain relief and a reduction in endometriotic lesions. Lupron is administered as a monthly (3.75 mg) or trimonthly (11.25 mg) IM injection. Synarel is administered as a nasal spray. Treatment with either is limited to six months. Both drugs appear to be better tolerated than the androgen danazol in the treatment of endometriosis.
Side effects of the GnRH agonists (menopausal symptoms) can include:

⚠ Hot flashes and diaphoresis

Vaginal dryness and vaginitis

! Headache and insomnia

Emotional or mood swings and reduced libido

Weight gain or loss and peripheral edema

Nasal congestion or irritation with Synarel

Acne

Precautions or contraindications include the following:

Not to be considered effective as a contraceptive; the patient should use a backup barrier method

Pregnancy or lactation

Diabetes (monitor the blood glucose level carefully)

Prolonged use creates a hypoestrogenic state that may lead to an increased risk of loss of bone density (monitor bone mineral density).

Patients must be fully informed of the benefits and risks of the use of GnRH analog drugs, and, generally speaking, the therapeutic values should outweigh any potential risks. Patient compliance is enhanced with adequate patient education, counseling, and support. See Table 24-6 for a summary of other gonadotropin-associated drugs.

TABLE 24-6 Other Gonadotropin-Associated Drugs

GENERIC NAME	TRADE NAME	DOSAGE	COMMENTS
nafarelin acetate	Synarel	Nasal spray, 200 mcg/spray; alternate nares, dose varies	For endometriosis, treatment not to exceed six months
leuprolide acetate	Lupron Depot, Eligard	IM, subcu, dose varies	For endometriosis, some cases of infertility, treatment not to exceed six months; also for prostate cancer (see Chapter 14—Antineoplastics)

CASE STUDY A

Reproductive System Drugs

Allison Cavanaugh is a 24-year-old female who has been experiencing painful and heavy-flow menses. At a recent visit to her gynecologist, she was diagnosed with endometriosis.

1. The physician writes a prescription for an oral contraceptive containing estrogen and progestin and explains that this might help Allison's condition by:
   a. Increasing the frequency of ovulation
   b. Increasing the amount or thickness of cervical mucus
   c. Decreasing the amount of pituitary hormones released
   d. Creating a thin, atrophic endometrium not conducive to sustaining a fertilized ovum

2. The physician explains that Allison might experience some minor side effects that should resolve after a few months of use. Which of the following is one of these possible side effects?
   a. Constipation   b. Weight gain   c. Painful joints   d. Pelvic pain

3. Prior to writing the prescription for the contraceptive, the physician reviews Allison's medical history. This is important because contraceptives are contraindicated in patients with a history of:
   a. Asthma   b. Thrombophlebitis   c. Peanut allergy   d. Breast augmentation

4. The nurse instructs Allison on how to take the contraceptive. Which of the following instructions is most likely to be included in her teaching plan?

   a. Use a backup contraceptive for three months.

   b. Take the oral contraceptive at the same time each day.

   c. Note that oral contraceptives protect against HIV.

   d. Take a drug holiday after taking the contraceptive for six months.

5. What symptom would be most important for Allison to report to her physician after starting the oral contraceptive?

   a. Chest pain   b. Urinary frequency   c. Breast tenderness   d. Rash on chest

CASE STUDY B

Reproductive System Drugs

Katrina Oosterlund is in her 31st week of pregnancy and has developed hypertension, 3+ edema in her ankles, and proteinuria. The OB physician is concerned that she may develop new-onset grand mal seizures related to eclampsia. She is admitted to the hospital and started on IV magnesium sulfate.

1. Katrina is reluctant to start on the IV because she is concerned about the drug magnesium sulfate. The physician explains that the medication is necessary for her condition and will produce an anticonvulsant effect by:

   a. Peripheral vasoconstriction

   b. An increase in circulatory volume

   c. Depressing the CNS and thereby causing cerebral vasodilation

   d. The induction of bradycardia and a subsequent reduction in blood pressure

2. The nurse notes a physician order for an antidote in case of an overdose of magnesium sulfate. The drug she will have on hand in case of an overdose is:

   a. Calcium carbonate   b. Glucagon   c. Calcium gluconate   d. Carboprost

3. Extreme caution should be exercised when administering magnesium sulfate because of its potential effects on the neonate. This includes the potential for:

   a. Hypotension

   b. Increased risk of seizure

   c. Respiratory depression

   d. Hypertension

4. What is one of the serious side effects of magnesium sulfate?

   a. Hypertension   b. Flaccid paralysis   c. Status asthmaticus   d. Severe dehydration

5. While Katrina is receiving IV magnesium sulfate, she will be monitored closely for:

   a. Vital signs and reflexes

   b. Blood glucose levels

   c. Hematocrit and hemoglobin

   d. Creatinine clearance

CHAPTER REVIEW QUIZ

Match the medications in the first column with the conditions they are used to treat. Conditions may be used more than once.

Medication

1. ___ Premarin
2. ___ Megace
3. ___ Depo-Testosterone
4. ___ Danocrine
5. ___ Covaryx
6. ___ terbutaline
7. ___ Cialis
8. ___ Levitra
9. ___ Pitocin

Condition

a. Endometriosis
b. Menopausal symptoms
c. Prostate cancer
d. Erectile dysfunction
e. Hypogonadism
f. Uterine inertia in labor
g. Infertility
h. Preterm labor
i. Cachexia of AIDS

Choose the correct answer.

10. What possible side effect should a patient taking tadalafil report to a physician?
    a. Insomnia
    b. Vision abnormalities
    c. Constipation
    d. Tingling in the feet

11. Which category of drugs has serious interactions with PDE inhibitors?
    a. Nitrates
    b. Anti-inflammatories
    c. Muscle relaxants
    d. Hypoglycemic agents

12. Women with a uterus should not use estrogen-alone therapy because it puts them at risk for which of the following?
    a. Blood clots
    b. Uterine cancer
    c. Stroke
    d. Osteoporosis

13. Estrogen therapy (i.e., estrogen alone) has been associated with an increased risk of endometrial cancer. Estrogen combined with which agent reduces this risk?
    a. Testosterone
    b. Androgens
    c. Progestin
    d. Progesterone agonist

14. A contraceptive preparation containing two sequences of progestin doses and less than 50 mcg of estrogen is called:
    a. Monophasic
    b. Biphasic
    c. Triphasic
    d. Four-phasic

15. Dinoprostone intravaginal gel or vaginal insert is indicated for:
    a. Premature labor
    b. Therapeutic abortion
    c. Induction of labor
    d. Cervical ripening

16. Oxytocin should be avoided for patients with a history of:
    a. Miscarriage
    b. Diabetes mellitus
    c. Endometriosis
    d. Placenta previa

17. A side effect of methylergonovine, given for the treatment of postpartum hemorrhage, can include:
    a. Fever
    b. Nausea and vomiting
    c. Urinary retention
    d. Peripheral vasodilation

18. A drug used primarily for pulmonary disorders but that can also be used for the management of preterm labor is:
    a. Oxytocin   **b.** Carboprost   **c.** Terbutaline   **d.** Misoprostol

19. Maternal side effects of terbutaline include:
    a. Hyperglycemia   **b.** Hypoglycemia   **c.** Hyperthryoidism   **d.** Hyperkalemia

20. Fetal side effects of terbutaline include:
    a. Hypercalcemia   **c.** Tachycardia
    b. Hypobilirubinemia   **d.** Intra-abdominal bleeding

21. Extreme caution is required with the administration of oxytocin, along with constant fetal and maternal monitoring, to prevent which side effect?
    a. Cervical stricture   **c.** Maternal seizures
    b. Maternal desaturation   **d.** Uterine rupture

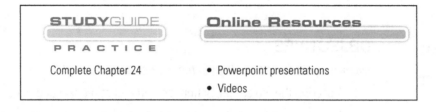

STUDYGUIDE   Online Resources

PRACTICE

Complete Chapter 24   • Powerpoint presentations
                             • Videos

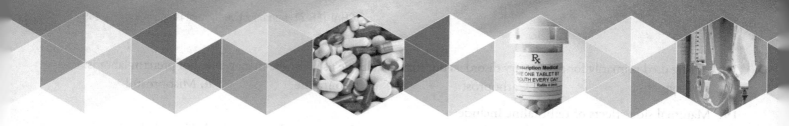

CHAPTER 25
CARDIOVASCULAR DRUGS

OBJECTIVES

Upon completion of this chapter, the learner should be able to

1. Describe the indication, action, and effects of digoxin and toxic side effects

2. Identify the different types of antiarrhythmics, general indications, side effects, and associated patient education

3. Identify the most commonly used antihypertensives, side effects, and required patient education

4. Describe the different types of coronary vasodilators with cautions, side effects, and patient education

5. Name the six antilipemic categories and describe their actions, common drugs, and patient education

6. Compare and contrast the three categories of antithrombotic agents in terms of administration, action, typical drugs, and antidotes

7. Explain appropriate and important patient education for all categories of antithrombotic therapy

8. Define the Key Terms and Concepts

Cardiovascular drugs include medications that affect the heart and blood vessels as well as anticoagulant and antiplatelet agents that prevent clotting. The drugs described in this chapter are divided into the following categories: cardiac glycosides, antiarrhythmic agents, antihypertensives, vasodilators, antilipemic agents, anticoagulants, platelet inhibitors, thrombolytics, and hematopoietic agents. Some of the drugs described in this chapter fall into more than one category because of their multiple actions and uses (e.g., propranolol, which is used to treat cardiac arrhythmias, hypertension, and angina). Diuretics, which also affect the blood vessels and reduce blood pressure, are discussed in Chapter 15. Autonomic nervous system effects of these drugs are explained in Chapter 13.

CARDIAC GLYCOSIDES (DIGOXIN)

FIGURE 25-1 Heart failure results in a decreased cardiac output, which leads to a lack of oxygenated blood from the lungs to be pumped throughout the body.

Cardiac glycosides occur widely in nature or can be prepared synthetically. These glycosides act directly on the myocardium to increase the force of myocardial contractions. Digoxin is the only clinical drug currently used in the cardiac glycoside family. Cardiac glycosides are used primarily in the treatment of **heart failure** in patients with symptoms that persist after optimization of treatment with an ACE inhibitor, a beta-adrenergic blocker, and/or a diuretic. They are sometimes also used alone or in conjunction with other medications (such as calcium channel blockers) to *slow* the ventricular response in patients with atrial fibrillation or flutter.

In patients with heart failure, the heart fails to adequately pump nutrients and oxygen to body tissues. Because the heart is failing, the body attempts to compensate by retaining salt and fluid, and this may result in both pulmonary and peripheral edema. The heart increases in size to compensate for the increased work load. Symptoms of heart failure include fatigue, weakness, dyspnea, cyanosis, increased heart rate, cough, and pitting edema. A small percentage of patients with heart failure will go on to develop atrial fibrillation. Two disabling and devastating complications of atrial fibrillation are ischemic stroke and systemic embolism.

In patients with heart failure, the cardiac glycosides act by *increasing the force of the cardiac contractions* without increasing oxygen consumption, thereby increasing cardiac output. Cardiac glycosides also lower norepinephrine levels, which are elevated in failure and are toxic to the failing heart. As a result of increased efficiency, the heart beats slower, the heart size shrinks, and the concurrent diuretic therapy decreases edema. Refer to Figure 25-1 to see how heart failure manifests in the body.

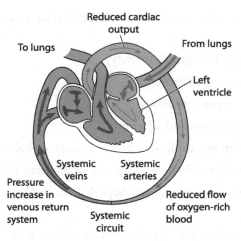

Reduced cardiac output

To lungs

From lungs

Left ventricle

Systemic veins

Systemic arteries

Pressure increase in venous return system

Reduced flow of oxygen-rich blood

Systemic circuit

CLINICAL CONNECTION

Patient Information Interviews

One of the most overlooked practices conducted by health care professionals is interviewing new or unfamiliar patients about their medications and disease states. This is important because medications can be used for multiple indications. Some disease states do not have medications that are unique to their treatment. Heart failure (HF) is a common condition that can result from other disease states and also cause complications. Although the diagnosis of HF is fairly straightforward, treatment can be complicated and vary drastically from patient to patient. HF patients are almost always prescribed three main classes of medications. (1) Certain beta-blockers (bisoprolol, carvedilol,

and metoprolol) are approved to treat HF and act to slow the heart rate; (2) angiotensin-converting enzyme (ACE) inhibitors and angiotensin receptor blockers (ARBs); and (3) diuretics.

Additional medications can be added on including digoxin, nitrates, or hydralazine (vasodilators) and aldosterone antagonists. All of these medication options are indicated in other disease states, so it may not be easy to recognize a person has heart failure with just a quick review of their medications, Therefore, it is important to be thorough during these patient interviews to avoid prescribing a drug that is contraindicated in clients with HF.

The most commonly used cardiac glycosides are digitalis products. Of these, digoxin (Lanoxin) is the only product still marketed for clinical use because it can be administered orally and parenterally and has an intermediate duration of action.

There is a very narrow margin between effective therapy with digoxin and dangerous toxicity, as discussed previously in chapter 23 this is considered a narrow therapeutic index (NTI) drug. Careful monitoring of cardiac rate and rhythm with EKG (electrocardiogram), cardiac function, side effects, and serum digoxin levels is required to determine the therapeutic maintenance dose. Checking the apical pulse before administering digoxin is an important part of this monitoring process. If the apical pulse rate is less than 60, digoxin may need to be withheld until the physician is consulted. The action taken should be documented.

Modification of dosage is based on individual requirements and response as determined by general condition, renal function, and cardiac function, monitored by EKG. When changing from tablets or intramuscular (IM) therapy to elixir or intravenous (IV) therapy, digoxin dosage adjustments may be required.

Toxic side effects of digoxin, which should be reported to the physician immediately, can include:

- Anorexia, nausea, and vomiting (early signs of toxicity)
  Abdominal cramping, distention, and diarrhea
- Headache, fatigue, lethargy, and muscle weakness
- Vertigo, restlessness, irritability, tremors, and seizures
- Visual disturbances including blurring, diplopia (double vision), or halos
- Cardiac arrhythmias of all kinds, especially bradycardia (rate less than 60)
- Electrolyte imbalance, especially potassium (either hyperkalemia or hypokalemia can cause arrhythmias)
- Insomnia, confusion, and mental disorders, especially with older adults

Treatment of digoxin toxicity includes:

Discontinuing the drug immediately (usually sufficient)

Monitoring electrolytes for hyperkalemia, hypokalemia, hypomagnesemia, and hypercalcemia

Drugs such as atropine for symptomatic bradycardia

Digoxin-specific Fab fragments (DigiFab) as an antidote in life-threatening toxicity

Precautions or contraindications apply to:

Severe pulmonary disease

Hypothyroidism

Acute myocardial infarction, acute myocarditis, and severe heart failure

Impaired renal function; hypokalemia and hypomagnesemia

Arrhythmias not caused by heart failure

Pregnancy and lactation

High doses in older adults

Interactions of digoxin may occur with:

Antacids, cholestyramine, neomycin, and rifampin (reduce the absorption of digoxin; administer far apart)

Diuretics, calcium, and corticosteroids (can increase the chance of arrhythmias)

Macrolides and antiarrhythmics (*especially* quinidine and verapamil; may potentiate digoxin toxicity)

Adrenergics (epinephrine, ephedrine, and isoproterenol; increase the risk of arrhythmias)

PATIENT EDUCATION

Patients taking digoxin should be instructed regarding:

Recognition and immediate reporting of side effects

Holding medication, if any side effects occur, until the physician can be consulted

Avoiding taking any other medication at the same time without physician approval

Avoiding all over-the-counter (OTC) medication, especially antacids and cold remedies

Avoiding abrupt withdrawal after prolonged use; must be reduced gradually under physician supervision

Checking heart rate (pulse) on a regular basis

ANTIARRHYTHMIC AGENTS

The term "arrhythmia" refers to any change from the normal sequence of electrical impulses of the heart. The electrical impulses may happen too fast, too slowly, or erratically—causing the heart to beat too fast (**tachycardia**), too slowly (**bradycardia**), or erratically (fibrillation). **Antiarrhythmic agents** include a variety of drugs that act in different ways to suppress various types of cardiac arrhythmias, including atrial or ventricular tachycardias, atrial fibrillation or flutter, and arrhythmias that occur with digoxin toxicity or during surgery and anesthesia. The choice of a particular antiarrhythmic agent is based on the careful assessment of many factors, including the type of arrhythmia; frequency; cardiac, renal, or other pathological condition; and current signs and symptoms.

The role of the health care professional is critical in this area in accurate and timely reporting of vital signs, pertinent observations regarding the effectiveness of medications and adverse side effects, and modification of precipitating causes. Adequate knowledge of drug action and effects, along with good judgment, is essential.

Side effects of the individual medications are discussed separately. However, keep in mind that most of the drugs given to counteract arrhythmias have the potential for lowering blood pressure and slowing heartbeat. Therefore, it is especially important to be alert for the signs of **hypotension** and bradycardia, which could lead to cardiac arrest. Although the antiarrhythmics commonly slow the heart rate, there are exceptions (e.g., procainamide and quinidine, which may cause *tachycardia*). When other cardiac drugs are administered concomitantly, cardiac effects may be additive or antagonistic. Antiarrhythmic agents can worsen existing arrhythmias or cause new arrhythmias, and therefore *careful monitoring is essential.*

Arrhythmia detection or monitoring can include EKG rhythm strips and 24-h Holter monitoring as indicated. Electrolyte surveillance, especially for disorders of potassium and magnesium, is very important for patients on antiarrhythmic agents. Nondrug therapy can include the insertion of a pacemaker or an automatic implantable cardioverter-defibrillator (AICD). The AICD has been widely accepted as the most effective treatment for patients with life-threatening ventricular tachycardia or fibrillation and for patients who have survived a cardiac arrest, and the AICD may also be effective in preventing sudden death in certain patients with heart failure.

Adenosine

Adenosine (Adenocard) is an injectable antiarrhythmic agent with multiple electrophysiological activities that complicate its placement into a single category. It restores normal sinus rhythm in paroxysmal supraventricular tachycardia (PSVT) by slowing conduction time through the atrioventricular (AV) node. Adenosine also has vasodilatory, antiadrenergic, and negative chronotropic (decrease in rate) properties, which act to decrease cardiac oxygen demand.

Adenosine is equal in effectiveness to diltiazem or verapamil in converting PSVT but is less likely to cause hypotension. Common side effects include facial flushing, lightheadedness, headache, dyspnea, and chest pressure. Adenosine is contraindicated in patients with a second- or third-degree heart block or symptomatic bradycardia (unless a functioning artificial pacemaker is present).

Amiodarone

Amiodarone (Cordarone) is an oral and injectable antiarrhythmic agent approved for the treatment of refractory life-threatening ventricular arrhythmias. Despite its problematic organ toxicity profile and black box warning, amiodarone is widely used for preventing the recurrence of atrial fibrillation. It is considered a broad-spectrum antiarrhythmic with multiple and complex electrophysiological effects. Amiodarone also relaxes both smooth and cardiac muscle, causing decreases in coronary and peripheral vascular resistance and systolic blood pressure.

Side effects of amiodarone, some of which are severe and potentially fatal, but may be less of a problem with lower doses (i.e., 200–400 mg per day), include:

Pulmonary fibrosis

❗ Cardiac arrhythmias, induction or worsening of heart failure, and hypotension

Nausea or vomiting, constipation, and anorexia

Hepatitis (rare)

Hyperthyroidism or hypothyroidism

Neurotoxicity (tremor, peripheral neuropathy, paresthesias [numbness, tingling, especially in extremities])

Visual disturbances; optic neuropathy and/or neuritis (may progress to permanent blindness)

Dermatological reactions, especially photosensitivity (avoid exposure, wear protective clothing)

Precautions or contraindications for amiodarone apply to:

Patients with a second- or third-degree heart block, marked sinus bradycardia because of severe sinus node dysfunction, and when bradycardia has caused syncope (unless a functioning artificial pacemaker is present); cardiogenic shock

Patients with thyroid disease (because of the large amount of iodine contained in amiodarone)

Iodine hypersensitivity

Older adults (more susceptible to thyrotoxic and neurotoxic adverse effects)

Interactions with amiodarone are numerous and significant, including:

Certain fluoroquinolones, macrolide antibiotics, systemic azole antifungals (QT prolongation)

⚠ Warfarin (can result in serious or fatal bleeding if warfarin dose is not reduced; effect may persist for months after discontinuation)

Certain antiarrhythmics, digoxin, and phenytoin (amiodarone increases serum concentrations of these drugs)

Protease inhibitors and grapefruit juice (increase amiodarone concentrations); beta-blockers, calcium channel blockers, and lidocaine (additive adverse cardiac effects)

Cholestyramine, phenytoin, and rifampin (serum concentrations of amiodarone are decreased, reducing its pharmacologic effect)

Beta-Adrenergic Blockers

Beta-adrenergic blockers, for example propranolol (Inderal), are antiarrhythmics, which combat arrhythmias by inhibiting adrenergic (sympathetic) nerve receptors. The action is complex, and the results can include a membrane-stabilizing effect on the heart. Propranolol (Inderal), a nonselective beta-blocker, is effective in the management of some cardiac arrhythmias and less effective with others. It is also used in the treatment of hypertension and some forms of chronic angina. Because it also blocks the beta$_2$ receptors in the lungs, it can lead to bronchospasm. *Low doses* of metoprolol (Lopressor), a selective beta$_1$-antagonist, may be used *with caution* in patients with lung conditions that cause bronchospasm. For additional use of beta-blockers, for example with migraine, see Chapter 13 and Table 13-2.

LEARNING HINT

Beta$_1$ receptors are found primarily in the heart and when stimulated cause an increase in the rate and force of contraction. Beta$_2$ receptors are found primarily in the lungs (when stimulated cause relaxation or bronchodilation of airways) and blood vessels (when stimulated cause vasodilation). A useful mnemonic is to think how many hearts you have (one) and how many lungs (two): The class of selective *beta$_1$-blockers* therefore would decrease the rate and force of contraction of the heart and if nonselective may also cause bronchospasm and mild vasoconstriction of blood vessels.

Side effects of beta-blockers, especially in patients over 60 years old and more commonly with the IV administration of the drug, can include:

- ⓘ Hypotension, with vertigo and syncope
- ⓘ Bradycardia, with rarely heart block and cardiac arrest
- ⓘ CNS symptoms (usually with long-term treatment with high doses), including dizziness, irritability, confusion, nightmares, insomnia, visual disturbances, weakness, sleepiness, lassitude, or fatigue
- GI symptoms, including nausea, vomiting, and diarrhea or constipation
- Rash or hematological effects (rare or transient)
- ⓘ Bronchospasm, especially with a history of asthma
- ⓘ Hypoglycemia
- Impotence (reported rarely)

Precautions or contraindications for the beta-blockers apply to:

Withdrawal after prolonged use (should always be gradual)

Withdrawal before surgery (weigh risk vs. benefits)

Diabetes (may cause hypoglycemia and mask the tachycardic response to hypoglycemia)

Renal and hepatic impairment

Asthma and allergic rhinitis (may cause bronchospasm)

Bradycardia, heart block, and congestive heart failure (CHF)

Pediatric use

Pregnancy and lactation

Chronic obstructive pulmonary disease (COPD)

Interactions include *antagonism* of beta-blockers by:

Adrenergics (e.g., epinephrine and isoproterenol)

NSAIDs and salicylates

Tricyclic antidepressants

Potentiation of the *hypotensive effect* of propranolol occurs with:

Diuretics and other antihypertensives, for example, calcium channel blockers

MAOIs; phenothiazine and other tranquilizers

Cimetidine (Tagamet), which slows metabolism of the drug

Certain antiarrhythmic drugs (e.g., adenosine, digoxin, and quinidine), which may potentiate toxic effects

Alcohol, muscle relaxants, and sedatives, which may precipitate hypotension, dizziness, confusion, or sedation

Calcium Channel Blockers

Of the calcium channel blockers available, only verapamil (Calan) and diltiazem (Cardizem) possess significant antiarrhythmic activity. These agents are indicated for the treatment of atrial fibrillation/flutter and PSVT. Verapamil and diltiazem counteract arrhythmias by slowing AV nodal conduction. Calcium channel blockers are also used in the treatment of angina and hypertension.

Side effects of calcium channel blockers can include:

- ! Hypotension, with vertigo and headache
- ! Bradycardia, with heart block
- ! Edema
- ! Constipation, nausea, and abdominal discomfort

Precautions or contraindications for calcium channel blockers apply to:

Heart block, heart failure, or angina

Hepatic and renal impairment

Pregnancy and lactation

Children

Hypotension and heart block

Certain arrhythmias and severe heart failure

> **Note**
>
> Do not drink grapefruit juice with certain calcium channel blockers because adverse effects may be potentiated.

Interactions of calcium channel blockers with other cardiac drugs, for example digoxin, can potentiate both good and adverse effects.

Antagonistic effects with calcium channel blockers include:

Barbiturates, cimetidine, phenytoin, ranitidine, and rifampin

Hypotensive effect potentiated with diuretics, ACE inhibitors, beta-blockers, and quinidine

Lidocaine

Local anesthetics (e.g., lidocaine) are administered for their antiarrhythmic effects and membrane-stabilizing action. Lidocaine has been historically used as a first-line antiarrhythmic agent for acute, life-threatening ventricular arrhythmias. However, it is now considered a second choice behind other alternative agents (e.g., IV amiodarone) for the treatment of ventricular arrhythmias.

Side effects of lidocaine are usually of short duration, are dose related, and can include:

- ! CNS symptoms, including tremors, seizures, dizziness, confusion, and blurred vision

! Hypotension, bradycardia, and heart block

! Dyspnea, respiratory depression, and arrest

EKG monitoring and availability of resuscitative equipment are necessary during the IV administration of lidocaine.

Precautions or contraindications with lidocaine apply to:

Patients hypersensitive to local anesthetics of this type (amide type)

Heart block and respiratory depression

Pregnancy and lactation

Children

Interactions of lidocaine with other cardiac drugs may be additive or antagonistic and may potentiate adverse effects. Other interactions may be of minor clinical significance because lidocaine is usually titrated to response.

Procainamide

Procainamide, quinidine, and disopyramide (Norpace) are antiarrhythmic agents. They act by decreasing myocardial excitability, inhibiting conduction, and may depress myocardial contractility. These agents possess anticholinergic properties. IV procainamide is a potential treatment alternative (to amiodarone) for the treatment of ventricular tachycardia during cardiopulmonary resuscitation. These agents are used orally primarily as prophylactic therapy to maintain normal rhythm after conversion by other methods.

Side effects of this class of antiarrhythmics are numerous and may necessitate cessation of treatment. They may include:

! Diarrhea, anorexia, nausea and vomiting, and abdominal pain (which are common)

! *Tachycardia*, QT prolongation, hypotension, and syncope

! Anticholinergic effects, including dry mouth, blurred vision, confusion, constipation, and urinary retention

! Vascular collapse and respiratory arrest with IV administration

Vision abnormalities or hearing disturbances (with quinidine)

Blood dyscrasias, including anemia, clotting deficiencies, and leukopenia (relatively rare)

Hepatic disorders; fever

! Dermatological effects, including rash, pruritis, urticaria

Precautions or contraindications with these agents apply to:

Atrioventricular block and conduction defects

Electrolyte imbalance

Digoxin toxicity

Heart failure and hypotension

Myasthenia gravis

Older adults—more susceptible to hypotensive and anticholinergic effects

Children

Pregnancy and lactation

Hepatic or renal disorders

Hypersensitivity to "ester-type" local anesthetics with procainamide

Systemic lupus erythematosus (SLE) with procainamide

Interactions with increased possibility of toxicity may occur with:

Muscle relaxants and neuromuscular blockers

Anticholinergics, tricyclic antidepressants, and phenothiazines

Other cardiac drugs, especially digoxin and antihypertensives

Interactions with increased possibility of *quinidine* toxicity may occur with:

Antiretroviral protease inhibitors

Antacids or sodium bicarbonate

Anticonvulsants (e.g., phenytoin and phenobarbital; cause decreased serum levels)

Anticoagulants (action can be potentiated by quinidine)

Propafenone

Propafenone (Rythmol) is an oral antiarrhythmic agent used to treat symptomatic supraventricular arrhythmias or severe, life-threatening ventricular arrhythmias. It is also useful in converting atrial fibrillation to sinus rhythm and maintaining it. Propafenone has local anesthetic effects, direct stabilizing action on myocardial membranes, and beta-adrenergic blocking properties.

Side effects of propafenone may include:

Dizziness and blurred vision

Nausea, vomiting, unusual taste, and constipation

Angina, heart failure, palpitations, arrhythmia, and dyspnea

Fatigue, weakness, and headache

Rash

Precautions or contraindications include:

Asthma or acute bronchospasm

Second or third-degree heart block (in the absence of a pacemaker), cardiogenic shock, heart failure, and bradycardia

Marked hypotension and electrolyte imbalance

Interactions of propafenone may occur with:

Quinidine, ritonavir, and certain SSRIs (may cause serum levels of propafenone to be elevated)

Beta-blockers, digoxin, and theophylline (may result in increased serum levels of the same)

PATIENT EDUCATION

Patients taking antiarrhythmics should be instructed regarding:

Immediate reporting of adverse side effects, especially palpitations, irregular or slow heartbeat, faintness, dizziness, weakness, respiratory distress, and visual disturbances

Holding the medication, if there are side effects, until the physician is contacted

Rising slowly from a reclining position

Modification of lifestyle to reduce stress

Mild exercise on a regular basis as approved by the physician

Not discontinuing the medicine, even if the patient feels well

Taking proper dosage of the medication on time, as prescribed, without skipping any dose

If the medication is forgotten, not doubling the dose

Taking the medication with a full glass of water on an empty stomach, 1h before or 2h after meals, so that it will be absorbed more efficiently (unless stomach upset occurs or the physician prescribes otherwise)

Avoiding taking any other medication, including OTC medicines, unless approved by the physician

Discarding expired medicines and renewing the prescription

Avoiding comparisons with other patients on similar drugs

Contacting the physician immediately with any concerns regarding medicines

See Table 25-1 for a summary of cardiac glycosides and the antiarrhythmics.

TABLE 25-1 Cardiac Glycosides and Antiarrhythmics

GENERIC NAME	TRADE NAME	DOSAGE	COMMENTS[b]
Cardiac glycoside			
digoxin	Lanoxin	PO: tablets, elixir, IM, IV, dosage varies	Monitor serum levels (0.5–0.8 mg/mL for heart failure; 0.8 –2 mg/mL for afib)
Antiarrhythmics (grouped by class)			
IA procainamide		IV	For VTach, afib, PAT, PSVT. Has anticholinergic properties
IB lidocaine	Xylocaine	IV diluted	Local anesthetic—amide type for Vfib, VTach. Check IV dilution directions
IC propafenone	Rythmol	PO, 150–300 mg q8h	For afib, PSVT, VTach
	Rythmol SR	PO, 225–425 mg q12h	For afib prevention
II metoprolol[a]	Lopressor	PO, 25–100 mg BID	Beta-blocker for heart rate control in afib
		IV, 2.5–5 mg IV bolus, repeat q5 min for three doses total	
III amiodarone	Cordarone, Pacerone	IV, PO; dose varies	For ventricular arrhythmias. Also a vasodilator; Medication Guide required
IV verapamil[a]	Calan	IV 2.5–10 mg; PO 240–480 mg daily in divided doses	Calcium channel blocker for afib and PSVT
adenosine	Adenocard	IV bolus 6 mg; then 12 mg PRN up to 30 mg	For PSVT; do not confuse with amiodarone

Note: Other antiarrhythmics are available. This is a representative sample by classification.

a. afib = atrial fibrillation; PAT = paroxysmal atrial tachycardia; PSVT = paroxysmal supraventricular tachycardia; Vfib = ventricular fibrillation; VTach = ventricular tachycardia.

b. Has other cardiac uses.

ANTIHYPERTENSIVES

Hypertension is a widespread epidemic that affects as many as one billion people worldwide and approximately 65 million adults in the United States. It is defined as systolic blood pressure (SBP) of 140 or greater or diastolic blood pressure (DBP) of 90 or greater. There is a strong, consistent relationship between blood pressure (BP) and the risk of cardiovascular disease (CVD). High blood pressure increases the risk of angina, myocardial infarction, heart failure, stroke, retinopathy, peripheral arterial disease, and kidney disease and thus requires aggressive treatment.

An additional 37% of adults in the United States are considered to have *prehypertension* (SBP range of 120–139 and DBP range of 80–89), a condition that may identify patients who are at a higher cardiovascular risk based on BP and a higher risk for developing sustained hypertension in later years. The purpose of this classification is to encourage patients to initiate or continue healthy lifestyle practices, rather than to begin antihypertensive drug therapy. Such practices include weight reduction (in patients who are overweight and obese), use of the *Dietary Approaches to Stop Hypertension* (DASH) eating plan, dietary sodium reduction, increased physical activity, modified alcohol use, and smoking cessation.

Antihypertensives do not cure hypertension; they only control it. After withdrawal of the drug, BP will return to levels similar to those before treatment with the medication, if all other factors remain the same. If antihypertensive therapy is to be terminated for some reason, the dosage should be gradually reduced, as abrupt withdrawal can cause rebound hypertension.

Side effects of antihypertensives are common. The most common side effect of antihypertensives is *hypotension*, especially postural hypotension. Another side effect common to many of the antihypertensives is *bradycardia*. Exceptions include hydralazine, which can cause tachycardia.

Thiazide Diuretics

Most patients meeting the criteria for drug therapy should be started on thiazide-type diuretics, either alone or in combination with a drug from one of the other drug classes: ACE inhibitors, ARBs, beta-blockers, or calcium channel blockers. Thiazide diuretics appear to be as effective as other antihypertensive agents and, in addition, are inexpensive. See Chapter 15 for a detailed discussion of these agents, especially side effects, precautions or contraindications, and interactions.

Beta-Adrenergic and Calcium Channel Blockers

Like thiazide diuretics, beta-adrenergic blockers such as carvedilol (Coreg) and metoprolol (Lopressor, Toprol XL) are generally well tolerated and are suitable for initial therapy in some patients with angina, post myocardial infarction, ischemic heart disease, heart failure, and certain arrhythmias. Only bisoprolol, carvedilol, and metoprolol extended-release have been proven to reduce mortality when used in patients with heart failure. Atenolol should not be used to treat hypertension because this drug has no effect in reducing cardiovascular events and mortality.

Calcium channel blockers such as diltiazem (Cardizem) and amlodipine (Norvasc) are an initial therapy option for hypertensive patients with diabetes or high coronary disease risk. They are more effective in treating African-American patients, older adults, and patients with higher pretreatment blood pressure readings. They may also be preferred in patients with obstructive airways disease. Based on historical data, *short-acting* calcium channel blockers should never be used to manage *hypertensive crisis* because of the reports of increased risks of myocardial infarction and mortality.

Because of their pharmacology, verapamil and diltiazem may be used to treat various arrhythmias. Refer to the discussion under "Antiarrhythmic Agents" earlier in this chapter for more information on these agents.

ACE Inhibitors (ACEIs)

Another class of antihypertensives is the ACE inhibitors, for example lisinopril or enalapril. Inhibition of ACE lowers blood pressure by *decreasing vasoconstriction*; there are not significant changes in heart rate or cardiac output. ACEIs are first- or second-line agents in the treatment of hypertension and are excellent alone, but also effective and synergistic in combination with other antihypertensives, including diuretics and calcium channel blockers.

ACEIs are especially good choices for patients who also have other serious conditions, including those with heart failure, following myocardial infarction, when high coronary disease risk exists, diabetes, renal disease, and cerebrovascular disease. For example, ACEIs can be considered drugs of choice for hypertensive patients with nephropathy because they slow the progression of the renal disease. They are more effective in younger and white populations and less effective in black patients, unless given in higher doses or in combination with a diuretic.

Side effects of ACE inhibitors (infrequent and usually mild) can include:

> ❗ Rash or photosensitivity
>
> Loss of taste perception; metallic taste
>
> Blood dyscrasias
>
> Renal impairment
>
> ❗ Severe hypotension
>
> ❗ Chronic dry cough or nasal congestion
>
> ❗ Hyperkalemia (monitor serum potassium levels periodically)

Precautions or contraindications with ACE inhibitors apply to:

> Collagen disease, for example lupus or scleroderma
>
> Heart failure
>
> Angioedema
>
> Pregnancy and lactation
>
> Children

Interactions of ACE inhibitors apply to:

> Diuretics (potentiate hypotension; watch BP closely)
>
> Vasodilators (watch BP closely)

Potassium-sparing diuretics and potassium supplements (hyperkalemia risk)

Nonsteroidal anti-inflammatory drugs (NSAIDs) and salicylates (antagonize effects of ACE inhibitors and increase deterioration of renal function in patients with compromised renal function)

Antacids (decrease absorption)

Digoxin (possible digitalis toxicity)

Lithium (risk of lithium toxicity)

Angiotensin Receptor Blockers (ARBs)

ARBs are similar to ACEIs and are generally used as alternatives. They block the angiotensin receptor that causes vasoconstriction when stimulated by angiotensin II. ARBs such as losartan (Cozaar) and valsartan (Diovan) block the effects of angiotensin II, decreasing blood pressure without a marked change in heart rate.

Compared to ACEIs, ARBs are associated with a lower incidence of drug-induced cough, rash, and/or taste disturbances and are used in those patients who cannot tolerate ACEIs. Like the ACEIs, African-American patients experience a smaller antihypertensive response with the ARBs compared to other ethnic populations. The addition of a low-dose thiazide diuretic to an ARB significantly improves hypertensive efficacy. ARBs are also good choices for patients with other serious conditions, including those with heart failure, diabetes, and renal disease.

Side effects are relatively uncommon with ARBs and include dizziness, orthostatic hypotension, upper respiratory tract infections, and hyperkalemia.

Precautions or contraindications for ARBs apply to:

Renal impairment

Pregnancy and lactation

Children

Interactions with ARBs are similar to those seen with ACEIs.

OTHER ANTIHYPERTENSIVES

Antiadrenergic Agents

Clonidine (Catapres) is a *central-acting* alpha-adrenergic blocking agent, used mainly in the treatment of hypertension. It is available as an oral preparation, a transdermal system, and an injection for epidural use. Clonidine has also been used successfully in a variety of other conditions including ADHD, nicotine/opiate withdrawal, vascular headaches, glaucoma, ulcerative colitis, Tourette's syndrome, and treatment of severe pain in cancer patients.

Prazosin (Minipress) is a *peripheral-acting* alpha-adrenergic blocker used primarily to treat hypertension. Other agents in this class are used to treat benign prostatic hyperplasia (BPH). Treatment with alpha-adrenergic blockers once was considered potentially favorable for the management of hypertension in patients with BPH to target both blood pressure and BPH symptoms. However, a study determined that patients treated with the alpha-blocker doxazosin, when compared with those treated with the diuretic chlorthalidone, had an increased risk for stroke and heart failure. Therefore, hypertension should not be managed with an alpha-blocker alone, and

BPH symptoms should be managed separately (see Chapter 15 for a discussion on the use of alpha-blockers in BPH).

Peripheral Vasodilator

Hydralazine, a peripheral vasodilator, is sometimes used in the treatment of moderate to severe hypertension, especially in patients with CHF, because it increases the heart rate and cardiac output. The drug is generally used in conjunction with a diuretic and another hypotensive agent, for example a beta-blocker. A fixed-dose combination of isosorbide dinitrate and hydralazine (BiDil) is available for the treatment of heart failure.

Side effects of hydralazine can include:

- **!** *Tachycardia* and palpitations
- Headache and flushing
- **!** Orthostatic hypotension
- GI effects, including nausea, vomiting, diarrhea, and constipation
- Blood abnormalities
- **!** Edema and weight gain

Precautions or contraindications for hydralazine apply to:

- Systemic lupus erythematosus (SLE)
- Renal disease
- Coronary artery disease and rheumatic heart disease
- Pregnancy, usually (however, many regard hydralazine as the antihypertensive of choice during preeclampsia)

See Figure 25-2, which illustrates the various mechanisms to reduce blood pressure and see Table 25-2 for a summary of the classifications and specific drug examples of antihypertensives.

TABLE 25-2   Antihypertensives

GENERIC NAME	TRADE NAME	DOSAGE
Beta-adrenergic blockers		
atenolol	Tenormin	25–100 mg PO daily
carvedilol	Coreg	6.25–25 mg PO BID with food (also has vasodilatory properties)
	Coreg CR	20–80 mg daily with food (SR)[a]
metoprolol	Lopressor	100–400 mg PO daily in divided doses
	Toprol XL	50–100 mg PO daily (SR)
nebivolol	Bystolic	5–40 mg PO daily (also has vasodilatory properties)
propranolol	Inderal	160–480 mg PO daily in two to three divided doses
	Inderal LA[a]	80–160 mg PO daily (SR)

(continued)

TABLE 25-2   **Antihypertensives (*continued*)**

GENERIC NAME	TRADE NAME	DOSAGE
Calcium channel blockers		
amlodipine	Norvasc	2.5–10 mg PO daily
diltiazem	(cap) Cardizem CD (tab) Cardizem LA	120–360 mg PO daily (SR); regular-release tabs are not approved to treat hypertension
	Diltiazem SR	120–180 mg PO BID (SR)
nifedipine	Procardia XL Adalat CC	30–90 mg PO daily (SR)
verapamil	Calan SR, Isoptin SR	120–240 mg PO one to two times per day (SR)
ACE inhibitors		
benazepril	Lotensin	10–20 mg one to two times per day
enalapril	Vasotec	5–20 mg PO BID
lisinopril	Prinivil, Zestril	5–40 mg PO daily
ramipril	Altace	2.5–20 mg PO one to two divided doses
trandolapril	Mavik	1–4 mg PO daily
ARBs		
losartan	Cozaar	25–100 mg PO one to two divided doses
olmesartan	Benicar	20–40 mg PO daily
telmisartan	Micardis	20–80 mg PO daily
valsartan	Diovan	80–320 mg PO daily
Other antihypertensives		
Antiadrenergic agents		
clonidine	Catapres	0.1–1.2 mg PO daily in divided doses
	Catapres TTS	Weekly patch (delivers 0.1–0.3 mg/24 h)
prazosin	Minipres	1–20 mg PO daily in two to three divided doses
Peripheral vasodilator		
hydralazine		10–50 mg PO two to four times per day; IM, IV dose varies

Note: This is only a representative list of the most commonly used drugs in this category. There are many others and many in combination with a diuretic.

a. All extended release products (ER/SR) must be swallowed intact! Quick release of the medication can cause the blood pressure to drop suddenly, sending the patient into shock. Caution is advised owing to potential confusion with various name extensions designating extended-release formulations (CC, CD, CR, LA, SR, and XL).

Drugs Used to Treat Hypertension

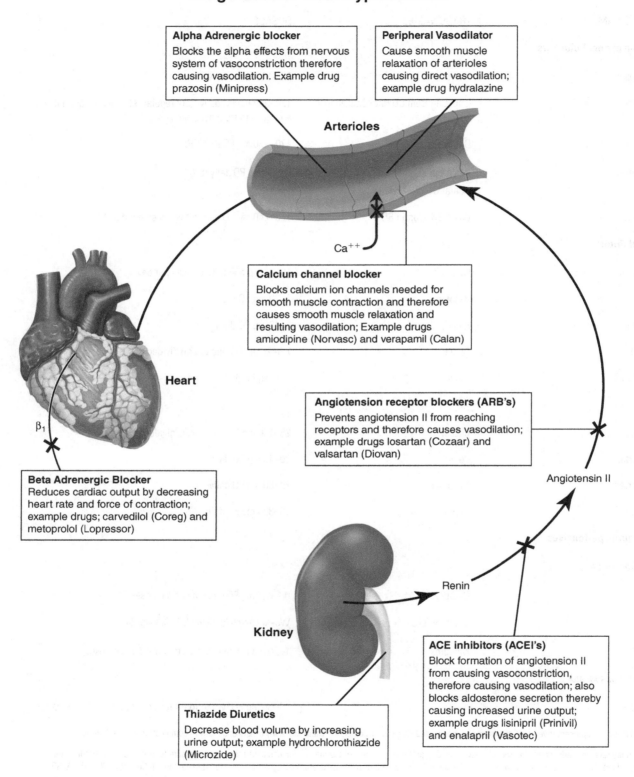

Alpha Adrenergic blocker
Blocks the alpha effects from nervous system of vasoconstriction therefore causing vasodilation. Example drug prazosin (Minipress)

Peripheral Vasodilator
Cause smooth muscle relaxation of arterioles causing direct vasodilation; example drug hydralazine

Arterioles

Ca^{++}

Calcium channel blocker
Blocks calcium ion channels needed for smooth muscle contraction and therefore causes smooth muscle relaxation and resulting vasodilation; Example drugs amiodipine (Norvasc) and verapamil (Calan)

Heart

β_1

Beta Adrenergic Blocker
Reduces cardiac output by decreasing heart rate and force of contraction; example drugs; carvedilol (Coreg) and metoprolol (Lopressor)

Angiotension receptor blockers (ARB's)
Prevents angiotension II from reaching receptors and therefore causes vasodilation; example drugs losartan (Cozaar) and valsartan (Diovan)

Angiotensin II

Kidney

Renin

ACE inhibitors (ACEI's)
Block formation of angiotension II from causing vasoconstriction, therefore causing vasodilation; also blocks aldosterone secretion thereby causing increased urine output; example drugs lisinipril (Prinivil) and enalapril (Vasotec)

Thiazide Diuretics
Decrease blood volume by increasing urine output; example hydrochlorothiazide (Microzide)

FIGURE 25-2 Various mechanisms of action of drugs used to treat hypertension.

LEARNING HINT

The ending of several drug names can help you determine their classification. Notice from Table 25-2 that all beta-adrenergic blockers end in "lol," all ACE inhibitors end in "pril," and all angiotension receptor blockers end in "sartan."

PATIENT EDUCATION

Patients taking antihypertensives should be instructed regarding:

Routinely monitoring blood pressure at home, keeping a log of their blood pressure readings, and sharing this information with their physician

Immediate reporting of any adverse side effects, especially slow or irregular heartbeat, dizziness, weakness, breathing difficulty, gastric distress, and numbness or swelling of extremities

Taking the medication on time as prescribed by the physician; *not* skipping a dose or doubling a dose; *not* discontinuing the medicine, even if the patient is feeling well, without consulting the physician first

Rising slowly from a reclining position to reduce lightheaded feeling

Taking care in driving a car or operating machinery if the medication causes drowsiness (ask the physician, nurse, or pharmacist about the specific medication, because medicines differ and individual reactions differ; older people are more susceptible to this effect)

Potentiation of adverse side effects by alcohol, especially dizziness, weakness, sleepiness, and confusion

Reduction or cessation of smoking to help lower blood pressure

Importance of lifestyle modifications, such as exercise, quitting smoking, limiting alcohol usage, and eating a healthy diet in control of blood pressure; following the physician's instructions regarding appropriate diet for the individual, which may include a low-salt or low-sodium or weight-reduction diet if indicated

Avoiding hot tubs and hot showers, which may cause weakness or fainting

Mild exercise on a regular basis as approved by the physician

Always swallowing the extended-release products intact. Quick release of the medication into the system can cause the blood pressure to drop suddenly, causing loss of consciousness and possible shock.

Avoiding grapefruit juice while taking calcium channel blockers, which can increase the risk of hypotension and other adverse cardiac effects.

CORONARY VASODILATORS

Coronary vasodilators are used in the treatment of angina. When there is insufficient blood supply (**ischemia**) to a part of the heart, the result is acute pain. The most common form of angina is angina pectoris, chest pain resulting from decreased blood supply to the heart muscle. Obstruction or constriction of the coronary arteries, which supply the heart muscle with oxygenated blood, results in angina pectoris. Vasodilators are administered to dilate these blood vessels (thus increasing myocardial oxygen supply) and stop attacks of angina or reduce the frequency of angina when administered prophylactically. Coronary vasodilators used in the treatment and prophylactic management of angina include nitrates, beta-blockers, and calcium channel blockers.

The nitrates used most commonly for relief of acute angina pectoris, as well as for long-term prophylactic management, are nitroglycerin and isosorbide (e.g., Isordil, Imdur). Nitroglycerin is available in several forms and can be administered in sublingual tablets allowed to dissolve under the tongue or a sublingual spray for the relief of acute angina pectoris. If chest pain is not relieved or worsens 5 min after a dose, EMS should be activated because unrelieved chest pain can indicate an acute myocardial infarction.

Although the traditional recommendation is for patients to take up to three SL nitroglycerin doses over 15 min *before* accessing the emergency system, recent guidelines suggest an alternative strategy to reduce delays in emergency care. New guidelines recommend instructing a patient with a prior prescription for nitroglycerin to call 911 immediately if chest discomfort or pain is persistent or worsened 5 min after *one* dose of nitroglycerin. Self-treatment with nitrates has been identified as a factor resulting in delays in emergency evaluation.

Nitroglycerin is also available in timed-release capsules and tablets and in an injectable formulation that must be diluted carefully according to the manufacturer's instructions for IV administration. Nitroglycerin tablets and capsules must be stored *only in glass containers* with tight-fitting metal screw tops away from heat. Plastic containers can absorb the medication, and air, heat, or moisture can cause loss of potency. Impaired potency of the SL tablets can be detected by the patient if there is an absence of the tingling sensation under the tongue common to this form of administration.

For the long-term prophylactic management of angina pectoris, nitroglycerin is frequently applied topically as a transdermal system. One type of nitroglycerin that is absorbed through the skin is Nitro-Bid ointment, applied with an applicator-measuring (Appli-Ruler) paper. Usual dosage is 0.5–2 inches applied every 8h. *Remove old paper first.* The ointment is spread lightly (not massaged or rubbed) over any hairless skin area, and the applicator paper is taped in place. Care must be taken to avoid touching the ointment when applying (accidental absorption through the skin of the fingers can cause headache). If nitroglycerin ointment is discontinued, the dose and frequency must be decreased gradually to prevent sudden withdrawal reactions. See Figure 9-1 in Chapter 9, "Administration," for ointment application technique.

Another topical nitroglycerin product, which has a longer action, is in transdermal form (e.g., Nitro-Dur). The skin patch is applied every 24h (on in a.m./off 12 h later in the p.m.) to clean, dry, hairless areas of the upper arm or body. Do not apply below the elbow or knee. *The sites should be rotated* to avoid skin irritation, and raw, scarred, or callused areas should be avoided. Patch dosage varies widely, from 0.1 to 0.8 mg/h daily. *Check prescribed dosage carefully. Remove old patch.*

Another nitrate used for the acute relief of angina pectoris and for the prophylactic long-term management is isosorbide. It is available in SL tablets, regular-release tablets, and timed-release capsules and tablets. When using long-acting nitrates, a 12–14h nitrate-free interval between the last dose of the day and the first dose of the following day is recommended to lessen the risk of nitrate tolerance.

Side effects of the nitrates can include:

- ❗ Headache (usually diminishes over time; analgesics may be given to alleviate pain)
- ❗ Postural hypotension, including dizziness, weakness, and syncope (*patients should be sitting during the administration of fast-acting nitrates*)

Transient flushing

Rash and skin irritation with transdermal forms

! Blurred vision and dry mouth (discontinue the drug with these symptoms)

! Hypersensitivity reactions, enhanced by alcohol, including nausea, vomiting, diarrhea, cold sweats, tachycardia, and syncope

Precautions or contraindications for nitrates apply to:

Glaucoma

GI hypermotility or malabsorption (with timed-release forms)

Intracranial pressure

Severe anemia

Hypotension

Interactions of nitrates may occur with alcohol, which potentiates hypotensive effects. Phosphodiesterase (PDE) inhibitors such as sildenafil (Viagra), used for erectile dysfunction, are contraindicated in men taking nitrates. The two drugs interact to cause a large, sudden, dangerous drop in blood pressure.

For the long-term prophylactic treatment of angina pectoris, beta-blockers such as metoprolol (Lopressor) and calcium channel blockers such as diltiazem (Cardizem) and verapamil (Calan) are frequently used (see "Antiarrhythmic Agents" for information on side effects, etc.). See Figure 25-3, which illustrates drugs used to treat angina.

Drugs Used to Treat Angina

Arterioles

Beta-blockers
Decrease rate and force of contraction of heart thereby reducing workload and oxygen demand. Example drug metoprolol (Lopressor)

β_1

Sympathetic nervous system

Ca^{++}

Calcium Channel Blockers
Dilates arterial smooth muscle causing vasodilation thereby decreasing blood pressure and cardiac oxygen demand. Example drugs diltiazem (Cardizem) and verapamil (Calan)

Sympathetic nervous system

Coronary Vasodilators
Dilate coronary arteries to increase blood supply and oxygen delivery to heart. In addition reduces venous blood return to heart. Example drugs Nitroglycerin (various forms including transdermal) and isosorbide (Isordil)

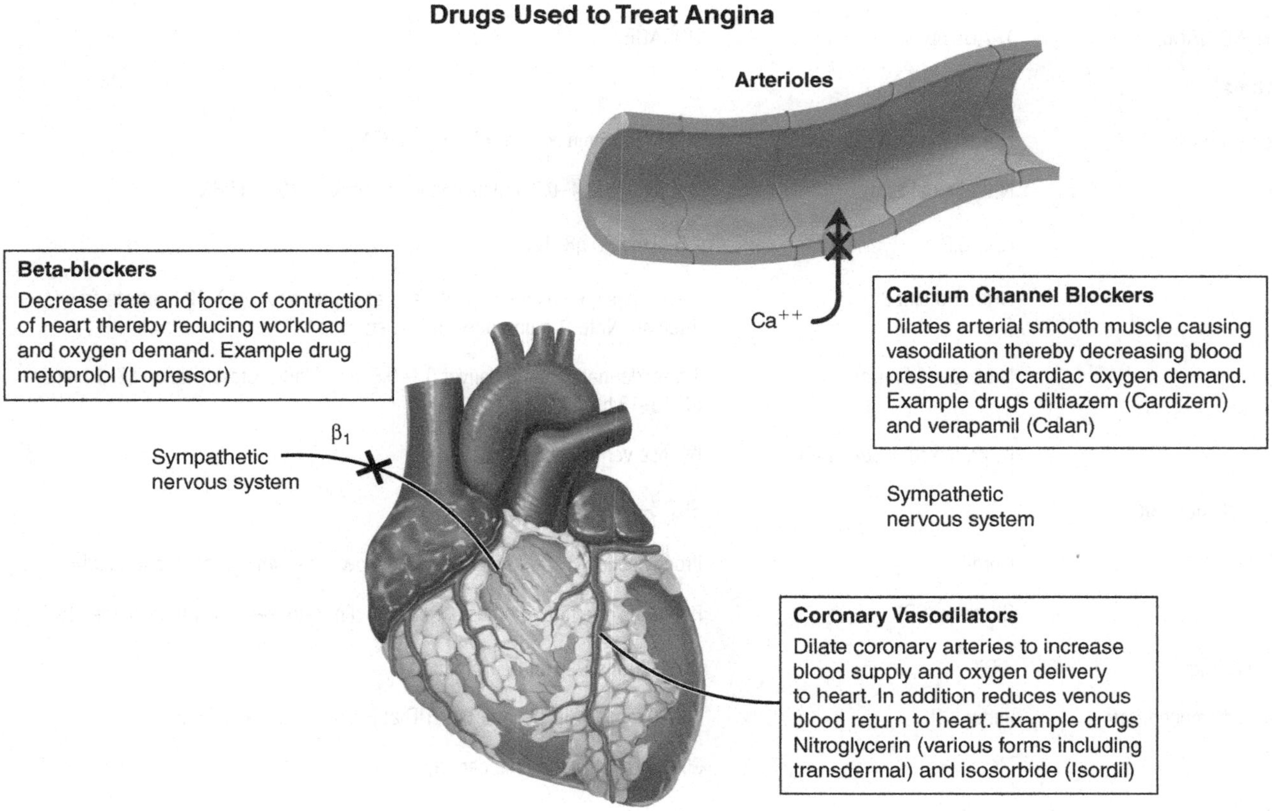

FIGURE 25-3 Various mechanisms of action of drugs used to treat angina.

PATIENT EDUCATION

Patients receiving coronary vasodilators (nitrates) should be instructed regarding:

Administering fast-acting preparations (sublingual tablets or spray) while sitting down because the patient may become lightheaded

Rising slowly from a reclining position

Not drinking alcohol or taking PDE inhibitors while taking these medicines, which can cause a serious drop in blood pressure

Using timed-release capsules or tablets to prevent attacks (they work too slowly to help once an attack has started)

The fact that nitrates taken for chronic angina may require periods of drug-free intervals to avoid the development of nitrate tolerance and lessening of antianginal effects

Taking timed-release capsules or tablets on an empty stomach with a full glass of water

Allowing sublingual tablets to dissolve under the tongue or in the cheek pouch and not chewing or swallowing them

Repeating sublingual tablets or spray in 5–10 min for a maximum of three tablets or sprays (if no relief or worsening of chest

pain within 5 min after the first tablet, activate EMS, or if EMS is unavailable, report to the emergency department); for patients known to have frequent angina, physicians may provide individualized instructions for the use of SL nitroglycerin, based on the characteristics of the patient's angina, time course, and response to the treatment

Not discontinuing the medication suddenly if administered for several weeks (dosage must be reduced gradually under the physician's supervision)

Sensations to be expected, including facial flushing, headache for a short time, and lightheadedness upon rising too suddenly (if these symptoms persist or become more severe, or other symptoms occur, such as irregular heartbeat or blurred vision, notify the physician at once)

Preventing attacks of angina by administering a sublingual tablet or spray before physical exertion or emotional stress (it is preferable to avoid physical or emotional stress when possible)

See Chapter 9 for patient education regarding the administration of nitroglycerin ointment or patch.

See Table 25-3 for a summary of coronary vasodilators.

TABLE 25-3   Coronary Vasodilators

GENERIC NAME	TRADE NAME	DOSAGE
Nitrates[a]		
nitroglycerin	Nitrostat tabs S.L.	1–3 tabs q5min × 3 max in 15 min PRN
	Nitrolingual spray	1–2 sprays (0.4–0.8 mg) SL q5min × 3 max in 15 min PRN
	caps E.R.	2.5–9 mg PO q8–12h
	Nitro-Bid oint 2%	1–2 inches q6–8h (while awake and at bedtime for a 10–12 h nitrate-free interval); Note: 1 g unit dose foilpac equiv to ~1"
	Nitro-Dur, Minitran	1 transdermal patch to deliver 0.1–0.8 mg/h daily, rotate site; on 12–14 h per off 10–12 h
	IV, premixed or sol for inj	IV dose varies
isosorbide dinitrate		SL 2.5–5 mg × 3 max in 15–30 min
	Isordil	Prophylactic PO 10–40 mg BID–TID (allow for a 14h nitrate-free interval)
	Dilatrate (SR)	PO 40 mg one to two times per day (18 h nitrate-free interval recommended)
with hydralazine	BiDil	PO 1–2 tabs TID (for heart failure)
isosorbide mononitrate	Imdur (SR)	10–20 mg PO BID (7h apart) or TID at 8 A.M., 1 P.M., and 6 P.M.
		30–120 mg PO one time per day

Note: Beta-blockers and calcium channel blockers are also administered prophylactically for angina pectoris and can be given concurrently with the nitrates.

a. For the prevention and treatment of angina pectoris.

ANTILIPEMIC AGENTS

It is estimated that nearly 50% of Americans have elevated total blood cholesterol levels above 200 mg/dL—a key risk factor for coronary heart disease (CHD). Cardiovascular disease is the leading killer of men and women in the United States (more deaths than cancer, diabetes, accidents, and chronic lung diseases combined). High cholesterol can lead to arterial blockage, hardening of the arteries, blood clots, heart attack, or stroke and may even play a role in dementia.

Lipoproteins are responsible for transporting cholesterol and other fats through the blood stream. *Low-density lipoproteins* (LDLs; "bad cholesterol") carry the largest amount of the cholesterol in the blood and are responsible for transporting and depositing it in the arterial walls. *Very low-density lipoproteins* (VLDLs; triglycerides) are precursors of the LDL and compose the largest proportion of lipids in the diet, adipose tissue, and the blood. Triglycerides (TGs) are a source of energy; excess dietary calories are converted to TGs and stored as fat in the adipose tissue for future energy needs. Excess TGs (greater than the normal 150 level) can be an independent risk factor leading to atherosclerosis and CHD, as well as pancreatitis.

High-density lipoproteins (*HDLs*; "good cholesterol") help transport LDL cholesterol from the walls of the arteries through the bloodstream to the liver for excretion. An HDL level of below 40 mg/dL is considered low, and each 1 mg/dL increase in the HDL level is associated with a 6% lower risk of cardiovascular disease. LDL cholesterol is the primary target of treatment in clinical lipid management. The use of therapeutic lifestyle changes (TLCs), including LDL-lowering dietary management (e.g., restriction of saturated and trans fats or cholesterol intake, including fiber and soy protein in diet), weight control, appropriate exercise, limiting alcohol intake, and smoking cessation, will achieve the therapeutic goal (LDL below 100 mg/dL) in many persons. If these measures are inadequate, drug therapy may be added. Drug therapy aimed at reducing cholesterol levels either reduces hepatic production or intestinal absorption of cholesterol. Six categories of antilipemic agents used to lower blood cholesterol levels are available: HMG-CoA reductase inhibitors (the *statins*), bile acid sequestrants, nicotinic acid (niacin), fibric acid derivatives, cholesterol absorption inhibitor, and omega-3 fatty acids.

Statins

HMG-CoA reductase inhibitors (statins) inhibit the enzyme for cholesterol synthesis. These agents are the most potent lipid-lowering medications available for monotherapy and are considered to be the first choice in managing high cholesterol. Statins (e.g., atorvastatin—Lipitor; simvastatin—Zocor) have been shown to be very effective in lowering LDL levels (up to 60%) and are modestly effective in reducing TG levels and increasing HDL levels, thereby reducing cardiovascular morbidity and mortality. Statins are generally well tolerated.

Because HMG-CoA is most active at night when dietary intake is low, most statins are generally given at bedtime to provide optimal decreases in LDL levels. Because of their longer half-lives, atorvastatin and rosuvastatin can be given at the same time each day, any time of day. Recently, the maximum dose of simvastatin was reduced from 80 to 40 mg (if using it for less than 12 months) because of the increased risk of myopathy from the higher dose.

Side effects of statins include:

Mild GI disturbances, headache, rash, fatigue

(!) Myalgia and muscle weakness (can try switching to a different statin if problematic)

(!) Rhabdomyolysis (destruction of the muscle tissue leading to renal failure; reported rarely)

(!) Elevated liver enzymes (the FDA recently revised statin labeling by removing the recommendation for periodic liver function tests; baseline tests are still suggested, but follow-up monitoring is necessary only if clinically indicated)

Increased risk (9% to 13%) of new-onset diabetes mellitus with high-dose statin use (benefits of statin therapy far outweigh the risk of statin-induced diabetes; be considerate of the risk and monitor the patient)

Precautions or contraindications for statins apply to:

Hepatic or renal disease

Existing myalgia or muscle weakness

Pregnancy and breast-feeding

Children

Gemfibrozil, HIV, and hepatitis C protease inhibitors (increased risk for myopathy and rhabdomyolysis)

Interactions of certain statins with amiodarone, dronedarone, immunosuppressive drugs, erythromycin, azole antifungals, diltiazem, verapamil, *grapefruit juice*, or other antilipemic drugs (fibrates and niacin) increase the risk of myopathy and renal failure. Recently, the maximum recommended dose for most statins, when taken with certain interacting drugs, was also reduced because of safety considerations.

Bile Acid Sequestrants

Cholestyramine (Questran) and colesevelam (WelChol), which are not absorbed from the GI tract, bind bile acids in the intestine, interrupting the process by which bile acids are returned to the liver for reuse. Because bile acids are formed from cholesterol, sequestrants reduce total body cholesterol. Bile acid sequestrants can be used as monotherapy when moderate reductions in LDL levels are required or as an add-on therapy to statins. They should not be used as a single agent in the presence of elevated TGs.

Side effects of bile acid sequestrants include:

(!) Constipation, gas, cramps, heartburn, nausea, anorexia, abdominal pain, and bloating (occurs frequently and may affect compliance)

Colesevelam is administered at lower doses because of its higher bile-binding capacity and is associated with fewer GI adverse effects.

Precautions or contraindications for bile acid sequestrants apply to:

Biliary cirrhosis and obstruction

GI obstruction or fecal impaction

Interactions with bile acid sequestrants can reduce the absorption of many drugs, including antibiotics, cardiac glycosides, fat-soluble vitamins, thiazide diuretics, and thyroid hormones (administer at least 1 h before or 4 h after the bile acid sequestrants).

Nicotinic Acid (Niacin)

Nicotinic acid reduces the hepatic synthesis of TGs and inhibits the mobilization of free fatty acids from the peripheral tissues. It lowers total and LDL cholesterol and TG levels in the serum and also raises HDL cholesterol levels. Niacin may be useful in combination with a statin in patients with diabetic dyslipidemia (abnormal levels of various blood lipid fractions).

Side effects of niacin can be troublesome and include:

> ⓘ GI upset, dyspepsia (indigestion), blurred vision, and fatigue
>
> ⓘ *Skin flushing*, itching, and irritation (more common with immediate-release preparations; pretreatment with aspirin or ibuprofen can diminish cutaneous reactions)
>
> Glucose intolerance and hyperuricemia (abnormal uric acid levels in blood) (higher doses)
>
> ⓘ Hepatotoxicity (especially with sustained-release products; monitoring hepatic function is recommended for all niacin formulations)

Precautions or contraindications of niacin include:

> Hepatic, gallbladder, or peptic ulcer disease; diabetes; glaucoma; or gout
>
> Pregnancy and lactation (high doses)
>
> Children (<10 years old)

Interactions of niacin occur with:

> Antihypertensives and vasodilators (potentiate hypotensive effects)
>
> Antidiabetic agents with the loss of blood glucose control
>
> Alcohol (worsens flushing)

Note

Regular- and extended-release formulations of niacin are not bio-equivalent and are not interchangeable.

Fibric Acid Derivatives (Fibrates)

The fibrates fenofibrate (TriCor) and gemfibrozil (Lopid) possess minimal LDL-reducing capacity but are especially effective in patients who have extremely high TG levels and elevated cholesterol levels, and in patients with combined forms of hyperlipidemia. They are a good choice for diabetics because they improve glucose tolerance. The mechanism by which fibrates reduce TGs is poorly understood. Fibrates may be used in combination with other antilipemics, because these agents appear to be additive in lowering LDL and raising HDL cholesterol. Fibrates are generally well tolerated.

Side effects of fibrates can include:

> ⓘ GI complaints (diarrhea, dyspepsia, nausea and vomiting, and abdominal pain)
>
> ⓘ Cholethiasis (gallstones in the gallbladder) because of the increased biliary excretion of cholesterol, jaundice, blood dyscrasias, myopathy (abnormal condition of skeletal muscles)

Hypersensitivity reactions (rare)

Increased risk of pulmonary emboli (PE)

Precautions or contraindications for fibrates apply to:

Gallbladder, hepatic, renal disease, or peptic ulcer

Pregnancy and lactation

Children

Gemfibrozil with statins (increased risk for myopathy and rhabdomyolysis)

Interactions of fibrates occur with:

Oral anticoagulants and hypoglycemic agents (potentiate effects)

Statins to increase the risk of serious muscle problems and elevated liver enzymes (use together only in the lowest effective doses and if benefits outweigh risks)

Ezetimibe is not advised (increased risk of cholethiasis)

Cholesterol Absorption Inhibitor

Ezetimibe (Zetia) moderately reduces LDL levels by inhibiting intestinal absorption of both dietary and biliary cholesterol, blocking its transport in the small intestine. It can be taken simultaneously with a statin (Vytorin, a combination product), allowing for lower doses of the statin to be used, and the LDL-lowering effects of the two drugs are additive. Ezetimibe is generally well tolerated, with abdominal pain, back pain, and arthralgia being reported. Patients with gallbladder disease and moderate to severe hepatic insufficiency should not take it.

> **Administer ezetimibe at least 1–2 h before or 2–4 h after administering antacids and bile acid sequestrants, respectively. Avoid use with cyclosporine (increases serum concentrations of both drugs) and fibrates (increased risk of cholethiasis).**

Omega-3 Fatty Acids

Omega-3 fatty acids include eicosapentaenoic acid (EPA) and docosahexaenoic acid (DHA), found in fatty cold-water fish, and alpha-linolenic acid (ALA), found in flaxseed, tofu, soybean oil, canola oil, and nuts. There is evidence that EPA and DHA may have a role in the prevention of primary and secondary heart disease and reduce TGs (as an adjunct to diet or simvastatin).

The best source of omega-3 fatty acids is fatty fish, like salmon, but fish oil capsules may be more convenient, especially if high doses are needed. A highly concentrated and purified form of omega-3 fatty acids is also available by prescription only as *Lovaza*. Fish oil can cause nausea, heartburn, or diarrhea. A fishy aftertaste can be reduced by refrigeration or freezing (Lovaza should not be frozen). Because omega-3 fatty acids inhibit platelet aggregation, caution is advised when used concurrently with anticoagulants, platelet inhibitors, and thrombolytic agents. The DHA component of omega-3 fatty acids may be responsible for the elevations in LDL levels seen with these products; patients should be monitored to ensure their LDL levels do not increase excessively.

See Table 25-4 for a summary of antilipemic agents.

TABLE 25-4   Antilipemic Agents

GENERIC NAME	TRADE NAME	DOSAGE
Antilipemic agents		
Statins		
atorvastatin	Lipitor	10–80 mg PO daily
lovastatin	Mevacor	20–80 mg PO at bedtime with food
pravastatin	Pravachol	10–80 mg PO at bedtime
rosuvastatin	Crestor	5–40 mg PO daily
simvastatin	Zocor	5–40 mg PO at bedtime (80 mg if already on it with no evidence of myopathy)
Bile acid sequestrants		
cholestyramine	Questran, Questran Light	4 g one to two times per day ac; mix powder with water, milk, or juice
colesevelam	Welchol	6 tabs (625 mg each) daily or 3 tabs BID with food and a full glass of water; max 7 tabs per day
Nicotinic Acid		
niacin	Niaspan (Rx) Slo-Niacin (OTC)	Dose varies with response; take after meals or a snack
Fibric acid derivatives		
fenofibrate	Antara, Lofibra, Tricor, Trilipix	43–200 mg PO daily with food depending on formulation/manufacturer
gemfibrozil	Lopid	600 mg PO BID ac
Cholesterol absorption inhibitor		
ezetimibe	Zetia	10 mg PO daily
Omega-3 fatty acids		
fish oil (OTC)		3–6 g per day
	Lovaza (Rx)	4 g per day
Combinations		
atorvastatin/amlodipine	Caduet	PO daily; dose varies with response
ezetimibe/simvastatin	Vytorin	PO daily evening; dose varies with response
lovastatin/niacin	Advicor	PO daily bedtime with food; dose varies with response

Note: Other antilipemic agents are available. Some reduce triglycerides as well.

PATIENT EDUCATION

Patients on antilipemic therapy should be instructed regarding:

Continuing diet (low-fat, low-cholesterol) and aerobic exercise

Taking the medicine with meals to reduce GI upset

Reporting side effects to the physician immediately, *especially muscle pain, tenderness, weakness, dark-stained urine, or bleeding*

With cholestyramine, the importance of a high-fiber diet and/or a stool softener, fat-soluble vitamin and folic acid supplements, and not taking other medication within 4h

Expecting facial flushing with niacin (unless extended-release formula is used)

Taking most statins in the evening (the body synthesizes most cholesterol at night)

Avoiding grapefruit juice while taking statins; adverse effects are potentiated

Giving their health care professional a list of all the medicines, herbs, nonprescription drugs, or dietary supplements they are taking so that potential interactions can be identified

The importance of initial liver function tests

If all the other factors remain the same, the medication will probably need to be taken throughout the patient's lifetime. Sometimes diet and exercise will eliminate the need.

ANTITHROMBOTIC AGENTS

Blood has the ability to flow freely through blood vessels yet clot when the need arises. Normal hemostasis or blood coagulation involves the formation of a fibrin clot or thrombus so a minor cut would not cause us to bleed profusely. However, inappropriate thrombus formation can be caused by vessel-wall injury, circulatory stasis, increased blood coagulability, immobilization, obesity, cigarette smoking, medication therapy, and other factors. The inappropriate thrombus formation or clot can dislodge and travel through the bloodstream (thromboembolism or TE) where it can fully or partially obstruct blood flow, leading to tissue damage. **Antithrombotic agents**, which interfere with or prevent thrombosis or blood coagulation, include anticoagulants, platelet inhibitors, and thrombolytics.

Anticoagulants

Anticoagulants prevent the formation of the fibrin clot by interfering with one of the steps leading to fibrin formation. They are divided into two general groups: oral (coumarin derivatives and the new oral anticoagulants) and injectable (heparins). The action of these two classes is quite different. However, their purpose is the same: to prevent the formation of clots or decrease the extension of existing clots in such conditions as venous thrombosis, stroke, pulmonary embolism, and coronary artery occlusion. Also, many patients with artificial heart valves, mitral valve disease, or chronic atrial fibrillation, or postsurgical patients (cardiac bypass, vascular surgery, and hip or knee replacement) receive anticoagulants to prevent embolism or thrombosis. Patients on anticoagulants, especially older patients, should be constantly observed for *bleeding complications*, such as cerebrovascular accidents (CVAs). The coumarin derivatives (warfarin) and heparin do not dissolve existing clots; they only interfere with the coagulation process preventing clot formation and/or propagation.

Warfarin

Warfarin (Coumadin) is administered *orally* (it is also available as an injectable preparation, which is rarely used). This medicine alters the synthesis of blood coagulation factors in the liver by interfering with the action of vitamin K. The *antidote for serious bleeding complications during warfarin therapy is prothrombin complex concentrate or fresh frozen plasma and vitamin K.* The action of warfarin is slower than that of heparin; therefore, warfarin is generally used as follow-up for long-term anticoagulant therapy, although warfarin may be started at the same time as heparin.

The most commonly used laboratory method of monitoring therapy with warfarin is the International Normalized Ratio (INR). The INR serves as a guide in determining the dosage. Dose adjustments made are based on INR and vary from patient to patient. For most patients taking warfarin an INR of 2.0–3.0 sec is desirable, although for higher risk patients the range raises to 2.5–3.5 sec. It is important when adjusting the dose to allow 3–5 days for the INR to adjust before making another dosing change.

Interactions of warfarin with *many* drugs have been reported. Concurrent administration of any other drug should be investigated, and the following drugs should be *avoided* if possible. Some of the drugs that may *increase* response to warfarin include:

> Anabolic steroids
>
> Alcohol (acute intoxication)
>
> Proton pump inhibitors
>
> All NSAIDs, including aspirin; thrombolytics
>
> Tricyclic antidepressants; SSRIs
>
> Thyroid drugs
>
> Amiodarone, propafenone, and quinidine
>
> Many anti-infective agents
>
> Many antilipemic agents
>
> Acetaminophen (large daily doses or long duration)
>
> Grapefruit juice, fish oil, vitamin E, many herbal supplements
>
> Some of the drugs that may *decrease* response to warfarin include:
>
> Alcohol (chronic alcoholism)
>
> Barbiturates
>
> Estrogen (including oral contraceptives)
>
> Antiretroviral protease inhibitors

Additionally, foods that are naturally high in vitamin K (leafy green vegetables), should be eaten by patients on warfarin with consistency, meaning they eat approximately the same amount of these types of food each day. There are many other interactions with warfarin. Always check before administering any other medicine.

New Oral Anticoagulants

Although warfarin was the mainstay of oral anticoagulation therapy for over 50 years, its significant limitations and interactions have led to the research and development for acceptable alternatives. In October 2009, dabigatran (Pradaxa) was the first oral anticoagulant (direct thrombin inhibitor) to be approved by the FDA in more than half a century. This was followed by the approval of two more oral anticoagulants (factor Xa inhibitors)—rivaroxaban (Xarelto) and most recently apixaban (Eliquis).

Compared to warfarin, the new oral anticoagulants have a rapid onset and predictable anticoagulant effects and fewer food and drug interactions; routine laboratory monitoring is not required.

However, anticoagulant effects cannot be monitored with standard laboratory testing, and there is currently no reversal agent in case of uncontrolled major bleeding or the need for emergency surgery (although some are in early clinical trials).

Dabigatran, rivaroxaban, and apixaban are all indicated for reducing the risk of stroke and systemic embolism in patients with nonvalvular atrial fibrillation. Rivaroxaban is also indicated for venous thromboembolism prevention, post-hip or -knee replacement, and DVT/PE treatment or prevention of recurrence.

Heparin and Low-Molecular-Weight Heparins

There are two types of heparin: the standard or unfractionated type (UFH) and the low-molecular-weight heparins (LMWHs).

Heparin is not absorbed from the GI tract, and the standard type (UFH) must be administered *intravenously* or *subcutaneously*. The LMWH type is usually only administered subcutaneously but may be given IV as well. Heparin acts on thrombin, inhibiting the action of fibrin in clot formation. The *antidote for serious bleeding complications during heparin therapy is protamine sulfate.* When administered IV, the action of heparin is immediate. A *dilute flushing* solution of heparin is also used to maintain the patency of indwelling venipuncture devices used to obtain blood specimens and of catheters used for arterial access (arterial lines). *Be sure to check that it is a dilute flushing solution before injection, and not full-strength heparin.* However, 0.9% sodium chloride (normal saline) injection alone is used to flush *peripheral* venipuncture devices, for example PRN adapters. Heparin is *not* normally used to flush these devices because of possible drug incompatibilities and laboratory test interferences.

The LMWHs include enoxaparin (Lovenox) and dalteparin (Fragmin). When administered subcutaneously, monitoring of anticoagulant effect is not necessary, but periodic complete blood counts (CBCs), stool occult blood tests, and platelet counts are recommended during treatment.

Unlike UFH, in the case of clinically significant bleeding, no agent fully reverses the activity of the LMWHs, although protamine has some activity and should be given for life-threatening bleeding along with packed red blood cells and fresh frozen plasma transfusions if indicated. Fondaparinux (Arixtra), a closely related pentasaccharide, is not generally classified as an LMWH (although often discussed with the same). It is an indirect clotting factor Xa inhibitor and lacks a specific antidote in the event of excessive anticoagulation.

Enoxaparin was the first LMWH to be approved in the United States. It is currently approved for the prevention of deep vein thrombosis (DVT) in patients undergoing hip or knee replacement or abdominal surgery, for the treatment of unstable angina and ST-elevation myocardial infarction (STEMI), and for the inpatient treatment of acute DVT and pulmonary embolism (PE). It is also used in the outpatient treatment of acute DVT not associated with pulmonary embolism and is combined with warfarin (until INR reaches 2–3).

When heparin is administered subcutaneously, especially if the patient is discharged and the medication will be administered at home, be sure to stress *patient education.* See also Chapter 9, "Administration by the Parenteral Route."

Measurement of the activated partial thromboplastin time (aPTT) is the most common laboratory test for monitoring heparin therapy. When long-term anticoagulant therapy is begun with warfarin, there is a short-term overlap period in which both heparin and warfarin are administered concurrently.

Interactions of all anticoagulants with other anticoagulants, for example aspirin and NSAIDs, platelet inhibitors, and fish oil, or with thrombolytic agents, for example alteplase (tPA), may increase the risk of hemorrhage.

Side effects of all anticoagulants can include:

- ! Major hemorrhage
- ! Thrombocytopenia
- ! Minor bleeding (e.g., petechiae, nosebleed, and bruising)
- ! Blood in the urine (hematuria) or stools (melena)
- ! Osteoporosis with long-term heparin use (less with the LMWHs; none with the other agents)

Precautions or contraindications for anticoagulants apply to:

GI disorders and ulceration of GI tract

Hepatic and renal dysfunction

Blood dyscrasias

Pregnancy (heparin can be used with caution as it does not cross the placenta)

Stroke (may increase the risk of fatal cerebral hemorrhage after stroke)

Patients with prosthetic heart valves (with the new oral anticoagulants)

Lumbar puncture and epidural anesthesia (could result in paralysis)

See Table 25-5 for a summary of the anticoagulants.

TABLE 25-5 Anticoagulants

GENERIC NAME	TRADE NAME	DOSAGE
Anticoagulants, oral		
Coumarin derivative		
warfarin	Coumadin, Jantoven	PO dose varies, based on PT/INR results. Initial starting dose for most adults is 5mg daily.
Factor Xa inhibitors		
apixaban	Eliquis	PO 2.5–5 mg two times per day
rivaroxaban	Xarelto	PO 20 mg one time daily with p.m. meal (stroke prevention)
		PO 15 mg two times daily for three weeks, and then 20 mg one time daily with food (DVT/PE treatment or prevention)
		PO 10 mg once daily for 35 days (post-hip replacement)
		PO 10 mg one time daily for 12 days (post-knee replacement)
Thrombin inhibitor		
dabigatran	Pradaxa	PO 150 mg two times daily (75 mg for creatinine clearance 15–30); store in original container only up to four months

(continued)

TABLE 25-5 **Anticoagulants (*continued*)**

GENERIC NAME	TRADE NAME	DOSAGE
Anticoagulants, injectable		
Unfractionated heparin		
heparin		IV, subcu dose varies
Low-molecular-weight heparins		
dalteparin	Fragmin	Subcu, in fixed or body-weight-adjusted doses one to two times daily
enoxaparin	Lovenox	One to two times daily subcu dose and duration varies; reduce dose for creatinine clearance <30 mL/min
Factor Xa Inhibitor		
fondaparinux	Arixtra	Daily subcutaneous dose varies; closely related to the LMWHs

Note: This is a representative sample; many other products are available.

PATIENT EDUCATION

It is very *important* that patients on anticoagulant therapy be instructed regarding:

- Reading the FDA-approved Medication Guide dispensed with the oral anticoagulants
- Importance of compliance with taking medications as prescribed and required laboratory monitoring (if any)
- The fact that this medication does not dissolve clots and that it decreases the clotting ability of the blood and helps prevent the formation of harmful blood clots in the blood vessels and heart
- Taking the medication as prescribed at the same time every day
- Not changing brands of the medication without the physician's approval
- Avoiding eating large amounts of grapefruit or drinking grapefruit juice or cranberry juice
- Avoiding shots such as flu shots, shingle vaccine, and pneumonia vaccine (Talk with your health care professional before getting shots.)
- Avoiding activities and contact sports that may cause injury, cuts, or bruises

- Using a soft toothbrush and an electric razor to shave to prevent cuts
- Always wearing closed-toe shoes
- Using a night light to prevent falls
- Immediately reporting unusual bleeding, bruising, brown spots, or blood-tinged secretions, injury, trauma, dizziness, abdominal pain or swelling, back pain, headaches, and joint pain and swelling to their physician
- If prescribed, carrying vitamin K for emergency use
- Using a reliable birth control method
- Reporting allergic reactions such as skin rash to their physicians
- Avoiding smoking, the use of alcohol, and OTC medications
- Wearing identifications and alerts at all times
- Keeping all follow-up appointments with their physician for laboratory work and for needed dosage changes

Note: Large amounts of vitamin K–rich foods can counteract warfarin therapy. Be consistent with your intake of foods high in vitamin K such as asparagus, broccoli, cabbage, Brussels sprouts, spinach, turnips, dried fruits, bananas, potatoes, peaches, and tomatoes to ensure a stable INR.

Platelet Inhibitor Therapy

Antiplatelet agents inhibit the aggregation (clumping) and release of thromboplastin from the platelets to begin the clotting process. **Platelet inhibitors** utilize a variety of mechanisms to interfere with activation pathways to prevent platelet clumping and are given as prophylactic therapy or as secondary prevention in patients with a history of recent stroke, recent MI, or established peripheral vascular disease. They are also used in the pharmacologic management of post-acute coronary syndrome (ACS), a spectrum of clinical conditions ranging from unstable angina to acute myocardial infarction, with or without ST-segment elevation. Platelet inhibitors are also used prior to and following percutaneous coronary intervention (PCI) with coronary stenting to prevent stent thrombosis.

In addition to drug therapy, patients should be educated on modifying risk factors for CHD and stroke, that is, abstinence from all forms of tobacco, weight control, low-fat and low-cholesterol diet, and aerobic exercise on a regular basis.

Dipyridamole (Persantine)

Dipyridamole (Persantine) is a non-nitrate coronary vasodilator that inhibits platelet aggregation. When used alone, it is ineffective as an antithrombotic for patients with AMI, DVT, or transient ischemic attacks (TIAs) and therefore must be combined with other anticoagulant drugs. Dipyridamole is used in combination with aspirin in the prevention of ischemic stroke.

Side effects of dipyridamole, usually transient, can include:

Headache, dizziness, and weakness

Nausea, vomiting, and diarrhea

Flushing and rash

Caution with older adults (more susceptible to orthostatic hypotension).

A combination of low-dose aspirin with extended-release dipyridamole (Aggrenox) is approved for stroke prophylaxis. Most adverse effects are mild and similar to those with either agent alone.

Aspirin

Because of its ability to inhibit platelet aggregation, aspirin has been studied extensively for use in the prevention of thrombosis. Aspirin therapy, usually 75–325 mg daily, has been used after myocardial infarction or recurrent TIAs to reduce the risk of recurrence. Aspirin has also been used to reduce the risk of myocardial infarction in patients with unstable angina.

Aspirin therapy is not recommended for low-risk patients because of an increased risk of hemorrhagic stroke associated with long-term aspirin therapy. Patients should be instructed not to start aspirin therapy without consulting a physician first. Because of *gastric irritation*, aspirin should be administered with food or milk. Film-coated tablets, enteric-coated tablets, and buffered aspirin preparations are available to reduce gastric irritation. Aspirin is *contraindicated* for anyone with bleeding disorders. See Chapter 19 for a description of other side effects, precautions or contraindications, and interactions.

Adenosine Diphosphate (ADP) Receptor Antagonists

ADP receptor antagonists block the activation of the platelet's receptor surface, thereby inhibiting platelet activation. Clopidogrel (Plavix) was the first agent approved in this class. It is used to reduce atherosclerotic events (myocardial infarction, stroke, and vascular death) in patients with a history of recent stroke, recent MI, or established peripheral vascular disease.

Clopidogrel is also used in combination with aspirin to prevent thrombosis of stents that are used to prop open diseased coronary arteries. Prasugrel (Effient) is a more potent antiplatelet agent with no clinically significant drug interactions identified to date.

The newest agent in this class, ticagrelor (Brilinta), is the first reversible oral ADP receptor antagonist. Its quicker onset of antiplatelet activity allows the platelet function to return to baseline quicker and may result in fewer coronary artery bypass surgery–related bleeding events in patients requiring emergent intervention. Ticagrelor's shorter half-life necessitates twice-daily dosing compared with once-daily dosing of clopidogrel and prasugrel. Ticagrelor is contraindicated in severe hepatic impairment.

All ADP receptor antagonists are ***contraindicated*** in patients with active pathological bleeding (such as peptic ulcer) or a history of intracranial hemorrhage. ***Interactions*** of all platelet inhibitors with other anticoagulants, for example aspirin and NSAIDs, other platelet inhibitors, or thrombolytic agents, may increase the risk of bleeding.

The use of certain PPIs (esomeprazole, omeprazole, including Prilosec OTC), azole antifungals, most macrolide antibiotics (except azithromycin), certain SSRIs (fluoxetine, fluvoxamine), and HIV NNRTIs may make clopidogrel less effective by inhibiting the enzyme that converts clopidogrel to the active form of the drug. The plasma concentrations of ticagrelor may be elevated by azole antifungals, HIV protease inhibitors, and some macrolide antibiotics; they may be reduced by carbamazepine, phenobarbital, phenytoin, and rifampin. Ticagrelor can increase digoxin concentrations (monitor levels) and increase lovastatin and simvastatin concentrations (avoid doses >40 mg).

THROMBOLYTIC AGENTS

The body maintains a process to dissolve clots (fibrinolysis) after they have formed. Tissue plasminogen activator (t-PA) is a natural peptide that initiates fibrinolysis. Thrombolytic agents actually dissolve and liquefy the fibrin of the existing clot. Thrombolytic drugs (e.g., reteplase and alteplase) potentiate t-PA, resulting in clot dissolution, reperfusion of organs, and restoration of blood flow to tissues.

Thrombolytic agents, given IV, reduce mortality when used as early as possible but within the first 12h after the onset of acute STEMI. Alteplase is also used to treat acute ischemic stroke (within 3–4.5 h of the onset of stroke symptoms) and acute pulmonary embolism. Administered in an ER or ICU setting, close monitoring of hemodynamics and vital signs is generally considered standard with thrombolytic therapy, particularly during the initial 24–48 h.

Intracranial hemorrhage is the most serious complication of thrombolytic therapy, but bleeding can occur at any site in the body. Bleeding occurs most commonly at access sites such as catheter insertion sites or venipuncture sites. Patients with preexisting coagulation problems, uncontrolled hypertension, severe chronic heart failure, and recent stroke are at the highest risk for developing bleeding complications during thrombolytic therapy.

Hemorrhage can result from concomitant therapy with heparin or other platelet-aggregation inhibitors. If severe bleeding occurs during therapy, the drug should be discontinued promptly. Rapid coronary lysis can result in the development of arrhythmias; however, they are generally transient in nature.

HEMATOPOIETIC AGENTS

Hematopoiesis is the formation, differentiation, and maturation of blood cells into specific cell lines. Hematopoietic agents to be discussed here include erythropoiesis-stimulating agents and the colony-stimulating factors. All hematopoietic agents are products of recombinant technology.

Erythropoiesis-Stimulating Agents

The erythropoiesis-stimulating agents (ESAs) such as epoetin alfa (Epogen or Procrit) are responsible for the regulation of the production and development of blood cells, normally in the bone marrow. Epoetin alfa stimulates the bone marrow to produce more red blood cells and is approved for the treatment of anemia in chronic renal failure, HIV infection, and anemia associated with chemotherapy. It also reduces the need for blood transfusions in anemic patients scheduled to undergo certain kinds of surgery. Darbepoetin alfa (Aranesp) is a *second-generation* agent that is dosed less frequently than epoetin alfa.

Before initiating ESA therapy, supplemental iron (folic acid, and/or vitamin B_{12} if necessary) is usually needed because adequate iron stores are necessary to incorporate iron into hemoglobin. Treatment of iron deficiency by regular use of iron improves erythropoiesis and response to ESA therapy. As of March 2010, prescribers and hospitals must enroll in and comply with the ESA APPRISE Oncology Program to prescribe and/or dispense epoetin alfa to patients with cancer. Recently, the FDA once again updated safety information in the black box warning regarding the use of ESAs: Use the lowest dose possible to gradually increase the hemoglobin (Hgb) concentration to avoid the need for transfusion.

Side effects of epoetin alfa (Epogen) include:

- **!** Hypertension (especially in dialysis patients)
- **!** Flu-like symptoms
- GI effects
- Rash
- Chest pain
- **!** Increased mortality, MI, stroke, thrombosis of vascular access, venous thromboembolic events, and increased risk of tumor progression or recurrence

Colony Stimulating Factors (CSFs)

A granulocyte colony-stimulating factor (G-CSF), filgrastim (Neupogen) is involved in the regulation and production of neutrophils in response to host defense needs. It lessens the severity of myelosuppression in patients with cancer and has allowed chemotherapy dose intensification or maintenance of dose intensity. Use with caution in patients with sickle cell disorders.

Side effects of filgrastim include:

- Bone pain (common)
- Headache
- Dermatological reactions

See Table 25-6 for a summary of platelet inhibitors, thrombolytic agents, and hematopoetic agents.

TABLE 25-6 Platelet Inhibitors, Thrombolytic Agents, and Hematopoetic Agents

GENERIC NAME	TRADE NAME	DOSAGE
Platelet inhibitors		
aspirin	Ecotrin, Ascriptin, others	75–325 mg PO daily
dipyridamole	Persantine	75–100 mg PO four times per day with warfarin or aspirin depending on indication
dipyridamole with aspirin	Aggrenox	1 cap PO BID
ADP receptor antagonists		
clopidogrel	Plavix	75 mg PO daily with or without food; 300 mg loading dose in ACS, usually with low-dose aspirin
prasugrel	Effient	60 mg PO loading dose and then 10 mg daily (5 mg if < 60 kg) with aspirin for ACS managed with PCI
ticagrelor	Brilinta	180 mg PO loading dose and then 90 mg twice daily with aspirin (100 mg max) for ACS
Thrombolytic agents		
alteplase, tPA	Activase	IV bolus and then IV infusion
	Cathflo Activase	2 mg injection one time (MR in 2h) for IV catheter occlusions
reteplase, r-PA	Retavase	IV bolus two times (30 min apart)
tenecteplase, TNK-tPA	TNKase	Rapid IV bolus
Hematopoetic agents		
ESAs		
darbepoetin alfa	Aranesp	IV, subcutaneous dose varies
epoetin alfa	Epogen, Procrit	IV, subcutaneous dose varies
CSFs		
filgrastim, G-CSF	Neupogen	IV, subcutaneous dose varies

Note: This is a representative sample; many other products are available.

CASE STUDY A

Cardiovascular Drugs

Isaac Doniego, a 77-year-old widower with heart failure, has been treated successfully with a combination of ACE inhibitors and diuretics. However, his symptoms worsen and became life threatening despite pharmacologic treatment, so he is hospitalized for evaluation and stabilization on a cardiac glycoside.

1. How will the cardiac glycoside act to lessen Isaac's heart failure?
   a. By increasing his heart rate
   b. By increasing the force of cardiac contraction
   c. By increasing his oxygen utilization
   d. By suppressing possible cardiac arrhythmias

2. What type of cardiac glycoside is Isaac's physician most likely to prescribe?
   a. Synthetic adenosine
   b. Lidocaine or a related drug
   c. Digitalis product
   d. Thiazide

3. Isaac's physician alerts him that cardiac glycosides should be avoided if he has which of the following conditions?
   a. Hyperthyroidism
   b. Hyperkalemia
   c. Hypermagnesemia
   d. Impaired renal function

4. Isaac should be advised to avoid certain medications because they can potentiate digoxin toxicity. Which of the following are in this category?
   a. Cholestyramine, neomycin, and rifampin
   b. Diuretics, calcium, and corticosteroids
   c. Macrolides and antiarrhythmics
   d. Adrenergics

5. Isaac should be cautioned about taking antacids because of the risk of:
   a. Reduced absorption of digoxin
   b. Arrhythmia
   c. Digoxin toxicity
   d. Increased force of cardiac contraction

CASE STUDY B

Cardiovascular Drugs

Dianna Whitfield, a 37-year-old African-American, has been diagnosed with hypertension. Her physician discusses various options for pharmacologic treatment.

1. What class of drugs is Dianna's physician most likely to prescribe first?
   a. Thiazides
   b. Beta-blockers
   c. ACE inhibitors
   d. Calcium channel blockers

2. What antihypertensives are known to be *more* effective in African-Americans and older adults?
   a. Thiazides
   b. Angiotensin receptor blockers
   c. Nonthiazide diuretics
   d. Calcium channel blockers

3. What antihypertensives are known to be *less* effective in African-Americans than in other groups?
   a. Beta-adrenergic blockers
   b. Antiadrenergics
   c. ACE inhibitors
   d. Peripheral vasodilators

4. Dianna also has lupus. What class of antihypertensive should be avoided?
   a. Beta-adrenergic blockers
   b. Antiadrenergics
   c. ACE inhibitors
   d. Thiazides

5. Suppose Dianna is pregnant and experiences preeclampsia. Under this circumstance, the antihypertensive of choice would likely be:
   a. Chlorthalidone
   b. Hydralazine
   c. Losartan
   d. Enalapril

CHAPTER REVIEW QUIZ

Match the medication in the first column with the condition in the second column that it is used to treat. Conditions may be used more than once.

Medication

1. _____ isosorbide

2. _____ Zetia

3. _____ Lovenox

4. _____ Cardizem

5. _____ Zocor

6. _____ Plavix

7. _____ Crestor

8. _____ hydralazine

9. _____ quinidine

10. _____ procainamide

Classification

a. Elevated cholesterol

b. Hypertension

c. Angina

d. Pulmonary emboli

e. Cardiac arrhythmia

f. Stroke prevention (platelet inhibitor)

Choose the correct answer.

11. Why is digoxin the only cardiac glycoside and digitalis product still marketed for clinical use?
    a. It is safe at higher doses.
    b. It is effective on cardiac arrhythmias.
    c. It is slow acting.
    d. It can be administered orally and parenterally.

12. About what percentage of adults in the United States are considered to have prehypertension?
    a. 27%
    b. 37%
    c. 47%
    d. 57%

13. Digoxin toxicity can usually be treated sufficiently by:
    a. Discontinuing digoxin
    b. Administering atropine
    c. Treating potassium and magnesium disturbances
    d. Administering digoxin-specific Fab fragments

14. Fibrillation refers to:
    a. Rapid heartbeat
    b. Irregular heart beat
    c. Slow heart beat
    d. Insufficient heart beat

15. Most drugs given to counteract arrhythmias have the potential for:
    a. Causing hypertensive crisis
    b. Deranging calcium levels
    c. Slowing the heart rate
    d. Increasing glucose metabolism

16. Which of the following is especially important to monitor in patients receiving antiarrhythmic drugs?
    a. Electrolytes
    b. Glucose
    c. Platelets
    d. Lipids

17. Which of the following has been widely accepted as the most effective treatment for patients with life-threatening ventricular tachycardia or fibrillation?
    a. Insertion of an AICD
    b. Amiodarone
    c. Adenosine
    d. Propranolol

18. Inhibition of ACE lowers blood pressure by:
    a. Decreasing cardiac output
    b. Increasing cardiac output
    c. Decreasing vasoconstriction
    d. Increasing vasoconstriction

19. Side effects from beta-blockers are most common in:
    a. Patients of age 50 or younger
    b. Patients receiving IV administration of the drug
    c. Patients with pre-existing arrhythmia
    d. Patients who suffer from migraines

20. Coronary vasodilators are used for the:
    a. Treatment of hypotension
    b. Reduction of intracranial pressure
    c. Prevention of tachycardia and resulting syncope
    d. Treatment of angina

21. Increased risk of new-onset diabetes mellitus is most associated with high doses of:
    a. Statins
    b. Cardiac glycosides
    c. Calcium channel blockers
    d. Bile acid sequestrants

22. Which drug is *least* effective in reducing the mortality associated with heart failure?
    a. Metoprolol
    b. Atenolol
    c. Bisoprolol
    d. Carvedilol

23. What is one purpose of International Normalized Ratio (INR) monitoring?
    a. To monitor warfarin therapy
    b. To monitor kidney function for persons on antilipemics
    c. To determine the need for pharmacologic treatment of angina
    d. To determine the effectiveness of antihypertensives

24. How are low-molecular-weight heparins usually administered?
    a. Orally
    b. Sublingually
    c. Subcutaneously
    d. As a skin patch

25. What is an advantage of the new oral anticoagulants?
    a. Slow onset for long-term therapy
    b. Fewer food and drug interactions
    c. Ability to monitor with standard laboratory equipment
    d. Availability of numerous reversal agents

STUDYGUIDE

PRACTICE

Complete Chapter 25

Online Resources

- Powerpoint presentations
- Videos

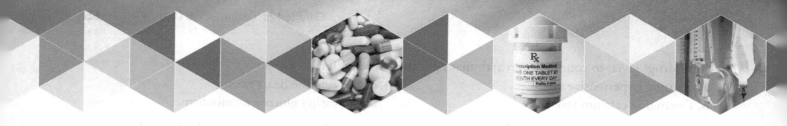

CHAPTER 26

RESPIRATORY SYSTEM DRUGS AND ANTIHISTAMINES

KEY TERMS AND CONCEPTS

Anticholinergics

Antihistamines

Antitussives

Asthma prophylaxis

Bronchodilators

Decongestants

Dry-powder inhalers (DPIs)

Expectorants

Maintenance medications

Metered-dose inhalers (MDIs)

Mucolytics

Rescue treatment

Small-volume nebulizers (SVNs)

Smoking-cessation aids

Sympathomimetics

Xanthine

OBJECTIVES

Upon completion of this chapter, the learner should be able to

1. Describe the uses of and precautions necessary with oxygen therapy

2. List the medications used as smoking-cessation aids and precautions for their use

3. Classify a list of respiratory system drugs according to their action

4. List the uses, side effects, and precautions or contraindications for bronchodilators and antitussives

5. Explain appropriate patient education for those receiving respiratory system drugs

6. Describe the action and uses of the antihistamines and decongestants

7. List the side effects, precautions or contraindications, and interactions of the antihistamines and decongestants

8. Describe the limitations for use and safety concerns associated with combination cough–cold–allergy products

9. Define the Key Terms and Concepts

RESPIRATORY DISEASES AND DISORDERS

According to the American Lung Association, lung disease is the third-leading cause of death in the United States. Respiratory diseases range from mild and self-limiting such as the common cold to life threatening such as bacterial pneumonia, pulmonary embolism, and lung cancer.

Chronic obstructive pulmonary disease (COPD) is a term that encompasses a group of progressive lung diseases—chronic bronchitis (inflammation of bronchial tubes, which leads to chronic mucus production and a wet cough) and emphysema (destruction of the tiny air sacs at the base of the lungs, diminishing the capacity and efficiency of the lungs to utilize oxygen, leading to shortness of breath and exercise intolerance). COPD is a progressive disease that worsens with time and has systemic manifestations, including muscle wasting. Cigarette smoking is the primary cause of COPD; less often, it is caused by long-term exposure to lung pollutants.

Therapeutic measures for respiratory distress include oxygen therapy, respiratory stimulants, bronchodilators, corticosteroids, mucolytics, expectorants, antitussives, and smoking cessation.

OXYGEN THERAPY

Oxygen is used therapeutically for hypoxia (insufficient oxygen supply to the tissues) and to decrease the workload of the heart and respiratory system, especially during distress. Some of the conditions for which oxygen therapy is indicated are heart and lung diseases such as COPD, smoke inhalation, carbon monoxide or cyanide poisoning, and some central nervous system (CNS) conditions with respiratory difficulty or failure. Oxygen may be administered by endotracheal intubation, nasal cannula, various masks, tents, or hoods.

Side effects of oxygen delivered at too high a concentration or for prolonged periods of time without proper monitoring can include:

Hypoventilation (particularly with COPD; may cause CO_2 retention and acidosis)

Confusion

Changes in the alveoli of the lungs

Blindness (in premature infants)

Precautions or contraindications apply to:

Patients with COPD (high O_2 concentrations may cause hypoventilation or apnea [cessation of breathing]).

After long-term oxygen therapy, patients should be reassessed periodically for the need of oxygen.

Danger of fire when oxygen is used. Oxygen is not flammable but does support combustion. Smoking, matches, cleaning aerosols, and electrical equipment that may spark (e.g., electric razors, hair dryers, curling irons) are not allowed in rooms where oxygen is in use.

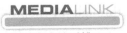

See it in Action! View a video on *Using Oxygen* on the Online Resources.

RESPIRATORY STIMULANTS

Respiratory stimulants include:

- Caffeine citrate in the treatment of neonatal apnea of prematurity (see Chapter 20)
- Theophylline administered IV and orally to stimulate respiration in infants (as an alternative to caffeine).

BRONCHODILATORS

Bronchodilators act by relaxing the smooth muscles of the bronchial tree, thereby relieving bronchospasm and decreasing the work of breathing. Bronchodilators are used in the symptomatic treatment of acute respiratory conditions such as asthma, as well as many forms of COPD. Classifications of bronchodilators include the sympathomimetics (adrenergics), the anticholinergics (parasympatholytics) (see Chapter 13, "Autonomic Nervous System Drugs"), and the xanthine derivatives.

Bronchodilator Administration

Bronchodilators can be given orally, parenterally, and by inhalation. The inhalation route of administration is preferred to minimize systemic adverse effects. Appropriate inhalation technique is essential to achieve optimal drug delivery and therapeutic effect of aerosol inhalant medications.

Metered-dose inhalers (MDIs) remain popular because of their ease of use, efficacy, and portability. In the past, all MDIs contained chlorofluorocarbon (CFC) as the propellant. Because of its detrimental effects on the ozone layer, the use of CFC was phased out by the end of 2013. Some manufacturers have reformulated their MDI to contain hydrofluoroalkane (HFA) as the propellant, which has not been linked to depletion of the ozone layer and is nonflammable. Other manufacturers are discontinuing production of MDIs and utilizing alternative formulations instead. MDIs are frequently used, and the use of a spacer or reservoir device assists in optimizing drug delivery within the lungs. (See Figure 26-1.)

MDI's and other inhalers need to be cleaned intermittently to avoid the buildup of medication at the mouthpiece that can inhibit drug delivery. Although it can be done more frequently, it is recommended that MDI inhalers be cleaned at least once per week. The following steps should be followed to ensure proper cleaning:

1. Remove the canister from the actuator, do not let the canister get wet.
2. Take the cap off the mouthpiece and wash the actuator by running warm water through the top for 30 seconds.
3. Turn the actuator upside down and run warm water through the mouthpiece for 30 seconds.
4. Shake the actuator off to remove as much water as possible and allow the actuator to dry overnight.
5. Replace the canister in the actuator and shake well, spray two sprays into the air away from your face, then replace the cap on the mouthpiece.

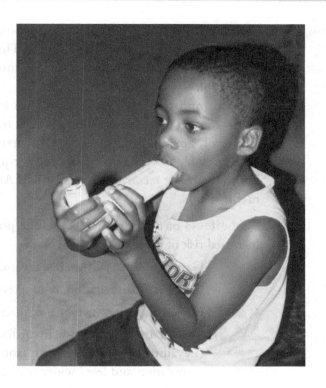

FIGURE 26-1 Child using a metered-dose inhaler (MDI) with a spacer and a mouthpiece.

Dry-powder inhalers (DPIs) provide the medication (especially corticosteroids and long-acting beta$_2$ agonists) only under the pressure of spontaneous inspiration rather than through compression of the valve. Therefore, the patient must be able to generate sufficient inspiratory effort on his or her own to deliver the medication, and therefore this device should not be used in acute respiratory distress. (See Figure 26-2.) This option is helpful for patients who are unable to coordinate inspiration with actuation of a conventional MDI.

Small-volume nebulizers (SVNs) will create an aerosol mist of a drug solution that can then be inhaled into the lungs through a mouthpiece or a mask. The aerosol is created by either compressed air or oxygen gas, and the optimal breathing pattern is a slow, deep breath, with a sustained breath hold; the aerosol should be delivered over an 8–12 min period. (See Figure 26-3.)

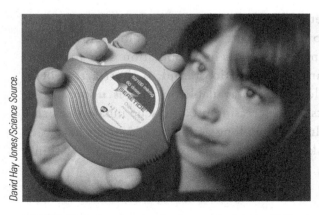

David Hay Jones/Science Source.

FIGURE 26-2 An example of a dry-powder inhaler (DPI).

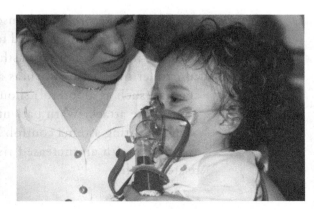

FIGURE 26-3 Child receiving a small-volume nebulizer (SVN) aerosol treatment with a mask.

Sympathomimetics

Sympathomimetics (adrenergics) are potent bronchodilators that increase vital capacity and decrease airway resistance. The adrenergics work on the smooth muscle in the lungs to cause relaxation. Examples include albuterol, epinephrine, and salmeterol.

An important classification system is differentiating between short-acting beta-agonists (SABAs) and long-acting beta-agonists (LABAs). SABAs, such as albuterol, are the drug of choice for managing acute exacerbations of asthma. LABAs, such as salmeterol, are used for prophylactic treatment. SABAs are also known as *rescue medications* versus the LABAs, which are known as maintenance medications.

Side effects of the adrenergics include potentiation of theophylline effects with increased risk of toxicity, especially:

Gastrointestinal (GI) (nausea, vomiting, and decreased appetite)

Cough, throat irritation, hoarseness, and sinusitis with inhaled preps

! CNS stimulation (nervousness, tremor, dizziness, and headache)

! Cardiac irregularities (tachycardia, palpitations, arrhythmias, and angina) (Levalbuterol [Xopenex], an isomer of albuterol, may cause less cardiac stimulation and less incidence of certain systemic adverse reactions such as tremor and nervousness compared to albuterol; the clinical significance of these small differences are unknown)

! Hypertension

! Hyperglycemia and hypokalemia (caution with loop or thiazide diuretics)

Precautions or contraindications for the adrenergics apply to:

First administration, which should be observed by medical personnel for hypersensitivity reactions

Contacting the physician if decreased effectiveness occurs

Close monitoring, if administering oral inhaled adrenergics with other oral inhaled bronchodilators, for cardiovascular effects

Patients with cardiovascular or kidney disorders, diabetes, seizure disorders, or hyperthyroidism

Because of a prolonged onset of action, long-acting beta$_2$ agonists (such as salmeterol) should not be used to treat an acute asthma attack or bronchospasm; these are indicated only for asthma prophylaxis in combination with an asthma controller medication such as an inhaled corticosteroid. A short-acting beta$_2$ agonist (such as albuterol) should always be available for the rescue treatment of an acute attack. Warn patients that increasing use of rescue inhalers is a sign of deteriorating asthma control. In addition, long-acting beta$_2$ agonists have been associated with an increased risk of severe asthma exacerbations and asthma-related deaths.

CLINICAL CONNECTION

Rescue inhaler use

Rescue inhalers, which are most commonly albuterol (SABA)-based MDI inhalers, are an effective way for patients who have asthma, COPD and other bronchospastic diseases to manage acute respiratory distress. These types of medications act very quickly, but also only provide temporary relief to patients. Overuse of SABA's can result in tachycardia, jitteriness, anxiousness, and insomnia. The recommended maximum dose for inhaled albuterol MDI's is 12 inhalations in any 24h period. Patients should be counselled that their rescue inhaler is intended for "as needed" use, and should not be taken if symptoms are not present. Even if a patient is not exceeding the max daily dose, it is important as

a health care practitioner to limit rescue inhaler use, as frequent use can be a sign of poor disease state control. Ideally, patients should only require the use of the rescue inhaler two days per week or less. If patients are using the rescue relief more frequently, there is a need for maintenance therapy initiation, adjustment, or addition of new medications. Maintenance medications for respiratory diseases include inhaled corticosteroids, LABA's, oral corticosteroids, and leukotriene inhibitors. The use of these medications can vary based on patient age, disease severity, and other factors. Additionally, patients can be instructed to limit activities or avoid environments that exacerbate their condition.

See Table 26-1 for selected sympathomimetic products and dosages.

Anticholinergics

Anticholinergics (*parasympatholytics*), for example Atrovent, achieve bronchodilation by decreasing the chemical that promotes bronchospasm. Anticholinergics block the parasympathetic nervous system and can cause drying of pulmonary secretions. Adequate hydration should be encouraged to avoid mucus plugging. Inhaled anticholinergics are the first-line therapy for COPD once symptoms become persistent. See Table 26-1 for dosage and other product names.

Side effects of anticholinergics can include:

- ! Cardiac effects (changes in heart rate and palpitations)
- ! CNS stimulation (headache, drowsiness, dizziness, confusion, and agitation)
- ! Thickened secretions and mucus plugging; dry mouth and metallic taste

  Constipation and abdominal pain

Cautions: Anticholinergics are not indicated for patients with unstable cardiac status, history of heart attacks, glaucoma, drug sensitivity, or prostatic hypertrophy.

Tiotropium (Spiriva), which is structurally similar to ipratropium (Atrovent), is administered daily as a maintenance drug in a dry-powder inhaler (vs. three to four times daily for ipratropium). It is more efficient than ipratropium for the maintenance treatment of COPD and may lead to a reduction in the use of sympathomimetics for rescue therapy.

PATIENT EDUCATION

Chapter 9 covered much of the needed information for proper inhaler technique and other inhaled medication use. Please refer to this chapter and review:

- Patient education for administration for various inhalation delivery systems to include MDI, DPI and SVN's.

- Instructions for cleaning nebulizer devices
- Instructions for taking more than one medication concurrently

Xanthines

The **xanthine** derivative theophylline, listed in Table 26-1, relaxes the smooth muscle of the bronchial airways and pulmonary blood vessels and may possess anti-inflammatory actions. Xanthines are no longer a first-line treatment because of the modest clinical effectiveness, the need for serum monitoring, their many adverse effects, and their drug interactions.

Theophylline is generally reserved for patients with COPD who do not respond to or cannot take inhaled long-acting bronchodilators. When used, xanthines are usually administered as sustained-release formulations with other respiratory system drugs such as adrenergics and anticholinergics for additive effects on symptom relief and breathing functions.

Side effects of theophyllines can be mild or severe with acute toxicity, including:

- (!) GI distress (nausea, vomiting, epigastric pain, abdominal cramps, anorexia, or diarrhea. To reduce gastric irritation, take with meals)
- (!) CNS stimulation (nervousness, insomnia, irritability, headache, tremors, and seizures; can be fatal)
- (!) Cardiac effects (palpitation, tachycardia, arrhythmias, *especially with rapid IV administration*)
- Urinary frequency (mild diuresis)
- (!) Hyperglycemia

Precautions and contraindications when administering theophylline apply to:

Sudden cessation of tobacco smoking (may result in reduced clearance of theophylline and increased serum theophylline concentrations)

Cardiovascular, kidney, pulmonary, or liver dysfunction

Diabetes, peptic ulcer, or glaucoma

Children and older adults (more prone to toxicity)

IV injection (*must be done slowly*—see cardiac side effects)

Patients undergoing influenza immunization or who have influenza

Pregnancy and lactation

Note

Roflumilast (Daliresp) is a drug that acts as a selective, long-acting inhibitor of the enzyme PDE-4, a contributor to inflammation, and therefore this drug has anti-inflammatory effects. Roflumilast is an *orally* administered drug for the prevention of inflammatory conditions of the lungs in chronic obstructive pulmonary disease but currently has many dose-limiting side effects, including nausea, diarrhea, and headache; it must be used with at least one long-acting bronchodilator.

Interactions occur with:

Cimetidine, allopurinol, erythromycins, quinolones, oral contraceptives, calcium channel blockers, and beta-blockers (increase theophylline levels)

Smoking, barbiturates, phenytoin, and rifampin (decrease theophylline effectiveness)

Roflumilast or PDE-4 inhibitor

PATIENT EDUCATION

Patients taking bronchodilators (e.g., adrenergics, anticholinergics, or the xanthines) should be instructed regarding:

Following the written directions on the package very carefully regarding dosage and administration because of the danger of serious side effects

The differences between rescue medications and long-term controllers

Proper technique for inhaler use; capsules used with DPIs must not be swallowed

Use of spacers for patients who have difficulty using MDIs

Watching closely for cardiac irregularities or CNS stimulation (e.g., nervousness, tremor, dizziness, confusion, and headache), and reporting these symptoms to the physician immediately

Other side effects possible with adrenergics and xanthines, for example gastric distress, insomnia, or hyperglycemia

Drinking adequate fluids to prevent mucus plugging, especially with anticholinergics

The importance of quitting smoking and avoiding second-hand smoke, fumes, or pollution

Asthma guidelines state that OTC bronchodilators are *not recommended* because the temporary relief provided may delay the patient from seeking medical care

Avoiding any new medications, including over-the-counter (OTC) drugs, without consulting the physician first, because of the danger of serious complications; many interactions are possible

Avoiding changing brands of medicine without consulting the physician or pharmacist

See Table 26-1 for a summary of the sympathomimetic, anticholinergic, and xanthine bronchodilators.

TABLE 26-1 Bronchodilators

GENERIC NAME	TRADE NAME	DOSAGE
Sympathomimetics		
Short-acting Beta$_2$ agonists (rescue medications)		
albuterol sulfate	Proair HFA, Proventil HFA, Ventolin HFA	MDI, 1–2 puffs (90–180 mcg) q4–6h
	Accuneb (Nebulizer solution) ProAir RespiClick	Inhal sol 2.5 mg q4–6h Oral sol, Tabs 2–4 mg q6–8h MDI, 1–2 puffs (90–180 mcg) q4–6h
	Vospire ER	Tabs ER 4–8 mg q12h
levalbuterol	Xopenex	Inhal sol 0.63–1.25 mg TID (q6–8h); max 3.75 mg per day
	Xopenex HFA	MDI, 1–2 inhal (45–90 mcg) q4–6h

(*continued*)

TABLE 26-1 Bronchodilators (*continued*)

GENERIC NAME	TRADE NAME	DOSAGE
Long-acting Beta₂ agonists* (maintenance medications)		
arformoterol	Brovana	Inhal sol 50 mcg q12h (for COPD only)
formoterol	Foradil Aerolizer	Powder for inhal, 12 mcg (contents of 1 cap) q12h
	Perforomist	Inhal sol 20 mcg BID
salmeterol	Serevent Diskus	Powder for inhal, 1 puff (50 mcg per blister) q12h
Others		
epinephrine	Adrenalin	IM/subcu 1:1,000 sol 0.3–0.5 mL; watch dose carefully!
racepinephrine	Asthmanefrin (OTC)	1–3 inhalations, max of 3 q3h
Anticholinergics		
Short-acting		
ipratropium bromide	Atrovent HFA	MDI, 1–2 puffs (17–34 mcg) three to four times per day (max 12 sprays per day)
	Atrovent	Inhal soln, 1 unit dose (500 mcg/2.5 mL NS) three to four times per day
		Nasal sol 0.03%–0.06%, 2 sprays each nostril three to four times per day (up to four days for cold, three weeks for rhinitis)
ipratropium/albuterol (combination of anticholinergic and sympathomimetic)	Combivent Respimat	Inhal soln, 1 puff four times per day (max 6 puffs per day)
	DuoNeb	Neb sol 1 vial (3 mL) four times per day (max 6 doses per day)
Long-acting		
tiotropium	Spiriva HandiHaler	Powder for oral inhal, 18 mcg daily (for COPD only)
aclidinium	Tudorza Pressair	1 puff (400 mcg) BID
Combination with LABA		
umeclidinium	Incruse Ellipta	1 puff (62.5 mcg) daily
umeclidinium and vilanterol	Anoro Ellipta	1 actuation daily (62.5 mg/25 mcg)
Xanthines		
theophylline	RTU infusion in D₅W	Dosage based on response and drug levels
	Elixophyllin	Elixir, 80 mg/15 mL
	Theo-24	Caps ER, 100–400 mg daily

*Note: Because of the delayed onset of action, long-acting beta² agonists should never be used to treat an acute attack and should be used in combination with an inhaled corticosteroid. This is a representative list. Other products are available.

CORTICOSTEROIDS

Synthetic corticosteroids are used to relieve inflammation, reduce swelling, decrease bronchial hyper-responsiveness to triggers, and suppress symptoms in acute and chronic reactive airway disease (asthma and some COPDs). Corticosteroids should be administered systemically (oral and injectable forms) for short-term "bursts" during exacerbations and occasionally at the beginning of treatment until symptoms are controlled.

Inhaled

Inhaled corticosteroids (SVN aerosol, DPI, and MDI) are considered a preferred drug therapy in long-term prophylactic management of persistent asthma of various severities. Regular long-term treatment reduces exacerbations, improves control of symptoms and lung function, and reduces hospital admissions and deaths from asthma. Inhaled corticosteroids with long-acting beta-agonists are also used on a regular, long-term, scheduled basis in patients with COPD to improve symptoms and quality of life. Inhaled corticosteroids have less systemic side effects than oral or injectable administration. They are often used in combination with LABAs. Patients should be counselled to rinse their mouth out with water after use and to not swallow medication. Failure to follow these instructions could result in oral thrush or irritation of the esophageal passage.

Intranasal

Nasal corticosteroids are increasingly considered first-line therapy for most *noninfectious* types of rhinitis and reduce congestion, edema, and inflammation. They should be started before symptoms occur and taken regularly throughout the period of exposure. Aerosol corticosteroid preparations seem to be more irritating (burning, sneezing) to the nasal mucosa. Aqueous preparations may drip into the throat, resulting in reduced deposition of drug in the nasal mucosa.

Side effects of inhaled corticosteroids

⚠ Throat irritation and dry mouth

Hoarseness

Coughing and dysphonia (hoarseness)

⚠ Oral fungal infections (patient should be encouraged to rinse mouth with mouthwash or water after administration)

⚠ Increased susceptibility to pneumonia

Precautions or contraindications with corticosteroids apply to:

Viral, bacterial, or fungal infections

Hypertension or congestive heart failure

Diabetes

Hypothyroidism or cirrhosis

Renal failure

See Chapter 23 for further information about corticosteroids, and see Table 26-2 for a summary of corticosteroids.

TABLE 26-2 Corticosteroids

GENERIC NAME	TRADE NAME	DOSAGE
Corticosteroids (inhaled and intranasal)		
beclomethasone	QVAR HFA	MDI, 1–2 puffs (40 or 80 mcg per puff) BID
	Beconase AQ	Spray (42 mcg) 1–2 inhal each nostril daily–BID
budesonide	Pulmicort Flexhaler	Powder for inhal, 180–360 mcg BID
	Pulmicort Respules	Neb susp, 0.25–1 mg daily or BID; indicated for children ≥8 years old
	Rhinocort Aqua	Aerosol 1–4 inhal each nostril daily (32 mcg per spray)
with formoterol	Symbicort	MDI, 2 puffs (80/4.5, 160/4.5) BID
fluticasone furoate	Arnuity Ellipta	MDI, 1 puff daily (100–200 mcg)
with vilanterol	Breo Ellipta	MDI, I puff daily (100–200 mcg/25 mcg)
fluticasone propionate	Flovent HFA	MDI, 2–4 puffs BID (88–880 mcg)
	Flonase	Spray (50 mcg) 1 inhal each nostril BID or 2 inhal daily
with salmeterol	Advair Diskus (100/50, 250/50, 500/50)	Powder for inhal, 1 inhal q12h
	Advair HFA (45/21, 115/21, 230/21)	MDI, 2 puffs q12h
mometasone	Asmanex Twisthaler	Powder for inhal, 220 mcg BID or 440 mcg qPM
	Nasonex	Spray 2 inhal each nostril daily (50 mcg per spray)
triamcinolone	Nasacort AQ (Rx)	Inhaler, 1–2 inhal each nostril daily (55 mcg/inhal)
	Nasacort Allergy 24HR (OTC)	Inhaler, once daily (age 2 and older), not to exceed two months a year; dosing varies per age group

Note: This is a representative list. Other products are available. Breo Ellipta comes with two foil blister strips, each dose contains one blister from each strip (one contains fluticasone furoate and the other contains vilanterol).

ASTHMA PROPHYLAXIS

Leukotriene Inhibitors

Zafirlukast (Accolate) and montelukast (Singulair) are oral leukotriene receptor antagonists for asthma prophylaxis, prevention of exercise-induced bronchoconstriction, and treatment of chronic asthma. Leukotriene receptor antagonists primarily help to control the inflammatory process of asthma caused by leukotriene production, thus helping to prevent asthma symptoms and acute attacks. They can be used as monotherapy or as add-on therapy in patients whose persistent mild to moderate asthma is inadequately controlled with inhaled corticosteroids. Montelukast can be used in children as young as 2 years old and has fewer drug interactions compared to zafirlukast.

Side effects of Singulair include:

> ❗ Headache

> ❗ Dizziness

> Nausea or dyspepsia

> Pain

> Fatigue

> Respiratory infections and fever

> Behavior or mood changes, sleep disturbances, and suicidal ideation (both drugs)

Precautions or contraindications apply to:

> Hepatotoxicity (zafirlukast)

> Pregnancy or lactation

> Treatment of acute episodes of asthma (these are *not* rescue medications)

Drug interactions occur with:

> Aspirin (increased levels of zafirlukast)

> Erythromycin and theophylline (decreased levels of zafirlukast)

> Warfarin and zafirlukast (increased prothrombin time)

> Phenobarbital and rifampin (decreased levels of montelukast)

Mast Cell Stabilizers

The rupture or degranulation of mast cells and the subsequent spilling of their chemical mediator contents cause an inflammatory response that can lead to asthma. Stabilizing the mast cell membrane has anti-inflammatory actions that modify the release of mediators from mast cells and eosinophils.

A prophylactic for asthma, cromolyn was one of the first classified mast-cell stabilizers. Cromolyn has no value in the treatment of acute attacks of asthma. It has also been used in the prevention of exercise-induced bronchospasm. Cromolyn is available as a solution for inhalation or a nasal solution (to treat seasonal allergic rhinitis) for use in adults and children as young as 2 years old. To be effective, the manufacturer's directions must be followed carefully.

Side effects of cromolyn can include:

> ❗ Throat irritation, cough, and bronchospasm

> ❗ Nose burning, stinging, and sneezing (with nasal solution)

> Nausea or headache

Caution applies to:

> Those with cardiovascular disorders

> Proper use on a regular schedule

See Table 26-3 for a summary of asthma prophylaxis.

TABLE 26-3 Asthma Prophylaxis Agents

GENERIC NAME	TRADE NAME	DOSAGE
Asthma prophylaxis and treatment of chronic asthma		
Mast cell stabilizers		
cromolyn sodium		Inhal sol, 20 mg per treatment four times per day
	NasalCrom (OTC)	Inhaler, 1 spray each nostril three to four times per day
Leukotriene inhibitors		
montelukast	Singulair	Tabs 10 mg qPM
		Chew tabs, 4–5 mg qPM
zafirlukast	Accolate	Tabs 10–20 mg BID on empty stomach

This is a representative list. Other products are available.

PATIENT EDUCATION

Patients treated with inhaled corticosteroids or the asthma prophylaxis agents should be instructed regarding:

The fact that these agents are *not* effective for acute exacerbations of asthma or immediate symptom relief

Proper technique for inhaler use

Side effects to expect, such as throat irritation, dry mouth, and cough (rinse mouth and gargle to minimize), and with products administered nasally; for example, nose burning, stinging, or sneezing are possible with cromolyn

Complications of inhaled corticosteroids without proper precautions, for example oral fungal infections (Patient should be encouraged to rinse mouth with mouthwash or water after treatment and to always rinse and air dry equipment after use.)

Administering bronchodilator before corticosteroid when the two inhaled medications are ordered at the same time

Reporting side effects to the physician, especially respiratory distress

The importance of not smoking

MUCOLYTICS AND EXPECTORANTS

Mucolytics, such as acetylcysteine, decrease the hypersecretion of and liquefy pulmonary secretions. Thick secretions can be a problem in patients with obstructive lung disease, but there is little evidence that *inhaled* acetylcysteine is more effective than adequate hydration for thinning or increasing the clearance of secretions.

Precautions or contraindications for mucolytics apply to:

Asthma or a history of bronchospasm (IV administration or inhalation may result in acute bronchospasm or anaphylaxis)

Respiratory insufficiency, inadequate cough mechanism, or gag reflex depression (liquefied pulmonary secretions can occlude the airway if the patient is unable to adequately clear the secretions)

Expectorants, such as guaifenesin (the only agent approved for use as an expectorant), increase secretions, reduce viscosity, and help to expel sputum but like mucolytics offer little clinical benefit for patients with obstructive lung disease. Adequate fluid intake is important to maintain normal fluid volume, but excessive fluid intake is of no value.

Guaifenesin is commonly combined in cough syrups for the symptomatic management of productive ("wet") coughs associated with upper respiratory tract infections, bronchitis, pharyngitis, influenza, and measles or coughs provoked by sinusitis, but evidence of benefit is lacking. It is also commonly used in combination with a cough suppressant, dextromethorphan, to reduce the incidence of dry cough, but still loosen mucus in the respiratory tract to allow for productive cough.

Expectorants should not be used for self-medication for persistent or chronic coughs such as those associated with smoking or COPD. A persistent cough may be indicative of a serious condition. If cough persists for more than a week, is recurrent, or is accompanied by a fever, a physician should be consulted.

Side effects of the expectorants are infrequent, usually not serious at recommended doses, and can include:

Nausea and vomiting and diarrhea

Drowsiness, dizziness, and headache

Precautions or contraindications for expectorants apply to:

Persistent or chronic cough

Some asthmatics (prone to bronchospasm)

Cardiovascular disease and hypertension, diabetes, glaucoma, hyperthyroidism, and prostatic hypertrophy, especially with combination products

Pregnancy or lactation

See Table 26-4 for a summary of the mucolytics and expectorants.

TABLE 26-4 Mucolytics and Expectorants

GENERIC NAME	TRADE NAME	DOSAGE
Mucolytic		
acetylcysteine	(Mucomyst)[a]	Neb soln, 3–5 mL 20% sol (diluted) or 6–10 mL 10% sol (undiluted) three to four times per day; give short-acting bronchodilator 10–15 min prior to dose
Expectorant		
guaifenesin	Mucinex	ER tabs 600–1,200 mg, daily BID; do not crush
	Robitussin	Sol 2–4 tsp q4h as needed

Note: Guaifenesin is frequently combined with other drugs, for example, analgesics, antihistamines, decongestants, and antitussives in OTC and prescription respiratory combination products.

a. This brand name is no longer marketed, but the name is still commonly used.

ANTITUSSIVES

Antitussives are medications to prevent coughing in patients not requiring a productive cough. Coughing, a reflex mechanism, helps eliminate secretions from the respiratory tract. A dry, nonproductive cough can cause fatigue, insomnia, and, in some cases, pain to the patient (e.g., pleurisy and fractured ribs).

Most antitussives produce cough suppression by acting centrally on the cough center located in the brainstem. Cough suppressants are divided into narcotic preparations such as codeine and hydrocodone and non-narcotic preparations such as dextromethorphan.

Codeine, a *narcotic antitussive,* is widely used as a cough suppressant owing to its reduced incidence of side effects (respiratory depressant action and bronchial constriction) at antitussive doses as compared to morphine. In some states, codeine is available behind the pharmacy counter as an OTC cough medication. Hydrocodone, another narcotic cough suppressant, has slightly greater antitussive activity compared to codeine but is more sedating. With the recent change from DEA Schedule III to DEA Schedule II, hydrocodone is prescribed less frequently as an antitussive.

Recently, a new boxed warning—FDA's strongest warning—was added to the drug label of codeine-containing products about the risk of codeine used to *manage pain* in children after a tonsillectomy and/or adenoidectomy. Some children died after being given codeine in amounts that were within the recommended dose range. Codeine is converted to morphine in the liver by an enzyme. Some people are ultra-rapid metabolizers who are more likely to have higher-than-normal amounts of morphine in their blood after taking codeine. High levels of morphine can result in breathing difficulty, which may be fatal. Although this warning applies to codeine as a pain reliever, it bears consideration when codeine is used as an antitussive.

Non-narcotic antitussives (e.g., dextromethorphan) are used more frequently because they do not depress respirations, do not cause dependence, and have few side effects at recommended doses. It is considered to have a similar antitussive effect as codeine at the same dose. Dextromethorphan should not be used in patients under the age of 4 (caution in age less than 6) because of the cough center in the brain not being full developed. Benzonatate (Tessalon), chemically related to the local anesthetic tetracaine, suppresses cough peripherally by anesthetizing receptors in the alveoli of the lungs, the bronchi, and the pleura; it also acts centrally like the other antitussives. Diphenhydramine (Benadryl), a first-generation antihistamine, is also used as a cough suppressant and is described in detail later in this chapter.

Side effects of antitussives can include:

> ❗ Respiratory depression (large doses or excessive use)
>
> Constipation
>
> Urinary retention with narcotic antitussives
>
> ❗ Sedation and dizziness
>
> Nausea and vomiting

Precautions or contraindications for antitussives apply to:

> Addiction-prone patients (refer also to the discussion on dextromethorphan abuse by adolescents in Chapter 20)
>
> Asthma; COPD
>
> Other CNS depressants (refer to Chapter 19 for opioid interactions)

Caution for antitussives with children can include:

Some CNS side effects, behavioral disturbances, and respiratory depression reported, especially with large doses

Ester-type anesthetic (e.g., tetracaine) hypersensitivity with *benzonatate*

Interactions with dextromethorphan can include:

Triptans used for migraine headache

Monoamine oxidase inhibitors (MAOIs), resulting in "serotonin syndrome" (applies to benzonatate as well)

The SSRIs fluoxetine and paroxetine (reduce dextromethorphan dose)

Memantine (Namenda)

The American College of Chest Physicians practice guidelines do not recommend the use of cough suppressants in coughs associated with upper respiratory infection (URI) because of their limited efficacy. It is recommended that patients experiencing a cough associated with the common cold or postnasal drip associated with a URI use a first-generation antihistamine and a decongestant to treat cough.

See Table 26-5 for a summary of the antitussives.

TABLE 26-5 Antitussives

GENERIC NAME	TRADE NAME	DOSAGE	COMMENTS
Narcotic			
codeine with guaifenesin	Cheratussin AC	Syrup 10–20 mg q4–6h	Antitussive dose is lower than that required for analgesia. Any cough medicine containing a controlled substance is not for extended use; can develop physical dependence and tolerance; watch for side effects
with promethazine	(Phenergan)[a] with codeine		
hydrocodone with homatropine[b]	Hydromet	Syrup or tabs 5 mg q4–6 h	
with chlorpheniramine	Tussionex	ER Susp, 5 mL q12h	
Non-narcotic			
benzonatate	Tessalon	Caps 100–200 mg TID	Related to tetracaine; swallow caps whole
dextromethorphan	Delsym	ER susp, 10 mL (60 mg) q12h	Note interactions
with guaifenesin	Robitussin DM	Sol 10–20 mg q4h or Sol 30 mg q6–8h	
	Mucinex DM	Tab (200-400/10-20mg) 1 to 2 taken BID	Extended release, do not crush or chew
diphenhydramine	Benadryl	Caps, liquid 25 mg q4–6h	Antihistamine with anticholinergic effects, especially drying

a. This brand name is no longer marketed, but the name is still commonly used.
b. An anticholinergic agent is added in subtherapeutic amounts to some hydrocodone products to discourage deliberate overdosage.

PATIENT EDUCATION

Patients taking antitussives should be instructed regarding:

- Reading and carefully following the directions on the product label
- Starting with a low dose of antitussives and increasing the dose only if cough suppression does not occur
- Avoid using with alcohol and other CNS depressants
- Taking care in operating machinery because of sedative effect

ANTIHISTAMINES

Antihistamines competitively antagonize the $histamine_1$ receptor sites. Through this action, the antihistamines combat the increased capillary permeability and edema, inflammation, and itch caused by sudden histamine release. Antihistamines are used to treat the symptoms of allergies (e.g., rhinitis, conjunctivitis, and rash). However, when antihistamines are used to reduce nasal secretions in the common cold, the consequent thickening of bronchial secretions may result in further airway obstruction, especially in those with COPD and asthma. H_1-blockers are grouped into two categories: the first-generation agents and the second-generation agents.

First Generation

These antihistamines, such as diphenhydramine (Benadryl), were the first group of medications available to treat symptoms of allergies. Diphenhydramine is also approved as an antitussive, nighttime sleep aid (see also hypnotics in Chapter 19), and antiemetic. It is also used as an adjunctive treatment of anaphylactic reactions after the acute symptoms (e.g., laryngeal edema and shock) have been controlled with epinephrine and corticosteroids. Some antihistamines are used in the symptomatic treatment of vertigo associated with pathology of the middle ear or in the prevention and treatment of motion sickness (see Chapter 16).

Side effects of the first-generation antihistamines are primarily anticholinergic in action and include:

- (!) Drying of secretions, especially of the eyes, ears, nose, and throat
- (!) Sedation, dizziness, tachycardia, and hypotension, especially in older adults
- Muscular weakness and decreased coordination; cognitive impairment
- Urinary retention and constipation
- Visual disorders
- (!) Paradoxical excitement, insomnia, and tremors, especially in children
- GI effects—nausea, vomiting, and anorexia
- Nasal irritation, epistaxis, and bitter taste with nasal spray

Precautions or contraindications for first-generation antihistamines apply to:

- COPD and asthma
- Persons operating machinery or driving a car
- Older adult patients (extended half-life with sedation)
- Closed-angle glaucoma

Cardiovascular disorders

Benign prostatic hyperplasia (BPH)

Children under the age of 6 years

Pregnancy and lactation

Seizure disorders

Interactions of first-generation antihistamines may occur with:

Potentiation of CNS depression with tranquilizers, analgesics, hypnotics, alcohol, and muscle relaxants

PATIENT EDUCATION

Patients taking first-generation antihistamines should be instructed regarding:

Avoiding frequent or prolonged use of antihistamines (may cause increased bronchial or nasal congestion and dry cough)

Not using antihistamines to sedate children

No self-medication (check with the physician first) in those with COPD or cardiovascular disorders, BPH, older adults, and children

Taking care in driving or operating machinery because of sedative effect

Not mixing with alcohol or any other CNS depressant drugs

Second Generation   The *second-generation antihistamines* include fexofenadine (Allegra), cetirizine (Zyrtec), levocetirizine (Xyzal), and loratadine (Claritin). These drugs are *selective* (have greater specificity for) histamine$_1$ receptor antagonists and have fewer CNS effects, for example less sedation, and less anticholinergic effects compared to the first-generation antihistamines. Although these agents cause little or no sedation, it is important to note that the incidence of sedation is not zero. They are used to provide symptomatic relief of seasonal allergic rhinitis, for example hay fever. The second-generation antihistamines are not effective in the treatment of cough.

Side effects of second-generation antihistamines, usually mild, can include:

Headache, dizziness, fatigue, and drowsiness (especially cetirizine)

Dry mouth and pharyngitis

Precautions or contraindications for second-generation antihistamines apply to:

Asthma

Renal and hepatic impairment

Hydroxyzine (Vistaril) allergy with Zyrtec

Driving or operating machinery

Pregnancy or lactation

Children less than 2 years of age

PATIENT EDUCATION

Patients taking second-generation antihistamines should be instructed regarding:

Avoiding any other drug, including OTC, without consulting the physician first

Reporting symptoms such as fainting, dizziness, or palpitations to the physician immediately

Using caution with driving or operating machinery until you know how these drugs affect you

DECONGESTANTS

Several adrenergic drugs, for example phenylephrine (Neo-Synephrine) or pseudo-ephedrine (Sudafed), act as **decongestants**. These drugs constrict blood vessels in the respiratory tract, resulting in the shrinkage of swollen mucous membranes (because of colds or allergies) and helping to open nasal airway passages. Given orally, they are less effective than topical decongestants and have the potential for systemic side effects, especially increasing blood pressure. However, these drugs, both oral and nasal, should be used only on a short-term basis because rebound congestion may occur within a few days.

Decongestants are frequently combined with antihistamines, analgesics, caffeine, and/or antitussives. Many of these products are available OTC, and by combining several drugs, the possibility of adverse side effects is increased, especially without adequate medical supervision.

As mentioned in Chapter 20, the Combat Methamphetamine Epidemic Act of 2005 (which took effect in 2006) banned OTC sales of ingredients commonly used to make methamphetamine. Psuedoephedrine (PSE), a popular and effective oral nasal decongestant, was the primary target of the act. PSE can now be stored and sold only in limited quantities under special conditions (behind the counter) by pharmacies in an attempt to limit its sale in large quantities Purchasers are limited to 3.6 g (15 days of the max daily dose) of PSE per day and 9 g per month. Pharmacies are limited in the amount that can be sold per day as well.

Side effects of decongestants can include:

> ❗ Anxiety, nervousness, insomnia, tremor, and seizures

> ❗ Palpitations, tachycardia, hypertension, headache, and cerebral hemorrhage

> Reduced cardiac output and reduced urine output

> Burning, stinging, sneezing, and dryness with nasal preparations

Precautions or contraindications for decongestants apply to:

> Cardiovascular disorders

> Hyperthyroid or diabetes

> Older adults—especially those with glaucoma or BPH

> Pregnancy or lactation

Interactions may occur with:

> Potentiation of adverse side effects with other adrenergics, ergot, tricyclics, MAOIs

Note

Saline nasal spray (i.e., Ocean) is a safe, effective treatment option for nasal congestion.

PATIENT EDUCATION

Patients taking decongestants should be instructed regarding:

Using decongestants for only a few days (three days for nasal; seven days for oral) to avoid rebound congestion

Avoiding when cardiac or thyroid conditions or diabetes are present

Discontinuing with side effects such as nervousness, tremor, palpitations, or headache

Avoiding combining with any other medications without consulting the physician

See Table 26-6 for a summary of the antihistamines and decongestants.

TABLE 26-6 **Antihistamines and Decongestants**

GENERIC NAME	TRADE NAME	DOSAGE
First-generation antihistamines		
azelastine (Rx)	Astelin, Astepro	1–2 sprays per nostril BID
chlorpheniramine	Chlor-Trimeton, Aller-Chlor	Liquid 2 mg/5 mL q4–6h
		Tabs 4 mg q4–6h
		ER caps, tabs 8 mg TID–12 mg BID
clemastine (Rx/OTC)	Tavist Allergy	Syrup, tabs 1.34–2.68 mg BID–TID
diphenhydramine (Rx/OTC)	Diphenhist	Liquid 25–50 mg q4–6h
	Benadryl Allergy	Tabs 25–50 mg q4–6h
	Benadryl	IM or IV 10–50 mg q4–6h
Second-generation antihistamines		
cetirizine	Zyrtec	Syrup, tabs 5–10 mg per day
desloratadine (Rx)	Clarinex	Syrup, tabs 5 mg daily
fexofenadine	Allegra	Susp, tabs 30–60 mg BID, 180 mg per day
levocetirizine (Rx)	Xyzal	Soln, tabs 2.5–5 mg per day
loratadine	Claritin, Alavert	Syrup, tabs 10 mg daily
Decongestants		
oxymetazoline	Afrin	Sol 1–2 of 0.05% sprays, drops q12h
phenylephrine	Neo-Synephrine	Sol 0.125%–1%, 2–3 drops/sprays q4h;
	Sudafed PE	Tabs 10 mg q4–6h
pseudoephedrine	Sudafed	Sol or tabs 30–60 mg q4–6h
		Tabs ER 120 mg q12h or 240 mg q24h

Rx = available by prescription only; Rx/OTC 5 availability depends on product labeling.

Note: This is a representative list. Many prescription and OTC drugs have combinations of antihistamines, decongestants, and/or antitussives. Many second generation antihistamines are available in combination products with a decongestant (pseudoephedrine), these products can be identified by being labeled with a capital D (example: Claritin D).

SAFETY OF COUGH–COLD–ALLERGY PRODUCTS

Many prescription and OTC cough and cold formulations are available that combine several drugs, for example antitussives with expectorants, antihistamines, and decongestants, to treat two or more simultaneous symptoms. Combination formulations should be used only if the corresponding symptom is present and each individual component is available in the proper strength and dosing interval a patient may need. Patients should be cautioned to seek advice from a health care professional familiar with each ingredient. The health care practitioner should thoroughly assess each patient's use of similar products (both OTC and Rx) to avoid duplication of therapy and the potential for inadvertent overdose. Some ingredients are contraindicated in certain medical conditions as detailed earlier.

In 2011, the FDA required removal of many *prescription* cough, cold, and allergy products from the market that were never approved by the FDA. Many of the unapproved drug products covered by the 2011 action contained the same ingredients as the *OTC* cough and cold preparations that were the subject of a 2008 public health advisory. The FDA's Nonprescription Drugs and the Pediatric Advisory Committee found there was no proof that these medications eased cold symptoms in children, whereas there were reports that they caused serious adverse effects, overdose, and even deaths. At that time, many manufacturers voluntarily removed from the market cough and cold products labeled for use in children under 2 years old, and some products were relabeled to state that they were not for use in children under 4 years old.

In addition to product labeling changes, new child-resistant packaging and measuring devices for the products were introduced. With the changing status of cough and cold medications, a website (www.otcsafety.org/Parents) is available for parents seeking information on the use of these medicines in children.

PATIENT EDUCATION

Patients taking respiratory system drugs should be instructed regarding:

- Use of appropriate nondrug measures for the patient's particular symptoms
- Care in taking medications only as prescribed and required; do not give children medicine labeled only for adults
- Use and safety concerns of combination products
- Avoiding combining respiratory system drugs with other prescription or OTC drugs or alcohol, which could potentiate CNS stimulation or depression, resulting in serious adverse side effects
- Choosing OTC cough and cold medications with child-resistant safety caps; using only measuring devices that come with the product or those made for measuring the medicine

- Avoiding self-medication when cardiac, thyroid, or CNS conditions are present
- Benefits from desensitization therapy and air-conditioned environmental control for patients with allergic conditions
- Avoiding air pollution (e.g., smoke-filled rooms)
- Exercises (e.g., swimming) that increase lung capacity and help reduce the necessity for the medication
- Importance of receiving (and safety of) inactivated influenza vaccinations in adults and children with asthma, which can reduce serious illness, complications, and mortality
- Proper use of inhalers when prescribed (see administration with inhalers in Chapter 9)
- Not crushing, chewing, or breaking extended-release preparations; swallow whole

SMOKING-CESSATION AIDS

Cigarette smoking is the leading cause of preventable disease and death in the United States. Most smokers fail to quit on their first try, and after experiencing how difficult quitting is, many will never try again. All **smoking-cessation aids** have been shown to help twice as many smokers quit versus quitting "cold turkey" when used properly and in conjunction with nonpharmacologic therapies (behavioral modification and social support system).

Nicotine Replacement Therapy

Nicotine replacement products (Table 26-7), including Nicorette gum, Commit lozenges, the Nicoderm CQ patch, and the Nicotrol inhaler and nasal spray, help to lessen withdrawal symptoms by slowly lowering the level of nicotine in the body. They let the smoker focus on breaking the social habits of nicotine and participating in a behavior modification program for smoking cessation without battling the withdrawal symptoms at the same time. The most effective method is for patients to use one long acting nicotine replacement method (e.g., patch) and one "rescue" nicotine replacement method (e.g., gum) for breakthrough cravings.

Electronic cigarettes (or e-cigarettes) are battery-powered devices that heat liquid nicotine into an inhaled vapor ("vaping"), which simulates tobacco smoking. E-cigarettes should *theoretically* have fewer toxic effects (because of fewer toxic chemicals) than traditional cigarettes, but concrete evidence is lacking. Although e-cigarettes have not yet been linked to any serious health issues, they have been in widespread use for such a short period of time, that there is no basis for determining if there are long-term risks.

Side effects of nicotine replacement products (which could also be related to nicotine withdrawal symptoms) can include:

Mechanical problems with chewing gum, especially if the patient has dentures

❗ Cardiac irritability

❗ Chewing too fast (may cause lightheadedness, nausea, heartburn, vomiting, and throat and mouth irritation)

Skin reaction at the application site

Precautions or contraindications for nicotine replacement products apply to:

Dental problems that might be exacerbated by chewing gum

Drug abuse and/or overdependence

Overdosage—studies have shown that combination therapy (nicotine patch plus one other form of nicotine replacement) is more effective if unable to quit using a single agent, but there is little safety data on this, and combination therapy may increase the risk of nicotine overdose

Pregnancy and lactation

Unstable cardiovascular disease

Patients *should be warned not to smoke*

Proper disposal to avoid accidental ingestion by children and pets

Bupropion

Bupropion is an oral antidepressant drug (Wellbutrin) that is also prescribed as an aid to smoking cessation (marketed as Zyban) and has been associated with decreases in cravings for cigarettes and lessening of nicotine withdrawal. Zyban is also indicated for use in combination with nicotine patches for treating the symptoms of nicotine withdrawal. (Refer to Chapter 20 for information on bupropion.)

Varenicline

Varenicline (Chantix) is a prescription-only partial nicotine receptor agonist– antagonist given orally and indicated for adults as an aid in smoking cessation. It alleviates the symptoms of nicotine craving and withdrawal through its agonist activity while inhibiting the effects of repeated nicotine exposure by its antagonist activity, thus eliminating the pleasurable feelings associated with smoking. Mild to moderate nausea and vomiting, sleep disturbance, and abnormal dreams are the most common side effects, with nausea and vomiting occurring in nearly one-third of patients (take after a meal with fluids). To date, no clinically significant drug interactions have been identified.

There have been reports of serious neuropsychiatric symptoms, such as changes in behavior, agitation, depressed mood, and suicidal ideation and behavior associated with varenicline. There is some controversy as to whether these were caused by complications owing to nicotine withdrawal or by the drug itself. The safety and efficacy of varenicline in patients with serious psychiatric disorders such as schizophrenia, bipolar, and major depression has not been established. Patients and caregivers should be aware of the need to monitor for these symptoms and report them immediately to the physician.

See Table 26-7 for a summary of smoking cessation aids.

TABLE 26-7 Smoking-Cessation Aids

GENERIC NAME	TRADE NAME	DOSAGE
nicotine	Nicorette	1 piece of gum (2 or 4 mg) whenever urge to smoke up to 24 pieces per day for up to 12 weeks
	Commit	1 lozenge (2 or 4 mg) after waking up; no more than 5 loz in 6 h/20 loz per day for up to 12 weeks
	Nicoderm CQ	First dose 21 mg patch per day, six weeks
		Second dose 14 mg patch per day, two weeks
		Third dose 7 mg patch per day, two weeks
	Nicotrol NS (Rx)	1 spray each nostril one to two times per hour; max 10 sprays/h or 80 sprays per day for up to 12 weeks. Taper doses over four to six weeks
	Nicotrol inhaler (Rx)	24–64 mg (6–16 cartridges) daily up to 12 weeks and then gradual reduction in dose lasting 6–12 weeks
bupropion	Zyban (Rx)	Tabs, SR 150 mg daily for three days and then 150 mg BID for 7–12 weeks for up to six months maintenance; start one to two weeks before quit date
varenicline	Chantix (Rx)	Tabs, 1 mg BID, following a one-week titration for 12 weeks with additional 12-week course if needed

Rx = available by prescription only.

CASE STUDY A

Respiratory Medications

Thirty-four-year-old Rohan Jackson has had asthma for four years. During his annual physical, he explains that he uses his rescue inhaler more than one time a day. The physician performs a physical exam with a focus on Rohan's respiratory system and reviews his plan of care, including his medications.

1. The physician decides to start Rohan on a new medication, montelukast. She explains that this medication works by:
   a. Controlling the inflammatory process caused by leukotrienes
   b. Producing an antihistamine effect
   c. Suppressing the cough associated with asthma
   d. Liquefying pulmonary secretions and thus promoting increased air flow

2. When starting montelukast, Rohan should be prepared for which potential side effect?
   a. Flushing of face and hands
   b. Dry cough
   c. Headache
   d. Tinnitus

3. One advantage of montelukast over other asthma medications is that it:
   a. Can be used as monotherapy or as an add-on therapy
   b. Has no drug interactions
   c. Can be taken during pregnancy and breastfeeding
   d. Can be used as a rescue drug

4. Montelukast belongs to which category of drugs?
   a. Asthma rescue
   b. Asthma curative
   c. Asthma prophylaxis
   d. Asthma acute exacerbation

5. What is a side effect of montelukast that Rohan should promptly report to his physician?
   a. Throat irritation
   b. Suicidal ideation
   c. Fatigue
   d. Double vision

CASE STUDY B

Respiratory Medications

During a visit to an urgent care clinic, 38-year-old Mariella Sanchez is diagnosed with a severe sinus infection. The nurse practitioner prescribes an antibiotic and an oral decongestant.

1. A decongestant's primary action in opening nasal passages is to:
   a. Reduce nasal irritation
   b. Anesthetize receptors in nasal passages
   c. Thicken bronchial secretions
   d. Constrict blood vessels in the respiratory tract

2. A potential systemic side effect of a decongestant is:
   a. Bradycardia
   b. Hypertension
   c. Sedation
   d. Hypotension

3. Prior to prescribing the decongestant, the nurse practitioner carefully reviews Mariella's chart because decongestants are contraindicated in individuals with:
   a. Pregnancy
   b. Depression
   c. Asthma
   d. Multiple sclerosis

4. To avoid the potential complications of rebound congestion, Mariella is cautioned to take the oral decongestant for no more than:

a. Three days

b. Seven days

c. Ten days

d. Thirty days

5. When Mariella goes to the pharmacy, how will she be able to purchase the decongestant pseudoephedrine?

a. OTC

b. By prescription only

c. From the pharmacist behind the counter

d. Only in combination with an antihistamine

CHAPTER REVIEW QUIZ

Match the medication in the first column with the condition in the second column that it is used to treat. Conditions may be used more than once.

Medication

1. ____ Allegra

2. ____ Commit

3. ____ guaifenesin

4. ____ Xopenex

5. ____ Spiriva

6. ____ Tessalon

7. ____ cromolyn sodium

8. ____ Accolate

9. ____ Zyban

Condition

a. Bronchospasm (anticholinergic)

b. Chronic asthma

c. Asthma (adrenergic)

d. Asthma (prophylactic)

e. Allergies

f. Smoking cessation

g. Bronchitis (unproductive cough)

Choose the correct answer.

10. What is the first-line therapy for noninfectious rhinitis?

a. Nasal corticosteroids

b. Oral corticosteroids

c. Aqueous preparations

d. Aerosol preparations

11. A potential side effect of inhaled corticosteroids is:

a. Staining of teeth

b. Throat irritation

c. Canker sores

d. Excessive salivation

12. When educating a patient prior to initiating an inhaled corticosteroid, which instruction is most important?

a. Expect an increased susceptibility to influenza.

b. Use only half of one dose if experiencing dry mouth.

c. Exhale immediately after inhaling the dose.

d. Rinse your mouth with water or mouthwash after administration.

13. What is an appropriate instruction for patients taking second-generation antihistamines?

a. Take OTC medications as needed—no restrictions.

b. Take laxatives in conjunction with an antihistamine to avoid constipation.

c. Use caution when driving or operating machinery.

d. Expect palpitations that will resolve over time.

14. How should bronchodilators be administered in conjunction with corticosteroids?

  a. Administer the bronchodilator immediately before the corticosteroid.

  b. Administer the corticosteroid immediately before the bronchodilator.

  c. Administer the medications 4h apart.

  d. Administer the medications 2h apart.

15. A mucolytic is contraindicated in patients:

  a. With pharyngitis

  b. With swollen lymph nodes

  c. Taking oral steroids

  d. With a depressed gag reflex

16. What cough medication is frequently used because it does not depress respirations?

  a. Dextromethorphan

  b. Codeine

  c. Guaifenesin

  d. Mometasone

17. What side effect is most likely to occur with large doses of antitussives?

  a. Urinary retention

  b. Constipation

  c. Respiratory depression

  d. Nausea

18. Antitussives frequently contain controlled substances. Which one of the following medicines is available OTC?

  a. Hyromet

  b. Delsym

  c. Tussionex

  d. Cheratussin AC

19. Cough and cold medications containing antihistamines are appropriate only when the cause of the cough is

  a. Asthma

  b. Allergic rhinitis

  c. Emphysema

  d. Smoking

20. Nicorette would be an appropriate treatment for one with which condition?

  a. Arrhythmia

  b. Dentures

  c. Pregnancy

  d. A smoker with COPD

21. Individuals taking first-generation antihistamines can expect anticholinergic side effects such as:

  a. Hypertension

  b. Drying of secretions

  c. Tearing of the eyes

  d. Bradycardia

22. If a patient currently using nicotine patches to quit smoking asks if he can use anything for breakthrough cravings, which of the following would be the appropriate response?

  a. Yes you can use nicotine gum, lozenges or the inhaler for cravings.

  b. Yes there is but only if you are having cravings more than 10x per day.

  c. You should never use two nicotine products concurrently for safety reasons.

  d. No there isn't because although you can use two nicotine products at the same time, it would be a waste of money to use both.

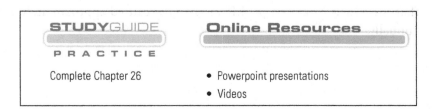

STUDYGUIDE

PRACTICE

Complete Chapter 26

Online Resources

- Powerpoint presentations
- Videos

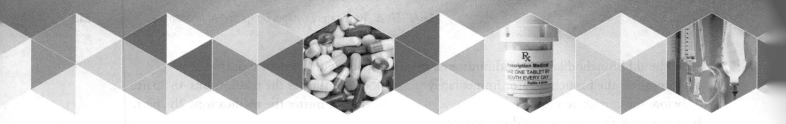

CHAPTER 27

DRUGS AND OLDER ADULTS

KEY TERMS AND CONCEPTS

Absorption

Beers list drugs

Comprehensive medication review (CMR)

Cumulative effects

Distribution

Excretion

Medication-related problems (MRPs)

Medication therapy management (MTM)

Mental impairment

Metabolism

Motor impairment

Nonadherence

Polypharmacy

Potentially inappropriate medications (PIMs)

OBJECTIVES

Upon completion of this chapter, the learner should be able to

1. List several drugs that are inappropriate for older adults and understand how to access updated information

2. Describe four factors that may lead to cumulative effects in older adults

3. Name at least five categories of drugs that frequently cause adverse side effects in older adults

4. List several drugs that can cause mental problems in older adults

5. Describe the dangers and side effects associated with NSAID therapy

6. List the side effects and cautions for gastrointestinal (GI) drugs

7. Name at least five categories of drugs that cause or contribute to syncope or falls

8. Describe patient education for all patients on long-term drug therapy

9. Describe the impact of polypharmacy on older adults

10. List the responsibilities of health care professionals in preventing complications of drug therapy in older adults

11. Define the Key Terms and Concepts

Today, people are living longer and are taking more medications. In the United States, almost 40% of people age 60 years and older take at least five prescribed medications, and many add OTC medications and supplements. Consequently, there has also been an increase in serious complications resulting from adverse drug reactions. It has been estimated that about 50% of hospitalizations because of adverse drug effects are in older adults. In 2012, it was estimated that **medication-related problems (MRPs)** caused approximately 100,000 deaths annually.

MRPs can be mistaken for what is often considered a normal consequence of aging or for progression of disease. Cognitive impairment and behavioral changes are frequently the result of drug therapy. Therefore, it is imperative that members of the health care community work together to reverse this dangerous trend.

The aging process is an individualized matter. Because of genetic or environmental factors or good health practices, for example exercise, healthy diet, and mental stimulation, some older adults may not feel or appear particularly different. However, we need to realize that there are gradual changes in our body composition and organ function as we grow older. These changes can affect the reaction to drugs and make the individual more sensitive to a wide variety of medications.

Harvard Medical School researchers investigated medicines prescribed for individuals over 65 years of age. The panel of experts in geriatrics and pharmacology found "a disturbingly high level of potentially inappropriate prescribing for older adults. Over the course of one year, almost one quarter of older Americans were unnecessarily exposed to potentially hazardous prescribing."

PHYSIOLOGIC CHANGES WITH AGE

Complex changes of aging involve both anatomic and physiological factors that affect how drugs are processed in the body (see Chapter 3). The four processes that drugs undergo in the body—that is, absorption, distribution, metabolism (biotransformation), and excretion—are all altered as the body ages. The end result of this slowed process can be exaggerated responses to medications, changes in drug levels, increased susceptibility to drug–drug interactions, and a 3- to 10-fold risk of adverse drug reactions compared with younger individuals.

Cumulative effects of drugs in older adults can be because of:

Inadequate absorption—slowed GI motility, reduced fluid intake, and/or relative achlorhydria (lack of stomach acid)

Impaired distribution—circulatory dysfunction, less muscle, and more fat

Slower metabolism—hepatic dysfunction

Impaired excretion—renal dysfunction, constipation, or poor exchange of gases in the lungs

Absorption

As we age, several changes happen to our GI tract. Not only does the gastric motility decrease, but gastric acid production diminishes, increasing the gastric pH, causing a more alkaline environment, which affects the absorption process. Many older adults also take medication that reduces gastric acid, for example ranitidine (Zantac) or omeprazole (Prilosec) (see Chapter 16, "Gastrointestinal Drugs").

Antacids are also used frequently by older adults. Calcium, magnesium, and aluminum, form insoluble and nonabsorbable complexes that are passed out of the body in the feces. Some of the drugs that are affected by antacids are quinolone antibiotics, tetracycline, iron salts, ketoconazole, and isoniazid. Therefore, it is recommended that these, and certain other drugs as well, not be taken within 2h of taking antacids.

Decreased gastric motility, especially when taking anticholinergic drugs, for example the tricyclic antidepressants or the antispasmodics, can cause adverse effects. Gastric slowing will lead to increased time for other drugs to be dissolved and absorbed.

Absorption by other routes of administration may be affected as well. Aging skin atrophies and becomes thinner, potentially impairing transdermal drug absorption of patches and gels because of reduced blood flow to the skin. Muscle mass may be significantly decreased in some older adult patients, which may alter drug absorption of IM and subcutaneous injections.

Distribution

Once drugs are absorbed and enter the circulation, many of them bind to proteins. Albumin is the principal protein used to bind drugs. As we age, the liver produces less albumin, especially in conditions such as malnutrition, cancer, diabetes, surgery, burns, and liver disease. This allows more of the drug to be unbound (free) to reach receptor sites and therefore have a greater than expected response.

Phenytoin (Dilantin) is an example of a drug that responds quite noticeably to drops in plasma albumin levels. Older adults need to be monitored frequently with laboratory studies, especially with symptoms such as sleepiness, confusion, nystagmus (involuntary back-and-forth eye movements), diplopia, and ataxia. Other drugs that are highly protein bound include warfarin, aspirin, naproxen, diazepam, and valproic acid (Depakote). When any of these drugs are used in the older adult, the best advice is to start at the lowest effective dose and increase slowly to avoid adverse effects. The frequency of administration may also need to be decreased.

Water accounts for approximately 60% of body weight in healthy young individuals but accounts for only 45% in healthy seniors. Because the older adult has less body water, drugs that are water soluble, such as digoxin, ethanol, lithium, morphine, and theophylline, may become concentrated and cause adverse reactions, with additive effects over time. Smaller doses would be needed to avoid potential toxicity.

Metabolism

The liver serves as a major site for drug metabolism. As we age, the mass of functional liver tissue and blood flow to the liver decreases. The ability of the liver to break down drugs declines, and drugs remain in the body longer. Repeated dosing can result in the accumulation of the drug and increases the risk for toxicity. Some drugs that can produce toxic effects when poorly metabolized are caffeine, diazepam, chlordiazepoxide, lidocaine, theophylline, meperidine, hydromorphone, warfarin, phenytoin, diphenhydramine, and propranolol.

All benzodiazepines increase the risk of cognitive impairment, delirium, falls, fractures, and motor vehicle accidents in older adults. Older adults have an increased sensitivity to all benzodiazepines and decreased metabolism of long-acting agents. These drugs build up with repeated administration and cause *side effects,* such as daytime sedation, dizziness, lethargy, and ataxia. Therefore, it may be necessary to consider SSRIs, SNRIs, or buspirone as alternatives for anxiety and short-term use of zolpidem (Ambien) as an alternative for hypnotics. If a benzodiazepine must be used, older adults should be given one of the "LOT" benzo's as they are more easily metabolized and do not accumulate as readily. LOT stands for lorazepam, oxazepam, and temazepam and they show these cognitive effects and risks to a lesser extent.

Omeprazole (Prilosec) and cimetidine (Tagamet) inhibit liver enzymes from breaking down the long-acting benzodiazepines and prolong the drug's duration of action. It may be preferable to use other PPIs or H$_2$ blockers such as pantoprazole (Protonix) or ranitidine (Zantac) rather than omeprazole or cimetidine.

Excretion

In the older adult, kidney size, blood flow, and glomerular filtration all decrease, resulting in a decline in creatinine clearance. Illnesses such as hypertension, heart failure, and diabetes add to the age-related loss and further reduce creatinine clearance. Consequently, drug by-products normally eliminated through the kidneys can accumulate, with toxic effects. For example, digoxin poses increased risks of adverse reactions (e.g., arrhythmias) to older adults with impaired renal function.

Nephrotoxic drugs, such as the aminoglycosides, can prove particularly dangerous to older people with reduced renal function. Acute renal failure and irreversible damage to the eighth cranial nerve (auditory and vestibular branches) are possible.

Seniors and Drug Development

Although age-related physiological changes affect how older adults process and tolerate medications, pharmaceutical research is frequently focused on younger individuals, whereas older adults are often excluded from or underrepresented in clinical trials. The study results may be inappropriately extrapolated to other populations with negative outcomes.

An example of this was a study in which spironolactone was found to reduce mortality in clinical trial patients who were around 60 years old. When this finding was extrapolated to the general population, where most patients with heart failure are older than 75 years, there was an increase in hyperkalemic deaths and no change in heart failure hospitalizations.

CLINICAL CONNECTION

The other end of the spectrum

Although this chapter focuses on the older adult, there are some special considerations for infants and pediatric patients that must be taken into consideration when prescribing medications that are primarily intended for adults. The ADME processes for children can vary greatly from that of an adult and if not accounted for can lead to potential side-effects or dangerous overdose. **Absorption:** Similar to older adults, infants and children have a lower gastrointestinal pH and a slower motility in the bowels. Additionally, they have a short GI tract and faster gastric emptying rate that can also decrease absorption. **Distribution:** Infants and children have a much higher body mass made up of water, so drugs that are water soluble may require higher doses. This volume of distribution changes throughout the child's early life and needs to be accounted for when a child is on a maintenance medication. Protein binding to drugs is also decreased in this population because of decreased albumin levels. **Metabolism:** In general drug metabolism via the liver is lower in infants and children when compared to adults. Although it can fluctuate throughout early life, it does not reach the same level until after the child is an adolescent. Drugs metabolized primarily by the liver should be used in lower doses. **Excretion:** In the early stages of life glomerular filtration rate (GFR), renal blood flow and tubular secretion are all decreased, which means drugs can stay in the body longer and have the potential to accumulate and therefore should be used at lower doses if they are primarily excreted via the kidneys. Although you will not be expected to know specific doses for children, it is important to be aware of these considerations as a health care professional.

Some medicines that are perfectly safe for a 30-year-old person may produce unexpected results in a person over age 50 or 60 years. An example is *digoxin* (*Lanoxin*). An older person still on the same dose that was appropriate 10 or 20 years earlier may experience *side effects* such as loss of appetite, weakness, personality changes, nightmares, confusion, or even hallucinations. In addition, digoxin can interact with many other drugs, sometimes slowing the clearance of the drug from the system, which could result in cumulative effects, including possible dangerous arrhythmias.

POTENTIALLY INAPPROPRIATE MEDICATION USE IN OLDER ADULTS

A group of physicians led by Dr. Mark Beers conducted a national survey of geriatric experts in 1991 to determine the most *inappropriate* drugs for ambulatory nursing home residents and adults 65 years or older. Medications were considered inappropriate if there was evidence in the literature to substantiate that the risk of drug use outweighed the clinical benefit when alternative therapy was available. The results of this survey came to be called the *Beers list* (**Beers list drugs**).

The Beers study was updated and revised by another panel of experts, and the results were published in 2003, 2012 and 2015 in the *Journal of the American Geriatrics Society* under the title "Updated Beers Criteria for Potentially Inappropriate Medication Use in Older Adults." The goal of this list is to improve care for older adults by reducing their exposure to **potentially inappropriate medications (PIMs)**. Keep in mind that the criteria are not applicable in all circumstances (e.g., patients receiving palliative and hospice care).

The complete article concerning the development of the Beers list and additional reference tables with rationale is available for free download from http://www .americangeriatrics.org.

Health care professionals treating older adults should have ready access to the Beers list and recognize the common classes of medications that can produce problems. For example, according to a recent study from the CDC, improper antidiabetic and antithrombotic drug therapy is responsible for more than two-thirds of drug-related hospitalizations in older patients. Focusing on improving the management of antithrombotic and antidiabetic drugs is most likely to have sizable, clinically significant, and measureable effects.

DRUGS TO AVOID WITH CERTAIN MEDICAL CONDITIONS

Many of the medications on the Beers list have anticholinergic properties and are not recommended for use in the older adult population. Older adults become very sensitive to drug actions and are more likely to have adverse drug reactions to *anticholinergics*. (See Chapter 13.) The resulting *side effects* are blurred vision, confusion, disorientation, dry mouth, dry eyes, constipation, palpitations, worsening of glaucoma, and urinary retention. Men with prostate problems are at extreme risk for acute urinary retention.

Drugs that produce significant anticholinergic effects include:

- Antipsychotic agents, such as the phenothiazines, chlorpromazine, fluphenazine, thioridazine, and perphenazine
- Antidepressants, such as the tricyclics amitriptyline, doxepin, imipramine (Tofranil), and nortriptyline (Pamelor)
- Antiparkinson agents, such as benztropine (Cogentin) and trihexyphenidyl
- Antispasmodics, such as dicyclomine (Bentyl) and hyoscyamine (Levsin)
- Antihistamines, such as diphenhydramine (Benadryl) and promethazine (Phenergan)

There are many other classes of medications (SSRIs, some atypical antipsychotics, H_2 blockers, certain cardiovascular drugs, corticosteroids, etc.) that exhibit subtle anticholinergic activity that becomes more pronounced in the older adults. Because the increase in the amount of a drug circulating in the system is often gradual, the consequences of an "overdose" may not be recognized. Family, friends, and even patients themselves may conclude that their symptoms are just because of aging.

Cognitive Impairment

Many medications can cause mental problems in older people. One government study found that more than 150,000 older adults had experienced *serious mental impairment either caused or worsened by drugs.* Many medications can have CNS *side effects,* such as anxiety, depression, confusion, disorientation, forgetfulness, hallucinations, nightmares, or impaired mental clarity, *especially in older adults.* Some drugs (this is a representative list) that can cause **mental impairment** (including dementia and delirium) in older adults include:

- Anticholinergics
- Antidepressants, tricyclic (TCAs)
- Antipsychotics (chronic and as-needed use)
- Benzodiazepines
- Corticosteroids
- H_2 receptor antagonists
- Meperidine
- Phenothiazines
- Sedative hypnotics

As discussed in Chapter 20, avoid taking antipsychotics for behavioral problems of dementia unless nonpharmacologic options have failed and the patient is a threat to him- or herself or others. Antipsychotics are associated with an increased risk of cerebrovascular accidents and mortality in persons with dementia. In addition, all antipsychotics can cause tardive dyskinesia and/or parkinsonism. When discontinuing many of the listed categories of drugs used chronically, *taper to avoid withdrawal symptoms.*

Syncope/Falls

Syncope (fainting or passing out) in seniors can be attributed to age-related physiological changes in conjunction with medications that result in decreased delivery of cerebral oxygen. Many CNS drugs and antihypertensives cause dizziness or **motor**

impairment, which increase the risk of falls. These drugs can also impair sexual functioning, reducing the quality of life for some older adults. Some drugs causing or contributing to syncope or falls include:

- Anticonvulsants (avoid except for treating seizures)
- Antidepressants (SSRIs and TCAs)
- Antipsychotics (especially chlorpromazine, thioridazine, and olanzapine, which increase the risk of orthostatic hypotension)
- Alpha-blockers (doxazosin, prazosin, and terazosin, which increase the risk of orthostatic hypotension and tachycardia)
- Benzodiazepines
- Nonbenzodiazepine hypnotics (e.g., Ambien)

Gastrointestinal Conditions

Many older people suffer from chronic and acute pain and take over-the-counter (OTC) nonsteroidal anti-inflammatory drugs (NSAIDs), frequently without adequate supervision. Anyone taking NSAIDs should be cautioned about the real danger of serious complications. Every year there are over 70,000 hospitalizations and more than 7,000 deaths from drug-induced bleeding ulcers or perforations. Particularly in older adults, there may be no warning signs of pain, and the first symptoms of trouble may be a "silent" bleed that could lead to fatal GI hemorrhage.

The COX-2 selective NSAID Celebrex has less *potential* for gastric problems, GI bleeding, or other bleeding problems than the other nonselective NSAIDs. However, more data is needed to confirm this. The use of PPIs and misoprostol (Cytotec) reduces but does not eliminate the risk of GI bleeding associated with NSAIDs. The risks of long-term use of PPIs are discussed in Chapter 16. The key to avoiding problems with NSAIDs is to use the lowest effective dose for the shortest period of time. Consideration should also be given to a trial of acetaminophen in place of NSAIDs.

Other GI problems, for example indigestion, heartburn, and constipation, are frequent complaints of older adults. Consequently, a common practice is the taking of OTC remedies without adequate awareness of potential side effects or implications. Side effects of antacids include constipation (with aluminum or calcium carbonate products); diarrhea (with magnesium antacids); and acid rebound, belching, or flatulence (with calcium carbonate). Avoid prolonged use (no longer than two weeks) of OTC antacids without medical supervision because of the danger of masking symptoms of GI bleeding or GI malignancy.

Constipation can be worsened by anticholinergics and oral antimuscarinics (e.g., oxybutynin, tolterodine) for urinary incontinence. Consider alternatives if constipation develops and avoid frequent use of strong cathartics, which can lead to laxative dependence and loss of normal bowel function. Instead, increase fluids and high-fiber diet and regular bowel habits. If laxatives are necessary, use bulk laxatives (e.g., psyllium), stool softeners, or sennosides (Senokot) or PEG 3350 (Miralax).

Cardiovascular Disease

Studies have indicated an *increased risk of cardiovascular problems* (thrombotic events, MI, and stroke) with the use of NSAIDs and COX-2 inhibitors. Consultation with the physician should include consideration of whether the benefits outweigh the potential risks.

Older adult patients with heart failure should avoid the calcium channel blockers diltiazem and verapamil, the antidiabetic glitazones (Actos, Avandia), cilostazol (Pletal), and dronedarone (Multaq). These agents have the potential to promote fluid retention and/or exacerbate heart failure.

PATIENT EDUCATION

Patients receiving NSAID therapy should be instructed regarding:

Administering the medication with food

Not exceeding the dosage prescribed by the physician

Not taking aspirin, alcohol, or any other drugs at the same time because they may potentiate GI or bleeding problems

The possibility of "silent" bleeding

Reducing the dosage of NSAIDs and substituting acetaminophen for pain, if possible, at least part of the time

Trying exercise and heat for pain control, as approved by the physician

POLYPHARMACY

Individuals at any age, but especially older adults, may experience **polypharmacy**, that is, the use of multiple drugs, whether they be OTC, herbals, or prescription, given at one time for the treatment of their medical conditions (see Figure 27-1). The fact that a patient is on multiple medications to treat multiple medical conditions may not necessarily be problematic.

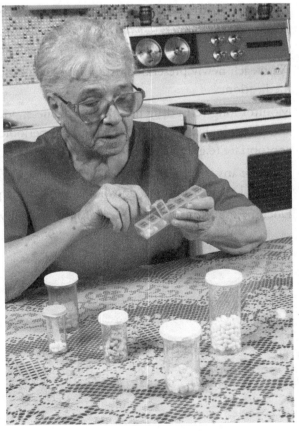

FIGURE 27-1 Polypharmacy: "My white pills are from my cardiologist and should be taken twice a day, my yellow pills are from my gastroenterologist for my stomach condition when needed, the pink pills are from my primary care physician for blood pressure and need to be taken in the morning...." In addition, many older adults add OTC medications and herbal and mineral supplements that can increase drug interactions and adverse effects.

Pinkcandy/www.Shutterstock.com

Polypharmacy becomes problematic when negative outcomes occur. Polypharmacy may result in unnecessary and/or inappropriate medication prescribing, an increase in the risk of dangerous interactions with potentially serious adverse side effects, and medication nonadherence. Health care professionals should take every opportunity to educate their patients regarding their medicines, the purpose for them, possible side effects, potential dangers, and interactions between medicines. Anyone receiving medicines should be monitored on an ongoing basis to determine the continuing effectiveness and possible cumulative or adverse effects. Medicines should be reviewed regularly to determine the feasibility of reducing dosage, possibly substituting a more effective or safer medicine or discontinuing some of the medicines.

To combat polypharmacy and the adverse effects that can result from it, medication therapy management (MTM) and comprehensive medication reviews (CMRs) are becoming common practice in pharmacies. Often times, the insurance provider of older adult patients will provide compensation for these services to help ensure safe and effective treatment of all disease states. **Medication therapy management** involves reviewing all a patient's medications, identifying potential or actual adverse effects or other medication related problems, and developing a plan to optimize therapy. Often, at the end of a MTM session, the patient will be provided with a **comprehensive medication review**, which is a document that lists their medications, how they are to take each one, and what indication they are taking each for.

All health care professionals must be aware of their responsibilities in preventing complications of drug therapy in patients of any age, but especially the old and the very young, who are more vulnerable. The following guidelines should be helpful:

- Educate yourself, your patients, and their families regarding adverse side effects, cumulative effects, and interactions. For example, have the American Geriatrics Society *Updated Beers Criteria for Potentially Inappropriate Medication Use in Older Adults* readily available for quick reference.

- With each newly prescribed drug, note diagnoses, allergies, and other medications.

- Monitor long-term drug use for effectiveness, potential for discontinuation, and physiological or mental changes. Do periodic laboratory tests as appropriate (e.g., digoxin levels).

- *Question* any inappropriate medicine or dosage. You have a moral, ethical, and legal responsibility to do what is best for the patient.

- Document all adverse side effects, calls to the physician, and action taken.

PATIENT EDUCATION

Older patients should be instructed regarding:

Making a list of *all* medicines (with dosage), including pain medicine, eye drops, OTC medicines, vitamins and herbal remedies, and topical medications (This list should be carried in the wallet or be readily available at all times.)

The purpose for their medicines, side effects, the best time to take each medication, and interactions

Asking the pharmacist for easy-to-hold and easy-to-open medication containers; proper storage and importance of keeping these types of containers out of children's sight and reach

Reporting side effects to the physician immediately

The importance of seeing their physician on a regular basis, every six months to a year or more often, to reevaluate the need for and effectiveness of the drug

Not stopping the medicine or changing the dose without consulting the physician (Abrupt withdrawal can be dangerous with some medicines.)

Asking the physician to prescribe a generic or less expensive alternative if the cost of the medicine is prohibitive. Sometimes social service departments can assist the patient in securing expensive medicines that are imperative to the patient's health. Also, some drug companies will help with costs for extremely expensive medications that patients cannot afford that they need. Suggest that the patient ask the pharmacist about this possibility

Asking the pharmacist to recommend a pillbox organizer or other memory aids if there is a problem with remembering to take medicines

Not taking another person's medication even if they think it is the same as theirs

Being sure all parties are informed of any issues if you use one or more physicians or pharmacies

ISSUES WITH ADHERENCE

Nonadherence is defined as not taking medications as prescribed on a regular basis. It can result for many reasons including side effects to a drug, lack of knowledge on how to take it, lack of understanding why it is important, forgetfulness, decreased cognitive function and many others. Older adult patients are often the most likely to be nonadherent and this can result in suboptimal therapy and worsening of disease states. The best way to combat nonadherence is to first identify the reason. In some cases, patient education or reinforcement is sufficient. In particular, older adult patients are often given weekly pill boxes (Figure 27-2), unit dose packs, or pill box alarms that can help aid those who are forgetful or have decreased cognitive function. Additionally, a caregiver can also help to increase overall patient adherence and can help report other reasons for nonadherence such as a side effect.

SUGGESTED READING

The American Geriatrics Society (2015). Beers Criteria Update Expert Panel. American Geriatrics Society Updated Beers Criteria for Potentially Inappropriate Medication Use in Older Adults. *Journal of the American Geriatrics Society.* (http://www.americangeriatrics.org)

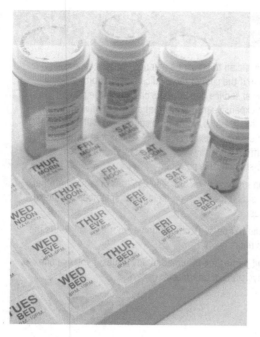
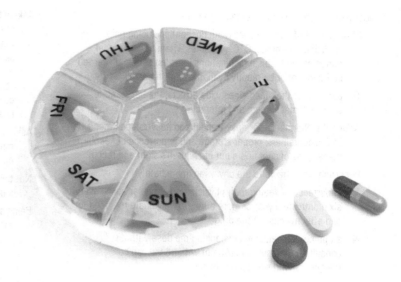

FIGURE 27-2 Pill boxes can help older adult patients remember to take medications.

CASE STUDY A

Drugs and Older Adults

Kita Wong is concerned that her 78-year-old mother, SuLyn, is not taking her medications correctly. SuLyn is on phenytoin, theophylline, digoxin, and a benzodiazepine.

1. What is the most likely age-related effect for SuLyn of the medications she takes every day?

a. High risk for periodic severe hypoglycemia

b. Frequent changes in the dose and schedule of her medications

c. Slowed clearance of drugs from her system, resulting in potentially cumulative effects

d. Increased clearance of drugs, resulting in the need for higher doses of the medication

2. How do benzodiazepines affect older adults as opposed to younger adults?

a. They have a decreased sensitivity to the drug.

b. They have largely the same reaction to the drug as young adults.

c. They require an increased dosage of the drug.

d. They have an increased sensitivity to the drug.

3. What is the best method for monitoring SuLyn's phenytoin therapy?

a. 24-h urine check

b. Patient reports of seizure activity

c. Serum phenytoin level

d. EEG

4. Consider that water accounts for only 45% of a senior's body weight. How will this most likely affect SuLyn's physiological response to theophylline?

a. SuLyn may need a larger dose.

b. SuLyn's vital signs may be critically affected.

c. SuLyn's response will not be affected by this.

d. SuLyn may need a smaller dose.

5. SuLyn has just been diagnosed with reduced renal function. What category of drugs may be particularly dangerous for her?

a. Aminoglycosides

b. Antihistamines

c. Salicylates

d. Calcium channel blockers

CASE STUDY B

Drugs and Older Adults

A visiting nurse is referred to Walter Jacobsen, an 89-year-old male living independently in a small apartment. During her intake interview, the nurse asks Walter about his medical history and his current medications. He reports his history to the nurse and then retrieves a large brown paper bag from the kitchen with numerous medications, explaining that he takes all of the medications in the bag.

1. Polypharmacy is the use of medication, more specifically defined as:
   a. Applying to prescription drugs only
   b. Taking two drugs at a time
   c. Taking one drug for at least 14 days
   d. The use of multiple drugs, either OTC or prescription

2. The nurse should instruct Walter, at a minimum, to keep a list of which medications?
   a. Only prescription drugs
   b. Prescription drugs and OTC drugs
   c. Prescription drugs, OTC drugs, and vitamins
   d. Prescription drugs, OTC drugs, vitamins, and herbal or mineral supplements

3. The nurse decides to set up a system for Walter. What method will be most beneficial for Walter to take the correct pills on the correct days?
   a. A note on his bathroom mirror
   b. Daily pillbox organizer
   c. A mailed reminder card from his primary care physician
   d. Monthly phone call reminders from the local pharmacy

4. The nurse decides to give Walter further instructions regarding his medications. Which item should she include in her teaching plan?
   a. In case of a missed dose, take two pills at the next scheduled dose.
   b. Memorize the purpose of each medication.
   c. Keep an updated list of all medications, including dose and frequency, in wallet.
   d. Always request a generic medication when filling a prescription.

5. When the nurse is reviewing Walter's medications, she is following a moral, ethical, and legal responsibility when she:
   a. Questions an inappropriate medication and/or dose
   b. Disregards Walter's concerns about a particular medication
   c. Discards pills that Walter did not take
   d. Changes the dose of a medication to better address his symptoms

Note

A Comprehensive Review Exam for Part II can be found at the end of the text following the Summary.

CHAPTER REVIEW QUIZ

Choose the correct answer. Please note that some questions require you to refer to the Updated Beer's Criteria for PIM use in older adults.

1. The aging process is:
   a. The same in individuals in similar decades of life
   b. Very individualized
   c. Different based upon ethnicity
   d. Slowed in males versus females

2. As an individual ages, the gastric pH:
- **a.** Stays at the same level
- **b.** Fluctuates over time
- **c.** Increases
- **d.** Decreases

3. You are educating an older adult who is taking a quinolone antibiotic in conjunction with an antacid. When should the patient be instructed to take the quinolone?
- **a.** Take with the antacid
- **b.** Take 1h prior to the antacid
- **c.** Take 1h post antacid
- **d.** Do not take within 2h of antacid

4. Cumulative effects of drugs in older adults can be because of:
- **a.** Increased GI motility
- **b.** Higher metabolism
- **c.** Inadequate absorption
- **d.** Improved renal function

5. What is an example of an antipsychotic drug that produces significant anticholinergic effects in older adults?
- **a.** Amitriptyline
- **b.** Benztropine
- **c.** Chlorpromazine
- **d.** Diphenhydramine

6. Which one of these is an appropriate medication to treat arthritis pain for older adults?
- **a.** Indocin
- **b.** Ketorolac
- **c.** Acetaminophen
- **d.** Talwin

7. Which one of these is an appropriate medication to treat allergies in older adults?
- **a.** Benadryl
- **b.** Claritin
- **c.** Chlor-Trimeton
- **d.** Vistaril

8. Which one of these is an appropriate pain medication for older adults after surgery?
- **a.** Morphine
- **b.** Indocin
- **c.** Demerol
- **d.** Talwin

9. When starting an older adult patient on a new drug, which is the best method of dosing?
- **a.** Allow the patient to titrate the dose to the desired effect
- **b.** Start with a high dose and then reduce to the desired effect
- **c.** Start with a moderate dose for the least risk with the most effectiveness
- **d.** Start at the lowest effective dose and increase slowly to avoid adverse effects

10. Which category of drugs is most likely to cause dizziness or motor impairment, increase the risk of falls, and impact sexual functioning in older adults?
- **a.** Anticoagulants
- **b.** Antihypertensives
- **c.** Anti-infectives
- **d.** Antidiabetics

11. Which of these cardiac drugs is *least* appropriate for older adults?
- **a.** Norpace
- **b.** Vasotec
- **c.** Procardia XL
- **d.** Hydralazine

12. Which one of these is an appropriate antidepressant to treat older adults with no history of seizure disorder?
- **a.** Prozac
- **b.** Amitriptyline
- **c.** Doxepin
- **d.** Wellbutrin

13. Which organ's function decreases with age, resulting in a decline of creatinine clearance?

    a. Liver   **c.** Small intestine

    b. Kidney   **d.** Large intestine

14. Which two categories of drug therapy are responsible for more than two-thirds of drug-related hospitalizations in older adult patients?

    a. Antidiabetic/antithrombotic   **c.** Antidiabetic/antihypertensive

    b. Antihypertensive/anticoagulants   **d.** Antidepressant/antihypertensive

15. Older adults are very sensitive to drug actions and are more likely to have adverse reactions to anticholinergics. What is one potential side effect of an anticholinergic?

    a. Drooling   **c.** Urinary frequency

    b. Constipation   **d.** Diarrhea

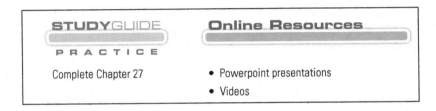

STUDYGUIDE	**Online Resources**
P R A C T I C E	
Complete Chapter 27	• Powerpoint presentations
	• Videos

Summary

The health care professional has a great responsibility in both the administration of medications and advising patients regarding drug therapy. As the older adult population increases many new drugs are developed and prescribed, requiring knowledge regarding their cumulative effects and interactions. The moral, ethical, and legal issues of drug therapy are being raised with increasing frequency. Therefore, it is imperative that the health care practitioner keep abreast of changes in drug therapy practices. Complete knowledge and good judgment are necessary for effective administration and adequate patient education.

The following guidelines should prove useful for safe drug therapy:

- Always research new drugs before administration to determine their side effects, interactions, and cautions.

- Always verify that you are administering the drug to the correct patient by whatever system your institution utilizes. If the patient is wearing a wrist band, this must always be checked.

- Assess the patient before administration for allergies, general condition, and possible contraindications and after administration for results and adverse effects.

- Question any inappropriate drugs, dosages, or possible interactions.

- Reduce the risk of medication errors by checking the spelling of each medicine very carefully. Many drug names look or sound alike, but the drugs act differently. Check the patient's diagnosis to be sure the medication is appropriate.

(Responsibilities of drug administration and medication errors are discussed in detail in Chapter 7.)

Comprehensive Exam For Part 1

Choose one correct answer and mark the appropriate letter.

1. Drug standards regulate the following factors in drug preparation:
   a. Strength, quality, purity
   b. Fillers, color, taste
   c. Color, taste, quality
   d. Quality, fillers, taste

2. The Pure Food and Drug Act:
   a. Requires warning labels on certain medications
   b. Sets limitations on prescription use
   c. Establishes consumer protection
   d. Was passed in 1976

3. The Food and Drug Administration regulates:
   a. Prescriber registration
   b. Creation of drug schedules
   c. Prescription labeling
   d. Establishment of drug regulations

4. Controlled substances include:
   a. Digoxin and Tylenol
   b. Benadryl and Cardizem
   c. Ampicillin and ibuprofen
   d. Valium and marijuana

5. Controlled drugs:
   a. Are listed by schedule
   b. Have no limitations on refills
   c. Do not cause dependence
   d. Are available over the counter

6. A good source of drug information is:
   a. News magazines
   b. Your colleagues
   c. Social networks
   d. PDR

7. The generic name of a drug is:
   a. Assigned by the drug company
   b. Written in capital letters
   c. The common name
   d. The same as the trade name

8. The term *OTC* refers to drugs that:
   a. Are often controlled
   b. Require a prescription.
   c. Are sold over the counter
   d. Are officially certified

9. Two conditions commonly listed as a *contraindication* for drug administration are:
   a. Obesity and glaucoma
   b. Hypersensitivity and pregnancy
   c. Psychosis and seizures
   d. Glaucoma and anemia

10. Before giving a new drug, you must know:
    a. Its absorption rate
    b. The distribution process it will follow
    c. Its excretion rate
    d. Its indication for use and side effects

11. An antibiotic with *photosensitivity* listed as a side effect could cause:
    a. Deafness
    b. Sunburn
    c. Blindness
    d. Kidney damage

12. Drugs have many sources. These sources include:
    a. Minerals and plants
    b. Inert gases
    c. Water
    d. Carbon monoxide

13. Drugs undergo biological changes in the body. One process affecting this is:
    a. Tolerance
    b. Dependence
    c. Metabolism
    d. Addiction

14. Patient characteristics affect the processing of drugs in the body. Two of these characteristics are:
    a. Hair color and gender
    b. Skin color and mental status
    c. Ethnicity and age
    d. Weight and age

15. Drug toxicity from cumulative effects may result from:
    a. Intracranial pressure
    b. Glaucoma
    c. Kidney malfunction
    d. High blood pressure

16. Idiosyncrasy means:
    a. An opposite effect from that expected
    b. An allergic response to a drug
    c. A unique, unusual, and unexpected response to a drug
    d. Having effect from a drug as the result of suggestion

17. The route of administration most often used is:
    a. Topical
    b. Sublingual
    c. Injection
    d. Oral

18. A form of parenteral administration is:
    a. Nasogastric tube
    b. Injection
    c. Oral
    d. Rectal

19. A type of medication that can be crushed and mixed with food to facilitate administration is:
    a. Timed-release capsule
    b. Lozenge
    c. Film-coated tablet
    d. Enteric-coated tablet

20. Topical administration includes which of the following?
    a. Nebulizer
    b. Cream
    c. Sublingual
    d. Inhalation

21. The most rapid form of administration is:
    a. PO
    b. IV
    c. IM
    d. Subcu

22. The least accurate system for measuring medication is:
    a. Metric
    b. Apothecary
    c. Household
    d. Standard

23. The most frequently used system for measuring medicine is:
    a. Apothecary
    b. Metric
    c. Household
    d. Standard

24. Medication orders must contain:
    a. Patient's address
    b. Alternate drugs
    c. Physician's address
    d. Drug name, dosage, and route

25. The prescription blank for a controlled substance must contain
    a. Name of the drug company
    b. Physician's DEA number
    c. Physician's address
    d. Lot number of the drug

26. The least accurate type of equipment for measuring medicine is a:

    a. Medicine cup

    b. Minim glass

    c. Teaspoon

    d. Syringe

27. Responsibilities of the health care professional in drug administration include:

    a. Assessing and evaluating patients

    b. Checking the order for accuracy

    c. Reporting adverse patient outcomes

    d. All the above

28. After administering medication, you should:

    a. Inform the patient's family

    b. Document drugs administered

    c. Complete additional treatments ordered

    d. Administer drugs to the next patient

29. The most helpful patient information to know when administering medication is:

    a. Patient's residence

    b. Patient's handicaps

    c. Patient's health history, including allergies

    d. Patient's occupation

30. If a medication error is made, once the patient is cared for you should:

    a. Immediately report the error to the physician

    b. File an incident report

    c. Note the error on the patient record

    d. Apologize to the patient

31. Before giving any medicine, it is essential to review the seven Rights of Medication Administration, including

    a. Right medication and right amount

    b. Right physician and DEA number

    c. Right drug company

    d. Right drug lot

32. Documentation of a controlled drug given PRN for pain requires:

    a. Review of pharmacy delivery record

    b. Note of the effectiveness in progress note

    c. Note of the trade name

    d. Review of the physician's comments

33. Administration by the gastrointestinal route includes which of the following?

    a. Nasogastric tube

    b. Oral inhaler

    c. Transdermal patch

    d. Eye drops

34. An advantage of the oral route over other routes is that it:

    a. Absorbs fastest

    b. Is the best route to treat emergencies

    c. Is economical, with few equipment costs

    d. Can be used for all patients all the time

35. If a medication is ordered PO and the patient is NPO, you should:

    a. Give the medication by injection

    b. Give the medication rectally

    c. Omit the medication and note on the chart

    d. Consult the person in charge

36. Oral medications are usually best administered with:

    a. Fruit juice

    b. Milk

    c. Water

    d. Hot tea

37. When preparing cough syrup, you should:

    a. Shake the bottle

    b. Dilute with liquid

    c. Hold the bottle with the label side down

    d. Hold the medicine cup at eye level

38. When administering a rectal suppository, you should:

    a. Assist the patient to self-administer

    b. Provide privacy and use disposable gloves

    c. Turn the patient onto the right side

    d. Warm suppository under warm water

39. The parenteral route *least* likely to be used for systemic effects is:
    a. Transdermal
    b. Topical
    c. Sublingual
    d. Inhalation

40. The route with the slowest action is:
    a. Transcutaneous
    b. Inhalation
    c. Sublingual
    d. Injection

41. After instilling eye drops, you should:
    a. Rub the eyelid vigorously
    b. Press the inner canthus
    c. Close the eyelid quickly
    d. Discard the eyedropper

42. For intradermal injection, you should:
    a. Use a tuberculin syringe
    b. Use a 21-gauge, 1-inch needle
    c. Pinch the skin
    d. Inject 1–3 mL of solution

43. Which of the following is *not* true for intramuscular injections?
    a. Pinch the skin
    b. Administer at a 45-degree angle of needle
    c. Use a 1½-inch needle for most patients
    d. Always administer Z-track for medications that are irritating to tissue

44. Which of the following IM injection sites can be used in all patients?
    a. Dorsogluteal
    b. Vastus lateralis
    c. Deltoid
    d. Ventrogluteal

45. Before administering medication via NG tube, you should verify placement by:
    a. Injecting 10 mL water
    b. Attaching NG to suction
    c. Having an X-ray of the abdomen taken
    d. Checking the pH of gastric aspirate

46. If a two-year-old accidentally swallows several children's aspirin tablets, you should:
    a. Administer ipecac
    b. Give activated charcoal
    c. Call Poison Control
    d. Give 8 oz of milk

47. If there is doubt about the type of poison ingested by an individual, toxicology tests will be done on body fluids including:
    a. Tears and saliva
    b. Blood and urine
    c. Stool and emesis
    d. Emesis and tears

48. The groups at greatest at risk of accidental poisoning are:
    a. Young children and older adults
    b. Adolescents and healthy adults
    c. Healthy adults and disabled adults
    d. Adolescents and dementia patients

49. Prevention is the key to preventing harm and death from poisoning. Key to prevention is
    a. Legislation
    b. Oversight
    c. Regulation
    d. Public education

50. Which of the following is the IV route used for?
    a. To correct body fluid imbalances
    b. Administer blood
    c. Administer medications
    d. All of the above

51. How many types of IV administration are there?
    a. 1
    b. 2
    c. 3
    d. 4

52. Which of the following is an isotonic fluid?

    a. Lactated ringers   **c.** D5W

    b. ½ NSS   **d.** D5LR

53. Which of the following is an important consideration when choosing the "Right Medication" for administration?

    a. What time it is?   **c.** The right dosage form

    b. How old the patient is?   **d.** The right route

Calculate the correct dosage for administration in the following problems. Label your answers. Remember that syringes are not marked in fractions; therefore, when computing dosages for administration, you must convert all fractions to decimals and round off to one decimal place.

54. You are to give 7,500 units of heparin subcu. The vial is labeled 10,000 units/mL. How many milliliters should you give?

55. You are to give 10 mL of guaifenesin cough syrup with codeine. The bottle is labeled 10 mg of codeine in 5 mL of cough syrup. How much codeine would the patient receive in each prescribed dose?

56. The medicine bottle label states that the strength of each tablet in the bottle is 0.25 mg. The physician has ordered that the patient is to receive 0.5 mg. How many tablets should you give?

57. The physician has ordered 20 mg of meperidine to be given. On hand is medication containing 50 mg/mL. How many milliliters should you give?

58. To convert pounds to kilograms (kg), you would divide the number of pounds by what number?

Comprehensive Exam For Part 2

Choose one correct answer and mark the appropriate letter.

1. Vitamin C aids in the absorption of:
   - **a.** Protein
   - **b.** Iron
   - **c.** Fat
   - **d.** Zinc

2. What is one side effect of taking an iron preparation?
   - **a.** Blood-tinged stools
   - **b.** Brown stools
   - **c.** White stools
   - **d.** Black stools

3. A side effect of niacin is:
   - **a.** Postural hypertension
   - **b.** Hypoglycemia
   - **c.** Decreased uric acid
   - **d.** Flushing of the face and neck

4. Which side effect may occur after prolonged use of a corticosteroid cream?
   - **a.** Hyperglycemia
   - **b.** Epidermal thinning with frequent skin tears
   - **c.** Immunodeficiency disorders
   - **d.** Systemic viral infection

5. Which type of preparation is topically used to soothe the skin and seal out wetness from diaper rash?
   - **a.** Keratolytics
   - **b.** Antipruritics
   - **c.** Protectants
   - **d.** Enzymatics

6. A yeast infection of the tongue is medically known as:
   - **a.** Tinea pedis
   - **b.** Varicella zoster
   - **c.** Tinea coporis
   - **d.** Candidiasis

7. A common topical antifungal medication used for athlete's foot would be?
   - **a.** Clotrimazole
   - **b.** Betamethasone
   - **c.** Mupirocin
   - **d.** Povidone–Iodine

8. Drugs that mimic the action of the sympathetic nervous system are known as:
   - **a.** Adrenergics
   - **b.** Cardiogenics
   - **c.** Adrenergic blockers
   - **d.** Cholinergics

9. Adrenergics should be used with caution in patients with:
   - **a.** Hypotension
   - **b.** Angina
   - **c.** Asthma
   - **d.** Diabetes

10. Cholinergic blockers would most likely cause which of the following side effects?
    - **a.** Hypotension
    - **b.** Photosensitivity
    - **c.** Dry mouth and constipation
    - **d.** Enhanced vision

11. What would be the best food choice for an individual undergoing treatment with an antineoplastic?
    - **a.** Spaghetti and meatballs
    - **b.** Orange juice
    - **c.** Mashed potatoes
    - **d.** Peppered steak

12. A clinician is reviewing an order sheet for a patient with breast cancer. Herceptin is ordered to be given orally. The clinician knows that this is an error and that instead the drug should be administered by which route?
    a. Intrathecal
    b. Intravenous
    c. Topical
    d. Intramuscular injection

13. Plant alkaloids can be fatal if administered by which route?
    a. Intrathecal
    b. Intravenous
    c. Oral
    d. Intraosseous

14. The main indication for the use of a diuretic is to:
    a. Reduce bladder spasm
    b. Promote excretion of uric acid
    c. Reduce urinary frequency
    d. Reduce the circulating fluid volume

15. Which of the following is common side effect of all the antineoplastic agents discussed?
    a. Photosensitivity
    b. Cardiotoxicity
    c. GI effects such as nausea and vomiting
    d. Extravasation

16. Bethanechol would be contraindicated in a patient with which condition?
    a. Hypothyroidism
    b. Crohn's disease
    c. Hemorrhoids
    d. Urinary tract obstruction

17. UTIs are commonly treated with?
    a. Antibiotics and Pyridium
    b. Steroids and fluids
    c. Antibiotics and ibuprofen
    d. Nothing, uncomplicated UTIs self-resolve

18. Long-term use of agents that reduce gastric acid can possibly result in a deficiency of which vitamin?
    a. Vitamin D
    b. Vitamin E
    c. Vitamin C
    d. Vitamin B_{12}

19. Mesalamine produces an anti-inflammatory effect in which section of the gastrointestinal tract?
    a. Stomach
    b. Colon
    c. Esophagus
    d. Duodenum

20. What instruction should be given with a prescription for esomeprazole (Nexium)?
    a. Take 2h after a meal.
    b. Take on an empty stomach.
    c. Take with water only.
    d. Take with meals.

21. What is the drug of choice for infective endocarditis prophylaxis?
    a. Penicillin
    b. Cefaclor
    c. Amikacin
    d. Amoxicillin

22. What is a potential hypersensitivity reaction caused by vancomycin?
    a. Red man's syndrome
    b. Lactic acidosis
    c. Flushing of hands
    d. Elevated CPK

23. Amphotericin B is administered by which route?
    a. Oral
    b. Intravenous
    c. Intramuscular
    d. Transdermal

24. What is the primary function of mydriatic eye preparations?
    a. Pupil constriction
    b. Pupil dilation
    c. Corneal anti-inflammatory
    d. Retinal anesthetic

25. Patients being treated with an anti-infective ophthalmic preparation should be instructed to:
    a. Avoid eye makeup
    b. Wear contact lenses for not more than 12h a day
    c. Instill into the upper eyelid area
    d. Use drops only until symptoms begin to improve

26. Which is a key guideline in educating a patient with an eye infection?
    a. Consider an eye patch as an effective alternative to an antibiotic for treatment.
    b. Engage in careful handwashing to prevent the spread of infection.
    c. Gently massage the upper eyelid after instillation of eye drops.
    d. When using more than one drop instill both drops at the same time.

27. Large doses of acetaminophen can cause which side effect?
    a. Gastric ulcer
    b. Petechiae
    c. Liver toxicity
    d. Splenic swelling

28. Opioids can tend to cause tolerance which is?
    a. When the drug is stopped withdrawal symptoms occur.
    b. When the person has a physical need to take the drug.
    c. When the drug is not tolerated in the body and side effects occur.
    d. When a larger dose of the drug is needed to achieve the same effect.

29. Why may a lidocaine patch be of benefit to a patient experiencing postherpetic neuralgia?
    a. It acts peripherally with little CNS action.
    b. It produces an anesthetic effect.
    c. It acts as a CNS depressant.
    d. It produces an anti-inflammatory effect.

30. What is the preferred first-step intervention in treating insomnia?
    a. Barbiturates
    b. Benzodiazepines
    c. Nondrug therapies
    d. Non-benzodiazepines

31. What is a possible side effect of an overdose of a tricyclic antidepressant?
    a. Hypertension
    b. Mania
    c. Hyperglycemia
    d. Tachyarrhythmias

32. Which antidepressant can be useful in a patient with severe depression, characterized by extreme fatigue, lethargy, and psychomotor retardation?
    a. Mirtazapine
    b. Bupropion
    c. Imipramine
    d. Trazodone

33. Which vital sign should be monitored continuously when administering midazolam to a patient?
    a. Blood pressure
    b. Pulse
    c. Temperature
    d. Respiratory rate

34. What is first-line therapy for children with ADHD?
    a. Stimulants such as Adderall or Ritalin
    b. Anti-depressants such as Celexa or Zoloft
    c. Nonpharmacological therapy
    d. All of the above

35. The use of skeletal muscle relaxants is of greatest concern, and should be avoided, in which population?
    a. Young children
    b. Older adults
    c. Pregnant or breast-feeding women
    d. Individuals with bone cancer

36. Individuals with a sulfonamide hypersensitivity should follow which guideline when taking celecoxib (Celebrex)?
    a. Take only three doses
    b. Take for one month
    c. Avoid taking the drug
    d. Wait 2h after aspirin ingestion

37. What is the IV drug of choice to treat status epilepticus?
    a. Diazepam
    b. Lorazepam
    c. Valproate
    d. Fosphenytoin

38. A patient taking entacapone (Comtan) may need assistance with getting out of bed due to which possible side effect?
    a. Muscular stiffness
    b. Peripheral neuropathy
    c. Orthostatic hypotension
    d. Tachycardia

39. Which anticonvulsant is considered "broad-spectrum" and is useful for the management of many seizure types?
    a. Phenytoin
    b. Oxcarbamazepine
    c. Valproic acid
    d. Clonazepam

40. Corticosteroids can be used to treat all of the following except for?
    a. Allergic reactions
    b. Respiratory disorders
    c. Malignancies
    d. Headaches

41. A patient taking thyroid replacement medication should be instructed to take it:
    a. Anytime during the day
    b. Only when they are having symptoms
    c. On an empty stomach in the morning
    d. Before bed with a snack

42. An overdosage of thyroid is manifested in which of the following ophthalmic conditions?
    a. Drooping eyelids
    b. Bulging eyeballs
    c. Dilated pupils
    d. Reddened conjunctive

43. Which oral medication for diabetes is considered first-line therapy?
    a. Metformin
    b. Januvia
    c. Lantus
    d. Victoza

44. Which of the following is a long-acting insulin?
    a. Novolog
    b. Novolin N
    c. Levemir
    d. Apidra

45. Insulin should be injected:
    a. In the largest muscle every time
    b. In various muscles with the patient rotating sites
    c. Subcutaneously with the patient rotating sites
    d. Subcutaneously in the back of the arm only

46. If a diabetic patient is hypoglycemic, what is a reasonable choice for acute treatment?
    a. 4 oz of orange juice
    b. Sugar-free candy
    c. A small portion of red meat
    d. 8 oz of diet soda

47. What hormone is responsible for the changes in the uterine endometrium during the second half of the menstrual cycle in preparation of implantation of the fertilized ovum?
    a. Estrogen
    b. Progesterone
    c. Gonadotropin-releasing hormone
    d. Testosterone

48. What is one side effect of continuous progestin?

   a. Breast size reduction
   b. Weight loss

   c. Constipation
   d. Amenorrhea

49. Postcoital contraception should be taken within how many hours of unprotected sex?

   a. 48h
   b. 24h

   c. 96h
   d. 72h

50. Which of the following is critical to monitor prior to administering digoxin?

   a. Blood pressure
   b. Radial pulse rate

   c. Apical heart rate
   d. Respiratory rate

51. Digoxin taken in conjunction with what type of medications can increase the chance of arrhythmias?

   a. Antacids
   b. Macrolides

   c. Benzodiazepines
   d. Diuretics

52. Which antiarrhythmic may cause tachycardia?

   a. Procainamide
   b. Adenosine

   c. Verapamil
   d. Metoprolol

53. Which medication could be used in replacement of an ACE inhibitor when a patient has problems with a dry cough as a side effect?

   a. Losartan
   b. Metoprolol

   c. Digoxin
   d. Atorvastatin

54. The most effective and most commonly used antilipemic medications are called:

   a. Bile acid sequestrates
   b. Statins

   c. Nicotinic acids
   d. Fibrates

55. Warfarin is monitored with what laboratory method?

   a. Complete blood work with differential
   b. LH levels

   c. TSH levels
   d. INR

56. Clopidogrel should not be taken with the following medication:

   a. OTC Zantac
   b. OTC Aspirin

   c. OTC Prilosec
   d. OTC Pepcid

57. In patients with COPD, what precaution should be taken when administering oxygen?

   a. Avoid smoking when in use
   b. Always use the highest concentration tolerable

   c. Only use a nasal cannula to delivery it
   d. Use for no more than 1 h continuously

58. What is the preferred route of administration of bronchodilators to minimize systemic adverse effects?

   a. Oral
   b. Injection

   c. Sublingual
   d. Inhalation

59. Which antitussive has the greatest effectiveness?

   a. Codeine
   b. Hydrocodone

   c. Benzonatate
   d. Dextromethorphan

60. What is one side effect of nicotine replacement products?

   a. Diarrhea
   b. Thickened secretions

   c. Hyperglycemia
   d. Nausea and vomiting

61. Why should older adults avoid taking over-the-counter (OTC) antacids for longer than two weeks without medical supervision?

    a. OTC antacids may mask GI bleed.

    b. OTC antacids may cause *C. difficile* infection.

    c. OTC antacids may cause excessive flatulence.

    d. OTC antacids may cause urinary incontinence.

62. Constipation is a concern for older adults. Which is a suggested first-line laxative for this population?

    a. Calcium carbonate

    b. Bismuth sulfate

    c. Magnesium citrate

    d. Sennosides

63. What is the key strategy to avoiding problems when taking NSAIDs?

    a. Take on an empty stomach.

    b. Take in conjunction with Tylenol.

    c. Take the lowest effective dose for the shortest time period with food or milk.

    d. Take for no more than 28 days continuously.

64. What is one potential side effect of a calcium carbonate antacid?

    a. Mild diuresis

    b. Constipation

    c. Diarrhea

    d. Nausea

65. Due to various reasons, older adult patients tend to:

    a. Take medications exactly as prescribed

    b. Be nonadherent to one or more medications

    c. Go to one pharmacy and one doctor for all their health care needs

    d. Be on few medications

Glossary

A

Absence seizure. Absence of convulsions characterized by a sudden 10–30 sec loss of consciousness with no falling; formerly called petit mal.

Absorption. Passage of a substance through a body surface into body fluids or tissues.

Acetylcholine. Chemical mediator of nerve impulses in the nervous system.

Achlorhydria. Lack of stomach acid.

Actions. A description of the cellular changes that occur as a result of a drug.

Addiction. Physical and/or psychological dependence on a substance, especially alcohol or drugs, with the use of increasing amounts (tolerance) and withdrawal reactions.

Adjunct. Addition to the course of treatment to increase the efficacy.

Adjuvant. A drug added to a prescription to hasten or enhance the action of a principal ingredient.

Adrenal glands. Glands located adjacent to the kidneys that secrete hormones called corticosteroids.

Adrenergic. Sympathomimetic drug that mimics the action of the sympathetic nervous system.

Adsorbent. Substance that leads readily to absorption.

Adverse drug reactions (ADRs). Unintended side effects from medications such as cough, headache, nausea, and so on.

Adverse effects. Harmful unintended reactions to a drug.

Adverse reactions. A list of possible unpleasant or dangerous secondary effects other than the desired effect.

Albuminuria. Albumin (proteins) in urine.

Allergic reaction. Response of the body resulting from hypersensitivity to a substance (e.g., rash, hives, and anaphylaxis).

Alopecia. Loss or absence of hair.

Alpha-blockers. Drugs that block the alpha-1 receptors found in the smooth muscle in the bladder neck and prostate, causing them to relax.

Alzheimer's disease. Dementia characterized by a devastating, progressive decline in cognitive function, followed by increasingly severe impairment in social and occupational functioning.

Aminoglycosides. Drugs used in combination with other antibiotics that treat many infections caused by gram-negative and gram-positive bacteria.

Amnesia. Loss of memory.

Ampule. Glass container with drug for injection; must be broken at the neck to withdraw (via a filter needle if necessary) the drug in solution.

Analeptic. A drug used to stimulate the central nervous system, especially with poisoning by CNS depressants.

Analgesics. Medications that alleviate pain.

Anaphylactic reaction. A life-threatening reaction to a drug, insect/jellyfish sting, snake bite, or foreign substance requiring immediate medical attention.

Anaphylaxis. Allergic hypersensitivity reaction of the body to a foreign substance or drug. Mild symptoms include rash, itching, and hives. Severe symptoms include dyspnea, chest constriction, cardiopulmonary collapse, and death.

Androgens. Male hormones that stimulate the development of male characteristics.

Angina pectoris. Severe chest pain resulting from decreased blood supply to the heart muscle.

Angiogenesis. Development of new blood vessels.

Anorexia. Loss of appetite.

Antacids. Agents that neutralize gastric hydrochloric acid.

Antagonism. Opposing action of two drugs in which one decreases or cancels out the effect of the other.

Antiandrogens. Gonadotropin-releasing hormone analogs that are used to treat prostate cancer.

Antiarrhythmic agents. Drugs that control or prevent cardiac irregularities.

Anticholinergics. Drugs that block the action of the parasympathetic nervous system.

Anticoagulants. Medications used to prevent the formation of clots or decrease the extension of existing clots in such conditions as venous thrombosis, pulmonary embolism, and coronary occlusion.

Anticonvulsants. Medications used to reduce the number or severity of seizures in patients with epilepsy.

Antidepressant. Medications used to treat patients with various types of depression; sometimes called mood elevators.

Antidiabetic. Medications used to lower blood glucose levels in those with impaired metabolism of carbohydrates, fats, and proteins.

Antidiarrhea. Medications that reduce the number of loose stools.

Antidote. Substance that neutralizes poisons or toxic substances.

Antiemetics. Drugs that prevent or treat nausea, vomiting, or motion sickness.

Antiepileptic drug (AED) therapy. Medical therapy aimed at treating and/or reducing seizure activity.

Antiflatulents. Medications used in the symptomatic treatment of gastric bloating or GI gas pain.

Antifungals. Medications used in the treatment of candidal and other specific susceptible fungi.

Antiglaucoma agents. Medications used to lower intraocular pressure.

Antihistamines. Medications that provide symptomatic relief of allergic symptoms caused by histamine release.

Antihypertensives. Medications used in the treatment and management of all degrees of hypertension.

Anti-infective. Medication used in the treatment of infections; includes antibiotics, antifungals, and antivirals.

Anti-inflammatory. Medication used to relieve inflammation.

Antilipemic agents. Drugs that lower the serum cholesterol and low-density lipoproteins (LDLs) and increase the high-density lipoproteins (HDLs).

Antimuscarinics. Drugs that block cholinergic stimuli at muscarinic receptors. A type of anticholinergic; also called parasympatholytics.

Antineoplastic. An agent that prevents the development, growth, or spreading of malignant cells.

Antioxidants. Agents that prevent or inhibit oxidation or cell destruction in damaged or aging tissues. Compounds that fight against the destructive effects of free radical formation.

Antiparkinsonian drugs. Medications used in the treatment of Parkinson's disease to relieve symptoms and maintain mobility but that do not cure the disease.

Antipruritics. Products applied topically to alleviate itching.

Antipsychotic. Major tranquilizers used to relieve the symptoms of psychoses or severe neuroses; sometimes called neuroleptics.

Antipyretic. Medication to reduce fever.

Antiretroviral (ARV) agents. Agents that act against retroviruses such as HIV.

Antiseptics. Substances that inhibit the growth of bacteria.

Antispasmodics. Medications used to reduce the strength and frequency of contractions of the urinary bladder and to decrease gastrointestinal motility.

Antithrombotic agents. Agents that interfere with or prevent thrombosis (clot formation).

Antithyroid. Medication used to relieve the symptoms of hyperthyroidism in preparation for surgical or radioactive iodine therapy.

Antituberculosis agents. Medications used to treat asymptomatic infection and to treat active clinical tuberculosis and prevent relapse.

Antitussives. Medications that suppress coughing.

Antiulcer. Drug that reduces gastric acid secretion or that acts to prevent or treat gastric or duodenal ulcers.

Antivenom injections. A serum that contains antitoxin specific for an animal or insect venom.

Antiviral agent. Medications used to treat viruses, for example HIV and herpes.

Anxiolytics. Antianxiety medications (tranquilizers) used for the short-term treatment of anxiety disorders, neurosis, some psychosomatic disorders, and insomnia.

Apnea. Cessation of breathing.

Appropriate. Reasonable under the circumstances for a specific patient.

Arteriosclerosis. A common arterial disorder characterized by the thickening and loss of elasticity of the arterial walls, resulting in a decreased blood supply, especially to the cerebrum and lower extremities.

Ascites. The abnormal accumulation of fluid in the pleura or peritoneal cavity.

Aspiration. The inhalation of a foreign substance or regurgitated gastric contents into the lungs.

Asthma prophylaxis. Medications used for prophylaxis and the treatment of chronic asthma. Bronchodilators are used for acute asthmatic attacks.

Asymptomatic. Showing no evidence of clinical disease.

Ataxia. Defective muscular coordination, especially with voluntary muscular movements (e.g., walking).

Atherosclerosis. A type of arteriosclerosis characterized by yellowish plaques of cholesterol, lipids, and cellular debris in the walls of large- and medium-sized arteries, resulting in reduced circulation, the major cause of coronary heart disease such as angina pectoris or myocardial infarction.

Atypical antipsychotics. A newer class of antipsychotics with less potential for adverse effects, such as extrapyramidal symptoms and tardive dyskinesia.

Autonomic. Automatic, self-governing, or involuntary nervous system.

B

Bactericidal. Destroying bacteria.

Bacteriostatic. Inhibiting or retarding bacterial growth.

Beers list drugs. The most inappropriate drugs for ambulatory nursing home residents and adults 65 years or older.

Benign. Not recurrent or progressive; nonmalignant.

Benign Prostatic Hyperplasia (BPH). Benign irregular growth of the prostatic glandular tissue that can cause issues with male urination.

Beta-adrenergic blocker. Agent that blocks the beta receptors such as those found in the heart, causing a decrease in the rate and force of cardiac contraction.

Beta-blockers. Drugs that block the action of the sympathetic nervous system.

Biotransformation. Chemical changes that a substance undergoes in the body.

Bipolar disorders. Manic-depressive mental disorders in which the mood fluctuates from mania to depression.

Bladder antispasmodics. Agents that treat urinary incontinence by relaxing the bladder and reducing frequent and uncontrolled urination.

Blood dyscrasia. A condition in which any of the blood constituents are abnormal or are present in abnormal quantity.

BPH. Benign prostatic hyperplasia.

BPH therapy. Drugs used to reduce prostate size and associated urinary obstruction and manifestations in patients with BPH.

Bradycardia. Abnormally slow heartbeat.

Bradykinesia. Abnormally slow movement.

Broad spectrum. Antibiotic effective against a large variety of organisms.

Bronchodilators. Medications that relax the smooth muscles of the bronchial tree, thereby relieving bronchospasm and increasing the vital capacity of the lungs.

Buccal. In the cheek pouch.

C

C & S. Culture and sensitivity test to identify a causative infectious organism and the specific medicine to which it is sensitive.

Cachexia. Condition of malnutrition and wasting in chronic conditions such as some malignancies or AIDS.

Calculating dosage. Using mathematical computation to determine the correct dosage to administer when a dosage ordered differs from the dose on hand.

Calculus. Stone.

Capsule. A special container made of gelatin sized for a single dose of drug.

Carbapenems. A class of broad-spectrum antibiotic drugs, derived from cephalosporins, that resist degradation by bacterial beta-lactamases.

Carbonic anhydrase inhibitors. Drugs that reduce the hydrogen and bicarbonate ions and have a diuretic effect (increasing the excretion of fluids from the body through the urine).

Cardiac glycosides. Medications used primarily in the treatment of heart failure.

Cardiotonic. Increasing the force and efficiency of contractions of the heart muscle.

Cardioversion. Correcting an irregular heartbeat (arrhythmia). Usually accomplished by electrical shock (e.g., defibrillation).

Catecholamines. Mediators released at the sympathetic nerve endings (e.g., epinephrine and norepinephrine).

Cautions. Precautions; steps to take to prevent errors.

Cephalosporins. Semisynthetic antibiotic derivatives produced by a fungus.

Cheilosis. Reddened lips with cracked corners.

Chemical dependency. Condition in which alcohol or drugs have taken control of an individual's life and affect normal functioning.

Chemoinformatics. Application of computer technology, statistics, and math to study information about the structure, properties, and activities of molecules.

Chemotherapy. Chemicals (drugs) with specific and toxic effects upon disease-producing organisms.

Chemotherapy-induced nausea and vomiting (CINV). Vomiting that occurs after the administration of drugs used to treat cancer.

Cholelithiasis. The presence of gallstones in the gallbladder.

Cholinergic drugs. Parasympathomimetic drugs that mimic the action of the parasympathetic nervous system.

Classifications. Broad subcategory for drugs that affect the body in similar ways.

Clone. A copy.

Clonic. Spasm marked by alternate contraction (rigidity) and relaxation of muscles.

Clostridium difficile (*C. difficile*). Species of bacteria that cause pseudomembranous colitis.

Coanalgesic. Nonopioid analgesic drugs that are combined with opioids for more effective analgesic action in relief of acute or chronic pain (e.g., NSAID or acetaminophen).

Coenzyme. Enzyme activator.

Comorbidities. Other serious conditions existing concurrently with the one under discussion.

Comprehensive Medication Review (CMR). A document provided to a patient by a health care provider that provides an inclusive list of their medications, indications, and directions for use.

Computerized physician order entry (CPOE). Prescriptions are typed into the computer by the prescriber, printed and signed or sent directly to the pharmacy.

Concomitant. Taking place at the same time.

Concurrent. Existing at the same time.

Continuous IV infusion. An IV solution that may or may not contain medication that is administered over long periods.

Contraceptives. Medications used for birth control.

Contraindications. Conditions or circumstances that indicate that a drug should not be given.

Controlled substances. Drugs controlled by additional prescription requirement because of the danger of addiction or abuse.

Conversion of units. Changing from one system of measurement to another.

COPD. Chronic obstructive pulmonary disease.

Coronary heart disease (CHD). Narrowing of the coronary arteries usually as a result of atherosclerosis.

Coronary vasodilators. Medications used in the treatment of angina. See Vasodilator.

Corticosteroids. Hormones secreted by the adrenal glands that act on the immune system to suppress the body's response to infection or trauma; medications given for their anti-inflammatory and immunosuppressant properties.

COX-2 inhibitor. Anti-inflammatory drug that does not inhibit clotting and causes fewer gastric problems and less GI bleeding than other NSAIDs.

Cryptorchidism. Undescended testicles.

Crystalluria. Crystals in the urine.

Culture and Sensitivity (C&S) tests. Performed by medical institutions to reveal what antibiotic class or specific antibiotic will be effective in treating a certain infective organism.

Cumulative effect. Increased effect of a drug that accumulates in the body.

Cushing's syndrome. Excessive production or administration of adrenal cortical hormones, resulting in edema, puffy face, fatigue, weakness, and osteoporosis.

Cutaneous. Pertaining to skin.

Cycloplegic. Drug that paralyzes the muscles of accommodation for eye examinations.

Cytotoxic. Substance that destroys cells.

D

Decongestants. Drugs that constrict blood vessels in the respiratory tract, resulting in the shrinkage of swollen mucous membranes and opened nasal airway passages.

Deficiency. Lacking adequate amount.

Demulcent. Medication used topically to protect or soothe minor dermatological conditions such as diaper rash, abrasions, and minor burns.

Dependence. Acquired need for a drug after repeated use; may be psychological with craving and emotional changes or physical with body changes and withdrawal symptoms.

Dietary Reference Intakes (DRIs). A system of nutrition recommendations from the Institutes of Medicine of the U.S. National Academy of Sciences.

Digitalization. The process of establishing a loading dose of digitalis for maintaining optimal functioning of the heart without toxic effects.

Diplopia. Double vision.

Direct toxicity. Drug that results in tissue damage; may or may not be permanent.

Distribution. Circulation of drugs, after absorption, to the organs of the body.

Diuresis. The secretion and passage of large amounts of urine.

Diuretics. Medications that increase urine excretion.

Documentation of drug administration. Recording the medication given to a patient on the patient's medical record, including the dose, time, route, and location of injections.

Dosage. Amount of a drug given for a particular therapeutic or desired effect.

Drug. Chemical substance taken into the body that affects body function.

Drug abuse. The use of a drug for other than therapeutic purposes.

Drug Enforcement Administration (DEA). A bureau of the Department of Justice that enforces the Controlled Substances Act.

Drug form. The type of preparation in which a drug is supplied.

Drug-induced parkinsonism (DIP). The inducement of Parkinson-like symptoms because of drug administration.

Drug interactions. Response that may occur when more than one drug is taken. The combination may alter the expected response of each individual drug.

Drug processes. Four biological changes that drugs undergo within the body.

Drug standards. Federally approved requirements for the specified strength, quality, and purity of drugs.

Dry-powder inhalers (DPIs). Self-generating devices that form a fine aerosol from a powdered drug solution that can then be inhaled using a fast, deep breath into the respiratory system.

Dyskinesia. An impairment of the ability to execute voluntary movements, frequently an adverse effect of prolonged use of some medications, for example phenothiazines.

Dyslipidemia. Abnormal levels of various blood lipid fractions.

Dysmenorrhea. Painful menstruation.

Dyspepsia. Indigestion.

Dysphagia. Difficulty in swallowing.

Dysphonia. Difficulty speaking or hoarseness

Dystonic reaction. Spasm and contortion, especially of the head, neck, and tongue, as an adverse effect of antipsychotic medication.

E

e-prescribing (eRX). The manner in which medications are ordered through the electronic medical record.

Effects of drugs. Physiological changes that occur in response to drugs.

Electrolytes. Minerals dissolved in the body fluids.

electronic medication administration record (eMAR). Medication administration record in the electronic medical record.

Elixir. A usually sweetened, aromatic liquid used in the compounding of oral medicines.

Emetic. Agent that induces vomiting.

Emollient. Medication used topically to protect or soothe minor dermatological conditions, such as diaper rash, abrasions, and minor burns.

Empiric. Best guess therapy based on history and available clinical information.

Emulsion. A mixture of two liquids not mutually soluble.

Endocrine. Internal secretion (hormone) produced by a ductless gland that secretes directly into the bloodstream.

Endogenous. Produced or originating within a cell or organism.

Endorphins. Endogenous analgesics produced within the body.

Enema. The introduction of a solution into the rectum and colon to stimulate bowel activity and cause emptying of the lower intestine.

Enteric-coated tablet. Tablet with a special coating that resists disintegration by the gastric juices and dissolves in the intestines.

Enuresis. Urinary incontinence; bed-wetting.

Enzymatics. Agents that promote the removal of necrotic or fibrous tissue.

Epidural anesthesia. Local anesthetic solution injected into the epidural space just outside the spinal cord.

Epilepsy. A recurrent paroxysmal disorder of brain function characterized by sudden attacks of altered consciousness, motor activity, or sensory impairment.

Epistaxis. Nosebleed.

Erectile dysfunction (ED). The inability to achieve or sustain a penile erection for sexual intercourse.

Estrogen/progestin therapy (EPT). The use of combined hormones for birth control and menopausal symptoms.

Estrogens. Female sex hormones responsible for the development of female secondary sexual characteristics; medications used for many conditions.

Estrogen therapy (ET). The use of the hormone estrogen for the prevention of diseases in woman and relief of menopausal symptoms.

Eunuchism. Lack of male hormone, resulting in high-pitched voice and absence of beard and body hair.

Euphoria. Exaggerated feeling of well-being and elation.

Euthyroid. Normal thyroid function.

Excretion. Elimination of by-products of drug metabolism from the body, essentially through the kidneys, some from the intestines and lungs.

Exogenous. Originating outside the body or an organ or produced from external causes.

Expectorants. Drugs that increase secretions, reduce viscosity, and help to expel sputum.

Extrapyramidal. Disorder of the brain characterized by tremors, Parkinson-like symptoms, dystonic twisting of body parts, or tardive dyskinesia, sometimes associated with prolonged use of antipsychotic drugs and some other CNS drugs.

F

Fat-soluble vitamins. Vitamins A, D, E, and K.

Febrile seizures. Seizures associated with high temperatures.

Flatulence. Excessive gas in the digestive tract.

Follicle-stimulating hormone (FSH). Hormone that stimulates development of ovarian follicles in the female and sperm production in the testes of the male.

Food and Drug Administration (FDA). An agency within the Department of Health and Human Services that enforces the provisions of the Federal Food, Drug, and Cosmetic Act and amendments of 1951 and 1962.

Free radicals. Unbound compounds that attack and damage the cells or initiate the growth of abnormal cells, resulting in conditions such as cancer or atherosclerosis.

G

Gastric tube administration. Medication administered through a tube in the abdomen to the stomach.

Gastroesophageal reflux disease (GERD). A backward flow of gastric secretions into the esophagus causing inflammation and discomfort. GERD is treated with drugs to accelerate gastric emptying.

Gastroparesis. Partial paralysis of the stomach.

Generic names. General, common, or nonproprietary names of drugs.

GERD. Gastroesophageal reflux disease.

GI antispasmodics. Medications used to help calm the bowel.

Gingivitis. Inflammation of the gums characterized by redness, swelling, and tendency to bleed.

Glaucoma. Abnormal condition of the eye with increased intraocular pressure (IOP) because of obstruction of the outflow of aqueous humor.

Glossitis. Inflammation of the tongue.

Glycosuria. Sugar in the urine.

Goiter. Enlargement of the thyroid gland.

Gout. A form of arthritis in which uric acid crystals are deposited in and around joints.

Grand mal seizures. A form of epilepsy characterized by loss of consciousness, falling, and generalized tonic, followed by clonic contractions of the muscles. Current term is tonic-clonic seizure.

Gray List. List of inappropriate drugs for nursing home residents based on a national survey of geriatric experts.

G-tube or peg tube. Gastric tube also known as a percutaneous endoscopic gastrostomy (PEG) tube inserted into the abdomen to administer medications.

Gynecomastia. Enlargement of breast tissue in males.

H

HAART. Highly active antiretroviral therapy for HIV infections.

HAIs. Hospital-acquired infections.

Heart failure. The inability of the heart to circulate blood effectively enough to meet the body's metabolic needs.

Hematological. Concerned with the blood and its components.

Hematopoiesis. Production of blood cells, normally in the bone marrow.

Hematuria. Blood in the urine.

Hepatotoxicity. Damage to the liver as an adverse reaction to certain drugs.

Herbal. Plants or other substances occurring naturally that are available over the counter and are non-FDA regulated.

Herbs. Any product intended for ingestion as a supplement to the diet.

Heterocyclic. Second-generation cyclic antidepressants with very different adverse effect profiles.

Hirsutism. Excessive growth of hair in unusual places, especially in women.

Histamine₂ blockers. Agents that block the histamine receptors found in the stomach to reduce gastric acid secretions.

Holter monitoring. Patient wears monitor, which records cardiac rhythms for 24h.

Homeostasis. Body balance; state of internal equilibrium.

Hormones. Substances originating from an organ, gland, or body part, conveyed through the blood to another body part, and chemically stimulating that part to increase or decrease its functional activity or to increase or decrease the secretion of another hormone.

Hormone replacement therapy (HRT). Estrogen with or without progestin used for osteoporosis prevention and treatment.

Hormone therapy (HT). The therapeutic use of hormones.

household system. The least accurate way of measuring medications, examples include teaspoons, ounces and pints.

Household system of measures. Any of the volumes represented by commonly used items as they are applied to administering medicines.

Hyperalimentation. The intravenous infusion of a hypertonic solution containing all of the necessary elements to sustain life. Usually infused through a subclavian catheter into the superior vena cava.

Hypercalcemia. Abnormally high blood calcium.

Hyperglycemia. Abnormally high blood glucose.

Hyperkalemia. Abnormally high potassium in the blood; can lead to cardiac arrhythmias.

Hyperlipidemia. High lipid levels in the blood.

Hyperosmotic. Laxative to draw water from the tissues and stimulate evacuation.

Hyperplasia. An increase in the number of normal cells.

Hyperpyrexia. Extreme elevation of body temperature.

Hypersensitivity. Allergic or excessive response of the immune system to a drug or chemical.

Hypertension. High blood pressure. One of the major risk factors for coronary artery disease, heart failure, stroke, peripheral vascular disease, kidney failure, and retinopathy.

Hypertriglyceridemia. High triglyceride level in the blood.

Hyperuricemia. Abnormal amount of uric acid in the blood.

Hypnotics. Drugs that promote sleep.

Hypocalcemia. Abnormally low blood calcium.

Hypoglycemia. Abnormally low blood glucose.

Hypokalemia. Abnormally low blood potassium; can lead to cardiac arrhythmias.

Hyponatremia. Decreased sodium in the blood.

Hypotension. Low blood pressure.

Hypotensive. Antihypertensive; medication used in the treatment of hypertension.

Hypothyroidism. Diminished or absent thyroid function.

Hypoxia. Deficiency of oxygen.

Idiopathic. Condition without a known cause.

Idiosyncratic reaction. Unusual reaction to a drug, other than that expected.

Immunosuppressant. An agent that decreases or inactivates the immune response to antigens.

Immunosuppressive. Decreasing the production of antibodies and phagocytes and depressing the inflammatory reaction.

Indications. List of conditions for which a drug is meant to be used.

Infiltration anesthesia. Local anesthetic solution injected into the skin, subcutaneous tissue, or mucous membranes of the area to be anesthetized.

Inflammatory bowel disease (IBD). The term for a number of chronic, relapsing inflammatory diseases of the gastrointestinal tract of unknown etiology.

Ingestion. To take into the body by mouth through swallowing.

Inhalation drug forms. Forms of a drug to be inhaled by the respiratory system usually through a specialized device such as a metered-dose inhaler (MDI).

Inhalation route. A route of drug administration through the respiratory system where the large surface area and high vascularity cause a rapid response.

Inhalation therapy. Medications administered through a metered-dose inhaler, small-volume nebulizer, dry-powder inhaler, or intermittent positive pressure breathing apparatus.

Injectable drug forms. Forms of drugs manufactured to be given via injections such as intravenous (IV) or intramuscular (IM).

Injections. The most common form of parenteral administration.

Interactions. Actions that occur when two or more drugs are combined or when drugs are combined with certain foods. See Drug interactions.

Intermittent IV infusion. A small amount (50-100ml) of IV fluid or medication administered over a short period in prescribed intervals. Sometimes referred to as IV piggyback.

Intra-articular (intracapsular). Injected into the joint.

Intradermal (ID). Injected into the layers of the skin.

Intramuscular (IM). Injected into the muscle.

Intraocular pressure. Pressure within the eyeball.

Intrathecal. Injection into the spinal canal.

Intravenous (IV). Injected into the vein.

Ischemia. Holding back of the blood; local deficiency of blood supply because of the obstruction of circulation to a part (e.g., the heart or extremities).

K

Keratolytics. Agents that promote loosening or scaling of the outer layer of the skin.

Keep Vein Open (KVO). A slow rate of IV fluid administration to maintain patency of the IV.

Korsakoff's psychosis. Disorder characterized by polyneuritis, disorientation, mental deterioration, and ataxia with painful foot drop, usually associated with chronic alcoholism.

L

Lability. State of being unstable or changeable.

Lacrimation. Discharge of tears.

Laxatives. Drugs that promote evacuation of the intestine.

Legend drug. Available only by prescription.

Leukopenia. Abnormal decrease in white blood cells, usually below 5,000.

Local anesthetic. Medications administered to produce temporary loss of sensation or feeling in a specific area.

Local effect. Affecting one specific area or part.

Lozenge (troche). Tablet that dissolves slowly in the mouth for local effect.

Luteinizing hormone (LH). Hormone that works in conjunction with FSH to induce the secretion of estrogen, ovulation, and development of corpus luteum.

Luteotropic hormone (LTH). Hormone that stimulates the secretion of progesterone by the corpus luteum and secretion of milk by the mammary gland.

M

Macrolides. A class of drugs used in many infections of the respiratory tract, for skin conditions such as acne, or for some sexually transmitted infections when the patient is allergic to penicillin.

Maintenance medications. Medications meant to preserve a desired condition. Drugs used to prevent recurrence or progression of an illness.

Major depressive disorder (MDD). Clinical depression characterized by episodes of all-encompassing low moods, low self-esteem, and loss of interest or pleasure in normally enjoyable activities.

Malignant. Growing worse, resisting treatment; said of cancerous growths.

Medical abbreviations. Symbols used for medication orders.

Medication Errors Reporting (MER) program. The United States Pharmacopeia established Medication Errors Reporting (MER) program.

Medication reconciliation. A method used to compare the medication the patient is taking at home to that ordered by the physician when there is a change in care.

Medication-related problems (MRPs). Serious complications resulting from adverse drug reactions.

Medication orders. The physician's prescription for the administration of a drug.

Medication therapy management (MTM). The process of a pharmacist or other health care provider reviewing a patient's medications, identifying potential or actual adverse effects or other medication-related problems, and developing a plan to optimize therapy.

MedWatch. A voluntary and confidential program of the Food and Drug Administration for monitoring the safety of drugs, biochemical and medical devices, and nutritional products.

Megadose. Abnormally large dose.

Melena. Blood in the stool.

Mental impairment. Decreased mental function in older adults frequently caused or worsened by drugs.

Metabolism. Physical and chemical alterations that a substance undergoes in the body.

Metered-dose inhalers (MDIs). Canisters containing a propellant used to deliver a fine mist (aerosol) of a drug into the respiratory system. Often used with a spacer device or reservoir to increase the effectiveness of drug delivery.

Metric system. International standard for weights and measures.

Minerals. Chemical elements occurring in nature and in body fluids.

Miotics. Drugs that cause the pupil to contract.

Mixed seizure. Having more than one type of seizure.

Monamine oxidase inhibitors (MAOIs). Antidepressant agents used to increase serotonin, norepinephrine, and dopamine levels.

Monoclonal antibodies. Chemotherapy designed to target only cancer cells, thereby sparing normal tissues.

Mortar and pestle. Glass cup with glass rod used to crush tablets.

Motor impairment. A loss or limitation of function in muscle control or movement.

Mucolytics. Medications that liquefy pulmonary secretions.

Myalgia. Tenderness or pain in the muscles.

Mydriatics. Drugs that dilate the pupil.

Myelosuppression. Inhibiting bone marrow function.

Myopathy. Abnormal condition of skeletal muscle.

N

Nasogastric tube administration. Medication administered through a tube inserted through the nose and extending into the stomach.

National Drug Code (NDC) Directory. Provides the FDA with a list of all drugs manufactured for commercial distribution.

Nebulizer (vaporizer). Apparatus for producing a fine spray or mist for inhalation.

Neoplasms. New growth or tumors.

Nephropathy. Disease of the kidneys.

Nephrotoxicity. Damage to the kidneys as an adverse reaction to certain drugs.

Neuroleptic malignant syndrome. Characterized by delirium, rigid muscles, fever, and autonomic nervous system instability.

Neuromuscular blocking agents (NMBAs). Muscle relaxants that cause a direct effect on the muscles including the diaphragm.

Neuropathy. Any disease of the nerves.

Neurotoxicity. Having the capability of harming nerve tissue.

Neurotransmitters. Substances that travel across the synapse to transmit messages between nerve cells.

Neutropenia. Abnormally small number of neutrophil leukocytes in the blood.

Nonadherence. When a patient does not take one or more medications as prescribed on a regular basis.

Nosocomial. Hospital-acquired infection.

NSAID. Nonsteroidal anti-inflammatory drug.

Nystagmus. Involuntary rhythmic movements of the eyeball.

O

Objective. Referring to symptoms observed or perceived by others.

Official name. Name of the drug as it appears in the official reference, the *USP/NF*; generally the same as the generic drug.

Oligospermia. Deficient sperm production.

Onychomycosis. Toenail fungus.

Oophorectomy. Excision of an ovary.

Opioid agonists. Analgesics; controlled substances whose action is similar to opium in altering the perception of pain; can be natural or synthetic.

Opioid antagonists. Drugs used in the treatment of opioid overdoses and in the operating room, delivery room, and newborn nursery for opiate-induced respiratory depression.

Opportunistic infections. Infections that occur because the immune system is compromised.

Oral drug forms. Drugs manufactured to be given via the oral route such as pills, solutions, and capsules.

Oral medications. Medication administered by mouth.

Oral medication administration. Administering medications by mouth.

Orphan drugs. Drugs or biological products used for the diagnosis, treatment, or prevention of a rare disease or condition, that is, one affecting less than 200,000 persons in the United States, or greater than 200,000 persons where the cost of developing the drug is probably not recoverable in the United States.

Osmotic agents. Medications used to reduce intracranial or intraocular pressure.

Osteomalacia. Softening of the bones because of inadequate calcium and/or vitamin D.

Osteoporosis. Softening of the bone seen most often in older adults, especially postmenopausal women.

Osteoporosis therapy. Medications used to prevent or treat osteoporosis by increasing bone mineral density.

Otitis Media. The most common type of otic infection, located in the middle region of the ear.

Ototoxicity. Damage to the eighth cranial nerve, resulting in impaired hearing or ringing in the ears (tinnitus); adverse reaction to certain drugs.

Overactive bladder (OAB). A sudden intense urge to urinate that may or may not lead to loss of the urine.

Overdose. A higher than normal amount sufficient to cause toxicity.

Over-the-counter (OTC) medication. Medication available without a prescription.

Oxytocin. Hormone that stimulates the uterus to contract, thus inducing childbirth.

P

Palliative. Referring to the alleviation of symptoms, but not producing a cure.

Paradoxical reaction. Opposite effect from that expected.

Paraphilia. A psychosexual disorder in which unusual or bizarre imagery or acts are necessary for the realization of sexual excitement.

Parasympatholytics. Anticholinergics; medications that decrease the chemical that promotes bronchospasm.

Parenteral. Any route of administration not involving the gastrointestinal tract (e.g., injection, topical, and inhalation).

Paresthesia. Numbness, tingling, or a "pins and needles" feeling, especially in the extremities.

Parkinsonism. A neurological disorder with symptoms resembling Parkinson's disease (e.g., muscle rigidity, tremor).

Parkinson's disease. A chronic neurological disorder characterized by fine, slowly spreading muscle tremors, rigidity and weakness of muscles, and shuffling gait.

Partial seizures. Also known as focal seizures. The onset is limited to one area of the brain.

Pedophilia. Sexual attraction to children.

Pellagra. A disease caused by the deficiency of niacin (nicotinic acid), characterized by skin, gastrointestinal, mucosal, neurological, and mental symptoms.

Penicillins. A class of antibiotics produced from certain species of a fungus.

Perioral. Around the mouth.

Peripheral. Away from the center. Usually refers to the extremities.

Peripheral nerve block. Local anesthetic solution injected into or around nerves or ganglia supplying the area to be anesthetized.

Pharmacogenomics. The study of the effects of genetic differences among people and the impact that these differences have on the uptake, effectiveness, toxicity, and metabolism of drugs.

Pharmacology. The study of drugs and their origin, nature, properties, and effects on living organisms.

Photosensitivity. Increased reaction, for example burn, from brief exposure to the sun or an ultraviolet lamp.

Physiological dependence. Physical adaptation of the body to a drug and withdrawal symptoms after abrupt drug discontinuation.

Phytoestrogen. A plant substance with estrogen-like properties.

Placebo. Inactive substance given to simulate the effect of another drug; physical or emotional changes that occur reflect the expectations of the patient.

Placebo effect. Relief from pain as the result of suggestion without active medication.

Platelet inhibitors. Class of drugs that inhibit platelet aggregation (clumping) to prevent clots.

Poison. A toxic substance that is taken into the body by ingestion, inhalation, injection, or absorption and that can cause illness, injury, or death.

Polypharmacy. Excessive use of drugs or prescription of many drugs given at one time.

Postherpetic neuralgia. Nerve pain following an episode of shingles.

Postoperative nausea and vomiting (PONV). One of the most commonly occurring post-operative complication. During the post-operative period, patients may experience considerable pain, difficulty moving, nausea, and vomiting.

Potentially inappropriate medications (PIMs). Medications listed under "Updated Beers Criteria for Potentially Inappropriate Medication Use in Older Adults."

Potentiation. Increased effect; action of two drugs given simultaneously is greater than the effect of the drugs given separately.

Precautions. List of conditions or types of patients that warrant closer observation for specific side effects when given a drug.

Prevention of medication errors. Rules to follow to avoid making mistakes.

Priapism. Prolonged penile erection.

Primary generalized seizure. A classification of seizures in which widespread electrical discharges occur in the brain, involving both sides of the brain.

Probiotics. Agents having favorable or health-promoting effect on living cells and tissues; for example, *Lactobacillus acidophilus*, present in the GI tract, is probiotic because its presence inhibits the growth of harmful bacteria.

Prodrugs. Inert drugs that exhibit their pharmacological activity only after biotransformation.

Progesterone. Hormone responsible for changes in uterine endometrium in the second half of the menstrual cycle in preparation for implantation of the fertilized ovum, development of maternal placenta after implantation, and development of mammary glands; medication with several uses.

Progestins. Synthetic drugs that exert progesterone-like activity.

Proliferation. Rapid reproduction.

Proportion. Two ratios that are equal.

Protectants. Medication used topically to protect or soothe minor dermatological conditions, such as diaper rash, abrasions, and minor burns.

Proton pump inhibitor (PPI). Gastric antisecretory agent unrelated to H_2 receptor antagonists used for short-term symptomatic relief of GERD, ulcers, heartburn, and erosive esophagitis.

Prototype. A model or type from which subsequent types arise (e.g., an example of a drug that typifies the characteristics of that classification).

Pruritis. Itching.

Psychomotor epilepsy. Also known as temporal lobe epilepsy or focal seizures because of the area in the brain that is involved; characterized by temporary impairment of consciousness, confusion, loss of judgment, and abnormal acts, even crimes and hallucinations, but no convulsions.

Psychotropic. Any substance that acts on the mind.

Pyrosis. Heartburn.

Q

Quinolones. A class of antibiotics used in adults for the treatment of some infections of the urinary tract, lower respiratory tract, gastrointestinal tract, skin, bones, and joints.

R

Ratio. A relationship between two numbers.

Reconstitution. The return of a substance previously altered for preservation and storage to its original state, as is done with dried blood plasma and powdered medications.

Rectal drug forms. Drugs manufactured to be administered via the rectal route, such as suppositories.

Rectal medications. Medication in suppository or liquid form administered as a retention enema.

Refractory. A disorder resistant to treatment.

REM. Rapid eye movement or dream phase of sleep.

Reporting of medication errors. Notifying the FDA of serious adverse events or product quality problems associated with medications (MEDWATCH).

Rescue treatment. Treatment used in the emergency situation, such as a severe asthma attack, to give quick relief of symptoms.

Resistance. An organism's lack of response to antibiotics when they are used too often or treatment is incomplete.

Responsibilities. Needed for safe and accurate administration of medication and include, knowledge, judgment and skill.

Responsibilities of drug administration. Duty to administer drugs safely and accurately.

Restless legs syndrome (RLS). A condition marked by an intolerable creeping sensation or itching in the lower extremities, causing almost irresistible urge to move the legs.

Retention enema. An enema that may be used to provide nourishment, medication, or anesthetic.

Reye's syndrome. Complication following acute viral infections in those under 18 years of age, characterized by rash, vomiting, and confusion about one week after the onset of a viral illness. May lead to respiratory arrest. Aspirin may induce Reye's syndrome when administered to children or adolescents with viral infections.

Rhabdomyolysis. An acute, sometimes fatal disease characterized by the destruction of muscle, leading to renal failure.

Route of delivery. The way that drugs are taken into the body.

S

Scurvy. A vitamin C deficiency disease usually resulting from a lack of fresh fruits and vegetables in the diet. Symptoms include ulcerated gums and mouth, loose teeth, muscle cramps and weakness, poor healing, and bruising.

Sedatives. Controlled substances used to promote sedation in smaller doses, and some may be used to promote sleep in larger doses.

Selective distribution. Affinity or attraction of a drug to a specific organ or cells.

Selective norepinephrine reuptake inhibitors (SNRIs). Antidepressants that block the reabsorption of the neurotransmitter norepinephrine, thus helping to restore the brain's chemical balance.

Selective serotonin reuptake inhibitors (SSRI). Antidepressants that block the reabsorption of the neurotransmitter serotonin, thus helping to restore the brain's chemical balance.

Serotonin syndrome. A potentially life-threatening reaction to excessive serotonin activity in the central nervous system.

Side effects. Unpleasant or dangerous secondary effects of medications.

Six "Rights" of medication administration. Guidelines for giving medication that include the right medication, right amount, right time, right route, right patient, and right documentation.

Skeletal muscle relaxants. Medications used to treat some musculoskeletal disorders associated with pain, spasm, abnormal contraction, or impaired mobility.

Small-volume nebulizers (SVNs). Devices that create a fine mist of a drug solution using a gas source (aerosolization). The aerosol is then inhaled via a mouthpiece or mask.

Smoking-cessation aids. Medications used to slowly lower the level of nicotine while the patient participates in a behavior modification program for smoking cessation.

Solution. A liquid containing a dissolved substance.

Somogyi effect. Hyperglycemic rebound, usually a result of frequent overdoses of insulin, which causes an accelerated release of glucagon.

Sources of drugs. Five ways that the drugs are obtained.

Spinal anesthesia. Local anesthetic solutions injected intrathecally (into the subarachnoid space of the spinal canal) either in the lumbar region or in the lower region (saddle block), depending on the area to be anesthetized.

Status asthmaticus. Persistent and intractable asthma.

Status epilepticus. Continual attacks of convulsive seizures without intervals of consciousness.

Stevens–Johnson syndrome. A severe, sometimes fatal inflammatory disease affecting children and young adults, characterized by ulcers on the skin and mucous membranes, fever, and painful joints.

STI. Sexually transmitted infection.

Stomatitis. Inflammation of the mucous membranes of the mouth.

Subcutaneous (subcu, SC, or SubQ). Beneath the skin.

Subjective. Perceived by the individual, not observable by others.

Sublingual (SL). Under the tongue.

Sulfonamides. A class of anti-infectives used in combinations with other drugs to slow the development of resistance; used in the treatment of urinary tract infections, enteritis, and opportunistic infections of AIDS.

Sulfonylureas. Oral antidiabetic drugs for the treatment of Type 2 diabetes.

Superinfection. A new infection with different resistant bacteria or fungi. Usually associated with certain types of antibiotic therapy.

Supplements. Products intended for ingestion as an addition to the diet.

Suppository. A semisolid substance for introduction into the rectum, vagina, or urethra, where it dissolves.

Suspension. A state of a solid when its particles are mixed with but not dissolved in a fluid or in another solid; also a substance in this state.

Sustained-release capsule or tablet. Capsule or tablet containing drug particles that have various coatings (often of different colors) that differ in the amount of time required before the coatings dissolve.

Sympathomimetic. Adrenergic drug that mimics the action of the sympathetic nervous system.

Symptoms of overdose. Symptoms caused by a higher than normal amount of drugs sufficient to cause toxicity.

Syncope. A brief lapse in consciousness; fainting.

Synergism. Action of two drugs working together for increased effect.

Synthetic. Prepared in the laboratory by artificial means.

Syrup. A concentrated solution of sugar in water to which specific medicinal substances are usually added.

Systemic effect. Affecting the whole body or system.

T

Tablet. Disk of compressed drug.

Tachycardia. Abnormally fast heartbeat.

Tachypnea. Abnormal rapidity of respiration.

Tall Man Lettering. A method of writing drug names to help differentiate between look-alike and sound-alike drugs. Example: CeleXA and CeleBREX.

Tardive dyskinesia (TD). Slow, rhythmical, stereotyped, involuntary movements such as tics.

Telephone order (TO). An order for treatment medication via the phone. Some agencies allow only certain health care practitioners to take telephone orders. All phone orders should be read back for accuracy, and a physician must sign the order within 24h.

Temporal lobe seizures. See Psychomotor epilepsy.

Teratogenic effect. Effect of a drug administered to the mother that results in abnormalities in the fetus.

Testosterone. Male hormone; medication used for replacement therapy and other purposes.

Tetracyclines. Broad-spectrum antibiotics used in the treatment of infections caused by rickettsia, chlamydia, or some uncommon bacteria.

Therapeutic range. A range of drug levels in the blood that will produce the desired effects without causing serious side effects.

Thrombocytopenia. Abnormal decrease in the number of blood platelets.

Thrombolytic agents. Medications used to dissolve clots after they have formed.

Timed-release capsules (sustained-release [SR] or extended-release [ER]). Capsules containing many small pellets that are dissolved over a prolonged period of time.

Tinnitus. Ringing in the ears.

Tocolysis. Suppression of uterine contractions in preterm labor.

Tolerance. Decreased response to a drug after repeated dosage; greater amounts of the drug are required for the same effect.

Tonic. Muscular tension resulting in *extension* of the trunk and extremities, sometimes followed by synchronous *contractions* of the muscles (clonic spasm).

Tonic-clonic seizure. Seizures characterized by an abrupt loss of consciousness and falling, with tonic extension of trunk and extremities.

Topical. Applied to a specific area for a local effect to that area only (e.g., applied to the skin or mucous membranes).

Topical drug forms. Drugs used for dermal and mucosal application.

Topical anesthesia. Application of a local anesthetic directly to the surface of the area to be anesthetized.

Toxicity. Condition resulting from exposure to a poison or a dangerous amount of a drug.

Toxicology. Study and detection of toxic substances, establishing treatment and methods of prevention of poisoning.

Trade names. Names by which a pharmaceutical company identifies its products; brand names.

Tramadol. A synthetic opioid used for the treatment of moderate to severe pain, it is a partial antagonist at the mu receptor which decreases its risk for abuse compared to other opioids.

Transcutaneous. Across the skin, as in transdermal medication delivery to the body by slow absorption through the skin.

Transdermal (transcutaneous) delivery system. Patch containing the medicine is applied to the skin; the drug is absorbed through the skin over a prolonged period of time.

Tricyclics. Antidepressants that elevate the mood, have a mild sedative effect, and increase appetite.

U

Unilateral seizures. Seizures that affect only one side of the body.

Unit-dose form. Each dose of the medicine is prepackaged in a separate packet, vial, or prefilled syringe.

Uricosuric agents. Promoting urinary excretion of uric acid.

Urinary analgesic. Medication used to relieve burning, pain, and discomfort in the urinary tract mucosa.

Urinary anti-infectives. Drugs used for initial or recurrent urinary tract infections caused by susceptible organisms, usually bacteriostatic instead of bactericidal.

Urticaria. Hives.

U.S. Recommended Dietary Allowances (U.S. RDAs). Vitamins and minerals necessary for the maintenance of good nutrition in the average healthy adults under normal living conditions in the United States.

V

Vaccines. Suspensions containing antigenic molecules derived from a microorganism, given to stimulate an immune response to an infectious disease.

Variables. Factors that affect the speed and efficiency of drugs processed by the body.

Vasoconstrictors. Drugs that narrow blood vessels, resulting in increased blood pressure; used in the treatment of shock.

Vasodilator. A drug that expands the walls of the blood vessels, improving blood flow and resulting in the lowering of blood pressure.

Verify your calculations. Confirm the result of calculations with another professional, such as an instructor.

Vertigo. Dizziness; lightheadedness.

Vial. Glass container with rubber stopper that must be punctured with a needle to withdraw a drug solution or to reconstitute a drug in powdered form.

W

Water-soluble vitamins. B-complex vitamins and vitamin C.

Wernicke's syndrome. Mental disorder characterized by the loss of memory, disorientation, and confusion; usually associated with old age or chronic alcoholism.

Withdrawal. Cessation of administration of a drug, especially an opioid or alcohol, to which a person has become physiologically and/or psychologically addicted; withdrawal symptoms vary with the drug used.

X

Xanthine. Medication that indirectly increases the chemical that causes bronchodilation; also a respiratory stimulant to increase the ventilatory drive.

Xerophthalmia. Dryness of the eyes.

Xerostomia. Dryness of the mouth.

Z

Z-track method A specific type of injection procedure used for medications that are irritating to the tissues such as iron injections.

Index

Note: Italicized page numbers indicate illustrations.

D

MindTap

Foster Student Progress

MindTap is the online learning platform that gives you complete control. Craft personalized, engaging learning experiences that boost performance and deliver access to eTextbooks, study tools, assessments and student performance analytics.

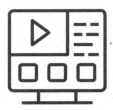

Access robust and organized course materials

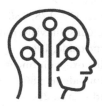

Increase student engagement

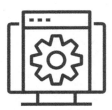

Personalize your course to support your goals

Connect with dedicated, live support

cengage.com/mindtap

Cengage Unlimited

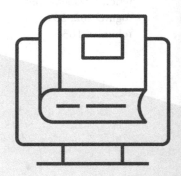

With Cengage Unlimited, a student receives access to an entire library of eTextbooks, online learning platforms, at least four free hardcopy rentals and hundreds of student success and career readiness skill-building activities. Only assigning textbooks for your course? Ask about Cengage Unlimited eTextbooks.

Available to all higher education and career students in the U.S., in bookstores and online. For customers outside the U.S., contact your local sales partner.

cengage.com/unlimited/instructor

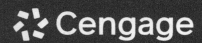